I0056088

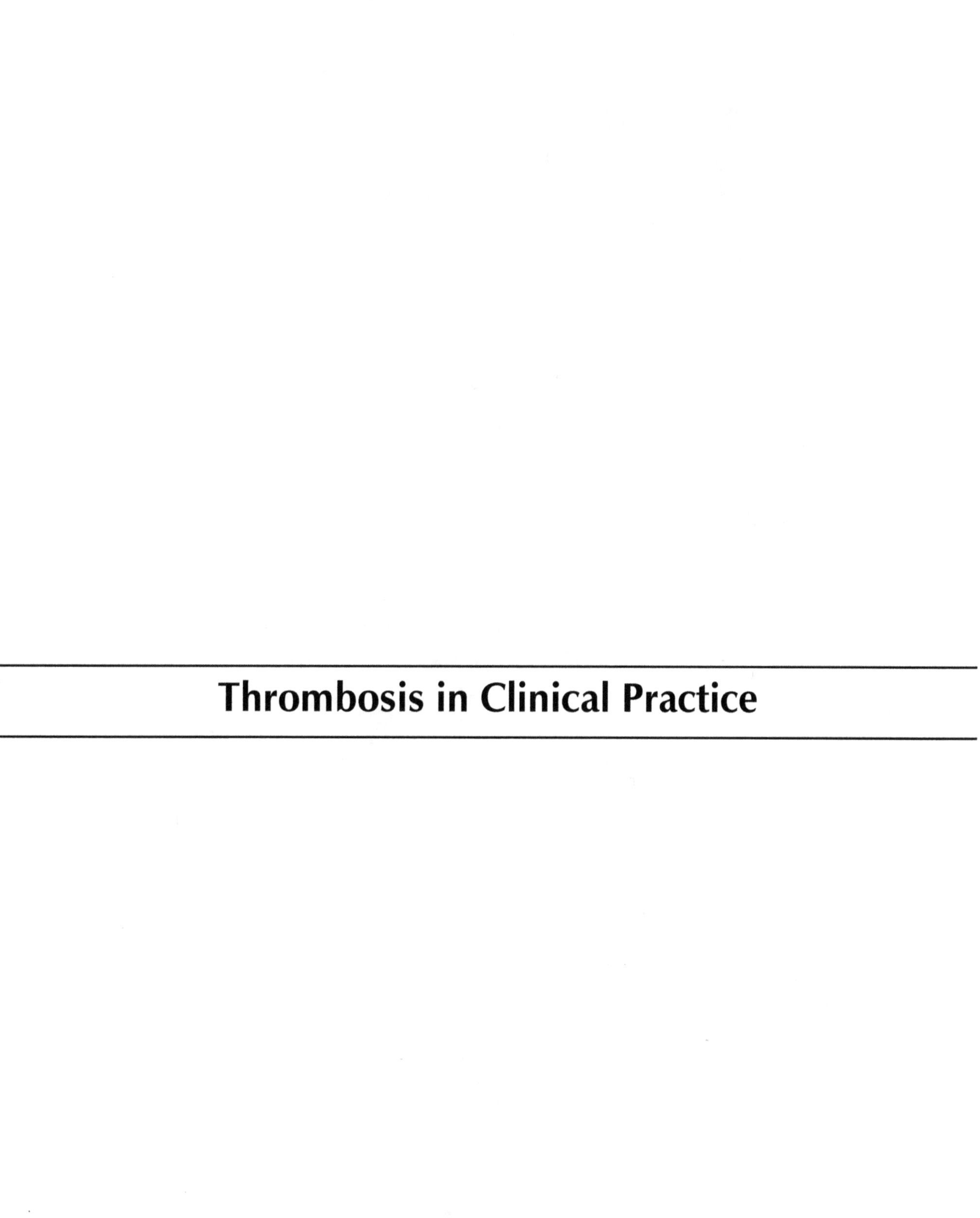

Thrombosis in Clinical Practice

Thrombosis in Clinical Practice

Editor: Morgan Bell

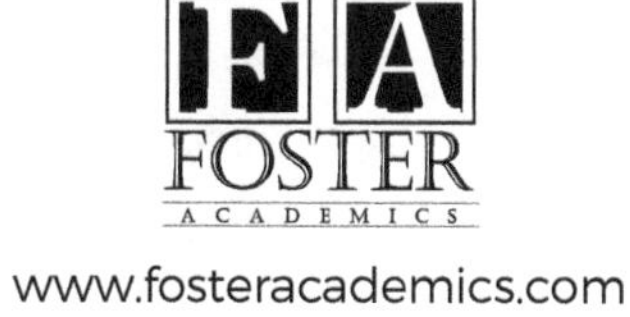

www.fosteracademics.com

www.fosteracademics.com

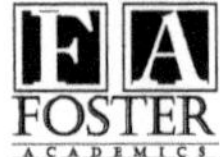

Cataloging-in-Publication Data

Thrombosis in clinical practice / edited by Morgan Bell.
p. cm.
Includes bibliographical references and index.
ISBN 978-1-63242-674-1
1. Thrombosis. 2. Thrombosis--Complications. 3. Blood--Coagulation.
4. Hematology. I. Bell, Morgan.
RC694.3 .T47 2019
616.135--dc23

Foster Academics,
118-35 Queens Blvd., Suite 400,
Forest Hills, NY 11375, USA

ISBN 978-1-63242-674-1 (Hardback)

Contents

Preface

The main aim of this book is to educate learners and enhance their research focus by presenting diverse topics covering this vast field. This is an advanced book which compiles significant studies by distinguished experts in the area of analysis. This book addresses successive solutions to the challenges arising in the area of application, along with it; the book provides scope for future developments.

The blood clot, which develops inside a blood vessel is known as thrombosis. In this condition the blood flow through the circulatory system is obstructed. This can occur in either veins or arteries. Atrial fibrillation is the most common cause of arterial thrombosis whereas venous thrombosis is majorly caused by a combination of hypercoagulability and venous stasis. In some cases a thrombus may get detached as an embolus and travel through circulation. This results in a type of embolism called thromboembolism. Low molecular weight heparin, insertion of a vena cava filter and mechanical calf compression are some of the methods used for its treatment. This book aims to shed light on some of the unexplored aspects related to thrombosis. It includes some of the vital pieces of work being conducted across the world, on various topics related to this medical condition. A number of latest researches have been included to keep the readers up-to-date with the global concepts in this area of study.

It was a great honour to edit this book, though there were challenges, as it involved a lot of communication and networking between me and the editorial team. However, the end result was this all-inclusive book covering diverse themes in the field.

Finally, it is important to acknowledge the efforts of the contributors for their excellent chapters, through which a wide variety of issues have been addressed. I would also like to thank my colleagues for their valuable feedback during the making of this book.

Editor

1

Evaluation of the chromogenic anti-factor IIa assay to assess dabigatran exposure in geriatric patients with atrial fibrillation in an outpatient setting

Luigi Brunetti[1*], Betty Sanchez-Catanese[2], Leonid Kagan[3], Xia Wen[4], Min Liu[5], Brian Buckley[5], James P. Luyendyk[6] and Lauren M. Aleksunes[4]

Abstract

Background: Dabigatran etexilate may be underutilized in geriatric patients because of inadequate clinical experience in individuals with severe renal impairment and post-marketing reports of bleeding events. Assessing the degree of anticoagulation may improve the risk:benefit ratio for dabigatran. The aim of this prospective study was to identify whether therapeutic drug monitoring of dabigatran anticoagulant activity using a chromogenic anti-factor IIa assay is a viable option for therapy individualization.

Methods: Plasma dabigatran concentration was assessed in nine patients with nonvalvular atrial fibrillation aged 75 years or older currently receiving dabigatran etexilate for prevention of stroke, using an anti-factor IIa chromogenic assay and HPLC-MS/MS. Trough concentrations were evaluated on two separate occasions to determine intrapatient variation.

Results: Blood was collected at 13.1 ± 2.3 h (mean ± SD) post dose from patients prescribed dabigatran etexilate 150 mg twice daily (5/9 patients) or dabigatran etexilate 75 mg twice daily (4/9 patients). Results from the anti-factor IIa chromogenic assay correlated with dabigatran concentrations as assessed by HPLC-MS/MS ($r^2 = 0.81$, $n = 16$). There was no correlation between dabigatran trough values taken at separate visits ($r^2 = 0.002$, $n = 7$). Furthermore, there was no correlation found between the drug concentrations and patients' renal function determined by both creatinine and cystatin-C based equations. None of the patients enrolled in the study were in the proposed on-therapy trough range during at least one visit.

Conclusion: The chromogenic anti-factor IIa assay demonstrated similar performance in quantifying dabigatran plasma trough concentrations to HPLC-MS/MS. Single measurement of dabigatran concentration by either of two methods during routine visits may not be reliable in identifying patients at consistently low or high dabigatran concentrations.

Keywords: Dabigatran, Atrial fibrillation, Geriatric, HPLC-MS/MS, Chromogenic anti-factor IIa

Background

Dabigatran possesses many of the attributes of an ideal anticoagulant for stroke prevention in nonvalvular atrial fibrillation (NVAF) including predictable pharmacokinetics and lack of the requirement for routine monitoring [1–3]. While routine monitoring may be unnecessary, assessment of degree of anticoagulation may be important in populations at risk of altered pharmacokinetics [4, 5]. Since the FDA approval of dabigatran etexilate in 2010, several regulatory agencies have issued warnings regarding the risk of bleeding, analogous to other target specific oral anticoagulants and vitamin K antagonists. The majority of hemorrhagic events linked to dabigatran have been reported in geriatric patients with renal dysfunction [6–9]. Although the landmark Randomized Evaluation of Long-Term Anticoagulation Therapy (RE-LY) trial found dabigatran etexilate 150 mg twice daily to be superior to

* Correspondence: brunetti@pharmacy.rutgers.edu
[1]Department of Pharmacy Practice and Administration, Ernest Mario School of Pharmacy, Rutgers, The State University of New Jersey, Piscataway, USA
Full list of author information is available at the end of the article

warfarin; it has been difficult to extrapolate the results to the geriatric population or to patients with severe renal impairment. A post-hoc analysis of the RE-LY trial revealed that patients ≥ 75 years of age had a greater incidence of gastrointestinal bleeding (but not intracranial) compared with patients on warfarin (1.85 %/year versus 1.25 %/year, respectively, $p < 0.001$) [10]. Furthermore, an increased risk of bleeding was identified in elderly patients irrespective of renal function [11]. Dabigatran etexilate is underutilized in geriatric patients because of insufficient clinical experience with dosing recommendations in severe renal impairment and post-marketing reports of bleeding complications [6–8, 12–18]. The mean age of RE-LY patients was 71.5 years old and the mean creatinine clearance (CrCl) was approximately 70 mL/min [19]. Patients with a CrCl < 30 mL/min were excluded from RE-LY. Moreover, the FDA approval of dabigatran etexilate dosing regimen for patients with severe renal dysfunction was supported by pharmacokinetic modeling based on data from middle-aged patients rather than actual clinical outcome [20–23]. The European Medicines Agency (EMA) considers dabigatran etexilate as contraindicated in patients with a CrCl < 30 mL/min and patients with a CrCl < 50 mL/min should receive 110 mg twice daily [24]. Collectively, these data suggest that the ability to gauge the degree of anticoagulation in the geriatric patient population may be beneficial.

There are a number of routine coagulation tests used in clinical practice; however, few are useful for quantitative assessment of dabigatran [5, 25]. The chromogenic anti-factor IIa assay has been successfully used for therapeutic drug monitoring of parenteral direct thrombin inhibitors and is insensitive to lupus anticoagulant or genetic coagulation deficiencies [26, 27]. Very little data have been published on the use of chromogenic anti-factor IIa assay and its correlation with HPLC-MS-MS measurement of dabigatran [28]. The aim of this prospective pilot study was to evaluate the utility of the chromogenic anti-factor IIa assay for monitoring dabigatran therapy and the intra- and interpatient variability of trough concentrations in elderly patients with atrial fibrillation.

Methods

A prospective study of nine geriatric patients was performed to assess dabigatran plasma trough concentrations using HPLC-MS/MS and the chromogenic anti-factor IIa quantification methods on two separate visits to the clinic. Male and female patients ≥ 75 years of age with NVAF currently receiving dabigatran etexilate mesylate (dabigatran prodrug) for the prevention of stroke were eligible for inclusion. Patients with a creatinine clearance of less than 15 mL/min were excluded since data are extremely limited and the use of dabigatran etexilate is contraindicated in this population (based on the United States product labeling) [29]. Patients with hemorrhagic disorders or baseline platelet count of less than 100,000 per liter, on hemodialysis, or with moderate or severe liver impairment (Child Pugh Score of B or greater) or those on strong P-glycoprotein inhibitors and inducers (i.e., amiodarone, clarithromycin, dronederone, ketoconazole, quinidine, rifampin, verapamil, and St. John's wort) were excluded. Dabigatran etexilate should be avoided with rifampin due to significant reduction in area under the curve (AUC) and maximum serum concentration (C_{max}) (66 and 67 %, respectively) [29]. While not contraindicated with P-glycoprotein inhibitors, the use of dabigatran etexilate with these agents should be carefully monitored due to increased AUC and C_{max}. Furthermore, in the setting of moderate-to-severe renal dysfunction and a P-glycoprotein inhibitor, dabigatran etexilate dose reductions should be considered [29]. The protocol was approved by the Rutgers University Institutional Review Board (Protocol # 13–503) and all patients signed an informed consent before participating in the study.

Patient dosing

The morning of study initiation, consenting patients were instructed to hold the morning dabigatran etexilate dosage until a blood sample was obtained at the physician's office. Once venous blood samples were drawn, the patient was instructed to take his/her dose. Patient demographics and concomitant medications were collected. The process was repeated on the patient's next scheduled visit, a minimum of 1 month apart.

Sample collection

Venous blood samples were taken just prior to the morning dose. Approximately 5 mL was collected in EDTA tubes for dabigatran plasma concentration measurement by HPLC-MS/MS. Another 5 mL was collected in 3.2 % tri-sodium citrate tubes (blood:citrate ratio 9:1) as recommended by the manufacturer for chromogenic assay. The samples were centrifuged at 2500 × g for 20 min and the plasma was kept on ice for a max of 1 h. Samples were kept frozen at −80 °C until assessment.

Quantitation of dabigatran

Dabigatran concentration in plasma samples was directly measured using a validated HPLC-MS/MS technique (modified from Delavenne et al.) [30] and estimated using a chromogenic anti-factor IIa assay (Hyphen Biomed, Neuville-sur-Oise, France). Plasma samples or standards (100 μL) were mixed with 10 μL of an internal standard ($^{13}C_6$-dabigatran 1 μg/mL). Analytes were isolated from plasma using protein precipitation with 400 μL methanol/0.1 N HCl (90:10). After centrifugation, a

100 μL aliquot of supernatant was taken for the injection, and the injection volume was 20 μL. A Thermo LTQ mass spectrometer was interfaced to a Finnigan Surveyor Autosampler plus and Finnigan Surveyor MS Pump plus for separation and quantitation of dabigatran. Separation was completed using Betasil Phenyl/Hexyl column (3 μm, 100 × 4.6 mm, Thermo Scientific) and a gradient flow of water and methanol with 0.1 % formic acid. Electrospray ionization source was used to ionize the dabigatran before introduction into the mass spectrometer. Quantification was performed by addition of 472.2– > 324.2 and 472.2– > 306.1 and 472.2– > 289.1 m/z for dabigatran and 478.3– > 330.2 and 478.3– > 295.1 m/z for the internal standard. The calibration curves were linear over a concentration range of 4–1000 ng/mL.

Chromogenic anti-IIa assay

Dabigatran activity was quantified using a BIOPHEN DTI kit (Aniara, West Chester, OH). Plasma samples, dabigatran calibrators or quality controls (50 μl) were mixed with 50 μl of thrombin chromogenic substrate at 37 °C for 1 min in a 96-well plate. The mixture was then incubated at 37 °C for 2 min after adding 50 μl of preheated purified human thrombin. Activity was measured spectrophotometrically at 450 nm (SpectraMax 5, Molecular Devices, Sunnyvale, CA) in the presence of 20 % of acetic acid and adjusted for sample blanks and extrapolated from a standard curve. Samples were run in duplicate. The limit of detection was 14.6 ng/mL and the dynamic range from 0 to 500 ng/mL.

Assessment of renal function

Both serum creatinine and cystatin-C were measured in order to estimate renal function using the Cockcroft-Gault ([140 − age [years] × total body weight]/0.72 × sCr (mg/dL)) × 0.85 [if female]) and CKD-EPI (127.7 × Cystatin $C^{-1.17}$ × $age^{-0.13}$ × 0.91 [if female] × 1.06 [if African American]) equations, respectively [31, 32]. Of note, Cockcroft-Gault was the method used to estimate renal function in RE-LY, [19] the landmark trial leading to the approval of dabigatran etexilate for prevention of stroke and systemic embolism in patients with NVAF. Serum creatinine levels were measured using a kit based on the Jaffe reaction (Pointe Scientific, Canton, MI). Briefly, 190 μl of pre-heated working reagent including 5 volumes of alkaline buffer and 1 volume of picric acid (40 mM) were added to 10 μl of samples, creatinine standard or blank serum. The mixture was incubated at 37 °C for 1 min and the change in optical density was measured at 510 nm over 3 min.

Cystatin C levels were quantified using a Quantikine ELISA kit according to the manufacturer's recommendations (R&D Systems, Minneapolis, MN). Samples or cystatin C standards (50 μl) were added to a 96-well plate coated with an antibody specific for human cystatin C and incubated at 2–8 °C for 3 h. After washing, cystatin C conjugate was then added to compete for binding with the antibody. Following incubation, washing and addition of substrate solutions (stabilized hydrogen peroxide and tetramethylbenzidine), the stop solution (2 N sulfuric acid) was added and the optical density was measured at 450 nm and 570 nm. Concentrations of cystatin C were extrapolated from the standard curve. Samples were run in duplicate. Renal function was assessed at each visit.

Data analysis

All data were analyzed using descriptive statistics. Categorical data were reported as proportions and continuous data as the mean or median as appropriate. Pearson correlation coefficients were calculated for the relationship between HPLC-MS/MS and chromogenic assay dabigatran trough levels and estimates of renal function. Bland-Altman analysis and linear regression were performed to assess the strength of agreement and proportionality bias between HPLC-MS/MS and chromogenic anti-IIa measures of dabigatran levels. Correlation of dabigatran trough levels between visits was also evaluated. Trough levels were also compared to proposed dabigatran on target range (30 ng/mL − 130 ng/mL) [33]. Analysis was performed using SAS 9.2 (SAS Institute, Cary, NC) or SPSS version 21 (IBM Corporation, Armonk, NY).

Results

Nine patients were enrolled, seven patients returned for a second visit. All patients were on dabigatran etexilate therapy for a minimum of one month before initiation of the study. Patient characteristics are summarized in Table 1. Blood was collected at 13.1 ± 2.3 h (mean ± SD) post dose from patients receiving dabigatran etexilate 150 mg twice daily (5/9 patients) or dabigatran etexilate 75 mg twice daily (4/9 patients). Results from the anti-IIa chromogenic assay correlated with dabigatran concentrations as assessed by HPLC-MS/MS ($r^2 = 0.81$, $n = 15$; Fig. 1). In addition, the Spearman's rho yielded similar results (rho = 0.91). The Bland-Altman plot shows a very high limit of agreement defined by the mean ± 1.96*SD (Fig. 2). The mean bias present was 0.86 and the limits of agreement were 93.0 and − 91.0. The linear regression of the Bland-Altman plot did not suggest any significant proportionality bias (equation; Y = 0.006545*X − 0.1945; $p = 0.9583$). High intrapatient variability in dabigatran trough plasma concentrations was observed ($r^2 = 0.002$, p = ns; $n = 7$; Fig. 3). All the patients enrolled in the study were not within the proposed on-therapy range [33] during at least one study visit. Seven patients had a dabigatran level exceeding

Table 1 Patient demographic and dabigatran dosing characteristics

Characteristic	Value
Mean Age ± SD (years)	81.3 ± 4.5
Female (%)	44.5
Mean time after last dabigatran dose ± SD (hours)	13.1 ± 2.3
Mean weight ± SD (kg)	83.0 ± 21.1
Body mass index ± SD (kg/m^2)	28.9 ± 4.7
Baseline Renal Clearance ± SD (mL/min)	
Cockcroft-Gault	68.4 ± 28.4
CKD-EPI	40.9 ± 12.3
Dabigatran dosage, n (%)	
75 mg twice daily	4 (44.4)
150 mg twice daily	5 (55.6)
Cormorbidities (n, %)	
Chronic obstructive pulmonary disease	3 (33.3)
Diabetes Mellitus	4 (44.4)
Heart Failure	3 (33.3)
Malignancy	2 (22.2)
Thyroid Disease	4 (44.4)
Coronary Artery Disease	2 (22.2)
Mean HPLC-MS/MS dabigatran level ± SD (ng/mL)[a]	161.1 ± 104.1
Mean chromogenic anti-IIa dabigatran level ± SD (ng/mL)[a]	161.9 ± 104.8

[a]Pooled data from all office visits

130 ng/mL and three patients had a level of less than 30 ng/mL during at least one of the recorded visits. Baseline creatinine based (Cockcroft-Gault) and cystatin-C based estimates (CKD-EPI) of renal function had no-to-poor correlation with plasma dabigatran concentrations ($r = 0.07$ and -0.26, $p =$ ns for both; respectively).

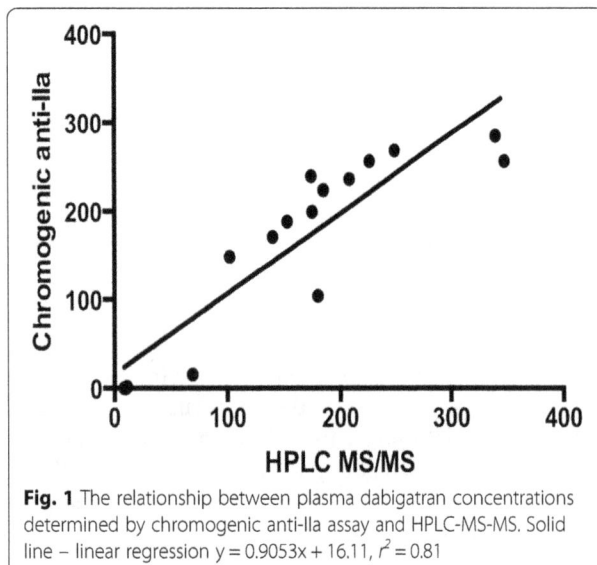

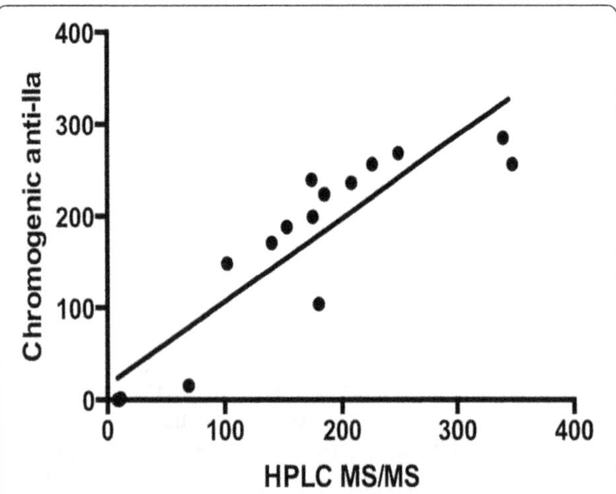

Fig. 1 The relationship between plasma dabigatran concentrations determined by chromogenic anti-IIa assay and HPLC-MS-MS. Solid line – linear regression y = 0.9053x + 16.11, $r^2 = 0.81$

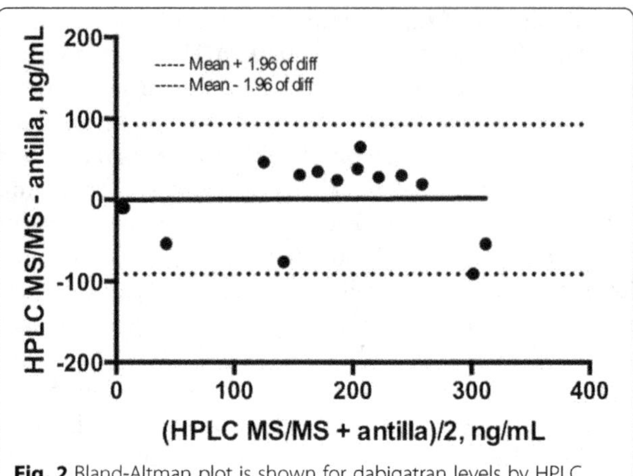

Fig. 2 Bland-Altman plot is shown for dabigatran levels by HPLC MS/MS and chromogenic anti-factor IIa (diff, difference; $n = 16$)

Discussion

There is a widely held view that the target specific oral anticoagulants, including dabigatran etexilate, have a predictable response and do not require monitoring; however, data suggest significant interpatient variability in pharmacokinetics [34, 35]. In addition, the landmark RE-LY trial suggests low trough concentrations (rapid decrease in the probability of stroke from a concentration of zero through approximately 70 ng/mL) [36, 37] were associated with reduced efficacy and high concentrations were associated with an increased risk of bleeding [4]. Chan and colleagues measured the Hemoclot® assay at baseline and every 2 months for up to 4 visits in 100 patients (mean age 69.9 years) with atrial fibrillation [35]. They reported a large intrapatient variability in Hemoclot® levels (geometric coefficient of variation 32 – 40 %). The authors concluded that a single Hemoclot® measurement is not reliable in identifying patients with consistently high or low dabigatran exposure. Some concerns have been raised regarding the large variation in trough dabigatran levels seen between visits in the Chan and colleagues study [38]. These concerns included timing of trough sample, stability of plasma stored at -80 °C, performance of the analysis on the same run, and lack of outcome data. Arguably, the most important concern is the lack of stringent timing of trough levels. While measuring trough levels at 12 ± 1 h is ideal, when relying on patient reported drug administration in clinical practice this criteria is difficult to enforce. Patient reported adherence is inherently a limitation and may result in measurement bias. Similar to the Chan and colleagues study, our pilot study found that in geriatric patients there was large intrapatient variability in dabigatran exposure as measured by chromogenic anti-IIa assay and HPLC MS/MS. Specifics on last dose intake in the current study may be found in Additional file 1.

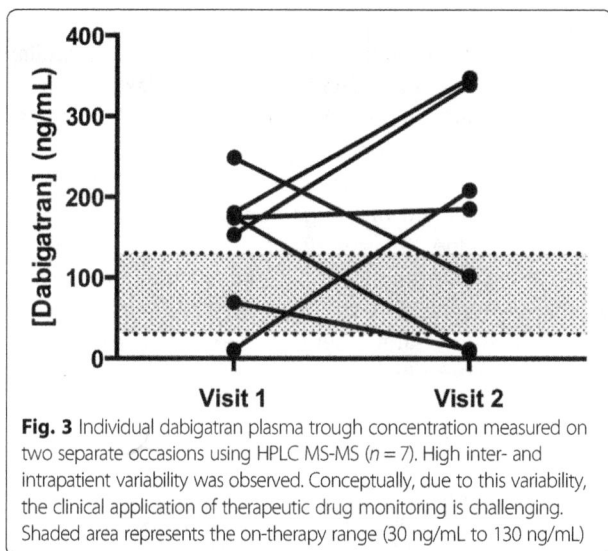

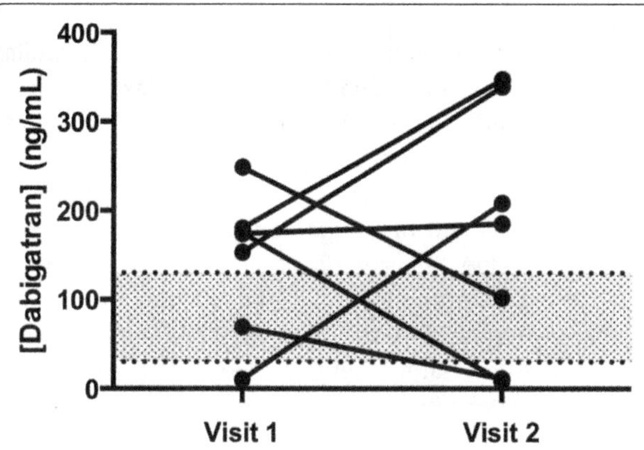

Fig. 3 Individual dabigatran plasma trough concentration measured on two separate occasions using HPLC MS-MS ($n = 7$). High inter- and intrapatient variability was observed. Conceptually, due to this variability, the clinical application of therapeutic drug monitoring is challenging. Shaded area represents the on-therapy range (30 ng/mL to 130 ng/mL)

Vulnerable populations such as the elderly and patients with renal impairment have the potential to exhibit exaggerated responses to dabigatran [11, 39, 40]. Dabigatran etexilate, a prodrug, completes its bioconversion in the liver and approximately 20 % is conjugated with glucuronic acid and excreted via the biliary system [2, 41]. Dabigatran etexilate requires conversion via esterase hydrolysis to the active form (dabigatran) [2]. Genetic factors, such as polymorphisms in carboxylesterase 1, may also be responsible for interpatient variability [42]. There may also be variability in drug exposure secondary to inhibition or induction of the efflux transporter P-glycoprotein, as dabigatran etexilate is substrate of this transport protein [29, 43]. While these factors explain the interpatient variability that may be present, they do not account for the intrapatient variability observed between clinic visits in this study.

No therapeutic range has been established for dabigatran; however, a target plasma dabigatran trough concentration of 30 – 130 ng/mL has been suggested by Chin and colleagues [33]. Some limitations to using this range include derivation from pharmacokinetic simulations and lack of prospective studies confirming that the range predicts clinical outcomes. However, with the lack of definitive data, this range provides a good starting point and there are data from landmark trials confirming dabigatran levels may be predictive of thrombosis and bleeding [4]. For example, patients in the RE-LY trial with any major bleeding had a higher dabigatran trough concentration (113 ng/mL) compared to patients without a bleeding event (72.8 ng/mL) [4]. Furthermore, age was the most important covariate. Collectively, these data may be used to construct a dabigatran concentration-to-assay result curve to predict drug exposure and predict risk of bleeding [44]. In our analysis, we found that all patients were not in the on-therapy range on at least one of the two visits. Furthermore, 4 out of 9 patients had dabigatran trough levels exceeding 200 ng/mL during at least one visit and trough levels above 200 ng/mL are associated with an increased risk of bleeding [45]. These results are concerning and suggest geriatric patients may be at an unecessary risk of treatment failure and/or bleeding.

Estimating renal function in the elderly is challenging and many of the currently available methods are inaccurate [46]. Unlike creatinine, cystatin C levels are unaffected by age, muscle mass, gender, and race [32]. We were not able to appreciate any significant correlation with either creatinine or cystatin C based estimates of renal function with dabigatran trough concentrations. Based on this finding, additional research is warranted to identify which estimate renal function leads to the selection of the most appropriate dose or if age alone is sufficient to suggest a dosage reduction [47, 48]. Current FDA and EMA recommendations for dosing dabigatran etexilate in renal disease advocate using the Cockcroft-Gault equation to estimate renal function and clinicians should not deviate from this strategy [24, 29]. Hellden and colleagues investigated the impact of using the Modified Diet in Renal Disease 4 (MDRD4 equation to estimate glomerular filtration rate and subsequent dose adjustment in the elderly population (defined as age > 65 years) [49]. Their findings suggest that the MDRD4 would result in higher recommended doses of dabigatran etexilate to elderly patients versus Cockcroft-Gault, particularly in women. The increased dose may increase the risk of toxicity, hence these findings suggest continued use of Cockcroft-Gault to estimate renal function for dabigatran etexilate dosing.

These data support further evaluation of strategies to individualize treatment. The literature on coagulation monitoring to guide dabigatran therapy is evolving with several studies and comprehensive reviews now published [4, 5, 34, 44, 50–55]. Evidence supports that dabigatran levels are correlated to bleeding risk and efficacy [4]. Furthermore, in an sub-analysis of the RE-LY trial, a plasma concentration at trough between 90 and 140 ng/mL provided the best benefit/risk ratio in patients with NVAF,[56] although other authors have suggested other on-target ranges [33, 57]. Tailoring dabigatran etexilate dose according to patient risk (i.e., age, renal function) is essential to balance the benefit:risk of thrombosis and bleeding [58]. Adding the ability to assess degree of anticoagulation has the potential to further improve the benefit:risk ratio of dabigatran and warrants consideration especially in special populations such as the geriatric population [59, 60].

This study provides important information obtained from 'real world' use of dabigatran etexilate in geriatric patients. Chromogenic anti-IIa assay correlates with

HPLC MS/MS measured dabigatran concentrations and may be useful for quantitative measurement; however, the intrapatient variability of dabigatran concentrations may make clinical application challenging. The frequency of patients outside a proposed therapeutic window suggests there may be opportunity for improvement of dosing strategy to further enhance the risk versus benefit ratio of dabigatran. Glucuronidation is the major metabolic pathway of dabigatran. The major metabolite of dabigatran, 1-O-acylglucuronide, and its isomers result in equipotent prolongation of the activated partial thromboplastin time [41, 61]. Acylglucuronides accounted for 2.0 % of the dose in plasma at 2 h and 4.3 % at 4 h post administration of intravenous dabigatran [41]. The acylglucuronide metabolites may contribute to the overall clinical effect of dabigatran and can explain some of the difference between HPLC-MS/MS detection of dabigatran and the chromogenic measurement of anti-IIa activity if there is interpatient variability in glucuronidation. Of note, previous studies suggest that age does not significantly influence glucuronidation [62, 63].

Certain limitations of our study should be acknowledged. Although the chomogenic anti-factor II assay may be performed manually or using an automated coagulometer as indicated in the assay specifications, manual methods may be a potential source of measurement bias. The timing of trough levels was often not within 1 h of the next scheduled dose due to patient availability, as suggeted to be optimal for pharmacokinetic studies [50]. Our data reflects a practical scenario that resembles the 'real world' clinical setting. Furthermore, data support that sampling within 6 h of the next scheduled dose will still provide a value within the 80 % confidence interval for the true trough value as was discussed by Chan and colleagues [22]. When planning to measure dabigatran levels it is paramount to educate the patient on the importance of accurately documenting the last intake of medication. In addition, scheduling patient visits according to their usual drug administration schedule may enhance the accuracy of trough levels. Another strategy involves collaboration of clinicians with laboratories or anticoagulation clinics. Patients can be instructed to hold their dabigatran etexilate dose until their office visit where administration can be directly observed. Following directly observed administration of dabigatran etexilate, the office staff can schedule an appointment for the patient to present to the laboratory or clinic for their blood to be drawn.

This study found no correlation between dabigatran trough levels taken at two different patient visits; however, the limited sample size requires future studies to confirm this finding. Ultimately, a large controlled study is necessary to confirm if a monitoring strategy will improve dosage selection and dabigatran treatment outcomes.

Conclusion

Chromogenic anti-factor IIa assay demonstrated similar performance in quantifying dabigatran plasma trough concentrations to HPLC-MS/MS. All geriatric patients were not within the on-therapy trough range during at least one visit. Routine adjustment of dosages based on a single measurement of trough concentration may not be appropriate due to significant intrapatient variation. Given the large proportion of patients falling outside the on-therapy range and the high variability observed in this pilot study, larger clinical studies can be recommended to determine the clinical utility of concentration monitoring in the outpatient setting.

Competing interests

JL Is the primary investigator on a research contract from Boehringer Ingelheim outside the scope of work described in this manuscript.

Authors' contributions

LB and BSC conceived, designed, enrolled subjects, and collected specimens from consenting subjects. LK was involved in the study design and data analysis. XW and LMA performed the chromogenic anti-IIa assay and serum creatinine and Cystatin-C measurement. ML and BB performed the HPLC MS/MS. JL provided input on study design and expertise on coagulation assays. LB drafted the manuscript and all authors read and approved the final draft.

Acknowledgements

This study was funded by the ANIARA Coagulation Grant and the National Institute of Environmental Health Sciences (NIEHS) Center for Environmental Exposures and Disease (grant ES005022).

Author details

[1]Department of Pharmacy Practice and Administration, Ernest Mario School of Pharmacy, Rutgers, The State University of New Jersey, Piscataway, USA. [2]Department of Medicine, Robert Wood Johnson University Hospital-Somerset, Somerville, USA. [3]Department of Pharmaceutics, Ernest Mario School of Pharmacy, Rutgers, The State University of New Jersey, Piscataway, USA. [4]Department of Pharmacology and Toxicology, Ernest Mario School of Pharmacy, Rutgers, The State University of New Jersey, Piscataway, USA. [5]Chemical Analytical Core Laboratory, Environmental and Occupational Health Sciences Institute, Rutgers, The State University of New Jersey, Piscataway, USA. [6]Pathology and Diagnostic Inv., Michigan State University, East Lansing, USA.

References

1. Hankey GJ. At last, a RE-LYable alternative to warfarin for atrial fibrillation. Int J Stroke. 2009;4(6):454–5. doi:10.1111/j.1747-4949.2009.00389.x.
2. Hankey GJ, Eikelboom JW. Dabigatran etexilate: a new oral thrombin inhibitor. Circulation. 2011;123(13):1436–50. doi:10.1161/CIRCULATIONAHA.110.004424.
3. Moore TJ, Cohen MR, Mattison DR. Dabigatran, bleeding, and the regulators. BMJ. 2014;349:g4517. http://dx.doi.org/10.1136/bmj.g4517.
4. Reilly PA, Lehr T, Haertter S, Connolly SJ, Yusuf S, Eikelboom JW, et al. The effect of dabigatran plasma concentrations and patient characteristics on the frequency of ischemic stroke and major bleeding in atrial fibrillation patients: The RE-LY Trial (Randomized Evaluation of Long-Term Anticoagulation Therapy). J Am Coll Cardiol. 2014;63(4):321–8. doi:10.1016/j.jacc.2013.07.104.

5. Brunetti L, Bandali F. Dabigatran: is there a role for coagulation assays in guiding therapy? Ann Pharmacother. 2013;47(6):828–40. doi:10.1345/aph.1R720.
6. Harper P, Young L, Merriman E. Bleeding risk with dabigatran in the frail elderly. N Engl J Med. 2012;366(9):864–6. doi:10.1056/NEJMc1112874.
7. Legrand M, Mateo J, Aribaud A, Ginisty S, Eftekhari P, Huy PT, et al. The use of dabigatran in elderly patients. Arch Intern Med. 2011;171(14):1285–6. doi:10.1001/archinternmed.2011.314.
8. Safouris A, Triantafyllou N, Parissis J, Tsivgoulis. The case for dosing dabigatran: how tailoring dose to patient renal function, weight, and age could improve the benefit-risk ratio. Ther Adv Neurol Disord. 2015;8(6):245-54. doi:10.1177/1756285615601360.
9. Cotton BA, McCarthy JJ, Holcomb JB. Acutely injured patients on dabigatran. N Engl J Med. 2011;365(21):2039–40. doi:10.1056/NEJMc1111095.
10. Eikelboom JW, Connolly SJ, Hart RG, Wallentin L, Reilly P, Oldgren J, et al. Balancing the benefits and risks of 2 doses of dabigatran compared with warfarin in atrial fibrillation. J Am Coll Cardiol. 2013;62(10):900–8. doi:10.1016/j.jacc.2013.05.042.
11. Eikelboom JW, Wallentin L, Connolly SJ, Ezekowitz M, Healey JS, Oldgren J, et al. Risk of bleeding with 2 doses of dabigatran compared with warfarin in older and younger patients with atrial fibrillation: an analysis of the randomized evaluation of long-term anticoagulant therapy (RE-LY) trial. Circulation. 2011;123(21):2363–72. doi:10.1161/CIRCULATIONAHA.110.004747.
12. Radecki RP. Dabigatran: uncharted waters and potential harms. Ann Intern Med. 2012;157(1):66–8. doi:10.7326/0003-4819-157-1-201207030-00467.
13. Anonymous. Bleeding with dabigatran (Pradaxa). Med Lett Drugs Ther. 2011;53(1379-1380):98.
14. Barton CA, McMillian WD, Sadi Raza S, Keller RE. Hemopericardium in a patient treated with dabigatran etexilate. Pharmacotherapy. 2012;32(5): e103–7. doi:10.1002/j.1875-9114.2012.01036.x.
15. Bene J, Said W, Rannou M, Deheul S, Coupe P, Gautier S. Rectal bleeding and hemostatic disorders induced by dabigatran etexilate in 2 elderly patients. Ann Pharmacother. 2012;46(6), e14. doi:10.1345/aph.1Q705.
16. Cano EL, Miyares MA. Clinical challenges in a patient with dabigatran-induced fatal hemorrhage. Am J Geriatr Pharmacother. 2012;10(2):160–3. doi:10.1016/j.amjopharm.2012.02.004.
17. Kernan L, Ito S, Shirazi F, Boesen K. Fatal gastrointestinal hemorrhage after a single dose of dabigatran. Clin Toxicol (Phila). 2012;50(7):571–3. doi:10.3109/15563650.2012.705290.
18. Lillo-Le Louet A, Wolf M, Soufir L, Galbois A, Dumenil AS, Offenstadt G, et al. Life-threatening bleeding in four patients with an unusual excessive response to dabigatran: implications for emergency surgery and resuscitation. Thromb Haemost. 2012;108(3):583–5. doi:10.1160/TH12-03-0149.
19. Connolly SJ, Ezekowitz MD, Yusuf S, Eikelboom J, Oldgren J, Parekh A, et al. Dabigatran versus warfarin in patients with atrial fibrillation. N Engl J Med. 2009;361(12):1139–51. doi:10.1056/NEJMoa0905561.
20. Hariharan S, Madabushi R. Clinical pharmacology basis of deriving dosing recommendations for dabigatran in patients with severe renal impairment. J Clin Pharmacol. 2012;52(1 Suppl):119S–25S. doi:10.1177/0091270011415527.
21. Lehr T, Haertter S, Liesenfeld KH, Staab A, Clemens A, Reilly PA, et al. Dabigatran etexilate in atrial fibrillation patients with severe renal impairment: dose identification using pharmacokinetic modeling and simulation. J Clin Pharmacol. 2011. doi:10.1177/0091270011417716.
22. Liesenfeld KH, Lehr T, Dansirikul C, Reilly PA, Connolly SJ, Ezekowitz MD, et al. Population pharmacokinetic analysis of the oral thrombin inhibitor dabigatran etexilate in patients with non-valvular atrial fibrillation from the RE-LY trial. J Thromb Haemost. 2011;9(11):2168–75. doi:10.1111/j.1538-7836.2011.04498.x.
23. Kowey PR, Naccarelli GV. The food and drug administration decision not to approve the 110 mg dose of dabigatran: give us a way out. Am J Med. 2012;125(8):732. doi:10.1016/j.amjmed.2011.10.035.
24. Pradaxa® European Medicines Agency. http://www.ema.europa.eu/docs/en_GB/document_library/EPAR_-_Product_Information/human/000829/WC500041059.pdf.
25. van Ryn J, Stangier J, Haertter S, Liesenfeld KH, Wienen W, Feuring M, et al. Dabigatran etexilate–a novel, reversible, oral direct thrombin inhibitor: interpretation of coagulation assays and reversal of anticoagulant activity. Thromb Haemost. 2010;103(6):1116–27. doi:10.1160/TH09-11-0758.
26. Salemi A, Agrawal YP, Fontes MA. An assay to monitor bivalirudin levels on cardiopulmonary bypass. Ann Thorac Surg. 2011;92(1):332–4. doi:10.1016/j.athoracsur.2010.12.064.
27. Salmela B, Joutsi-Korhonen L, Saarela E, Lassila R. Comparison of monitoring methods for lepirudin: impact of warfarin and lupus anticoagulant. Thromb Res. 2010;125(6):538–44. doi:10.1016/j.thromres.2010.02.002.
28. Adcock DM, Gosselin R, Kitchen S, Dwyre DM. The effect of dabigatran on select specialty coagulation assays. Am J Clin Pathol. 2013;139(1):102–9. doi:10.1309/AJCPY6G6ZITVKPVH139/1/102.
29. Boehringer Ingelheim. Pradaxa (dabigatran etexilate mesylate) prescribing information. http://docs.boehringer-ingelheim.com/Prescribing%20Information/PIs/Pradaxa/Pradaxa.pdf. (Accessed 2016 Apr 26).
30. Delavenne X, Moracchini J, Laporte S, Mismetti P, Basset T. UPLC MS/MS assay for routine quantification of dabigatran - a direct thrombin inhibitor - in human plasma. J Pharm Biomed Anal. 2012;58:152–6. doi:10.1016/j.jpba.2011.09.018.
31. Dowling TC, Wang ES, Ferrucci L, Sorkin JD. Glomerular filtration rate equations overestimate creatinine clearance in older individuals enrolled in the Baltimore longitudinal study on aging: impact on renal drug dosing. Pharmacotherapy. 2013. doi:10.1002/phar.1282.
32. Hojs R, Bevc S, Ekart R, Gorenjak M, Puklavec L. Serum cystatin C-based equation compared to serum creatinine-based equations for estimation of glomerular filtration rate in patients with chronic kidney disease. Clin Nephrol. 2008;70(1):10–7.
33. Chin PK, Wright DF, Patterson DM, Doogue MP, Begg EJ. A proposal for dose-adjustment of dabigatran etexilate in atrial fibrillation guided by thrombin time. Br J Clin Pharmacol. 2014. doi:10.1111/bcp.12364.
34. Freyburger G, Macouillard G, Labrouche S, Sztark F. Coagulation parameters in patients receiving dabigatran etexilate or rivaroxaban: two observational studies in patients undergoing total hip or total knee replacement. Thromb Res. 2011;127(5):457–65. doi:10.1016/j.thromres.2011.01.001.
35. Chan NC, Coppens M, Hirsh J, Ginsberg JS, Weitz JI, Vanassche T, et al. Real-world variability in dabigatran levels in patients with atrial fibrillation. J Thromb Haemost. 2015;13(3):353–9. doi:10.1111/jth.12823.
36. US Food and Drug Administration, Center for Drug Evaluation and Research. Dabigatran etexilate; deputy office director decisional memo application 22-512. October 19, 2010. http://www.Accessdata.Fda.Gov/drugsatfda_docs/nda/2010/022512orig1s000sumr.pdf Accessed 30 Oct 2013).
37. US Food and Drug Administration, Center for Drug Evaluation and Research. Dabigatran etexilate. Advisory committee briefing document, August 27, 2010. http://www.Fda.Gov/downloads/advisorycommittees/committeesmeetingmaterials/drugs/cardiovascularandrenaldrugsadvisorycommittee/ucm226009.pdf Accessed 30 Oct 2013.
38. Douxfils J, Chatelain B, Dogne JM, Mullier F. Real-world variability in dabigatran levels in patients with atrial fibrillation: comment. J Thromb Haemost. 2015;13(6):1166–8. doi:10.1111/jth.12880.
39. Stangier J, Stahle H, Rathgen K, Fuhr R. Pharmacokinetics and pharmacodynamics of the direct oral thrombin inhibitor dabigatran in healthy elderly subjects. Clin Pharmacokinet. 2008;47(1):47–59.
40. Stangier J, Rathgen K, Stahle H, Mazur D. Influence of renal impairment on the pharmacokinetics and pharmacodynamics of oral dabigatran etexilate: an open-label, parallel-group, single-centre study. Clin Pharmacokinet. 2010; 49(4):259–68. doi:10.2165/11318170-000000000-000004.
41. Blech S, Ebner T, Ludwig-Schwellinger E, Stangier J, Roth W. The metabolism and disposition of the oral direct thrombin inhibitor, dabigatran, in humans. Drug Metab Dispos. 2008;36(2):386–99. doi:10.1124/dmd.107.019083..
42. Pare G, Eriksson N, Lehr T, Connolly S, Eikelboom J, Ezekowitz MD, et al. Genetic determinants of dabigatran plasma levels and their relation to bleeding. Circulation. 2013;127(13):1404–12. doi:10.1161/CIRCULATIONAHA.112.001233.
43. Nutescu E, Chuatrisorn I, Hellenbart E. Drug and dietary interactions of warfarin and novel oral anticoagulants: an update. J Thromb Thrombolysis. 2011;31(3):326–43. doi:10.1007/s11239-011-0561-1.
44. Avecilla ST, Ferrell C, Chandler WL, Reyes M. Plasma-diluted thrombin time to measure dabigatran concentrations during dabigatran etexilate therapy. Am J Clin Pathol. 2012;137(4):572–4. doi:10.1309/AJCPAU7OQM0SRPZQ.
45. Huisman MV, Lip GY, Diener HC, Brueckmann M, van Ryn J, Clemens A. Dabigatran etexilate for stroke prevention in patients with atrial fibrillation: resolving uncertainties in routine practice. Thromb Haemost. 2012;107(5): 838–47. doi:10.1160/TH11-10-0718.
46. Spruill WJ, Wade WE, Cobb 3rd HH. Comparison of estimated glomerular filtration rate with estimated creatinine clearance in the dosing of drugs requiring adjustments in elderly patients with declining renal function. Am J Geriatr Pharmacother. 2008;6(3):153–60. doi:10.1016/j.amjopharm.2008.07.002.

47. Cockcroft DW, Gault MH. Prediction of creatinine clearance from serum creatinine. Nephron. 1976;16(1):31–41.
48. Chin P, Vella-Brincat J, Walker S, Barclay M, Begg E. Dosing of dabigatran etexilate in relation to renal function and drug interactions at a tertiary hospital. Intern Med J. 2013. doi:10.1111/imj.12170.
49. Hellden A, Odar-Cederlof I, Nilsson G, Sjoviker S, Soderstrom A, Euler M, et al. Renal function estimations and dose recommendations for dabigatran, gabapentin and valaciclovir: a data simulation study focused on the elderly. BMJ Open. 2013;3(4):e002686. doi:10.1136/bmjopen-2013-002686.
50. Douxfils J, Lessire S, Dincq AS, Hjemdahl P, Ronquist-Nii Y, Pohanka A, et al. Estimation of dabigatran plasma concentrations in the perioperative setting. An ex vivo study using dedicated coagulation assays. Thromb Haemost. 2015;113(4):862–9. doi:10.1160/TH14-09-0808.
51. He S, Wallen H, Bark N, Blomback M. In vitro studies using a global hemostasis assay to examine the anticoagulation effects in plasma by the direct thrombin inhibitors: dabigatran and argatroban. J Thromb Thrombolysis. 2013;35(2):131–9. doi:10.1007/s11239-012-0791-x.
52. Eikelboom JW, Weitz JI. Dabigatran monitoring made simple? Thromb Haemost. 2013;110(3):393–5. doi:10.1160/TH13-07-0576.
53. Douxfils J, Mullier F, Robert S, Chatelain C, Chatelain B, Dogne JM. Impact of dabigatran on a large panel of routine or specific coagulation assays. Laboratory recommendations for monitoring of dabigatran etexilate. Thromb Haemost. 2012;107(5):985–97. doi:10.1160/TH11-11-0804.
54. Samama MM, Guinet C. Laboratory assessment of new anticoagulants. Clin Chem Lab Med. 2011;49(5):761–72. doi:10.1515/CCLM.2011.134.
55. Stangier J, Feuring M. Using the HEMOCLOT direct thrombin inhibitor assay to determine plasma concentrations of dabigatran. Blood Coagul Fibrinolysis. 2012;23(2):138–43. doi:10.1097/MBC.0b013e32834f1b0c.
56. Boehringer Ingelheim. An idea for a mid to long term strategy for Pradaxa, showing EMA range comparisons. 2014. Available from: http://journals.bmj.com/site/bmj/dabigatran/compared_ema.pdf [Cited 15 March 2016].
57. Chin PK, Vella-Brincat JW, Barclay ML, Begg EJ. Perspective on dabigatran etexilate dosing - why not follow standard pharmacological principles? Br J Clin Pharmacol. 2012. doi:10.1111/j.1365-2125.2012.04266.x.
58. Rosencher N, Albaladejo P. A new approach with anticoagulant development: tailoring anticoagulant therapy with dabigatran etexilate according to patient risk. Expert Opin Pharmacother. 2012;13(2):217–26. doi:10.1517/14656566.2012.648614.
59. Cohen D. Dabigatran: how the drug company withheld important analyses. BMJ. 2014;349:g4670. doi:http://dx.doi.org/10.1136/bmj.g4670.
60. Douxfils J, Mullier F, Dogne JM. Dose tailoring of dabigatran etexilate: obvious or excessive? Expert Opin Drug Saf. 2015;14(8):1283–9. doi:10.1517/14740338.2015.1049995.
61. Ebner T, Wagner K, Wienen W. Dabigatran acylglucuronide, the major human metabolite of dabigatran: in vitro formation, stability, and pharmacological activity. Drug Metab Dispos. 2010;38(9):1567–75. doi:10.1124/dmd.110.033696.
62. Herd B, Wynne H, Wright P, James O, Woodhouse K. The effect of age on glucuronidation and sulphation of paracetamol by human liver fractions. Br J Clin Pharmacol. 1991;32(6):768–70.
63. Court MH. Interindividual variability in hepatic drug glucuronidation: studies into the role of age, sex, enzyme inducers, and genetic polymorphism using the human liver bank as a model system. Drug Metab Rev. 2010;42(1):209–24. doi:10.3109/03602530903209288.

2

Effects of Ramadan fasting on platelet reactivity in diabetic patients treated with clopidogrel

W. Bouida[1,10], H. Baccouche[1,10], M. Sassi[2,10], Z. Dridi[3], T. Chakroun[4], I. Hellara[5,10], R. Boukef[6,10], M. Hassine[5,10], F. Added[7,10], R. Razgallah[9], I. Khochtali[8,10], S. Nouira[1,10*] and On behalf of the Ramadan Research Group

Abstract

Background: The effects of Ramadan fasting (RF) on clopidogrel antiplatelet inhibition were not previously investigated. The present study evaluated the influence of RF on platelet reactivity in patients with high cardiovascular risk (CVR) in particular those with type 2 diabetes mellitus (DM).

Methods: A total of 98 stable patients with ≥2 CVR factors were recruited. All patients observed RF and were taking clopidogrel at a maintenance dose of 75 mg. Clinical findings and serum lipids data were recorded before Ramadan (Pre-R), at the last week of Ramadan (R) and 4 weeks after the end of Ramadan (Post-R). During each patient visit, nutrients intakes were calculated and platelet reactivity assessment using Verify Now P2Y12 assay was performed.

Results: In DM patients, the absolute PRU changes from baseline were +27 (p = 0.01) and +16 (p = 0.02) respectively at R and Post-R. In addition, there was a significant increase of glycemia and triglycerides levels with a significant decrease of high-density lipoprotein. In non DM patients there was no significant change in absolute PRU values and metabolic parameters. Clopidogrel resistance rate using 2 cut-off PRU values (235 and 208) did not change significantly in DM and non DM patients.

Conclusions: RF significantly decreased platelet sensitivity to clopidogrel in DM patients during and after Ramadan. This effect is possibly related to an increase of glycemia and serum lipids levels induced by fasting.

Keywords: Fasting, Platelet aggregation inhibitors, Diabetes mellitus, Platelet activation, Clopidogrel

Background

Each year, during the Ramadan month, millions of Muslims with cardiovascular risk factors observe obligatory fasting from early down to dusk. Ramadan fasting (RF) has been shown to be associated with vascular and metabolic disorders including glycemic control and lipid profile [1–3]. It may also alter pharmacologic properties of some medications resulting from the change in eating patterns and physiologic parameters disturbances [4–8]. Although patients with coronary artery disease (CAD) under antiplatelet therapy may be exempted from RF, many of them still insist to observe strictly their fasting. Clopidogrel is widely used and plays a pivotal role in reducing recurrent thrombotic events in patients with CAD, but the wide response variability of patients to this agent could lead to pharmacodynamics failure [9, 10]. Clopidogrel resistance has been documented in the range of 5–44% across the world and has been associated with adverse thrombotic events [11–13]. This is particularly true in patients type 2 with diabetes mellitus (DM) known for their suboptimal response to antiplatelet agents [14–16]. Consequently, accurate assessment of clopidogrel response during RF may have potential implications with regard to the delicate balance between thrombosis and bleeding in the monitoring of patients under antiaggregating agents. Investigating this issue is

* Correspondence: Semir.nouira@rns.tn
[1]Emergency Department, Fattouma Bourguiba University Hospital, 5000 Monastir, Tunisia
[10]Research Laboratory (LR12SP18), University of Monastir, 5000 Monastir, Tunisia
Full list of author information is available at the end of the article

now possible as several assays are available to measure platelet reactivity in order to better predict ischemic and/or bleeding complications [17]. Currently, it is not clear whether RF affects platelet reactivity in patients already treated with clopidogrel. This study was planned to assess the effects of RF on clopidogrel resistance in patients at high cardiovascular risk and especially those with DM.

Methods

Participants

This was a prospective observational study that was carried out in a group of patients having at least two currently accepted cardiovascular risk factors classification [18]. Patients were recruited from academic and non-academic medical centers serving a population of 500.000 Tunisian inhabitants. Participants were screened in outpatient clinics (cardiology, endocrinology, internal medicine, family medicine) when they presented for scheduled follow-up. Selection was based on the participant's decision to fast, while taking clopidogrel therapy for at least 6 months. Exclusion criteria included patients under 40 years or those with unstable diabetes, acute coronary syndrome within the past year prior to enrollment, current or previous (14 days) use of glycoprotein IIb/IIIa, inability to give informed consent, baseline platelet count $<100 \times 10^6$/L, current use of antidepressants, and chronic disease with <1 year expected mortality. The study was approved by the Institutional Review Board of Fattouma Bourguiba University Hospital and all patients provided written informed consent. After screening, the study design and requirements were thoroughly explained to the participants.

Methods

The study was conducted during 4 years (2010–2014) with three separate assessment visits in each year: 1) the last week before Ramadan (Pre-R) which represented the baseline period; 2) the last week of Ramadan (R); 3) and during the last week of the month following Ramadan (Post-R). Each patient served as his own control and was required to take the prescribed clopidogrel dose daily and chart the intake in a dosing diary. The duration of fasting was approximately 12 h from sunrise to sunset (the time of abstinence from food) during a 30 day period. The assessment in each of the three visits involved clinical exam and blood sampling for hematologic and metabolic tests.

Clinical assessment

Body weight and height were performed by a well-trained staff member. Weight was measured while the subjects were minimally clothed without shoes using digital scales and recorded to the nearest 0.1 kg. Body mass index (BMI) was calculated as body weight (kg) divided by squared height in meters (m2). Physical examination was carried out in all participants including systolic (SBP), diastolic (DBP) blood pressure, and heart rate. The visit is completed by a questionnaire on diet beginning 2 days before the blood sampling. No special nutritional regimen was applied to the participants during the study. All subjects were encouraged to continue their usual lifestyle and activities. The rate of hypoglycemic (symptomatic and non-symptomatic) and hyperglycemic episodes requiring ED admission was recorded within the three periods of the study. Hypoglycemia was defined as blood glucose <3.5 mmol/l. Compliance to current treatment (clopidogrel, oral hypoglycemic agents, statins...) was assessed by the attending physician based on interview and pill count. Venous blood samples were collected from the enrolled participants during the three time points. The time of blood sampling in the study was 9–10 a.m., at which all participants were fast. For the purpose of the study, we asked our patients to take clopidogrel treatment as late as possible. As Ramadan month during the study period has coincided with summer season, clopidogrel was generally taken between midnight and 1 am. We added this detail in the paper.

Hematological parameters and clopidogrel response assays

Blood samples were analyzed directly for hemoglobin, hematocrit, and platelet cell count. Prothrombin time and (PT) activated partial thromboplastin time (APTT) were studied in fresh samples. Platelet reactivity was assessed by the Verify Now P2Y12 point-of-care assay (Accumetrics, San Diego, CA, USA) using venous blood samples collected in tubes containing 3.2% sodium citrate. Verify Now P2Y12 specifically evaluates clopidogrel effect on P2Y12 receptor by optical turbidimetry. Results are reported as P2Y12 reaction units (PRU); the lower the PRU value the higher the platelet aggregation inhibition by clopidogrel. High platelet reactivity after clopidogrel (clopidogrel resistance) was defined at two cutoff values (PRU ≥ 235 [19] and ≥208 [20]). Reading recorded by the study team was not revealed to patients and their primary physician.

Metabolic measurements

An automated analyzer (Beckman Coulter DXC 600, UK) measured the concentrations of biochemical parameters using the appropriate reagents (Beckman Coulter, UK). Glucose, uric acid, total cholesterol (TC) and triglycerides (TG) were determined using an enzymatic colorimetric method (glucose oxidase, uricase, lipoprotein lipase-glycerol kinase reactions, cholesterol esterasecholesteroloxidase reactions, respectively).High-density lipoprotein cholesterol (HDL-C) concentrations were determined by immuno-inhibition. Low-density lipoprotein cholesterol (LDL-C) was calculated using the Friedewald formula: LDL-C (mmol/L) = TC – HDL-C – TG: 2.2.

Statistical analysis

All continuous data are presented as either the median with interquartile range (IQR) or the mean with SD according to the distribution of the data. The categorical data are presented as the percentage frequency of occurrence. The Kolmogorov-Smirnov test was performed to assess the normal distribution. Each subject served his own control by comparing his/her values before Ramadan with those during and after Ramadan. Differences between results were analyzed using paired samples t test for normally distributed parameters and Wilcoxon signed Rank test for not normally distributed parameters. Statistical significance was considered at $p < 0.05$ for all tests. Comparison was performed between patients with and without DM. Statistical analyses were conducted by using SPSS statistical software (version 11.5, SPSS Inc. Chicago, IL).

Results

One hundred eighteen patients under clopidogrel were included. From these, 20 patients (16.9%) were excluded from the analysis due to incomplete data at follow-up (n = 10), stop fasting (n = 6), and noncompliance with clopidogrel treatment (n = 4). At the completion of the study, 98 participants had been followed up throughout the study (Fig. 1). Demographic and clinical characteristics of the participants are summarized in Table 1. The mean age was 59.1 ± 10 years and 87,7% were men (n = 86). Most of the participants had at least 2 to 3 cardiovascular risk factors mainly dyslipidemia (77.5%) and DM (64.3%). Dual therapy with clopidogrel and aspirin was prescribed in 90 patients (91.8%) (Table 1). Mean blood pressure and heart rate did not change significantly between the three periods. Weight and BMI decreased significantly during RF and returned to baseline values at post-R period (Table 2). Caloric

Table 1 Baseline Characteristics

	Total n = 98
Age years (mean ± SD)	59.1 ± 10
Male gender; n (%)	86 (87.7%)
Cardiovascular risk factors n (%)	
Dyslipidemia	76 (77.5)
Diabetes	63 (64.3)
Arterial hypertension	61 (62.2)
Smoking	58 (59.2)
Coronary artery disease	48 (48.9)
Number	
2	60 (61.2)
3	27 (27.5)
≥ 4	11 (11.3)
Treatment n (%)	
Aspirin	90 (91.8)
Statins	81 (82.6)
Oral antidiabetics	63 (64.2)
Enzyme converting inhibitors	59 (60.2)
Beta-blockers	42 (42.8)
Diuretics	20 (20.4)
Angiotension receptor antagonists	12 (12.2)
Vitamin K antagonists	5 (4.9)
Clopidogrel indications	
Coronary artery disease	90 (91.8)
Peripheral artery disease	8 (8.2)

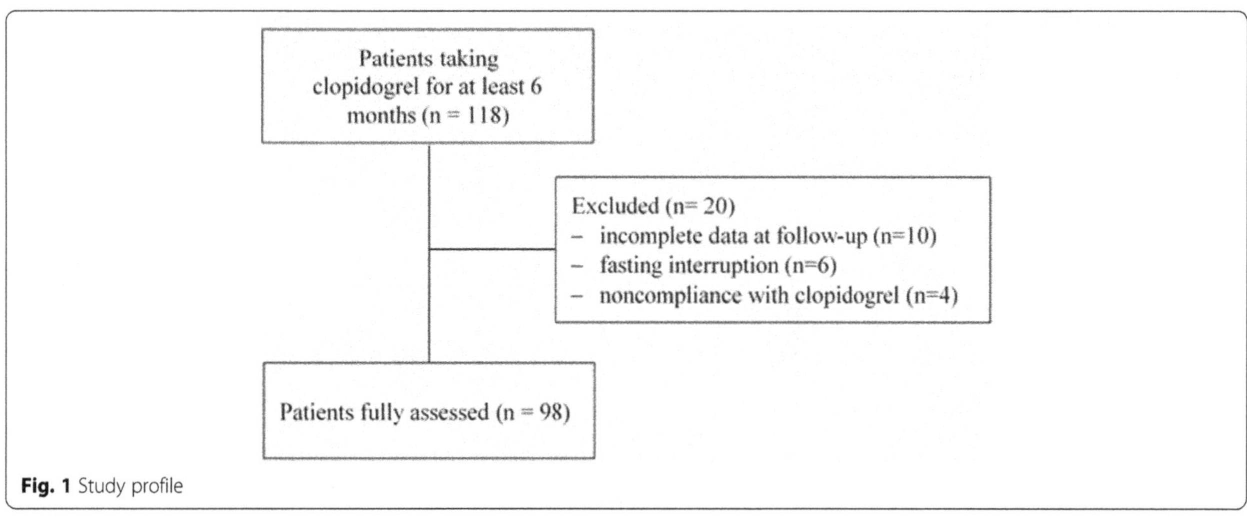

Fig. 1 Study profile

intake decreased slightly during RF and increased thereafter but all00these changes were not significant as was the distribution of caloric intake between glucids, lipids and proteins. Mean time intervals between clopidogrel taking and Verify Now testing was 9 ± 1 h at pre-R, 10 ± 1 h at R, and 10.5 ± 2 h at post-R. The time intervals were similar for the three visits (p = 0.68). Results of platelet reactivity at each time point for each period are presented in Table 3. Overall, PRU values increased significantly from pre-R to R and post-R periods (absolute increase +13 and +11 respectively; p = 0.03). In patients with DM, the absolute increase of PRU values from baseline was +27 during RF (p = 0.01) and +16 at post-R period (p = 0.02) (Fig. 2). Conversely, in non DM participants changes of PRU values were not significant between the three periods. In the overall group, the rate of clopidogrel resistance did not change significantly between the three periods whether using a PRU cutoff at 235 or 208 (Table 3). Using the cut off 208, the rate of patients with DM who were resistant during Ramadan and post-Ramadan periods compared with baseline was respectively 60.3% and 55.5 vs 52.3%, (p = 0.22). In the overall population no significant differences were observed during the three periods regarding hemoglobin, hematocrit, platelet count, prothrombin time, and activated partial thromboplastin time (Table 4). Glycemia was significantly higher during Ramadan (10.4 ± 4.7 mmol/L) compared to baseline (9.6 ± 4.9 mmol/L) (p = 0.003). Glycemia decreased after Ramadan fasting to 9.9 ± 4.8 mmol/L. Similar changes of glycemia were observed in patients with DM. With regard to serum lipid in DM patients, the following changes were observed: serum TG levels also increased significantly from 1.65 ± 0.87 mmol/L at baseline to 2.26 ± 1.91 mmol/L at Ramadan period (p = 0.002) and 1.74 ± 0.90 at post-R period (p = 0.01); HDL cholesterol decreased during Ramadan period from 1.01 ± 0.27 mmol/l at baseline to 0.93 ± 0.22 mmol/L (p = 0.001) during Ramadan, and returned to baseline values at post Ramadan period (1.02 ± 0.15 mmol/l). Serum lipids did not change significantly in non-DM patients. The other metabolic parameters (serum cholesterol, LDL cholesterol and uric acid) did not show significant changes between the three periods in patients with and without DM (Table 4). Non-symptomatic hypoglycemic events were reported in one participant before Ramadan, in three participants during Ramadan (two in DM and one in non DM patients), and in two participants after Ramadan. None of these events required ED admission. No participant was hospitalized for hyperglycemic complication.

Table 3 Platelet reactivity and clopidogrel resistance in patients with and without diabetes mellitus

	All n = 98	DM n = 63	Non DM n = 35
Pre-Ramadan			
PRU median (IQR)	199 (157–251)	200 (157–253)	196 (157–248)
Clopidogrel resistance n (%)			
PRU > 235	36 (36.7)	23 (36.5)	13 (37.1)
PRU > 208	48 (48.9)	33 (52.3)	15 (42.8)
Ramadan			
PRU median (IQR)	212 (169–257)	227 (176–261)*	200 (159–252) £
Clopidogrel resistance n (%)			
PRU > 235	39 (39.7)	27 (42.8)	12 (34.2)
PRU > 208	54 (55.1)	38 (60.3)	16 (45.7)
Post-R (n = 109)			
PRU median (IQR)	210 (166–251)	216 (176–247)*	202 (153–254)
Clopidogrel resistance n (%)			
PRU > 235	39 (39.7)	23 (36.5)	16 (45.7)
PRU > 208	52 (53.0)	35 (55.5)	17 (48.5)

DM diabetes mellitus
*p < 0.05 compared to Pre-Ramadan.
£p < 0.05 compared to patients with DM

Table 2 Clinical and caloric intake changes during the three protocol periods

	Pre-Ramadan mean (SD)	Ramadan mean (SD)	Post-Ramadan mean (SD)
Systolic arterial pressure (mmHg)	139 (24)	137 (24)	136 (24)
Diastolic arterial pressure (mmHg)	79 (12)	77 (12)	78 (12)
Pulse (b/min)	78 (12)	81 (14)	79 (14)
Weight (kg)	83.2 (11.2)	81.7 (11.1)*	82.9 (13.9)£
Body mass index (kg/m^2)	29.5 (3.7)	29.0 (3.6)*	29.6 (3.7)£
Caloric total intake (kcal/j)	2156 (449)	2035 (455)	2209 (551)
Carbohydrate intake (%)	55.2 (8.3)	56.8 (7.3)	55.1 (8.8)
Protein intake (%)	17.4 (3.9)	17.3 (3.4)	17.3 (4.8)
Fat intake (%)	27.4 (7.8)	25.7 (6.7)	27.6 (8.3)

*p < 0.05 between Pre-Ramadan and Ramadan, £p < 0.05 between Ramadan and post-Ramadan

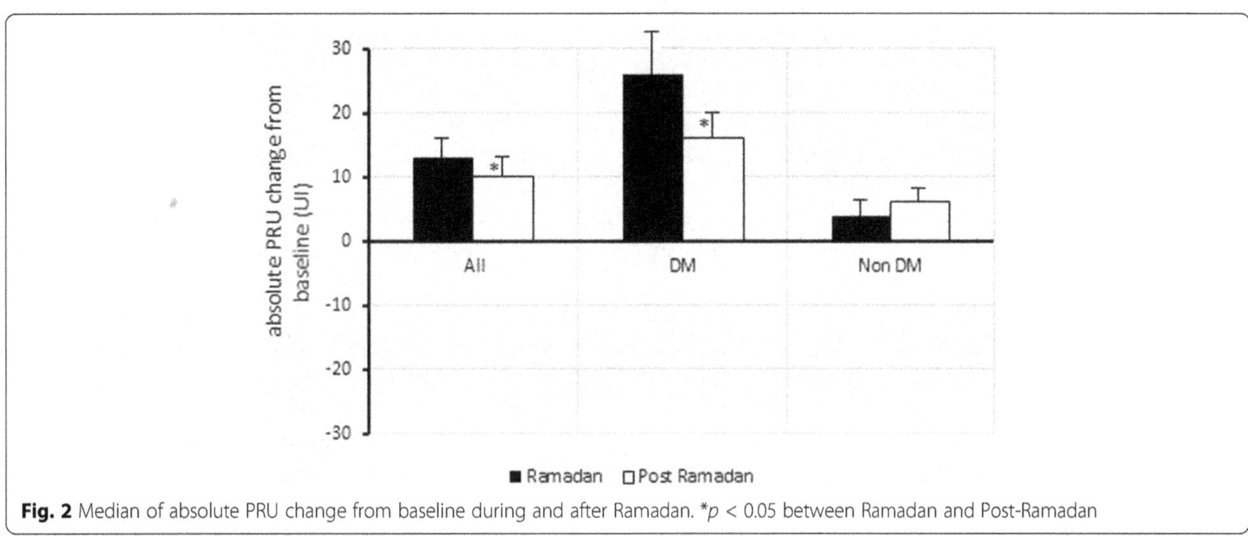

Fig. 2 Median of absolute PRU change from baseline during and after Ramadan. *$p < 0.05$ between Ramadan and Post-Ramadan

Discussion

Our results showed that platelet reactivity increased significantly during RF essentially in patients with DM and persisted 1 month later. These effects were associated with a significant increase in glycemia and serum TG levels and decrease of HDL cholesterol. In patients without DM, no significant changes were observed. No significant clinical event related to RF was reported during this study.

Antiplatelet agents are one of the most frequently used drugs in clinical practice. With regard to their wide pharmacodynamic variability, RF could significantly modify the response to these drugs. Multiple factors including changes in glycemic control and lipid profile may influence platelet reactivity and response to antiaggregating agents during RF. Patients with DM are particularly exposed to this hazard given their adverse metablolic features and comorbidities that could affect

Table 4 Biological changes during the three protocol periods

	All			Patients with DM n = 63			Patients without DM n = 35		
	Pre-Ramadan mean (SD)	Ramadan mean (SD)	Post-Ramadan mean (SD)	Pre-Ramadan mean (SD)	Ramadan mean (SD)	Post-Ramadan mean (SD)	Pre-Ramadan mean (SD)	Ramadan mean (SD)	Post-Ramadan mean (SD)
Hematological									
Hemoglobin g/dl	13.3 (1.2)	13.6 (1.5)	13.4 (1.3)	13.1 (1.1)	13.3 (1.3)	13.1 (1.2)	13.8 (1.1)	14.1 (1.4)	14.0 (1.1)
Hematocrit %	41 (5)	41 (4)	40 (4)	41 (4)	40 (4)	39 (4)	42 (7)	42 (4)	41 (4)
Platelets count × 10^3/ml	216 (22)	214 (21)	216 (24)	214 (24)	212 (24)	209 (23)	214 (22)	216 (23)	225 (22)
Prothrombin time (sec)	10.8 (0.6)	10.9 (0.6)	10.9 (0.5)	10.9 (0.5)	11.1 (0.5)	11.1 (0.6)	11.1 (0.7)	11.0 (0.5)	10.9 (0.5)
APTT (sec)	36.6 (1.6)	37.0 (1.8)	37.4 (1.7)	38.0 (2.5)	39.9 (4.2)	40.7 (4.7)	39.2 (2.5)	40.1 (3.8)	39.0 (2.8)
Biochemical									
Glycemia mmol/l	9.6 (4.9)	10.4 (4.7)*	9.9 (4.8)	11.40 (5.05)	12.23 (4.81)*	11.50 (4.77)	6.49 (2.39)	7.04 (1.55)	6.78 (3.01)
Cholesterol mmol/l	3.82 (1.19)	3.87 (1.26)	3.90 (1.21)	3.76 (1.13)	3.82 (1.33)	3.86 (1.21)	4.02 (1.35)	4.15 (1.19)	4.28 (1.24)
Triglycerides mmol/l	1.76 (1.04)	2.23 (1.16)*	1.90 (1.17)£	1.65 (0.87)	2.26 (1.91)*	1.74 (0.90)£	1.95 (1.28)	2.16 (1.46)	2.20 (1.52)
LDL cholesterol mmol/l	2.02 (0.97)	2.98 (0.97)	2.0 (0.98)	1.86 (0.87)	1.99 (0.87)	2.06 (0.95)	2.12 (1.20)	2.20 (1.06)	2.25 (1.06)
HDL cholesterol mmol/l	1.01 (0.27)	0.93 (0.22)*	1.02 (0.15)£	1.01 (0.29)	0.90 (0.23)*	0.97 (0.27)	1.01 (0.23)	1.0 (0.2)	1.05 (0.23)

DM diabetes mellitus, *$p < 0.05$ between Pre-Ramadan and Ramadan, £$p = 0.001$between Ramadan and Post-Ramadan
APTT activated partial thromboplastin time, *LDL/HDL* low-density/high-density lipoprotein

platelet function [21, 22]. Although the mechanisms for clopidogrel resistance related to RF are probably multiple in diabetic patients, inadequate metabolic control might be one of the contributor factors [23, 24]. Major glycemic excursions associated with RF may lead to non-enzymatic glycosylation of platelet membrane proteins changing their structure and conformation and consequently their function [25, 26]. Hyperglycemia may also affect platelet clopidogrel response through an increase of superoxide production or inflammatory markers discharge [20]. Geisler et al. [27] reported that diabetic patients with hyperglycemia had increased amounts of inflammatory markers in comparison to normoglycemics and non-diabetic patients. They showed that higher levels of inflammatory markers correlated with decreased response to aspirin and clopidogrel dual therapy, and found that hyperglycemia positively correlated with increased thrombus formation. In the present study, we showed that higher PRU values related to fasting was associated with a significant increase of serum triglycerides and decrease of HDL cholesterol which suggest that RF may have a lipid-related prothrombotic action. The fact that these parameters increased in the same time does not prove of course that the higher PRU values are caused by metabolic changes during Ramadan. Decrease in fish and olive oil consumption with increase of fatty acids mobilization from adipose tissue during RF could have a detrimental effects on serum lipid composition and may contribute to promote suboptimal response to antiplatelet agents. Although we demonstrated an increase of PRU values during and after RF, we did not observe higher rate of clopidogrel resistance as defined by the two cut-offs currently accepted. Early studies suggested that optimal threshold is between 230 and 240 PRU [28, 29], while post-hoc analysis of GRAVITAS suggested a somewhat lower cut-off, 208 PRU [30]. In our study, we used both PRU values and we demonstrated similar results and a trend to award a resistance increase with RF in DM patients. As optimal antiplatelet inhibition is essential in DM patients with CAD, we believe that those with borderline PRU values should be considered at increased risk of clopidogrel resistance during and after RF and should be managed on this basis.

Limitations

First, the number of DM patients is almost twice the number of non-DM patients. The fact that no differences in platelet reactivity during Ramadan fasting found in non-DM patients, could be explained by the lower number of patients. Of note, predominance of patients with DM could be expected since many participants were recruited from outpatient endocrinology clinic.

Second, although we attempted to verify compliance to clopidogrel and the treatment regimens during the three study periods, we cannot absolutely rule out inadequate compliance. Third, only the VerifyNow P2Y12 assay was used in our study to evaluate platelet function. We should note that except for a few, there are no head-to-head comparison studies between the most commonly used tests. Based on available evidence, diagnostic performance of VerifyNow assays is comparable to light transmission aggregometry which is the most widely accepted test of platelet function both in terms of biological and clinical endpoints. In addition, the Verify Now was validated in sufficiently large sample size for prediction of stent thrombosis and bleeding which justify our choice. Finally, this pilot study was not designed (size, limited follow up) to assess associations with clinical outcomes. Larger prospective studies may be warranted to elucidate the clinical regenace of our findings.

Hence, the clinical relevance of our results is unknown. Specific clinical studies are needed to define whether the decrease of clopidogrel antiplatelet activity may provide biological support for RF detrimental outcome of RF in diabetic patients.

Conclusions

In conclusion, the present study demonstrated that RF could induce an increase in clopidogrel resistance that seems to be related to a transient disturbance of glycemic control and lipid profile. The selective decrease response to antiplatelet agents during RF in diabetic patients in our study means that this population are at increased risk. This population might benefit from diagnostic testing of platelet function for whom we should better control lipid and glucose levels to adapt the dose of current medications such as statins and antidiabetics.

Abbreviations

APTT: Activated partial thromboplastin time; BMI: Body mass index; CAD: Coronary artery disease; CVR: Cardiovascular risk; DBP: Diastolic blood pressure; DM: Diabetes mellitus; HDL-C: High-density lipoprotein cholesterol; LDL-C: Low-density lipoprotein cholesterol; Post-R: After Ramadan; Pre-R: Before Ramadan; PRU: P2Y12 reaction units; PT: Prothrombin time; R: Ramadan; RF: Ramadan fasting; SBP: Systolic blood Pressure; TC: Total cholesterol; TG: Triglycerides

Acknowledgements

This work was supported in part by a grant from Medis Laboratories Tunisia.

Funding

Medis Laboratories provided Verify Now device and clopidogrel tests kits.

Authors' contributions

SN designed the study, performed data analysis, and wrote the manuscript. WB, HB, MS, ZD, TC and IH performed data collection and reviewed the manuscript. RB, FA and MH interpreted the data and critically reviewed the manuscript. RR and IK revised the intellectual content of the manuscript. All authors approved the final version of the manuscript.

Competing interests
Dr.W. Bouida, and Dr. H. Baccouche, and Dr.M. Sassi, and Dr.Z. Dridi, and Dr. T. Chakroun, and Dr.I. Hellara, and Dr.R. Boukef, and Dr.M. Hassine, and Dr. F. Added, and Dr. I. Khochtali, and Dr. S Nouira, and Dr.R. Razgallah report no competing interests.

Author details
[1]Emergency Department, Fattouma Bourguiba University Hospital, 5000 Monastir, Tunisia. [2]Laboratory of Biology, Maternity and Neonatal Medicine Center, 5000 Monastir, Tunisia. [3]Cardiology Department, Fattouma Bourguiba University Hospital, 5000 Monastir, Tunisia. [4]Regional Blood Transfusion Center, Farhat Hached University Hospital, 4004 Sousse, Tunisia. [5]Hematology Department, Fattouma Bourguiba University Hospital, 5000 Monasitr, Tunisia. [6]Emergency Department, Sahloul University Hospital, 4011 Sousse, Tunisia. [7]Cardiology Department, Abderrahman Mami University Hospital, 1080 Ariana, Tunisia. [8]Endocrinology and Internal Medicine Department, Fattouma Bourguiba University Hospital, 5000 Monastir, Tunisia. [9]Medis Laboratories, 1053 Tunis, Tunisia. [10]Research Laboratory (LR12SP18), University of Monastir, 5000 Monastir, Tunisia.

References
1. Barkia A, Mohamed K, Smaoui M, Zouari N, Hammami M, Nasri M. Change of diet, plasma lipids, lipoproteins, and fatty acids during Ramadan: a controversial association of the considered Ramadan model with atherosclerosis risk. J Health Popul Nutr. 2011;29:486–93.
2. Benaji B, Mounib N, Roky R, Aadil N, Houti IE, Moussamih S, et al. Diabetes and Ramadan: review of the literature. Diabetes Res Clin Pract. 2006;73:117–25.
3. Salti I, Bénard E, Detournay B, Bianchi-Biscay M, Le Brigand C, Voinet C, et al., EPIDIAR study group. A population-based study of diabetes and its characteristics during the fasting month of Ramadan in 13 countries: results of the epidemiology of diabetes and Ramadan 1422/2001 (EPIDIAR) study. Diabetes Care. 2004;27:2306–11.
4. Aslam M, Assad A. Drug regimens and fasting during Ramadan: a survey in Kuwait. Public Health. 1986;100:49–53.
5. Rashed AH. The fast of Ramadan. BMJ. 1992;304:521–2.
6. Addad F, Amami M, Ibn Elhadj Z, Chakroun T, Marrakchi S, Kachboura S. Does Ramadan fasting affect the intensity of acenocoumarol-induced anticoagulant effect? Br J Haematol. 2014;166:792–4.
7. Lai YF, Cheen MH, Lim SH, Yeo FH, Nah SC, Kong MC, et al. The effects of fasting in Muslim patients taking warfarin. J Thromb Haemost. 2014;12:349–54.
8. Farooq S, Nazar Z, Akhtar J, Irfan M, Subhan F, Ahmed Z, et al. Effect of fasting during Ramadan on serum lithium level and mental state in bipolar affective disorder. Int Clin Psychopharmacol. 2010;25:323–7.
9. Sharma RK, Voelker DJ, Sharma R, Reddy HK, Dod H, Marsh JD. Evolving role of platelet function testing in coronary artery interventions. Vasc Health Risk Manag. 2012;8:65–75.
10. Tantry US, Gesheff M, Liu F, Bliden KP, Gurbel PA. Resistance to antiplatelet drugs: what progress has been made? Expert Opin Pharmacother. 2014;15: 2553–64.
11. Siller-Matula JM, Trenk D, Schrör K, Gawaz M, Kristensen SD, Storey RF, et al., EPA (European Platelet Academy). Response variability to P2Y12 receptor inhibitors: expectations and reality. JACC Cardiovasc Interv. 2013;6:1111–28.
12. Gurbel PA, Bliden KP, Hiatt BL, O'Connor CM. Clopidogrel for coronary stenting: response variability, drug resistance, and the effect of pretreatment platelet reactivity. Circulation. 2003;107:2908–13.
13. Matetzky S, Shenkman B, Guetta V, Shechter M, Beinart R, Goldenberg I, et al. Clopidogrel resistance is associated with increased risk of recurrent atherothrombotic events in patients with acute myocardial infarction. Circulation. 2004;109:3171–5.
14. Schuette C, Steffens D, Witkowski M, Stellbaum C, Bobbert P, Schultheiss HP, et al. The effect of clopidogrel on platelet activity in patients with and without type-2 diabetes mellitus: a comparative study. Cardiovasc Diabetol. 2015;14:15.
15. Angiolillo DJ, Suryadevara S. Aspirin and clopidogrel: efficacy and resistance in diabetes mellitus. Best Pract Res Clin Endocrinol Metab. 2009;23:375–88.
16. Price MJ. Diabetes mellitus and clopidogrel response variability. J Am Coll Cardiol. 2014;64:1015–8.
17. Aradi D, Collet JP, Mair J, Plebani M, Merkely B, Jaffe AS, et al., Study Group on Biomarkers in Cardiology of the Acute Cardiovascular Care Association of the European Society of Cardiology, Working Group on Thrombosis of the European Society of Cardiology. Platelet function testing in acute cardiac care - is there a role for prediction or prevention of stent thrombosis and bleeding? Thromb Haemost. 2015;113:221–30.
18. Grundy SM, Pasternak R, Greenland P, Smith S Jr, Fuster V. Assessment of cardiovascular risk by use of multiple-risk-factor assessment equations: a statement for healthcare professionals from the American Heart Association and the American College of Cardiology. Circulation. 1999; 100:1481–92.
19. Price MJ, Endemann S, Gollapudi RR, et al. Prognostic significance of post-clopidogrel platelet reactivity assessed by a point-of-care assay on thrombotic events after drug-eluting stent implantation. Eur Heart J. 2008;29:992–1000.
20. Price M, Angiolillo D, Teirstein P, et al. Platelet reactivity and cardiovascular outcomes after percutaneous coronary intervention: a time dependent analysis of the Gauging Responsiveness with a VerifyNow P2Y12 assay: impact on thrombosis and safety (GRAVITAS) trial. Circulation. 2011;124:1132–7.
21. Ferroni P, Basili S, Falco A, Davì G. Platelet activation in type 2 diabetes mellitus. J Thromb Haemost. 2004;2:1282–91.
22. Grant PJ. Diabetes mellitus as a prothrombotic condition. J Intern Med. 2007;262:157–72.
23. Demirtunc R, Duman D, Basar M, Bilgi M, Teomete M, Garip T. The relationship between glycemic control and platelet activity in type 2 diabetes mellitus. J Diabetes Complicat. 2009;23:89–94.
24. Singla A, Antonino MJ, Bliden KP, Tantry US, Gurbel PA. The relation between platelet reactivity and glycemic control in diabetic patients with cardiovascular disease on maintenance aspirin and clopidogrel therapy. Am Heart J. 2009;158:784.e1–6.
25. Watala C, Golanski J, Pluta J, Boncler M, Rozalski M, Luzak B, et al. Reduced sensitivity of platelets from type 2 diabetic patients to acetylsalicylic acid (aspirin)-its relation to metabolic control. Thromb Res. 2004;113:101–13.
26. Winocour PD, Watala C, Perry DW, Kinlough-Rathbone RL. Decreased platelet membrane fluidity due to glycation or acetylation of membrane proteins. Thromb Haemost. 1992;68:577–82.
27. Geisler T, Mueller K, Aichele S, Bigalke B, Stellos K, Htun P, et al. Impact of inflammatory state and metabolic control on responsiveness to dual antiplatelet therapy in type 2 diabetics after PCI: prognostic relevance of residual platelet aggregability in diabetics undergoing coronary interventions. Clin Res Cardiol. 2010;99:743–52.
28. Breet NJ, van Werkum JW, Bouman HJ, Kelder JC, Ruven HJ, Bal ET, et al. Comparison of platelet function tests in predicting clinical outcome in patients undergoing coronary stent implantation. JAMA. 2010;303:754–62.
29. Price MJ, Endemann S, Gollapudi RR, Valencia R, Stinis CT, Levisay JP, et al. Prognostic significance of post-clopidogrel platelet reactivity assessed by a point-of-care assay on thrombotic events after drug-eluting stent implantation. Eur Heart J. 2008;29:992–1000.
30. Stone GW, Witzenbichler B, Weisz G, Rinaldi MJ, Neumann FJ, Metzger DC, et al., ADAPT-DES Investigators. Platelet reactivity and clinical outcomes after coronary artery implantation of drug-eluting stents (ADAPT-DES): a prospective multicentre registry study. Lancet. 2013;382:614–23.

3

Low-molecular-weight-heparin can benefit women with recurrent pregnancy loss and sole protein S deficiency: a historical control cohort study from Taiwan

Ming-Ching Shen[1†], Wan-Ju Wu[2,3†], Po-Jen Cheng[4], Gwo-Chin Ma[3], Wen-Chu Li[5], Jui-Der Liou[6], Cheng-Shyong Chang[1], Wen-Hsiang Lin[3] and Ming Chen[2,3,7,8*]

Abstract

Background: Heritable thrombophilias are assumed important etiologies for recurrent pregnancy loss. Unlike in the Caucasian populations, protein S and protein C deficiencies, instead of Factor V Lieden and Prothrombin mutations, are relatively common in the Han Chinese population. In this study we aimed to investigate the therapeutic effect of low molecular weight heparin upon women with recurrent pregnancy loss and documented protein S deficiency.

Methods: During 2011–2016, 68 women with recurrent pregnancy loss (RPL) and protein S deficiency (both the free antigen and function of protein S were reduced) were initially enrolled. All the women must have experienced at least three recurrent miscarriages. After excluding those carrying balanced translocation, medical condition such as diabetes mellitus, chronic hypertension, and autoimmune disorders (including systemic lupus erythematosus and anti-phospholipid syndrome), coexisting thrombophilias other than persistent protein S deficiency (including transient low protein S level, protein C deficiency, and antithrombin III), only 51 women with RPL and sole protein S deficiency were enrolled. Initially they were prescribed low dose Aspirin (ASA: 100 mg/day) and unfortunately there were still 39 women ended up again with early pregnancy loss (12 livebirths were achieved though). Low-molecular-weight-heparin (LMWH) was given for the 39 women in a dose of 1 mg/Kg every 12 h from the day when the next clinical pregnancy was confirmed to the timing at least 24 h before delivery. The perinatal outcomes were assessed.

Results: Of 50 treatment subjects performed for the 39 women (i.e. 11 women enrolled twice for two pregnancies), 46 singletons and one twin achieved livebirths. The successful live-birth rate in the whole series was 94 % (47/50). Nineteen livebirths delivered vaginally whereas 28 delivered by cesarean section. The cesarean delivery rate is thus 59. 57 %. Emergent deliveries occurred in 3 but no postpartum hemorrhage had been noted.

Conclusions: Our pilot study in Taiwan, an East Asian population, indicated anti-coagulation therapy is of benefit to women with recurrent pregnancy loss who had documented sole protein S deficiency.

Keywords: Anticoagulation, Protein S deficiency, Thrombophilia, Recurrent miscarriages, Low-molecular-weight-heparin

* Correspondence: mchen_cch@yahoo.com; mingchenmd@gmail.com
†Equal contributors
[2]Department of Obstetrics and Gynecology, Changhua Christian Hospital, Changhua, Taiwan
[3]Department of Genomic Medicine, Changhua Christian Hospital, 500 Changhua, Taiwan
Full list of author information is available at the end of the article

Background

Habitual abortion (defined as at least three recurrent miscarriages), namely recurrent pregnancy loss (RPL), is a condition caused by heterogeneous etiologies such as hormonal (luteal defect), chromosomal (carriers of balanced translocation), structural (Mullerian anomalies such as didelphys, bicornuate, or septate uterus), immunological (anti-phospholipid antibody or aberrations involving nature killer cells), and thrombophilia [1, 2]. Among them, heritable thrombophilias are treatable theoretically despite most published studies, including some but very limited well-conducted randomized trials, in the literature did not observe an apparent benefit by using anticoagulants to enhance the livebirth rate in women with RPL [3–9].

Heritable thrombophilias ever reported with clinical significance include protein S deficiency, protein C deficiency, anti-thrombin III deficiency, Factor V Leiden mutation, and prothrombin mutation, however, there are ethnic differences: The most common heritable thrombophilias in the Caucasian populations are Factor V Leiden mutation and prothrombin mutation whereas in Taiwan, protein S, protein C, and antithrombin III deficiencies are the most common [10–14]. Despite most published reports in the literature failed to observe a beneficial effect of anti-coagulants to enhance the livebirth rates in women with RPL, it may be inappropriate to extrapolate those results, mainly based on other ethnic groups, into an East Asian population (Taiwan is a multi-ethnic group country with a predominance of Han Chinese). According to our previous studies, the most common heritable thrombophilias in the thromboembolic patients in Taiwan are protein S and protein C deficiencies [13, 14]. Meanwhile, the selection criteria and treatment protocol varied across different studies and thus we should be cautious when reading reviews based upon meta-analysis [3–5, 15].

We are keen to explore if there is any role of using anticoagulants in this group of patients in Taiwan. In order to better define the enrollment criteria, those with other confounding factors such as anti-phospholipid antibody syndrome, underlying medical conditions including autoimmune diseases, diabetes mellitus, chronic hypertension, and previous history of thromboembolism are excluded. Only nulliparous women with protein S deficiency and suffered from RPL are enrolled in this pilot study. We intended to include women with in whom protein S deficiency is the only attributable etiology, and from another point of view, to include women with protein S deficiency who were otherwise healthy (that is, without previous thromboembolic events) until adult life except suffering from RPL. In addition, in order to simplify and better understand the actual effect of anticoagulants in the enrolled cases, we only included those receiving low-molecular-weight-heparin as the sole therapy. The livebirth rate is the primary outcome we aimed to observe in this historical cohort. Attributable causes of the failed cases, if any, will be assessed by examinations including fetal/placental pathology, immunological and genetic investigations.

Methods

Patient enrollment

During 2011–2016, women suffered from at least three recurrent miscarriages who came to our clinic received a series of investigation including karyotyping, thrombophilia profile (antithrombin III, protein C, Protein S levels), and immune profile (lupus anti-coagulant to explore if she has anti-phospholipid antibody syndrome). Only those women with sole protein S deficiency, and naturally conceived, were enrolled. They were prescribed low dose Aspirin (ASA, 100 mg per day) when another new pregnancy was achieved and in those ended up again with early pregnancy loss (less than 12 complete weeks of gestation), these patients were enrolled in this cohort and would be given daily anti-coagulant treatment in the injection starting from when next pregnancy is established. It is noteworthy that since the level of protein S may decrease physiologically during pregnancy due to the estrogen effect, only those with persistent low protein S level in the non-gestational period (we enrolled only those with low levels in both protein S function and free protein S antigen (Ag)), were included. Assays adopted for protein S measurement used the functional assay by clotting based kits (the reference ranges: protein S function 63.5~149 %; free protein S antigen: 54.7~123.7 %) according to the method reported by Moraes and colleagues in 2000 [16]. Women with other heritable thromobophilias (Protein C and antithrombin III deficiency), immune problems (such as systemic lupus erythematosus, anti-phospholipid antibody syndrome), other pre-conceptional underlying medical conditions (such as diabetes mellitus and chronic hypertension), or carrying balanced translocation, were excluded. The institutional review board (IRB) of Changhua Christian Hospital had approved the study (CCH-IRB-151209).

Clinical management protocol

Low-molecular-weight-heparin (enoxaparin) was given in a dose of 1 mg/Kg every 12 h from the day being enrolled to the timing a few days (at least 24 h) before delivery. Standard antenatal care was unaffected otherwise and the perinatal outcome was assessed. The patients received both the antenatal care from two of the coauthors (M Chen, an obstetrician who specializes in high-risk pregnancy, and MC Shen, a hematologist who specializes in thrombosis and hemostasis). In order to avoid the risk of postpartum hemorrhage due to emergent deliveries, which often occurs unexpectedly, the patients were either arranged for induction of labor if she chose to deliver vaginally, or scheduled cesarean section if there are obstetric indications or by their autonomous choice to choose elective cesareans. The anticoagulants were ought to be stopped at least 24 h before delivery in the ideal situation. The risk of postpartum hemorrhage as well as other side effects that may occur because of this treatment protocol were discussed and explained in great details to these patients and the informed consents were obtained. The blood coagulation profiles such as prothrombin time (PT), activated partial thromboplastin time (aPTT), or other assays to assess the status of the molecules involving the coagulation cascade were not regularly monitored. The livebirth rate is the primary outcome indicator. Secondary outcome indicators are also recorded for the obstetric complications such as premature births, low birth weight, and pre-eclampsia. The whole investigation period reported in this historical control cohort study ended at 22, May, 2016.

Results

A total of 68 patients with at least three recurrent miscarriages and having protein S deficiency (both the free antigen and the function of protein S) went to our clinics. In these 68 patients, 17 of them were further filtered out because these patients were found with heritable thromobophilias other than protein S deficiency (protein C deficiency ($n = 1$), antithrombin III ($n = 1$), immune problems (e.g., systemic lupus erythematosus ($n = 2$), anti-phospholipid antibody syndrome ($n = 1$)), or with other underlying medical conditions (e.g., diabetes mellitus ($n = 1$) and chronic hypertension ($n = 1$)), or carrying balanced translocation ($n = 1$). Another 9 women who only had transient low level of protein S during pregnancy were also excluded. Therefore, 51 women entered the cohort initially (12 of them enjoyed livebirths simply by being given low dose Aspirin in a dose with 100 mg per day). Of the remaining 39 women, 11 had two pregnancies being enrolled. Consequently, 50 treatment subjects were performed for the 39 women and 47 livebirths were achieved (Fig. 1). Only 3 pregnancies failed, two of which were later proved to be an aneuploidy pregnancy (trisomy 22 and monosomy X respectively) and one was ectopic pregnancy ended with tubal abortion. Of the 11 women with two pregnancies enrolled, 10 had successful two livebirths and one had one livebirth with one abortion due to trisomy 22. In 47 successful livebirths, 48 live babies were born (because there were one twin pregnancy), 19 of them delivered vaginally (40.43 %), and 28 of them delivered by cesarean section (59.57 %). Notably only 4 of the cesarean group demanded elective cesarean section due to the concern about the risk of natural births, and all the remaining 24 out of the 28 women in the cesarean group had obstetric indications. The indications include previous uterine surgery ($n = 5$, two are both repeated sections and entered the group twice and the first cesareans were elective), placenta previa ($n = 2$), prolonged labor ($n = 2$), fetal malpresentation ($n = 6$, one case is twin pregnancy with one fetal malpresentation), non-reassuring fetal heart rate tracings ($n = 8$), and severe pre-eclampsia ($n = 1$). All the successful live babies were born after gestational age (GA) 28 weeks (Table 1), with the patient numbers (percentage) delivered at GA 36 weeks or greater, between GA 32 and 35^{+6} weeks, between GA 28 and 31^{+6} weeks and less than 28 weeks were 33 (70.21 %), 12 (25.23 %), 2 (4.26 %), and 0 (0 %). The distribution of the percentiles (calculated by Hadlock chart) regarding birth body weights of these babies was 27.08 % ($n = 13$, < 10th percentile, "small for gestational age (SGA)" by definition), 41.67 % ($n = 20$, 10th–25th percentile), 22.92 % ($n = 11$, 25th–50th percentile), and 8.33 % ($n = 4$, > 50th percentile) (Table 2). Nine of the babies born with SGA were in the cesarean section group (exactly those whose indications for cesareans were non-reassuring fetal heart rate tracings ($n = 8$) and severe-preeclampsia ($n = 1$)). Only 3 of the entire cohort delivered emergently (two vaginal births and one cesarean birth) and no postpartum hemorrhage occurred. Pathological examination of the placentae belonging to the SGA babies all showed gross hypoplasia and histological vascular lesions.

In summary, the rate of successful livebirth was thus 94 % (47/50). If by comparing to their historical cohort (the livebirth rate before being enrolled into the treatment group is theoretically zero) themselves, the benefit to this group of patients is clear ($p = 0$ by Fisher's exact test).

Discussion

Recurrent pregnancy loss (RPL), or recurrent miscarriages, is a serious problem in women's health. It affects 1–2 % of women of reproductive age if 3 or more first trimester pregnancy losses (less than 12 complete gestational weeks) and 5 % of women of reproductive age if 2 or more first trimester pregnancy losses (less than 12 complete gestational weeks) [7]. The causes of RPL are varying and complicated. Etiologies that had been reported included structural (e.g., mullerian anomalies), hormonal (e.g., luteal defect), chromosomal (e.g., balanced translocation carriers), immune-related (e.g., anti-phospholipid antibody syndrome), thrombophilias (e.g., factor V Lieden mutations and prothrombin mutations in the caucasian populations), and others. Strategies to combat these putative causative factors were therefore developed, with varying efficacies [17, 18]. For example, some advocated anti-coagulation therapy (such as aspirin or low-molecular-weight-heparin) is effective in improving the pregnancy outcome in women

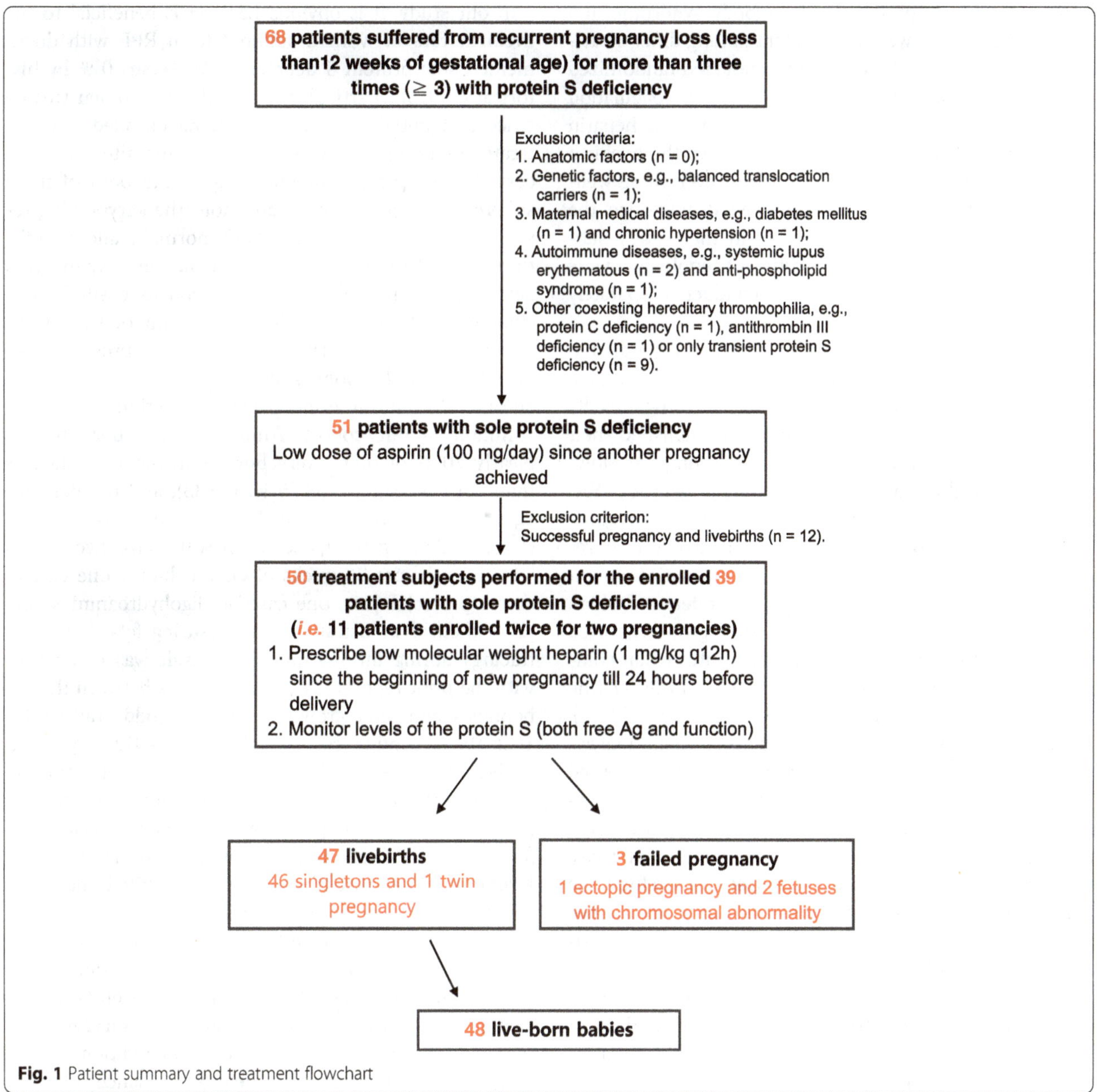

Fig. 1 Patient summary and treatment flowchart

Table 1 Summary of the gestational age (GA) at delivery and mode of delivery of the 47 livebirths

	% (= *n*/47)
GA at delivery	
≥ 36 weeks	70.2 (33/47)
32–35^{+6} weeks	25.23 (12/47)
28–31^{+6} weeks	4.26 (2/47)
< 28 weeks	0 (0/47)
Mode of delivery	
Normal spontaneous delivery	40.43 (19/47)
Cesarean section	59.57 (28/47)

Table 2 Percentile distributions of the birth body weight of the 48 live-birth babies

Percentile of birth body weight (Hadlock)	% (= *n*/48)
SGA (<10th percentile)	27.08 (13/48)
10th–25th percentile	41.67 (20/48)
25th–50th percentile	22.92 (11/48)
>50th percentile	8.33 (4/48)

SGA small for gestational age

suffered from anti-phospholipid antibody syndrome and RPL but the results were inconsistent among different trials [6, 19–21]. Most of the recently conducted randomized trials failed to show significant benefit of anti-coagulation therapy (either aspirin or low molecular weight heparin alone or if both were combined) to improve the livebirth rates in women with RPL [6, 7, 15]. However, these well-conducted trials actually did not well characterize the underlying possible causative factors in their study subjects, the subgroups due to different etiologies were pooled and no specific analyses were conducted separately on each subgroup.

There are at least three randomized trials conducted in earlier times dealing with women with RPL and a concomitant heritable thrombophilia and the results were varying. In 2004, the French group published their result of the randomized trial to compare low-molecular-weight heparin (LMWH) versus aspirin (ASA) and reported that LMWH was superior to ASA regarding the livebirth rates. In 2008, the Jordan group reported a similar beneficial effect of anticoagulant therapy (LMWH versus placebo, please refer to Qubian et al., 2008 [22]). However, the Canadian group reported there seemed no benefit to the livebirth rates when comparing LMWH plus ASA and ASA alone in 2009 (the HepASA Trial, please refer to Laskin et al., 2009 [23]). Tan and colleagues therefore conducted a meta-analysis and concluded that no obvious benefit can be attributed to the anti-coagulation therapy regarding the improvement of livebirth rates in women with RPL and a heritable thrombophilia [5]. However, the mixture of those three randomized trials is too arbitrary to exclude the possibility of real benefit in this group of women since the three randomized trails had different inclusion criteria and even different therapeutic regimens.

It is noteworthy that there are some recently well-conducted randomized trials being published and all of these trials failed to demonstrate the benefit of anticoagulant therapy in women with RPL (but not aiming solely at women with heritable thrombophilias). The Netherland study published in NEJM 2010 did included some women with heritable thrombophilas (even included protein S deficiency) but the authors also admitted the study lacked the power to study the effect in the subgroups of the study population [6]. The Scottish Pregnancy Intervention study (SPIN) also included some women with heritable thrombophilia but admitted their result did not exclude the possible benefit in women with a particular thrombophilia disorder as well [7]. A recent multi-center with minimized randomization scheme conduced in Germany and Austria actually excluded the women with constitutional thrombophilia disorders and therefore the trial result is of no reference value to our study [15].

In our study, it is obvious LMWH is beneficial to the livebirth rate in women suffered from RPL with documented sole protein S deficiency (94 versus 0 % by historical control). Particularly, 2 of the 11 women treated twice had initially decided not being enrolled into the treatment group receiving anticoagulants after one successful birth and got pregnant again and both of them suffered from spontaneous abortion (the karyotyping results of the abortion were both normal), and thereby they entered the study for the second time when again getting pregnant and successful livebirths ensued. Such experience strengthened the justification of this study. However, it seems LMWH was unable to prevent other obstetric complications such as placental insufficiency and therefore intrauterine growth restriction (IUGR) are common in our cohort. Among 48 live born babies, Nearly 70 % of them were born with birth weight less than 25th percentile (68.75 %; $n = 33$), and the percentage of small for gestational age (SGA) was 27.08 % ($n = 13$). Among the babies born with SGA, five infants were born before 36 weeks of GA, including one case of severe pre-eclampsia, one case of oligohydroamnios, and all of them demonstrated non-reassuring fetal heart rate tracings during intrapartum. The result was compatible with the prior reports [24], showed a link between thrombophilias and fetal growth restriction (odds ratio (OR) 10.2; 95 % confidence interval (CI) 1.1–91.0) by meta-analysis. However, available evidences in the literature do not support the prophylactic use of anticoagulants can prevent obstetric complications, including preeclampsia, fetal growth restriction, or abruption in women with any form of inherited thrombophilias [25], despite it may of be benefit in women with recurrent implantation failures when receiving in vitro fertilization [26]. It is still under debate if thrombophilias truly associated, or simply it is only by chance a coincidence, with the placental insufficiency [27]. Further investigations and surveys were required to establish causality. Hence, in addition to anticoagulation therapy, frequent fetal surveillance is necessary for pregnant women with thrombophilia to prevent adverse neonatal outcomes. The American Congress of Obstetricians and Gynecologists (ACOG) did not suggest special management in thrombophilia patients in the absence of obstetric complications such as preeclampsia, abruption or IUGR. Weekly fetal assessment with non-stress test beginning at ≥36 weeks of gestation and delivery at 39 weeks of gestation is still the recommended standard of care when managing these patients [28].

We admit the evidence level of historical control is much lower than prospective randomized control trials. Many inherent defects underlying the historical control study hampered its use. The most frequently cited defects of this historical control conducted by patients as their own controls included different diagnostic criteria, differences in the concomitant standard of care, and missing records across different times along the time period (especially if the time spans very long such as 10 or 20 years). However, the credibility of historical control study may be better if there is a large treatment effect, or it is very difficult to bias outcome assessment, or it follows the pair availability design (proposed by Baker and Lindeman in 1994) [29–32].

Conclusion

In this study, a strikingly high 94 % successful livebirth rate, straight-forward outcome indicators (livebirth rate and pregnancy complications), and the short time period (within 5 years), all indicated that our result is of better power, despite the limitations of historical control discussed above, to convince us that such intervention did benefit this group of patients in Taiwan. Our study clearly demonstrated a potential benefit of daily anticoagulation therapy in women suffered from RPL and had documented sole protein S deficiency. Future prospective randomized studies are needed to further prove its efficacy.

Abbreviations

ACOG: The American Congress of Obstetricians and Gynecologists; ASA: Aspirin; CI: Confidence interval; GA: Gestational age; IUGR: Intrauterine growth restriction; LMWH: Low-molecular-weight heparin; OR: Odds ratio; RPL: Recurrent pregnancy loss; SGA: Small for gestational age

Acknowledgements

The expenses of the medical care of the patients, however, were compensated and supported by the National Health Insurance System of Taiwan.

Funding

This study received a research fund from Changhua Christian Hospital (grant number: 105-CCH-PRJ-004) to M. Chen.

Authors' contributions

MCS, WJW, GCM, WHL, and MC wrote the paper. MCS, PJC, WCL, JDL, CSC, and MC conceived the idea and designed the study. MCS, WJW, and MC recruited the patients and analyzed the results. All authors read and approved the final manuscript.

Competing interests

The authors declare that they have no competing interests.

Author details

[1]Department of Internal Medicine, Changhua Christian Hospital, Changhua, Taiwan. [2]Department of Obstetrics and Gynecology, Changhua Christian Hospital, Changhua, Taiwan. [3]Department of Genomic Medicine, Changhua Christian Hospital, 500 Changhua, Taiwan. [4]Department of Obstetrics and Gynecology, Chang-Gung Memorial Hospital Linkou Medical Center and Chang-Gung University, Taoyuan, Taiwan. [5]Department of Obstetrics and Gynecology, Puli Christian Hospital, Nantou, Taiwan. [6]Department of Obstetrics and Gynecology, Taipei Chang-Gung Memorial Hospital, Taipei, Taiwan. [7]Department of Obstetrics and Gynecology, and Department of Medical Genetics, College of Medicine, and Hospital, National Taiwan University, Taipei, Taiwan. [8]Department of Life Science, Tunghai University, Taichung, Taiwan.

References

1. Saravelos SH, Regan L. Unexplained recurrent pregnancy loss. Obstet Gynecol Clin North Am. 2014;41(1):157–66.
2. Kupferminc M. Thrombophilia and pregnancy. Reprod Biol Endocrinol. 2003; 1:111.
3. de Jong PG, Kaandorp S, Di Nisio M, Goddijn M, Middeldorp S. Aspirin and/ or heparin for women with unexplained recurrent miscarriage with or without inherited thrombophilia. Cochrane Database Syst Rev. 2014;7: CD004734.
4. de Jong PG, Goddijn M, Middeldorp S. Antithrombotic therapy for pregnancy loss. Human Reprod Update. 2013;19(6):656–73.
5. Tan WK, Lim SK, Tan LK, Bauptista D. Does low-molecular-weight heparin improve live birth rates in pregnant women with thrombophilic disorders? A systematic review. Singapore Med J. 2012;53(10):659–63.
6. Kaandorp SP, Goddijn M, van der Post JA, Hutten BA, Verhoeve HR, Hamulyák K, Mol BW, Folkeringa N, Nahuis M, Papatsonis DN, Büller HR, van der Veen F, Middeldorp S. Aspirin plus heparin or aspirin alone in women with recurrent miscarriage. New Engl J Med. 2010;362(17):1586–96.
7. Clark P, Walker ID, Langhorne P, Crichton L, Thomson A, Greaves M, Whyte S, Greer IA, Scottish Pregnancy Intervention Study (SPIN) collaborators. SPIN (Scottish Pregnancy Intervention) study: a multicenter, randomized controlled trial of low-molecular-weight heparin and low-dose aspirin in women with recurrent miscarriage. Blood. 2010;115(21):4162–7.
8. Kaandorp S, Di Nisio M, Goddijn M, Middeldorp S. Aspirin or anticoagulants for treating recurrent miscarriage in women without antiphospholipid syndrome. Cochrane Database Syst Rev. 2009;1:CD004734.
9. Di Nisio M, Peters L, Middeldorp S. Anticoagulants for the treatment of recurrent pregnancy loss in women without antiphospholipid syndrome. Cochrane Database Syst Rev. 2005;2:CD004734.
10. Udry S, Aranda FM, Latino JO, de Larraanga JF. Paternal factor V Leiden and recurrent pregnancy loss: a new concept behind fetal genetics? J Thromb Haemost. 2014;12(5):666–9.
11. MacCallum P, Bowles L, Keeling D. Diagnosis and management of heritable thrombophilias. BMJ. 2014;349:g4387.
12. Battinelli EM, Marshall A, Connors JM. The role of thrombophilia in pregnancy. Thrombosis. 2013;2013:516420.
13. Shen MC, Lin JS, Tsai W. Protein C and protein S deficiencies are the most important risk factors associated with thrombosis in Chinese venous thrombophilic patients in Taiwan. Thromb Res. 2000;99(5):447–52.
14. Shen MC, Lin JS, Tsai W. High prevalence of antithrombin III, protein C and protein S deficiency, but no factor V Leiden mutation in venous thrombophilic Chinese patients in Taiwan. Thromb Res. 1997;87(4):377–85.
15. Schleussner E, Kamin G, Seliger G, Rogenhofer N, Ebner S, Toth B, Schenk M, Henes M, Bohlmann MK, Fischer T, Brosteanu O, Bauersachs R, Petroff D, ETHIG II group. Low-molecular-weight heparin for women with unexplained recurrent pregnancy loss: a multicenter trial with a minimization randomization scheme. Ann Intern Med. 2015;162(9):601–9.
16. Moraes C, Lofthouse E, Eikelboom J, Thom J, Baker R. Detection of protein S deficiency: a new functional assay compared to an antigenic technique. Pathology. 2000;32(2):94–7.

17. Regan L, Rai R. Epidemiology and the medical causes of miscarriage. Baillieres Best Pract Res Clin Obstet Gynaecol. 2000;14:839–54.
18. Kutteh WH. Novel strategies for the management of recurrent pregnancy loss. Semin Reprod Med. 2015;33(3):161–8.
19. Empson M, Lassere M, Craig J, Scott J. Prevention of recurrent miscarriage for women with antiphospholipid antibody or lupus anticoagulant. Cochrane Database Syst Rev. 2005;2:CD002859.
20. Farquharson RG, Quenby S, Greaves M. Antiphospholipid syndrome in pregnancy: a randomized, controlled trial of treatment. Obstet Gynecol. 2002; 100:408–13.
21. Rai R, Cohen H, Dave M, Regan L. Randomised controlled trial of aspirin and aspirin plus heparin in pregnant women with recurrent miscarriage associated with phospholipid antibodies (or antiphospholipid antibodies). BMJ. 1997;314:253–7.
22. Qublan H, Amarin Z, Dabbas M, Farraj AE, Beni-Merei Z, Al-Akash H, Bdoor AN, Nawasreh M, Malkawi S, Diab F, Al-Ahmad N, Balawneh M, Abu-Salim A. Low-molecular-weight heparin in the treatment of recurrent IVF-ET failure and thrombophilia: a prospective randomized placebo-controlled trial. Hum Fertil (Camb). 2008;11(4):246–53.
23. Laskin CA, Spitzer KA, Clark CA, Crowther MR, Ginsberg JS, Hawker GA, Kingdom JC, Barrett J, Gent M. Low molecular weight heparin and aspirin for recurrent pregnancy loss: results from the randomized, controlled HepASA Trial. J Rheumatol. 2009;36(2):279–87.
24. Alfirevic Z, Roberts D, Martlew V. How strong is the association between maternal thrombophilia and adverse pregnancy outcome? A systematic review. Eur J Obstet Gynecol Reprod Biol. 2002;101(1):6.
25. Bates SM, Greer IA, Middeldorp S, Veenstra DL, Prabulos AM, Vandvik PO, American College of Chest Physicians. VTE, thrombophilia, antithrombotic therapy, and pregnancy: Antithrombotic Therapy and Prevention of Thrombosis, 9th ed: American College of Chest Physicians Evidence-Based Clinical Practice Guidelines. Chest. 2012;141(2 Suppl):e691S.
26. Potdar N, Gelbaya TA, Konje JC, Nardo LG. Adjunct low-molecular-weight heparin to improve live birth rate after recurrent implantation failure: a systematic review and meta-analysis. Hum Reprod Update. 2013;19(6):674–84.
27. Rodger MA, Paidas M, McLintock C, Middeldorp S, Kahn S, Martinelli I, Hague W, Rosene Montella K, Greer I. Inherited thrombophilia and pregnancy complications revisited. Obstet Gynecol. 2008;112(2 Pt 1):320–4.
28. ACOG Practice Bulletin No. 111. Inherited thrombophilias in pregnancy. Obstet Gynecol. 2010;115(4):877–87.
29. Walton MK, Powers 3rd JH, Hobart J, Patrick D, Marquis P, Vamvakas S, Isaac M, Molsen E, Cano S, Burke LB. International Society for Pharmacoeconomics and Outcomes Research Task Force for Clinical Outcomes Assessment: Clinical Outcome Assessments: Conceptual Foundation-Report of the ISPOR Clinical Outcomes Assessment–Emerging Good Practices for Outcomes Research Task Force. Value Health. 2015;18(6): 741–52.
30. Castillo RC, Scharfstein DO, MacKenzie EJ. Observational studies in the era of randomized trials: finding the balance. J Bone Joint Surg Am. 2012;94(Supp 1):112–7.
31. Baker SG, Lindeman KS. The pair availability design: a proposal for evaluating epidural analgesia during labor. Stat Med. 1994;13:2269–78.
32. Baker SG, Lindeman KS. Rethinking historical controls. Biostatistics. 2001;2(4): 383–96.

4

Edoxaban versus enoxaparin for the prevention of venous thromboembolism after total knee or hip arthroplasty: pooled analysis of coagulation biomarkers and primary efficacy and safety endpoints from two phase 3 trials

Yohko Kawai[1*], Takeshi Fuji[2], Satoru Fujita[3], Tetsuya Kimura[4], Kei Ibusuki[4], Kenji Abe[5] and Shintaro Tachibana[6]

Abstract

Background: The objective of this analysis was to assess the effects of edoxaban compared with enoxaparin on key coagulation biomarkers and present pooled primary efficacy and safety results from phase 3 STARS E-3 and STARS J-V trials for prevention of venous thromboembolism (VTE) after total knee arthroplasty (TKA) or total hip arthroplasty (THA).

Methods: In the randomized, double-blind, double-dummy, multicenter, STARS E-3 and STARS J-V trials, patients received edoxaban 30 mg or enoxaparin 2000 IU (20 mg) twice daily for 11 to 14 days. The studies were conducted in Japan and Taiwan; enoxaparin dosing was based on Japanese label recommendations. The primary efficacy endpoint was incidence of VTE; the safety endpoint was major or clinically relevant nonmajor (CRNM) bleeding. Blood samples were taken at presurgical evaluation, pretreatment (postsurgery), predose on day 7, predose on completion of treatment, and at a follow-up examination 25 to 35 days after the last dose of study drug for D-dimer, prothrombin fragment 1 + 2 (F_{1+2}), and soluble fibrin monomer complex (SFMC) measurement.

Results: A total of 716 patients enrolled in STARS E-3 and 610 patients enrolled in STARS J-V; 1326 patients overall. This analysis included 657 patients who received edoxaban 30 mg QD and 650 patients who received enoxaparin 20 mg BID. Incidence of VTE was 5.1 and 10.7% for edoxaban and enoxaparin, respectively (P <0.001). Incidence of combined major and CRNM bleeding was 4.6 and 3.7% for edoxaban and enoxaparin, respectively ($P = 0.427$). On day 7, mean D-dimer (4.4 vs 5.5 μg/mL), F_{1+2} (363 vs 463 pmol/L), and SFMC (5.7 vs 6.8 μg/mL) were lower in edoxaban-treated patients relative to enoxaparin-treated patients, respectively (P <0.0001 for all). At end of treatment, mean D-dimer (5.4 vs 6.2 μg/mL), F_{1+2} (292 vs 380 pmol/L), and SFMC (6.2 vs 7.2 μg/mL) were lower in edoxaban-treated patients relative to enoxaparin-treated patients (P <0.0001 for all).

Conclusions: Edoxaban was superior to enoxaparin in prevention of VTE following TKA and THA, with comparable rates of bleeding events. Relative to enoxaparin, edoxaban significantly reduced D-dimer, F_{1+2}, and SFMC.

Keywords: DOAC, Total knee arthroplasty, Total hip arthroplasty, Biomarker, VTE prophylaxis

* Correspondence: yohko@iuhw.ac.jp
[1]International University of Health and Welfare, 8-10-16 Akasaka, Minato-ku, Tokyo 107-0052, Japan
Full list of author information is available at the end of the article

Background

Patients undergoing orthopedic surgery such as total knee arthroplasty (TKA) or total hip arthroplasty (THA) are at high risk for venous thromboembolism (VTE) [1, 2]. Anticoagulation therapy and/or mechanical prophylaxis, including compression stockings or intermittent pneumatic compression, are recommended for prevention of VTE after orthopedic surgery [1, 2]. In Japan, edoxaban [3], a direct oral anticoagulant (DOAC) selective inhibitor of activated factor Xa (FXa), and enoxaparin [4], an injectable low-molecular-weight heparin (LMWH), are both indicated for prophylaxis of deep vein thrombosis (DVT) following TKA, THA, or hip fracture surgery. The approval of edoxaban for the primary prevention of VTE after lower limb orthopedic surgery was based on evidence collected during three phase 3 studies evaluating the safety and efficacy of edoxaban compared with enoxaparin for prevention of VTE in Japanese or Taiwanese patients following TKA [5], THA [6], and hip fracture surgery [7]. In these studies, edoxaban demonstrated significantly reduced or comparable rates of VTE and similar rates of bleeding events relative to enoxaparin.

This report presents a post hoc pooled analysis of coagulation biomarkers in the TKA/THA studies as well as pooled results of the primary efficacy (VTE) and safety (bleeding events) endpoints. Coagulation biomarkers include D-dimer, prothrombin fragments 1 + 2 (F_{1+2}), and soluble fibrin monomer complex (SFMC). D-dimer, which has a high negative predictive value for VTE, is formed upon cleavage of cross-linked fibrin polymers by plasmin [8–10]. F_{1+2} is a marker of thrombin generation and represents coagulation activity [11]. Fibrin monomers result from cleavage of fibrinogen by thrombin [8]. Soluble fibrin in plasma is also a marker of coagulation activity and is seen to increase rapidly during and after hip replacement surgery [12]. Assessment of coagulation biomarkers can provide information on the effect of anticoagulants in relation to dose and clinical response.

Methods

Detailed descriptions of the methodology of these trials are available in the primary publications (STARS E-3 [5] and STARS J-V [6]). The trial designs for patients undergoing TKA (STARS E-3; NCT01181102) or THA (STARS J-V; NCT01181167) were similar. In the randomized, double-blind, double-dummy, multicenter trials, patients received oral edoxaban 30 mg or edoxaban placebo once daily within 6 to 24 h after surgery, and subcutaneous enoxaparin 2000 IU (equivalent to 20 mg) or enoxaparin placebo twice daily within 24 to 36 h after surgery, each for 11 to 14 days. Enoxaparin 20 mg is the usual recommended dose for adults in Japan due to the lower body weight of Japanese patients [13]; standard of care is administration of enoxaparin 24 to 36 h postsurgery.

Concomitant use of anticoagulants, antiplatelet agents, thrombolytic agents, or other agents that affect thrombus formation was not allowed from the day of surgery until 24 h after the final dose of study drug, unless treatment of deep vein thrombosis or pulmonary embolism (PE) was required. Mechanical prophylaxis (eg, elastic stockings or intermittent pneumatic compression therapy of the foot sole or lower leg and thigh) was permitted from the day of surgery to venography. Venography of the operated lower limb in the TKA trial STARS E-3 and of both lower limbs in the THA trial STARS J-V was performed within 24 h of the last dose of study drug or within 96 h in exceptional cases such as difficulty establishing an intravenous line.

The studies were performed in accordance with the provisions of the Declaration of Helsinki, Guidelines for Good Clinical Practice, and other related regulations. The protocols were approved by institutional review boards at each study center, and written informed consent was obtained from all patients prior to randomization.

Patients

Men and women 20 to <85 years of age undergoing unilateral TKA or THA (both excluding revision arthroplasty) were included. Presurgical exclusion criteria included risk for bleeding, risk for thromboembolism, previous TKA, weight <40 kg, severe renal impairment (creatinine clearance <30 mL/min) [14], evidence of hepatic dysfunction (serum aspartate aminotransferase or serum alanine aminotransferase levels ≥2 times the upper limit of normal or total bilirubin ≥1.5 times the upper limit of normal), previous treatment with edoxaban, and current antithrombotic therapy for another complication. Postsurgical exclusion criteria included abnormal bleeding from the puncture site during spinal anesthesia, need for repeat surgery before the start of study treatment, abnormal or excessive bleeding experienced during surgery, and inability to take oral medication.

Assessments

Thromboembolic events included asymptomatic or symptomatic DVT—confirmed by venography at the end of study treatment—and symptomatic and diagnosed PE. Additional imaging techniques used to confirm suspected DVT or PE included ultrasonography, computerized tomography scanning, pulmonary scintigraphy, or pulmonary arteriography.

Major bleeding was defined as fatal bleeding; clinically overt bleeding accompanied by a decrease in hemoglobin of >2 g/dL or requiring transfusion with >800 mL of blood; retroperitoneal, intracranial, intraocular, or intrathecal bleeding; or bleeding requiring repeat surgery. Clinically relevant nonmajor (CRNM) bleeding was defined as bleeding that did not meet the criteria for major bleeding, but was characterized by hematoma ≥5 cm in diameter, epistaxis or gingival bleeding in the absence of external factors lasting ≥5 min, gastrointestinal bleeding, gross hematuria persistent after 24 h of onset, or any other bleeding deemed clinically significant by the investigator. Minor bleeding was any bleeding event that was not considered a major or CRNM bleeding event. Thromboembolic events were assessed by the blinded Thromboembolic Event Assessment Committee and bleeding events by the Bleeding Event Assessment Committee.

Blood sampling was performed at presurgical evaluation, pretreatment (postsurgery), predose on day 7, predose on completion of treatment, and at a follow-up examination 25 to 35 days after the last dose of study drug. All biomarker assessments for D-dimer, F_{1+2}, and SFMC were performed and measured at a central laboratory (SRL Inc., Tokyo, Japan). D-dimer was measured by a latex agglutination assay using the LATECLE D-dimer test kit (Kainos Laboratories, Inc., Tokyo, Japan; upper limit of detection, 1.0 μg/mL); data were expressed as D-dimer units. Assessment of F_{1+2} was performed via ELISA (Fibinostika, Organon Teknika BV, The Netherlands; normal detection range 69–229 pmol/L) [15] and assessment of SFMC was performed via a latex immunoturbidimetric assay (upper limit of detection, 6.1 μg/mL) [16].

Treatment compliance was assessed by clinical interview with patients and by remaining drugs collected.

Statistical analysis

The primary efficacy endpoint—the proportion of patients who experienced at least 1 thromboembolic event from the start of treatment to venography—was assessed in the full analysis set of patients, those who received ≥1 dose of study drug and who underwent interpretable venography. Baseline data and safety results were analyzed in the safety set—patients who received ≥1 dose of study drug and had safety data collected after the start of treatment. Biomarker results were analyzed in the pharmacodynamic set—patients who received ≥1 dose of study drug, had no protocol violations, had compliance rates of ≥80%, and had ≥1 biomarker measurement (Fig. 1).

The number of VTE events and number of bleeding events across the 2 trials were added. The Farrington-Manning method [17] was used to derive the difference in VTE incidence. The SCORE method [18] was used to calculate 95% confidence intervals (CIs) for both VTE and bleeding events. For analysis of coagulation biomarkers, summary statistics were calculated by group and time.

Paired comparisons between groups were performed using chi squared or Wilcoxon rank sum testing with a

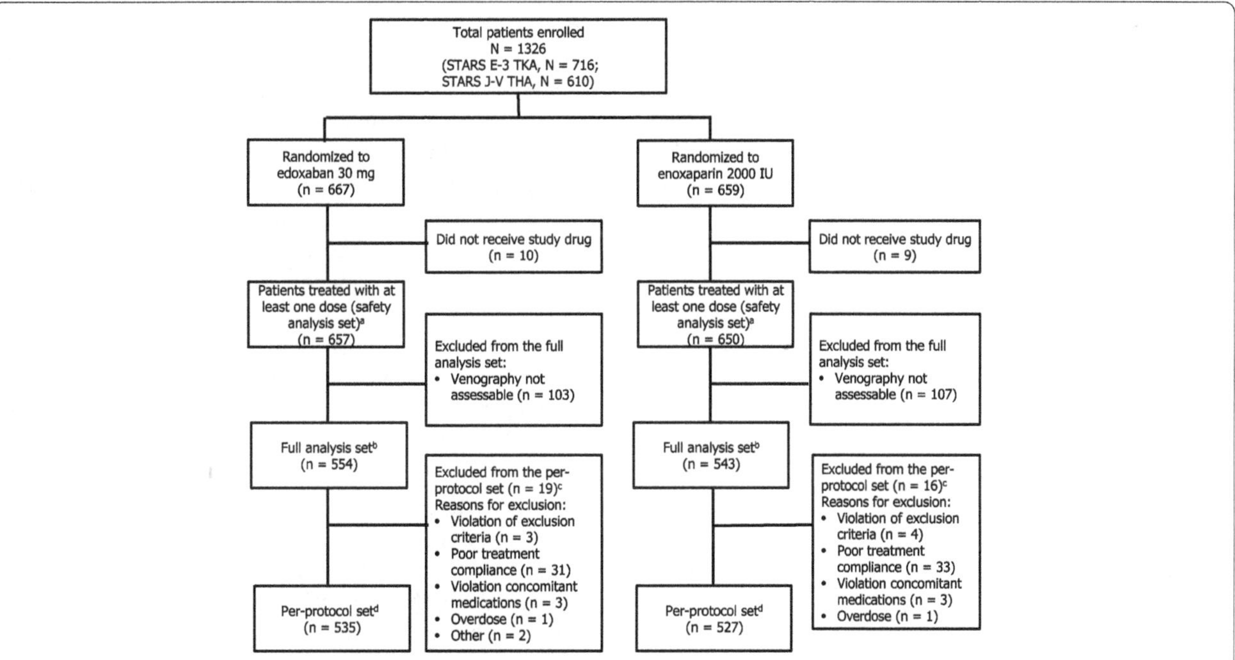

Fig. 1 Distribution of patients in the pooled data analyses. [a]The safety analysis set included all enrolled patients who received study drug, had posttreatment safety data, and did not have significant GCP violations. [b]The full analysis set included all patients receiving ≥1 dose of study drug and excluded patients with significant GCP violations or with inadequate venography. [c]Multiple answers were allowed; patients falling under multiple categories were counted once for each category. [d]The per-protocol set included patients in the FAS and excluded patients with violations of inclusion or exclusion criteria, violation of rules for prohibited concomitant drugs/treatment, or <80% compliance with study drug. GCP = good clinical practice; FAS = full analysis set; THA = total hip arthroplasty; TKA = total knee arthroplasty

significance level set to 5%. All statistical tests were conducted as 2-sided tests.

Results

Patients

There were no significant differences in baseline characteristics between the combined treatment groups from the 2 trials (Table 1). Overall, patients were predominantly women (83%) of a mean age of 68 years. The primary disease was most frequently osteoarthritis (88%). A total of 1326 patients were enrolled; this analysis included 657 patients who received edoxaban 30 mg once daily and 650 patients who received enoxaparin 20 mg twice daily. Patient disposition was similar between the 2 trials (Fig. 1).

Primary efficacy endpoint

The composite of asymptomatic DVT and symptomatic DVT or PE occurred in 28 of 554 patients who received edoxaban (5.1%) and 58 of 543 patients who received enoxaparin (10.7%), P <0.001 (Fig. 2). Thromboembolic events were primarily asymptomatic DVT.

Biomarkers

Plasma levels of the coagulation biomarker D-dimer are shown in Fig. 3a and Table 2. Mean D-dimer concentrations substantially increased after surgery but before treatment. After treatment, mean D-dimer levels (standard deviation [SD]) decreased significantly more in the edoxaban-treated than the enoxaparin-treated patients, respectively, both on day 7 (4.4 [2.1] vs 5.5 [2.6] μg/mL) and at the end of treatment (days 11–14) (5.4 [2.5] vs 6.2 [3.1] μg/mL), P <0.0001 for both. Median values and ranges are provided in Additional file 1: Table S1.

Table 1 Patient demographics and baseline characteristics

Variable	Edoxaban 30 mg QD $N=657$	Enoxaparin 20 mg BID $N=650$	P value
Female, n (%)	552 (84.0)	527 (81.1)	0.161[a]
Age, years, mean (min–max)	68.3 (36–84)	68.1 (24–84)	0.760[b]
Body weight, kg, mean (min–max)	58.7 (40–124)	58.8 (40–98)	0.848[b]
Creatinine clearance, mL/min, mean (min–max)	82.1 (30.6–242.9)	81.7 (31.0–209.7)	0.804[b]
Primary disease, n (%)			
Osteoarthritis	582 (88.6)	563 (86.6)	0.270[c]
Rheumatoid arthritis	42 (6.4)	46 (7.1)	
Other	35 (5.0)	41 (6.3)	

BID twice daily, *QD* once daily
[a]Chi square test
[b]t test
[c]Wilcoxon test

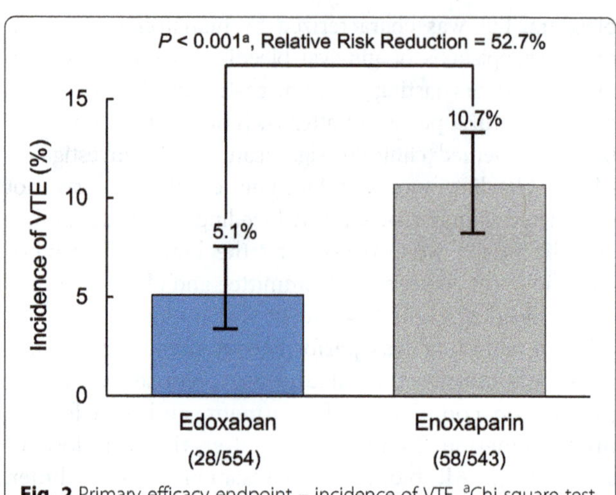

Fig. 2 Primary efficacy endpoint – incidence of VTE. [a]Chi square test. VTE = venous thromboembolism

Mean F_{1+2} concentrations increased after surgery and decreased following treatment with edoxaban or enoxaparin. The observed decrease in F_{1+2} following edoxaban treatment was larger relative to the decrease observed with enoxaparin treatment (Fig. 3b and Table 2). The mean F_{1+2} concentrations (SD) in edoxaban-treated and enoxaparin-treated patients, respectively, on day 7 of treatment were 363 (164) vs 463 (186) pmol/L and at the end of treatment were 292 (168) vs 380 (174) pmol/L, P <0.0001 for both. Median values and ranges are provided in Additional file 1: Table S1.

Mean SFMC concentrations rose after surgery and showed a larger decrease following edoxaban treatment relative to enoxaparin treatment (Fig. 3c and Table 2). The mean SFMC concentrations (SD) in edoxaban and enoxaparin patients, respectively, on day 7 were 5.7 (9.8) vs 6.8 (14.0) μg/mL and at the end of treatment were 6.2 (10.7) vs 7.2 (11.8), P <0.0001 for both. Median values and ranges are provided in Additional file 1: Table S1.

Assessment of plasma concentrations of biomarkers was performed in patients stratified by the presence or absence of VTE and the presence or absence of major or CRNM bleeding. Values followed a similar trend for patients with and without VTE and for edoxaban and enoxaparin treatment for D-dimer and F_{1+2} (Table 3). Values for SFMC were similar between edoxaban and enoxaparin treatments and were numerically elevated for patients with VTE relative to those who did not have VTE. Values for D-dimer, F_{1+2}, and SFMC followed a similar trend for patients with and without CRNM and for treatment with edoxaban and enoxaparin (Table 4).

Safety

There were no significant differences in the incidence of bleeding events during the trial between groups treated

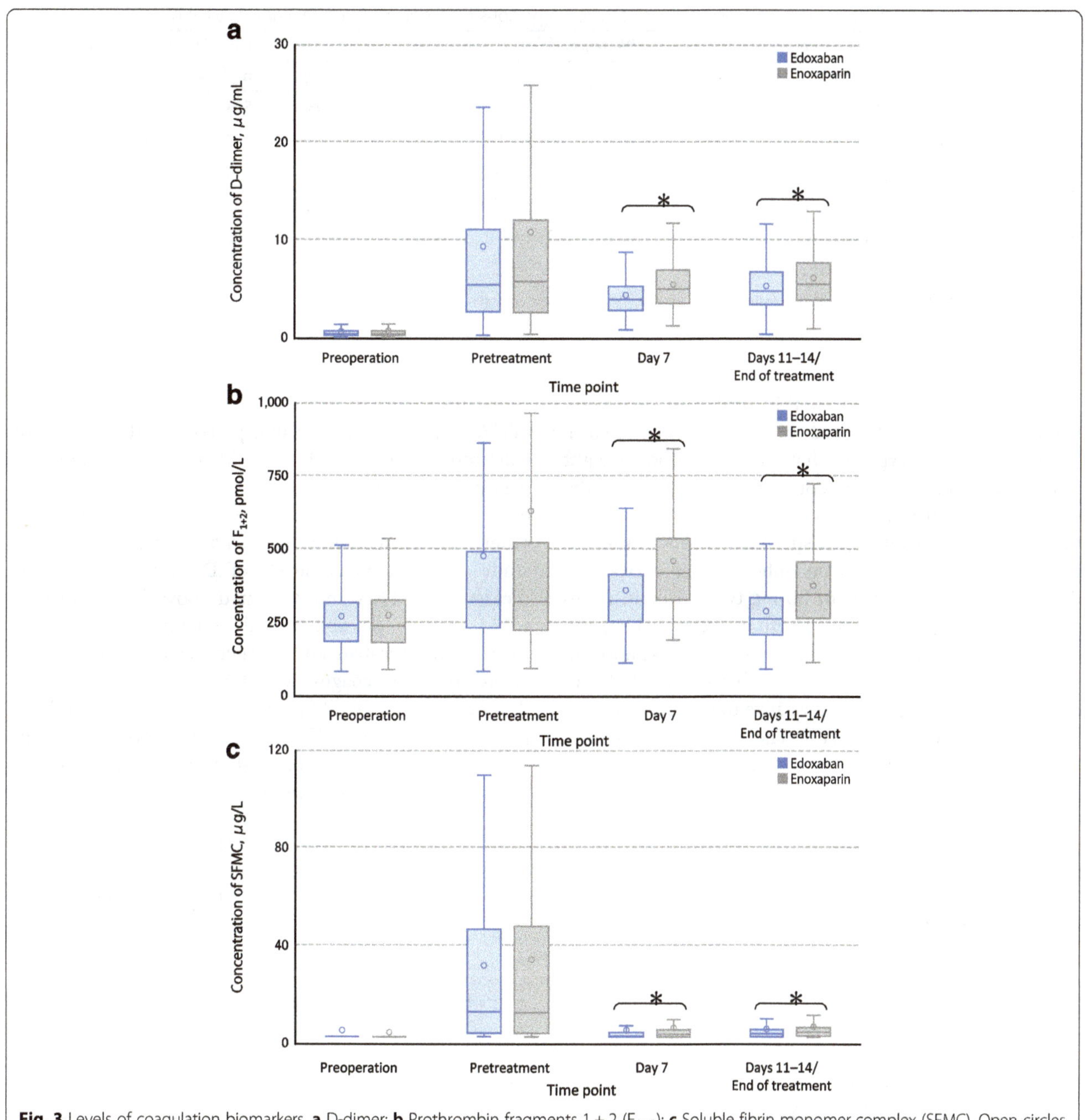

Fig. 3 Levels of coagulation biomarkers. **a** D-dimer; **b** Prothrombin fragments 1 + 2 (F_{1+2}); **c** Soluble fibrin monomer complex (SFMC). Open circles mark mean; horizontal lines indicate median; boxes represent 25–75%; capped lines represent 10 and 90%; * = P <0.001 (Wilcoxon test)

with edoxaban or enoxaparin (Fig. 4). Combined major and CRNM bleeding events occurred in 4.6% of edoxaban-treated and 3.7% of enoxaparin-treated patients ($P = 0.427$). The incidence of adverse events (AEs) was slightly lower in the edoxaban group (66%) than the enoxaparin group (75%). There were no differences in the frequency of serious AEs between the treatment groups [5, 6].

Discussion

The risk of VTE increases after knee or hip arthroplasty [1, 2]. As shown in this pooled analysis of two phase 3 trials 11 to 14 days after surgery for TKA or THA, the incidence of VTE was significantly lower in patients administered once-daily oral edoxaban 30 mg (5.1%) than in those receiving twice-daily subcutaneous enoxaparin 20 mg (10.7%), P <0.001. Coagulation biomarkers D-dimer, F_{1+2}, and SFMC each increased immediately after surgery. Over the course of 11 to 14 days, levels of the coagulation biomarkers were significantly lower after treatment with the DOAC edoxaban relative to the LMWH enoxaparin. In contrast, the frequency of bleeding events in the pooled results did not significantly differ.

Table 2 Mean plasma concentrations of coagulation biomarkers at various time points after total knee or total hip arthroplasty

		Preoperation		Pretreatment		Day 7[a]		End of treatment (days 11–14)[a]	
		n	Mean (SD)	n	Mean (SD)	n	Mean (SD)	n	Mean (SD)
D-dimer (μg/mL)	Edoxaban	535	0.73 (0.82)	535	9.42 (12.56)	532	4.43[b] (2.08)	528	5.37[b] (2.52)
	Enoxaparin	527	0.78 (0.96)	527	10.92 (16.23)	480	5.53 (2.56)	472	6.23 (3.12)
F_{1+2} (pmol/L)	Edoxaban	535	273.9 (150.6)	535	479.7 (741.8)	532	362.8[b] (164.2)	528	292.1[b] (167.6)
	Enoxaparin	527	277.8 (160.9)	527	633.2 (3234.9)	480	463.3 (185.6)	472	379.6 (174.4)
SFMC (μg/mL)	Edoxaban	535	5.62 (17.86)	535	32.25 (40.47)	532	5.71[b] (9.76)	528	6.15[b] (10.72)
	Enoxaparin	527	4.81 (8.42)	527	34.72 (45.62)	480	6.82 (13.99)	472	7.23 (11.78)

F_{1+2} thrombin fragments 1 + 2, *SD* standard deviation, *SFMC* soluble fibrin monomer complex
[a]Predose
[b]*P* vs enoxaparin <0.0001 (Wilcoxon test)

Doses and timing used in this study are consistent with the Japanese standard of care for enoxaparin. Japanese patients typically have a lower body weight relative to their Western counterparts. Although the dose of enoxaparin used was low (2000 IU, twice daily), this is the recommended dose specific to Japan for prevention of VTE [4]. Prophylactic, subcutaneous enoxaparin doses of 40 mg once daily or 30 mg twice daily in males weighing >57 kg are associated with increased enoxaparin exposure and increased bleeding risk. Administration of LMWH 2 to 4 h postoperatively has been associated with higher rates of major bleeding relative to administration at 12 to 48 h postoperatively [19]. The Japanese standard of care calls for initiation of enoxaparin 24 to 36 h following surgery.

The results of STARS E-3 (TKA) [5] and STARS J-V (THA) [6] followed the same pattern as the pooled results reported here, with an incidence of VTE after surgery of 7.4 and 2.4% for edoxaban and 13.9 and 6.9% for enoxaparin in the 2 trials, respectively, and no significant differences in bleeding events. In a phase 2, dose-finding study in Japan, mean levels of D-dimer and F_{1+2} increased after TKA and remained above baseline for 11 to 14 days in placebo-treated patients, whereas treatment with edoxaban after surgery significantly reduced levels of the coagulation biomarkers in a dose-dependent manner [20]. In a retrospective study of patients undergoing TKA in Japan, patients treated with edoxaban 15 mg once daily showed significant reductions in D-dimer relative to enoxaparin 20 mg twice

Table 3 Mean plasma concentrations of coagulation biomarkers at various time points after total knee or total hip arthroplasty in patients with and without VTE

		Preoperation		Pretreatment		Day 7[a]		End of treatment (days 11–14)[a]	
		n	Mean (SD)	n	Mean (SD)	n	Mean (SD)	n	Mean (SD)
Patients without VTE									
D-dimer (μg/mL)	Edoxaban	526	0.73 (0.84)	526	9.33 (12.54)	521	4.40 (2.09)	511	5.35 (2.49)
	Enoxaparin	485	0.77 (0.94)	485	10.28 (14.82)	443	5.38 (2.32)	430	6.00 (2.96)
F_{1+2} (pmol/L)	Edoxaban	526	273.6 (150.3)	526	478.6 (748.6)	521	361.5 (164.6)	511	293.5 (169.3)
	Enoxaparin	485	273.9 (139.3)	485	614.6 (3357.3)	443	457.9 (183.8)	430	372.6 (166.6)
SFMC (μg/mL)	Edoxaban	526	5.38 (17.34)	526	31.21 (39.32)	521	5.55 (9.04)	511	6.31 (11.22)
	Enoxaparin	485	4.33 (6.04)	485	31.87 (43.53)	443	6.22 (11.68)	430	6.94 (10.80)
Patients with VTE									
D-dimer (μg/mL)	Edoxaban	28	0.75 (0.86)	28	8.40 (9.17)	24	4.56 (1.52)	23	5.46 (2.88)
	Enoxaparin	58	0.90 (0.97)	58	16.96 (24.17)	47	7.06 (3.86)	49	8.41 (3.78)
F_{1+2} (pmol/L)	Edoxaban	28	258.4 (117.4)	28	483.3 (220.5)	24	352.9 (128.3)	23	248.7 (86.31)
	Enoxaparin	58	309.8 (273.2)	58	824.8 (959.3)	47	531.2 (213.6)	49	444.5 (222.0)
SFMC (μg/mL)	Edoxaban	28	8.90 (21.23)	28	52.19 (48.89)	24	8.10 (18.70)	23	4.77 (2.38)
	Enoxaparin	58	8.36 (18.17)	58	63.67 (56.12)	47	12.31 (26.32)	49	9.85 (17.73)

F_{1+2} thrombin fragments 1 + 2, *SD* standard deviation, *SFMC* soluble fibrin monomer complex, *VTE* venous thromboembolism
[a]Predose

Table 4 Mean plasma concentrations of coagulation biomarkers at various time points after total knee or total hip arthroplasty in patients with and without major or clinically relevant nonmajor bleeding

		Preoperation		Pretreatment		Day 7[a]		End of treatment (days 11–14)[a]	
		n	Mean (SD)	n	Mean (SD)	n	Mean (SD)	n	Mean (SD)
Patients without major or CRNM bleeding									
D-dimer (μg/mL)	Edoxaban	627	0.75 (0.99)	627	9.75 (12.95)	597	4.43 (2.07)	578	5.38 (2.49)
	Enoxaparin	626	0.78 (0.92)	626	10.72 (15.39)	552	5.47 (2.53)	517	6.15 (3.00)
F_{1+2} (pmol/L)	Edoxaban	627	275.4 (148.0)	627	484.7 (736.0)	597	361.1 (162.2)	578	291.7 (163.2)
	Enoxaparin	626	276.4 (153.3)	626	617.3 (2975.3)	552	463.4 (192.4)	517	378.2 (171.4)
SFMC (μg/mL)	Edoxaban	627	5.72 (17.49)	627	32.69 (40.46)	597	5.66 (9.50)	578	6.30 (11.18)
	Enoxaparin	626	4.80 (8.14)	626	34.71 (45.40)	552	6.88 (13.49)	517	7.12 (11.43)
Patients with major or CRNM bleeding									
D-dimer (μg/mL)	Edoxaban	30	0.52 (0.27)	30	8.73 (11.84)	15	4.53 (1.70)	9	6.29 (3.52)
	Enoxaparin	24	0.89 (1.29)	24	8.95 (9.28)	14	5.24 (1.86)	10	8.40 (6.20)
F_{1+2} (pmol/L)	Edoxaban	30	264.5 (108.3)	30	440.3 (430.4)	15	371.5 (141.5)	9	325.0 (140.9)
	Enoxaparin	24	265.8 (113.4)	24	526.2 (714.4)	14	470.3 (143.3)	10	449.0 (120.6)
SFMC (μg/mL)	Edoxaban	30	3.41 (1.82)	30	30.28 (44.24)	15	4.03 (1.06)	9	6.42 (3.20)
	Enoxaparin	24	5.05 (4.38)	24	26.66 (32.86)	14	4.08 (1.49)	10	7.84 (4.31)

CNRM clinically relevant nonmajor, F_{1+2} thrombin fragments 1 + 2, *SD* standard deviation, *SFMC* soluble fibrin monomer complex
[a]Predose

daily or fondaparinux 1.5 mg once daily over a 2-week period following surgery [21].

Edoxaban directly and selectively inhibits FXa, which is part of both the intrinsic and extrinsic coagulation pathways that lead to generation of thrombin and clot formation [22, 23]. One molecule of FXa can catalyze the formation of approximately 1000 thrombin molecules [23]. In contrast, LMWHs target FXa indirectly and affect multiple targets in the coagulation pathway [23]. The direct and selective targeting of FXa by edoxaban may account for the significantly greater reduction in coagulation biomarkers, which translates to reduced rates of VTE.

Limitations of this analysis include that it is post hoc and that it combines data from 2 different studies. However, the studies were very similar in anticoagulant treatment regimens and patient characteristics. In addition, for the coagulation biomarker results, pooling of results was required to obtain sufficient data to perform statistical comparisons between treatments. It also should be noted that edoxaban is approved only in Japan for VTE prophylaxis and is not approved for this indication in Europe or the United States.

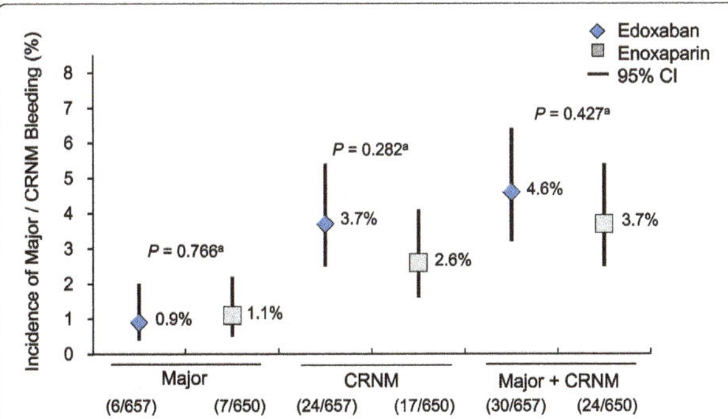

Fig. 4 Incidence of major and CRNM bleeding events. [a]Chi square test; CI = confidence interval; CRNM = clinically relevant nonmajor

Conclusions

In conclusion, the biomarker results for the pooled analysis of the TKA and THA trials may suggest stronger anticoagulant activity with once-daily oral edoxaban 30 mg than twice-daily, subcutaneous enoxaparin 20 mg following lower limb orthopedic surgery, although the initial timing of edoxaban or enoxaparin administration differed. The 2 treatments were associated with similar rates of bleeding events.

Abbreviations

AE: Adverse event; CRNM: Clinically relevant nonmajor; DOAC: Direct oral anticoagulant; DVT: Deep vein thrombosis; F_{1+2}: Prothrombin fragments 1 + 2; FXa: Factor Xa; LMWH: Low-molecular-weight heparin; PE: Pulmonary embolism; SD: Standard deviation; SFMC: Soluble fibrin monomer complex; THA: Total hip arthroplasty; TKA: Total knee arthroplasty; VTE: Venous thromboembolism

Acknowledgements
Daiichi Sankyo, the study sponsor, was involved in the design of the study and the collection and analysis of the data. Medical writing and editorial support was provided by Elizabeth Rosenberg, PhD; and Terri Schochet, PhD; of AlphaBioCom, LLC (King of Prussia, PA).

Funding
This study was sponsored by Daiichi Sankyo Co., Ltd. (Tokyo, Japan).

Authors' contributions
YK, TF, SF, TK, KI, and ST were involved in the concept and design of the study, interpretation of the data, critical revising of the manuscript, and provided final approval to submit the manuscript for publication. KA was involved in analysis of the data, critical review of the mansucript, and provided final approval to submit the manuscript for publication.

Competing interests
YK has been a consultant for Daiichi Sankyo and Toyama Chemical. TF has been a consultant for Daiichi Sankyo, Bayer, Astellas, GlaxoSmithKline, Kaken, and Ono Pharmaceutical Company; served on the speakers' bureau for Daiichi Sankyo; and received royalties from Century Medical and Showa Ikakogyo. SF has been a consultant for Daiichi Sankyo, Astellas, and GlaxoSmithKline. ST has been a consultant for Daiichi Sankyo and GlaxoSmithKline. TK, KI, and KA are employees of Daiichi Sankyo Co., Ltd.

Author details
[1]International University of Health and Welfare, 8-10-16 Akasaka, Minato-ku, Tokyo 107-0052, Japan. [2]Department of Orthopaedic Surgery, Japan Community Healthcare Organization Osaka Hospital, 4-2-78, Fukushima, Fukushima-ku, Osaka 553-0003, Japan. [3]Department of Orthopaedic Surgery, Takarazuka Daiichi Hospital, 19-5 Kogetsu-cho, Takarazuka 665-0832, Japan. [4]Daiichi Sankyo Co., Ltd, 3-5-1, Nihonbashi Honcho, Chuo-ku, Tokyo 103-8426, Japan. [5]Clinical Data & Biostatistics Department, Daiichi Sankyo Co. Ltd, 1-2-58, Hiromachi, Shinagawa-ku, Tokyo 140-8710, Japan. [6]Department of Orthopaedic Surgery, Mishuku Hospital, 5-33-12 Shimomeguro, Meguro-ku, Tokyo 153-0051, Japan.

References

1. Geerts WH, Bergqvist D, Pineo GF, Heit JA, Samama CM, Lassen MR, et al. Prevention of venous thromboembolism: American College Of Chest Physicians Evidence-Based Clinical Practice Guidelines (8th edition). Chest. 2008;133:381S–453.
2. JCS Joint Working Group. Guidelines for the diagnosis, treatment and prevention of pulmonary thromboembolism and deep vein thrombosis (JCS 2009). Circ J. 2011;75:1258–81.
3. Lixiana(R) Tablets [package insert]. Daiichi Sankyo Co. Ltd.; Tokyo. 2014.
4. Lovenox(R) (enoxaparin sodium injection) for subcutaneous and intravenous use. [Package insert]. Sanofi-Aventis U.S. LLC; Bridgewater. 2013.
5. Fuji T, Wang CJ, Fujita S, Kawai Y, Nakamura M, Kimura T, et al. Safety and efficacy of edoxaban, an oral factor Xa inhibitor, versus enoxaparin for thromboprophylaxis after total knee arthroplasty: the STARS E-3 trial. Thromb Res. 2014;134:1198–204.
6. Fuji T, Fujita S, Kawai Y, Nakamura M, Kimura T, Fukuzawa M, et al. Efficacy and safety of edoxaban versus enoxaparin for the prevention of venous thromboembolism following total hip arthroplasty: STARS J-V. Thromb J. 2015;13:27.
7. Fuji T, Fujita S, Kawai Y, Nakamura M, Kimura T, Kiuchi Y, et al. Safety and efficacy of edoxaban in patients undergoing hip fracture surgery. Thromb Res. 2014;133:1016–22.
8. Adam SS, Key NS, Greenberg CS. D-dimer antigen: current concepts and future prospects. Blood. 2009;113:2878–87.
9. Pulivarthi S, Gurram MK. Effectiveness of d-dimer as a screening test for venous thromboembolism: an update. N Am J Med Sci. 2014;6:491–9.
10. Wells PS, Anderson DR, Rodger M, Forgie M, Kearon C, Dreyer J, et al. Evaluation of D-dimer in the diagnosis of suspected deep-vein thrombosis. N Engl J Med. 2003;349:1227–35.
11. Aronson DL, Stevan L, Ball AP, Franza Jr BR, Finlayson JS. Generation of the combined prothrombin activation peptide (F1-2) during the clotting of blood and plasma. J Clin Invest. 1977;60:1410–8.
12. Misaki T, Kitajima I, Kabata T, Tani M, Kabata C, Tsubokawa T, et al. Changes of the soluble fibrin monomer complex level during the perioperative period of hip replacement surgery. J Orthop Sci. 2008;13:419–24.
13. Clexane® for Subcutaneous Injection Kit 2000IU [Package Insert (Ver. 8), in Japanese]. Sanofi-Aventis K.K; Tokyo. 2012.
14. Cockcroft DW, Gault MH. Prediction of creatinine clearance from serum creatinine. Nephron. 1976;16:31–41.
15. MacCallum PK, Thomson JM, Poller L. Effects of fixed minidose warfarin on coagulation and fibrinolysis following major gynaecological surgery. Thromb Haemost. 1990;64:511–5.
16. Hamano A, Umeda M, Ueno Y, Tanaka S, Mimuro J, Sakata Y. Latex immunoturbidimetric assay for soluble fibrin complex. Clin Chem. 2005;51:183–8.
17. Farrington CP, Manning G. Test statistics and sample size formulae for comparative binomial trials with null hypothesis of non-zero risk difference or non-unity relative risk. Stat Med. 1990;9:1447–54.
18. Newcombe RG. Interval estimation for the difference between independent proportions: comparison of eleven methods. Stat Med. 1998;17:873–90.
19. Strebel N, Prins M, Agnelli G, Buller HR. Preoperative or postoperative start of prophylaxis for venous thromboembolism with low-molecular-weight heparin in elective hip surgery? Arch Intern Med. 2002;162:1451–6.
20. Fuji T, Fujita S, Tachibana S, Kawai Y. A dose-ranging study evaluating the oral factor Xa inhibitor edoxaban for the prevention of venous thromboembolism in patients undergoing total knee arthroplasty. J Thromb Haemost. 2010;8:2458–68.
21. Sasaki H, Ishida K, Shibanuma N, Tei K, Tateishi H, Toda A, et al. Retrospective comparison of three thromboprophylaxis agents, edoxaban, fondaparinux, and enoxaparin, for preventing venous thromboembolism in total knee arthroplasty. Int Orthop. 2014;38:525–9.
22. Furugohri T, Isobe K, Honda Y, Kamisato-Matsumoto C, Sugiyama N, Nagahara T, et al. DU-176b, a potent and orally active factor Xa inhibitor: in vitro and in vivo pharmacological profiles. J Thromb Haemost. 2008;6: 1542–9.
23. Turpie AG. Oral, direct factor Xa inhibitors in development for the prevention and treatment of thromboembolic diseases. Arterioscler Thromb Vasc Biol. 2007;27:1238–47.

5

Pre-analytical issues in the haemostasis laboratory: guidance for the clinical laboratories

A. Magnette[1], M. Chatelain[1], B. Chatelain[1], H. Ten Cate[2] and F. Mullier[1*]

Abstract

Ensuring quality has become a daily requirement in laboratories. In haemostasis, even more than in other disciplines of biology, quality is determined by a pre-analytical step that encompasses all procedures, starting with the formulation of the medical question, and includes patient preparation, sample collection, handling, transportation, processing, and storage until time of analysis. This step, based on a variety of manual activities, is the most vulnerable part of the total testing process and is a major component of the reliability and validity of results in haemostasis and constitutes the most important source of erroneous or un-interpretable results.

Pre-analytical errors may occur throughout the testing process and arise from unsuitable, inappropriate or wrongly handled procedures. Problems may arise during the collection of blood specimens such as misidentification of the sample, use of inadequate devices or needles, incorrect order of draw, prolonged tourniquet placing, unsuccessful attempts to locate the vein, incorrect use of additive tubes, collection of unsuitable samples for quality or quantity, inappropriate mixing of a sample, etc. Some factors can alter the result of a sample constituent after collection during transportation, preparation and storage.

Laboratory errors can often have serious adverse consequences. Lack of standardized procedures for sample collection accounts for most of the errors encountered within the total testing process. They can also have clinical consequences as well as a significant impact on patient care, especially those related to specialized tests as these are often considered as "diagnostic". Controlling pre-analytical variables is critical since this has a direct influence on the quality of results and on their clinical reliability. The accurate standardization of the pre-analytical phase is of pivotal importance for achieving reliable results of coagulation tests and should reduce the side effects of the influence factors. This review is a summary of the most important recommendations regarding the importance of pre-analytical factors for coagulation testing and should be a tool to increase awareness about the importance of pre-analytical factors for coagulation testing.

Keywords: Haemostasis assays, Pre-analytical phase, Coagulation assays, Recommendations, Dabigatran, Idarucizumab, Microparticles, Centrifugation

Background

The term "pre-analytical phase" describes all actions and aspects of the medical laboratory diagnostic procedure that occurs prior to the analytical phase [1].

This phase is part of the total laboratory procedure consisting of several stages and beginning with the physician requesting the performance of a laboratory investigation on a patient. It is the most vulnerable part of the total testing process, where most laboratory errors occur [2, 3]. It encompasses all procedures, starting with the formulation of the medical question, and includes patient preparation, sample collection, handling, transportation, processing, and storage until time of analysis.

Pre-analytical laboratory errors can arise throughout the pre-analytical phase, because this phase comprises a lot of manual activities and accounts for most of the errors

* Correspondence: francois.mullier@uclouvain.be
[1]Université catholique de Louvain, CHU UCL Namur, Namur Thrombosis and Hemostasis Center (NTHC), NARILIS, Haematology Laboratory, B-5530 Yvoir, Belgium
Full list of author information is available at the end of the article

encountered within the testing process as a whole. Unsuitable, inappropriate or wrongly handled procedures during collection and handling of specimens are very likely to lead to pre-analytical errors [3].

Problems may arise during the collection of blood specimens such as misidentification of the sample, use of inadequate devices or needles, incorrect order of draw, prolonged tourniquet placing, unsuccessful attempts to locate the vein, incorrect use of additive tubes, collection of unsuitable samples for quality (e.g. contaminated, haemolysed) or quantity (e.g. insufficient amount of blood or inappropriate blood-to-anticoagulant ratio), inappropriate mixing of a sample, etc. Some factors can alter the result of a sample constituent after collection during transportation, preparation and storage. The side effects of such factors of influence can be reduced by standardizing the pre-analytical process [4–6].

This review aimed at summarizing recommendations with regard to the pre-analytical phase and provides some guidance to reduce the effects of biological factors that can have a significant impact on patient care.

Methods

A systematic review was conducted following the recommendations of the French Study Group on Haemostasis and Thrombosis (GFHT), the World Health Organization (WHO), the Clinical and Laboratory Standards Institute (CLSI) guidelines, the International Society on Thrombosis and Haemostasis (ISTH), the European Federation of Clinical Chemistry and Laboratory Medicine (EFLM) and the British Committee for Standard in Haematology (BCSH) about the pre-analytical phase and the pre-analytic variables which can have an impact on the quality of medical laboratory results and about the procedures for sample collection, processing, transportation, and storage in haemostasis testing.

The development of the present literature review was carried out using the PubMed database records including analysis of references from selected articles from 1991 to 2016 based on the following key-words: 'pre-analytical phase', 'pre-analytic variables', 'pre-analytical quality', 'preoperative/ pre-operative tests', 'order of draw', 'phlebotomy', 'screening tests', 'routine tests', 'screening testing', 'hemostasis/haemostasis', 'coagulation tests', 'bleeding history', 'preoperative bleeding questionnaire', 'preoperative evaluation', 'bleeding risk', 'haemorrhage/hemorrhage', 'surgery', 'von Willebrand disease', 'von Willebrand factor', 'inherited bleeding disorders', 'bleeding score', 'quality', standardization', 'collection of blood', 'sample collection', 'tourniquet', 'samples', 'transportation', 'preparation', 'storage', 'recommendations', 'discard tubes', 'activated partial thromboplastin time, PTT, aPTT', 'prothrombin time, PT', 'international normalized ratio, INR', 'bleeding time', 'platelet count', 'platelet function testing', 'PFA-100', 'blood sampling', 'sample tubes', 'anticoagulant', 'order of filling the tubes', 'sampling process', 'processing of samples', 'transportation of samples', 'centrifugation', 'storage conditions', 'freezing', 'thawing'. Only articles in English or French were analysed. The database was searched for studies, clinical practice recommendations and literature reviews.

The findings of our search have been grouped into different subtopics. The first one is devoted to the clinical history, bleeding score and physical examination to demonstrate the importance of the patient's history regarding various diseases such as thrombotic diseases in case of haemorrhagic diathesis or preoperative assessment. The following chapters concern the sample collection and sequence of drawing blood. The last subtopics concern the sampling process, transportation and storage conditions.

The first step before considering laboratory testing; Clinical history and physical examination

Prior to any type of haemostatic testing a bleeding history is a prerequisite for the diagnosis of any bleeding disorder and should guide further laboratory investigations [7, 8].

If this is done diligently, it can be considered as one of the best screening tests of the risk of bleeding [7, 9, 10]. It allows the detection of pathology known to cause abnormal primary haemostasis (malnutrition, haematologic disease, liver failure, etc.). In case of acquired haemostatic disorders, family history can be seen as a family tree of the types of haemorrhage observed as well as their spontaneous or provoked features. As far as a person's bleeding history is concerned, it is important to know the terms of appearance of haemorrhages, their frequency and their source, and whether bleeding is aggravated after taking aspirin and/or other medications like antiplatelet therapy, NSAIDs, etc. Regarding the surgical and obstetrical history, it is important to note the number of interventions that resulted in bleeding complications (new intervention due to complication, transfusion, admission to intensive care, etc.), but also the number of times that trauma was not associated with haemorrhagic complications. Antecedents of anemia, iron supplementation, hospitalization or blood transfusion can also guide the clinician [11, 12]. The patient's blood group provides relevant information related to haemostatic activity (e.g. activity levels of VWF). Patients with blood group O are known to have lower levels of VWF. The presence of the *H*-antigen (O group) promotes the cleavage of VWF by ADAMTS13 metalloprotease, and, moreover, a higher hepatic clearance of VWF [13, 14].

In order to prevent disturbing pre-analytical influences, any interfering drugs should be administered after collecting a blood sample. A record of all the drugs that the subject took during the week prior to testing should be collected [15]. Treatment with desmopressin, in treating or preventing bleeding episodes in patients with von Willebrand disease, haemophilia A and platelet function defects, should be noted [16]. It is important to know if the patient is pregnant. Pregnancy is associated with increase in fibrinogen, factors VII, VIII, X, VWF, D-dimer concentration and with increase in levels of prothrombin fragments 1 + 2 and thrombin-antithrombin III complexes. There is a decrease in physiological anticoagulants manifested by acquired activated protein C (APC) resistance. Free protein S is decreased secondary to increased levels of its binding protein, the complement component C4b [17–19]. The overall fibrinolytic activity is impaired during pregnancy, but returns rapidly to normal following delivery. This is largely due to placental derived plasminogen activator inhibitor type 2 (PAI-2), which is present in substantial quantities during pregnancy [19]. Microparticles derived from maternal endothelial cells and platelets, and from placental trophoblasts may contribute to the procoagulant effect [19].

Hormonal contraceptives can be responsible for interferences in coagulation testing and may lead to increased concentrations of fibrinogen, prothrombin and factors VII, VIII and X, and reduction in coagulation inhibitors, such as antithrombin (AT), protein S and tissue factor pathway inhibitor (TFPI) [17, 20, 21]. Use of combined oral contraceptives is associated with a three-to six-fold increased risk of venous thrombosis. This increased risk depends on the estrogen dose as well as the progestogen type of oral contraceptives [22]. These changes tend to me more pronounced in women taking third generation combined oral contraceptives than on second generation [21]. Women using combined oral contraceptives with the highest risk of venous thrombosis (e.g. containing desogestrel, cyproterone acetate or drospirenone), have lower levels of PS and TFPI than women using the combined oral contraceptive with the lowest risk of venous thrombosis (i.e. contraceptives containing levonorgestrel) [22, 23].

Reduced concentrations of protein S can be caused by functional impairment of this protein by differences in modulation of its activity by other plasma proteins that change during the oral contraceptives use or by changes induced in the protein S molecule that impair its anticoagulant activity [24]. For platelet function assays, treatment with drugs known to reversibly inhibit platelet function (e.g. NSAIDs) should be stopped at least 3 days before sampling, and treatment with drugs known to irreversibly inhibit platelet function (e.g. aspirin, thienopyridines) should be stopped at least 10 days before sampling, if possible [8, 15]. As it oftentimes impossible to stop all medication before being sampled for coagulation studies, drug-induced effects on platelet function should be considered when interpreting results [15]. Treatment continuation is also sometimes recommended to assess the efficacy and safety of antithrombotic drugs [9].

The referring physician should also have done a proper physical examination in order to detect signs of coagulopathy. In case of primary haemostatic abnormalities, it is common to seek a cutaneo-mucous type of haemorrhage. Elements usually seen in haemorrhagic syndrome are bruising, purpura, or haemarthrosis. In case of testing for thrombophilia, signs of previous venous thrombosis including post-thrombotic syndrome (venous insufficiency, corona phlebectatica etc.) can be informative. Moreover, it is very important that the clinician and the laboratory exchange all relevant information as much as possible [25].

Bleeding score

To collect the bleeding history, in case of haemorrhagic diathesis or preoperative assessment of bleeding risk, and to obtain the resulting bleeding score (BS), standardized and validated clinical tools are necessary [10].

a) haemorrhagic diathesis: In an attempt to standardize the diagnostic criteria of von Willebrand disease (VWD), the most prevalent congenital bleeding disorder which occurs with equal frequency among men and women and affecting up to 1% of the general population, a BS has been developed [26]. This one is useful for the identification of subjects requiring laboratory evaluation for VWD and for assessing the clinical severity of the disorder in patients with type 1 VWD [7, 27–29]. This BS, related to the number and the severity of bleeding symptoms, is based on a standardized questionnaire and used to evaluate haemorrhagic symptoms [7, 29]. The questionnaire has proven to be useful for diagnostic purposes, allowing the establishment of quantitative cut-offs discriminating healthy subjects and carriers of VWD [7]. The BS is proposed as a predictor of clinical outcomes of inherited VWD, and may also help to identify cases at higher risk of frequent and severe bleeds requiring more intensive prophylactic regimens [30].

Other BS have been developed for the large population of patients with atrial fibrillation (AF) that require oral anticoagulant therapy (e.g. HAS-BLED, ATRIA, ORBIT risk scores, etc.) [31].

The combination of the standardized bleeding questionnaire and an interpretation grid has been referred to as a Bleeding Assessment Tool (BAT) [7]. Although existing BS have limitations (e.g. dependence on clinician interpretation regarding patient recall, inability to distinguish among bleeding events occurring at different anatomical sites, etc.) their use is strongly encouraged, as BATs have proven validity in assessment of symptom severity and help identify patients needing further investigations [10, 32, 33].

To ensure reliability and reduce the time load, the questionnaire should be performed by a physician or other health professional experienced in assessing a (mild) bleeding disorder (MBD), particularly in patients who have abnormal clotting screening test results requiring invasive procedures or elective surgery [7, 34].

The ISTH/SSC Joint Working Group agreed to establish a single BAT to standardize the reporting of bleeding symptoms which would be useful for both paediatric and adult populations. More quantitative BATs have been proposed to improve the diagnostic criteria for MBD because most patients with an MBD do not show a definitive bleeding history, and are difficult to distinguish from normal subjects [7].

This revised BAT could be more generally applicable to the investigation of other inherited bleeding disorders with variable expressivity (e.g. mild platelet function disorders) to avoid the bias of subjective investigator evaluation of haemorrhagic symptoms and to reduce the need for expensive laboratory investigations [7, 8, 29]. Even if the ISTH-BAT has not been evaluated sufficiently in inherited platelet function disorders to allow a firm recommendation of its use, it could also be potentially useful for the diagnosis of platelet function disorders [32, 33].

b) pre-operative assessment: For preoperative investigations, some guidelines are available. Recently the French Society of Anaesthesia and Intensive Care issued recommendations for the prescription of routine preoperative testing before a surgical or non-surgical procedure, requiring any type of anaesthesia [9]. The aim of pre-anaesthetic screening, based on detailed patient interviews and on physical examination, is to identify patients with an increased risk of perioperative bleeding to minimise perioperative haemorrhagic complications.

Routinely haemostasis testing has very little therapeutic impact and lacks prognostic utility. Hence, haemostasis testing should not be systematically used in patients whose history and clinical examination results do not suggest any haemostatic disorders. Conversely, in patients with a positive history of haemorrhagic diathesis, haemostasis testing should be requested depending on the suspected disease [9].

These recommendations are in line with those issued in the United States and in the United Kingdom by the National Institute for Health and Clinical Excellence (NICE). Only the Italian SISET recommendations (Società Italiana per lo Studio dell'Emostasi et della Trombosi) suggest performing systematic haemostasis testing with aPTT, PT and platelet count prior to any intervention, even in patients with no bleeding diathesis history [9].

Variables during sample collection

During the pre-analytical phase, in case of haemostasis testing for patients with a positive history of haemorrhagic diathesis, certain steps regarding the preparation of patients and the execution of sampling (specimen collection, transportation, sample preparation and storage) are of special importance. Providing patients with the appropriate instructions before blood sampling and proper training of those persons involved in sampling procedures can reduce or prevent negative influences on laboratory results and their misinterpretation [4, 35].

In order to minimize misinterpretation of laboratory results, blood samples should be collected from fasting subjects in the morning between 7 and 9 a.m. and from subjects who have refrained from smoking for at least 30 min [4, 8, 15, 36, 37]. Consumption of caffeine should be discouraged within the 2 h prior to sampling [4, 15]. Physical activity within the 2 h prior to sampling is not recommended. Blood samples should be collected after the subject has rested for a short period (at least 5 min) [15].

Diet and drinking are major factors influencing a number of analyses. Before blood sampling, the disturbing influences of food and drink should be excluded. Patients should not be studied after meals associated with a high fat content, so as to avoid the formation of chylomicrons in plasma, which will interfere with light transmission aggregometry [15, 37]. A light meal does not influence the laboratory coagulation tests. However, to completely metabolize the lipids intake, sampling after at least 8 h (better 12 h) fasting and reduced activity (bed rest) is recommended [4, 38]. It is also advisable not to eat dark chocolate [39].

Stress should be avoided under all circumstances (e.g. restless child), because stress increases acute phase proteins of which von Willebrand factor (VWF), factor VIII and fibrinogen [40] are most important (in particular in the workup for haemophilia or VWD). Smoking around the time of phlebotomy enhances platelets aggregability, and induces a procoagulant state in plasma [41, 42]. Studies have reported an increase in blood coagulability but impaired fibrinolysis in habitual smokers when compared with nonsmokers [42]. It seems that higher plasma levels of fibrinogen and viscosity are the main contributors to higher coagulability found in smokers, whereas the lower fibrinolytic potential is mainly attributed to an increase in PAI-1 activity and possibly also a decrease in tPA activity and lower plasminogen levels [41, 42]. Smokers may have impaired acute substance P-induced endothelial release of active tPA in vivo related to impaired endothelial function, which suggests a possible direct link among impaired endogenous fibrinolysis, endothelial dysfunction, and arterial atherothrombosis in smokers [42].

Caffeine enhances fibrinolytic potential as whole blood fibrinolysis time is shortened and PAI-1 levels are decreased, whereas tPA activity increases after consumption of coffee and such effects are blunted during caffeine abstinence [42]. About dark chocolate, platelet aggregation is modulated by a flavanol-independent mechanism that is likely due to theobromine which is containing by cocoa products [39].

Physical activity may cause an increase in leukocyte count and activation of coagulation (decrease of prothrombin time (PT) and fibrinolysis). It can also activate partial thromboplastin time (aPTT), cause an increase in D-dimer, tissue plasminogen activator (tPA) and plasminogen activator inhibitor (PAI), an exercise-induced adrenaline release on platelet aggregation and an increase in platelets [4, 15, 36]. Strenuous exercise also promotes the release of microparticles by platelets and triggers a transient procoagulant condition, which is mirrored by increased thrombin generation, platelet hyperreactivity, increased activity of clotting factors, compounded by an increased fibrinolytic activity [41, 43].

Training in phlebotomy

Phlebotomy is the act of puncturing a vein for the purpose of withdrawing blood and is one of the most critical parts of the entire pre-analytical phase [44]. Training of phlebotomists is a pre-analytical challenge and requires continuous educational updates as equipment is changed in the healthcare institutions [45].

All staff members should be trained in phlebotomy, to prevent unnecessary risk of exposure to blood and to reduce adverse events for patients [46]. If the phlebotomist is a member of the laboratory staff, he/she will be aware of the impact of the quality of sampling on the quality of results. If he/she is external to the laboratory, the laboratory must provide all information necessary about good sampling practices [6, 36].

Blood sampling

According to the recommendations of the EFLM, tube labelling must be done, before or after venipuncture, in the presence of the patient. The phlebotomist should label each drawn tube with the patient's full name, patient's date of birth, identification number [6, 38]. Of course, the use of prebarcode tubes may facilitate collecting this information. The sampling equipment must be sterile and nonpyrogenic. The expiry dates of the needle and the integrity of the sterile seal should be checked. The phlebotomy procedure provided by the CLSI requires wearing gloves, cleansing the venipuncture site and drying of skin before applying the tourniquet and selecting the venipuncture site and vein [47]. The venipuncture should be ideally collected directly from a peripheral vein (antecubital vein). If a tourniquet needs to be used, it should immediately be released when the first tube starts to fill [48]. The diameter of the needle should preferably be comprised between 19 and 22 gauge [34, 49].

It is important to take samples so as to reduce platelet activation in-vitro and to restrict the use of the tourniquet [15, 36, 49]. Extended tourniquet application might produce unnecessary venous stasis or in-vitro haemolysis, which could introduce spurious and clinically meaningful biases in the measurement of several haematologic parameters [47]. Hence, the tourniquet should be placed tightly but less than one minute in order to prevent haemoconcentration, increased fibrinogen and factors VII, VIII, XII as well as activation of endothelial cells and therefore fibrinolysis [47, 48]. Some special coagulation assays, such as those that measure thrombin generation markers (e.g., thrombin antithrombin complex (TAT) and prothrombin fragment 1 + 2), should be drawn without the use of a tourniquet because that may lead to spurious elevation of these markers, particularly if the tourniquet is left in place for more than one minute [5]. A quality laboratory manager should verify the length of tourniquet application and forearm clenching in order to eliminate this source of laboratory error and safeguard quality throughout the total testing process [48].

Venipuncture may be necessary, on occasion, to obtain blood from an existing vascular access device such as an intravenous (IV) line or a central line [5]. If an IV line is present, the sample site selected is distant from the line.

Butterfly devices and 23 gauge needles can be used on patients with difficult veins (geriatrics, oncology and paediatrics), provided that the tubing is short (length <6 cm and air volume <150 μL) [36, 45].

However, owing to costs and the risk of obtaining unsuitable samples, the use of butterfly needles and IV catheters has generally been discouraged, because haemolysis, activation of the contact system, initiated by activation of factor XII, can occur when blood comes into contact with the surface of a biomaterial [2]. Blood samples should be obtained in a relatively atraumatic fashion, and during collection the blood should flow freely into the collection container [4]. In case of difficult sampling, at least this information should be recorded for adequate interpretation of haemostasis assays [50]. Blood sampling should be performed without generating foam or bubbles in the sample and with as little shear stress as possible [4].

The passage of blood through butterfly tubing and IV catheters might cause increased haemostatic alterations in comparison to blood collection using a conventional straight needle, directly into the tube [2].

The direct transfer of blood specimens from syringes to blood collection tubes by piercing of the rubber stopper of the tube is a practice that should be avoided. This may cause haemolysis when cells under pressure from the plunger collide with the tube wall [4].

The investigation of platelets is highly vulnerable to a broad series of pre-analytical variables [8]. In particular, the vacuum aspiration of blood into primary collection tubes could have an influence on platelet function testing. A syringe system permitting slow manual drawing of blood may be superior [4]. For the Platelet Function Analyser (PFA-100), which replaces the bleeding time in many laboratories, the lower shear stress generated by manual aspiration of blood into the primary collection tube would prevent spurious hyper-activation of platelets, thus, preserving the integrity of their function for subsequent testing on PFA-100 [8, 27, 51].

Optimally, blood sampling is done in the laboratory performing the analyses, which allows for verifying many of the above mentioned steps including when needed getting additional data on medical history, medication, fasting state etcetera. Patient identification and tube labelling are the most critical steps during phlebotomy, providing an essential safety barrier to prevent patient identity mix-up.

Labelling blood tubes in the absence of the patient is a potentially life threatening error. According to CLSI, patient identification is the responsibility of the phlebotomist to ensure that blood is drawn from the individual designated on the request form [6] (Table 1).

Sample tubes and anticoagulant

Blood samples for coagulation analyses should be drawn into siliconized glass tubes, or plastic (polypropylene) tubes [35, 49]. Vacuum tubes must be sealed and CE marked [15, 36]. Care must be taken to follow manufacturer's expiry dates. Sample tubes for haemostasis analyses generally contain an anticoagulant. The CLSI guidelines on the collection of blood specimens for coagulation testing recommend the use of sodium citrate in 105–109 mmol/L (3.2%) tubes. The use of mmol/L should be preferred to %. The pH of the anticoagulated plasma should be comprised between 7.3 and 7.45 [35, 36].

Table 1 Summary of key pre-analytical recommendations about blood sampling

Blood sampling	Use siliconized glass or plastic (polypropylene) tubes.
	Blood samples should be drawn into 105–109 mmol/L sodium citrate, buffered anticoagulant.
	The pH of the anticoagulated plasma should be comprised between 7.3 and 7.45.
	Perform blood collection from fasting subjects in the morning (between 7 and 9 a.m.).
	The patient should be relaxed. Stress should be avoided.
	Label each drawn tube with the patient's full name, patient's date of birth, identification number.
	Collect venipuncture directly from a peripheral vein (antecubital vein).
	The diameter of the needle should preferably be comprised between 19 and 22 gauge.
	Release the tourniquet immediately when the first tube starts to fill (<1 min).
	The order of drawing blood during phlebotomy should be blood culture/sterile tubes, then coagulation tubes, then plain tubes/gel tubes, then tubes containing additives.
	Draw a discard tube when citrated plasma is obtained using butterfly systems or other IV catheter devices.
	Discard tube may be considered to ensure correct filling of sample tubes for coagulation tests.
	Ensure correct filling of tubes (>90% filling).
	Respect the required ratio of sodium citrate to whole blood (1:9).

The vast majority of the samples should be collected into trisodium citrate, buffered anticoagulant to help keep the pH stable during processing and testing [15, 36]. The anticoagulant effect of sodium citrate is attributed to its ability to bind calcium, making the calcium unavailable to promote clot formation [4]. However there may also be higher citrate concentration (i.e., 3.8% or 129 mmol/L) leading to greater calcium binding and longer clotting times. Specimens collected in 3.8% buffered sodium citrate may prolong the PT and aPTT and underestimate fibrinogen if the normal range is based on 3.2% citrated samples [4, 47]. Due to the variation in clotting times and sodium citrate concentration, the consensus recommendation suggests that laboratories should standardize to one citrate concentration and develop appropriate reference intervals [4, 5, 35, 36, 47].

For some analyses, especially platelet function assays, buffered citrate solution or other anticoagulants are used. Citrate, theophylline, adenosine and dipyridamole (CTAD) is a cocktail of additives that prevent in-vitro platelet activation recommended for measurement of platelet-activation markers such as β-thromboglobulin or platelet factor 4 (PF4). These tubes allow for more reliable measurement of unfractionated heparin (UFH) and are useful for the study of membrane glycoproteins platelet by flow cytometry. They should be kept away from light [36]. Sampling these tubes allows a delay in analysis until 4 h before centrifugation [52].

It is easy to ensure that the anticoagulant is consistent when working on the primary tube; vigilance is therefore required in case of analysis performed on an aliquot [53].

Sequence of drawing blood

A standardized sequence of blood sampling must be respected in order to avoid carry-over between tubes [3]. National and international (WHO, CLSI) guidelines recommended that the order of draw of blood during phlebotomy should be blood culture/sterile tubes, then coagulation tubes, then plain tubes/gel tubes, then tubes containing additives [3–5]. According to the CLSI, a first discard tube (or a non-additive tube) is unnecessary for routine coagulation assays [47]. A discard tube (or a citrate tube if the sampling is difficult) must be drawn when citrated plasma is obtained using butterfly systems or other IV catheter devices because the air volume contained in the tubing partially fills the vacuum tube, leading to insufficient filling of the tube with citrate. A discard tube is also recommended when samples are subject to platelet function analysis and for thrombin generation measurements [2, 4, 8, 47].

Published studies have demonstrated that for routine coagulation testing, the use of a discard tube is not necessary because there was no significant difference in the aPTT and PT results between the first and second tubes drawn [2, 4, 5, 36, 44, 54]. Some studies evaluated the need for discard tubes in a variety of others coagulation tests (e.g. fibrinogen, D-dimer, factors II, V, VII, VIII, IX, X, XI, proteins C and S and AT, ...) and suggested that discard tubes are not necessary when drawing samples for specialized coagulation testing [2, 5, 54, 55]. There are no data to support the need for a discard tube for specialized haemostasis assays [5]. However, due to lack of sufficient evidence, the practice of drawing a discard tube should still be recommended [5].

Contamination can occur through contact from micro drops from caps with a compress, or from contact with the interior of the tube with the syringe and from the anticoagulant of the first tube to the second tube [4]. Contamination of coagulation assay tubes is possible if coagulation tubes are drawn following an additive tube like certain serum collection tubes containing clot activators [36]. In case of contamination, the results will be erroneous and a re-collection will be necessary, leading to a delay in subsequent medical decisions.

For platelet function assays and coagulation factors, we suggest numbering each tube according to the sample collection order. If a defect is observed on one tube, it could be useful to check this number and verify on another tube.

Sampling process

Filling the tubes

Sodium citrated tubes must be filled up to 90% of the nominal volume or to the mark noted on the tube if provided [41, 47]. The required ratio of sodium citrate to whole blood is 1:9 [35, 49].

Under-filling of tubes is another important source of error and severely affects laboratory results. An insufficient volume for testing greatly modifies the fixed blood-to-anticoagulant ratio. Under-filling increases the dilution of the sample due to the volume of liquid anticoagulant, and may increase the clotting time due to the excess calcium-binding citrate present [4, 5, 47].

It has been reported that when tubes are drawn at less than 89% of total fill, a clinically significant bias exists in test results for aPTT, less than 78% for fibrinogen, and less than 67% for coagulation factor VIII, whereas PT and activated protein C resistance remain relatively reliable even in tubes drawn at 67% of the nominal volume [41]. Similar results were obtained in further studies [45, 56]. Instead of rejecting a sample tube, it may be useful to note the sample volume and to adapt the result depending on the additional dilutional (e.g. for factor assays, fibrinogen). In case of high haematocrit, the citrate volume may be adjusted because this may also impact the citrate-calcium ratio. It may be necessary to remove part of the citrate solution from the sampling tube prior to drawing blood [35, 36, 44] (Table 2).

Mixing the samples

Following collection, blood should be adequately and promptly mixed by three to six complete end-over-end inversions of the tubes in order to ensure complete distribution of anticoagulant [8, 36, 47, 49, 57].

Mixing samples is an important way to prevent in-vitro clot formation. Sometimes samples are inappropriately mixed or left unmixed for a long time, thereby avoiding full contact of the blood with the anticoagulant, which determines partial clotting.

Vigorous shaking, vortexing or agitation of blood samples should be avoided in order to prevent inducing haemolysis or spurious platelet and factor activation that may result in shortened clotting times or false elevation of clotting factor activity in specimen tests (e.g. factor VII) [4, 8, 48, 58].

Examination of samples

When obtaining plasma for coagulation testing and prior to processing, samples must be examined for the presence of a clot, precipitates and signs of haemolysis.

In-vitro clots may develop in samples where the blood is slow to fill the collection container, where there is prolonged use a tourniquet, or when considerable manipulation of the vein by the needle has occurred. These situations must be avoided.

Several causes may induce in-vitro haemolysis, such as slow or difficult specimen collection; prolonged tourniquet placing; use of incorrect devices (e.g., butterfly needles or IV catheters) or needles (e.g., small gauge needles); unsuccessful attempts to locate the vein; inappropriate mixing of the sample; inappropriate centrifugation speed (e.g., > 1500g); inappropriate transportation procedures (pneumatic tube systems, duration, temperature and humidity), ... [2, 4, 5].

Table 2 Summary of key pre-analytical recommendations about sample processing

Sample processing	Blood should be adequately and promptly mixed by 3 to 6 complete end-over-end inversions of the tubes in order to ensure complete distribution of anticoagulant.
	Avoid vigorous shaking, vortexing or agitation of blood samples.
	Adjust the citrate volume in case of high haematocrit (remove part of the citrate solution from the sampling tube prior to drawing blood).
	Check tubes for presence of clots, precipitates or haemolysis.

Haemolysis can affect some tests of haemostasis, either because of the presence of thromboplastic substances or interference of haemoglobin pigment with photo-optical systems [2, 49].

Lysis of the red cell membranes induces the release of red cells contents (many intracellular enzymes, ADP ...) into plasma and may lead to activation of the plasma sample altering coagulation parameters and activation of other bloodlines (leucocytes, platelets).

Haemolysed samples may lead to early flow obstruction in the PFA, presumably due to platelet activation, fragmentation of platelet and red blood cells and the presence of micro-thrombi [4]. Haemolysis may lead to statistically significant increases in PT and D-dimer. The aPTT can be falsely prolonged or shortened and AT and fibrinogen decreased by in vitro haemolysis [5, 49, 59, 60].

Plasmas that are lipemic and icteric may also affect analytic results by interfering with optical absorbance or impeding light transmittance [49]. Mechanical and/or electromechanical methods for clot detection should be utilized when possible for these plasma samples [5]. Because the presence of lipid particles can still bias the measurement for biologic interference, the CLSI currently recommends the removal of excess triglycerides by ultracentrifugation [61]. This kind of equipment being unavailable in most routine laboratories due to high costs and incompatibility with daily practice and because ultracentrifugation may cause precipitation of the large molecular proteins such as fibrinogen or factor VIII/VWF complex, an alternative approach entails high speed microcentrifugation (e.g., double centrifugation at >20,000 g for 15 min) or lipid extraction by means of organic solvents or lipid-clearing agents [45, 61].

Transportation of samples

Samples should be transported non-refrigerated at ambient temperature (15–25 °C) in as short a time as possible [8, 49, 57].

Before transport, samples should be tested regarding identification, safety conditions and stability. Errors in either sample identification, sample preparation before or after transport may have an adverse effect on patients if they are not detected on time [4, 6].

When possible, samples should be drawn directly in a laboratory. Immediately after drawing, whole blood should remain capped for transport both for safety reasons and to minimize loss of CO2, which causes pH to increase, leading to prolongation of PT and/or aPTT [44]. Tubes should be stored at ambient temperature until centrifugation [4, 5, 36]. Temperature control is recommended in rooms where samples are kept for analysis [2]. If tubes need to be transported this should be done with care in order to avoid unnecessary agitation. During transportation, samples should be transferred vertically in the shortest possible time [36].

Delays between sample collection and analysis can cause in-vitro degradation of coagulation proteins [2].

Ideally, samples for coagulation assays should be performed in the laboratory that performs the assays. If not, specimens should be shipped from peripheral collection facilities to the core laboratory utilizing current CLSI guidelines (non-refrigerated at ambient temperature in as short a time as possible, preferably within the first hour after collection) [5, 57]. Blood samples for coagulation analyses should not be shaken. Any sample that has been dropped should be discarded. For the transport, a box maintaining blood tubes in a steady vertical position should be used. Transporting blood tubes in a vertical rather than a horizontal position limits the extent of in vitro microparticles (MP) generation [62, 63].

The temperature during transport is of special relevance. Extreme temperatures should be avoided in order to maintain sample integrity [5]. Temperatures higher than room temperature can lead to degradation of factor V and factor VIII [64].

The use of pneumatic tube systems (PTS) for transport of samples is problematic and could have a significant influence on platelet function testing [8, 45]. Rapid acceleration and deceleration may induce excessive vibration, denature proteins and result in haemolysis, platelet activation, and other effects [4, 35, 63]. Clinical decisions regarding platelet function and aspirin responsiveness should not be based on blood specimens transported by a PTS [65–68] (Table 3).

Specimen rejection

Each laboratory should have guidelines for rejection of samples; some criteria are obligatory: inappropriate collection tubes and additives, outdated tubes, error in patient identification or lack of identification, insufficient volume, haemolysed specimens, identification of a clot, inadequate volume, haematocrit >50% or <30% for the

Table 3 Summary of key pre-analytical recommendations about transportation of samples

Transportation of samples	Before transport, test samples regarding identification, safety conditions and stability.
	Transport samples at ambient temperature (15–25 °C) in as short a time as possible.
	Draw samples directly in a laboratory.
	Immediately after drawing, whole blood should remain capped for transport.
	Temperature control is recommended in rooms where samples are kept for analysis.
	Transfer samples vertically.
	Do not use pneumatic tube systems (PTS) for transport of samples used for platelet function analysis.

PFA, platelet count <100,000/µL for PFA and platelet aggregation ... All samples deemed unacceptable due to pre-analytic handling and unfulfilled transport requirements should be rejected [4–6, 8].

Haemolysed blood is the most common reason for rejecting specimens in the laboratory and, therefore, in-depth knowledge on how to properly access the vein with the correct blood collection equipment to avoid haemolysis in the collected specimens is a must for the phlebotomist [45].

In case of reception of an aliquot without information about the anticoagulant used, this one must be rejected because serum and all types of plasma have virtually identical visual appearance. Because samples that are rejected must be recollected, which gives potential delay in patient management, phlebotomists must be fully aware of the common reasons why specimens are rejected (Table 4).

Centrifugation

Whenever a delay in transport is expected, it might be advisable to perform local centrifugation and separation. Plasma is generally prepared by centrifugation of a whole blood sample. A temperature-controlled centrifuge is required for processing routine coagulation assays. Centrifugation should take place at room temperature (15–25 °C) [36]. The effect of centrifugation temperature on MP determination is still unknown [37].

It is recommended to use a centrifuge that has a rotor with swing-out buckets to facilitate the separation of plasma from the cellular components and to minimize re-mixing of plasma and red cells [5, 36, 44]. It is recommended to centrifuge the primary tube for coagulation testing at 1500g for no less than 15 min with a centrifuge brake set off [8, 36, 47]. The centrifuge should be validated before use, every 6 months or after modifications, in order to assure that platelet-poor plasma (PPP) is achieved [47].

Use of the rotor brake may lead to higher residual microparticles and platelet counts, which also has an effect on PT and fibrinogen concentration [69]. Therefore, it seems feasible to centrifuge samples for coagulation analyses with the rotor brake set to off [4, 62]. However, according to our personal experience, this should be validated in appropriate studies. Our experience shows it is important to check the absence of vibration (during acceleration/deceleration processes) due to lack of centrifuge maintenance.

Table 4 Summary of key pre-analytical recommendations about specimen rejection

Specimen rejection	All samples deemed unacceptable due to pre-analytic handling and unfulfilled transport requirements should be rejected.
	Inappropriate collection tubes and additives.
	Outdated tubes.
	Error in patient identification or lack of identification.
	Insufficient volume (depending on the assay). An alternative may be to adapt the result depending on the additional dilutional (e.g. for factor assays, fibrinogen).
	Haemolysed specimens (depending on the assay).
	Identification of a clot.

Using relative centrifugal forces greater than 1500g is not recommended as this may induce platelet activation, haemolysis or other unwanted effects [4, 5, 47]. However, in case of emergency, for general haemostasis parameters performed on fresh plasma, higher centrifugation force (greater than 1500g) and shorter time (less than 10 min) can be used [36, 47].

Some studies have evaluated the impact of high acceleration centrifugation conditions on routine coagulation testing (including especially PT, aPTT and fibrinogen; no data were found for the thrombin time) and concluded that rapid centrifugation does not modify results and contributes, by decreasing duration of the pre-analytical variable, to reduce the turnaround time for these tests [70–76]. Note that in the REVERSE-AD study conducted to evaluate the efficacy and safety of Idarucizumab, the reversal agent for dabigatran [77], the centrifugation (i.e. 3 min at 1000g) used before performing dilute thrombin time and ecarin clotting time, was not validated [78]. Both tests were used as primary endpoints and they should thus be interpreted cautiously.

a) For analysis in platelet-poor plasma For analysis in PPP, which is the standard material required for PT, aPTT, fibrinogen, single coagulation factor assays, functional protein S and C assays, activated protein C resistance, lupus anticoagulant (LA) assays, antiphospholipid antibody testing, thrombin generation, microparticles measurements, homocysteine, VWF assays, tPA, PAI, plasminogen and antiplasmin, or monitoring of unfractioned heparin therapy, and many other tests, sample tubes require a second centrifugation and should be centrifuged in capped tubes within 4 h after drawing blood [2, 36, 37, 79]. For thrombin generation measurements, whole blood is best centrifuged immediately, to prevent activation or degradation of coagulation proteins. In order to eliminate platelet debris and microparticles from plasma, which may contribute to the variability in thrombin generation results, a second centrifugation step at 10,000g is recommended [2].

Double centrifugation significantly reduces the residual amount of platelets in a sample and can be performed to produce PPP such that the post centrifugation plasma platelet count is less than or equal to $10x10^9$/L. Residual platelets in plasma have been known to affect phospholipid-dependent coagulation tests through the exposure from platelet membranes of anionic phospholipids that quench LA activity. This effect leads to shorter coagulation time and is particularly evident, especially in test plasmas that undergo freezing and thawing before analysis. Adequate plasma preparation for LA testing is an essential prerequisite for reliable diagnosis [80].

The generation of PPP should be prepared for all coagulation parameters if there is a possibility that measurement is not performed immediately after centrifugation, or if samples are going to be frozen [5, 63].

Following initial centrifugation, the plasma is carefully transferred to a nonactivating plastic centrifuge tube using an automatic pipette, and then centrifuged again for about 15 min. When pipetting, 1 cm of plasma must remain above the buffy layer.

It is important to use an automatic pipette because it permits slow and linear suction, unlike plastic pipettes that pose a risk of getting a high rate of residual platelets. The plasma is aliquoted to a secondary tube, taking care not to include the residual platelets that may have precipitated at the bottom of the centrifuge tube. It has been demonstrated that a high platelet count (>200 × 10^9/L) does not affect results of PT, D-dimer, fibrinogen and aPTT assays, when samples are tested fresh and analyzed immediately after centrifugation [36, 79]. These samples should not be stored for later analyses [47].

b) For analysis in platelet-rich plasma The preparation of platelet-rich plasma (PRP) for platelet function analysis requires that centrifugation is performed at 200–250 g for 10 min without application of a rotor brake [8, 15]. These centrifugal forces appear to be the best condition for preparing PRP for light transmission aggregometry (LTA) studies, both in terms of the degree of contamination of PRP by other blood cells and of platelet reactivity [15]. The recommendation to avoid using a rotor brake is based on expert opinion and should be demonstrated in appropriate studies.

Centrifugation with less than 150 g does not yield a sufficient volume of PRP. The PRP should then be transferred to a capped polypropylene tube and a platelet count performed.

For LTA, the platelet count of PRP samples should not be adjusted to a standardized value by addition of autologous PPP, unless the platelet count is >600x10^9/L [8, 15]. However, the results of LTA studies could be inaccurate when the platelet count in the PRP samples is lower than 150x10^9/L [8, 15].

All assays using whole blood or PRP need to be performed within a maximum of 4 h after blood sampling [4, 15].

If the pre-analytical phase of the laboratory is supported by an automated system, vigilance must be in order to test and validate the centrifugation conditions meeting the requirements of haemostasis but also the requirements of chemistry and immunology analysis [36] (Table 5).

Table 5 Summary of key pre-analytical recommendations about centrifugation

Centrifugation	Use a temperature-controlled centrifuge for processing routine coagulation assays.
	Validate the centrifuge before use, every 6 months or after modifications, in order to assure that platelet-poor plasma (PPP) is achieved.
	Check the absence of vibration (during acceleration/deceleration processes) due to lack of centrifuge maintenance.
	Centrifuge the primary tube for coagulation testing at 1500g, 15 min
	In case of emergency, for PT, APTT and fibrinogen performed on fresh plasma, higher centrifugation force (greater than 1500g) and shorter time (less than 10 min) can be used. The preparation of PPP require a double centrifugation to obtain a residual platelet count lower than 10x10^9/L.
	Following initial centrifugation, transfer carefully the plasma to a nonactivating plastic centrifuge tube using an automatic pipette, and then centrifuged again for about 15 min.
	The preparation of platelet-rich plasma (PRP) for platelet function analysis requires a centrifugation performed at 200–250 g for 10 min without application of a rotor brake.

Storage conditions

a) conditions for the interval from sampling to analysis: For routine coagulation testing like the PT and the aPTT, storage of uncentrifuged samples at room temperature up to 6 h may yield acceptable results. However, a shorter delay is desirable. Whole blood assays should be performed within 4 h after blood sampling and centrifugation should ideally be taken within 1 h [4, 41, 47, 49, 79, 81]. During storage, samples should remain capped [5]. Extremes of temperature (e.g., both refrigerated or high) should be avoided.

Cold storage of citrated whole blood prior to centrifugation, by placing samples either in an ice bath or in refrigerated (2–8 °C) storage, is no longer recommended. Improper storage of whole blood at cold temperature may cause VWF and factor VIII values to fall below normal reference threshold levels, which may potentially lead to a false suspicion of haemophilia A or VWD due to inappropriate pre-analytical handling of blood [4, 5, 25, 44, 82].

Once the blood sample has been centrifuged, plasma can remain on the cells in a capped primary tube until testing, or it can be aliquoted and stored in a secondary tube. When aliquoting the plasma, care must be taken so that the buffy coat (the layer of cells between the red cells and plasma) is not disturbed or that this cellular component is not introduced back into the plasma. Aliquoted plasma is stable for 4 h when refrigerated, except for plasma for PT-INR and PT-sec, which should not be refrigerated [2, 5, 47]. This is due to the potential for cold activation of a sample. This may strongly influence some of the coagulation assays and may lead to platelet activation, activation of factor VII, which in turn can give shorter clotting times and hence lower PT-INR and PT-sec results.

Delays in transport may affect in particular the labile factors (FV, FVIII), leading to prolonged clotting times and in vitro loss of factor activity [2, 83].

The time frame for analysis depends upon the stability of the analysis, which depends on storage temperatures and conditions. As far as the stability of citrated whole blood, plasma on cells and aliquoted plasma is concerned, more studies are needed, because there are large differences between the conclusions of different studies and partially missing studies.

b) short term plasma storage: PPP should be stored at room temperature (20–25 °C) or at −80 °C until analysis. External influences (like temperature, light ...) may be of major impact (Table 6).

Samples for PT/INR have longer stability (24 h) at room temperature. Samples can be stored as whole blood or stored following centrifugation [81].

Samples for aPTT testing should be stored at room temperature and be performed using fresh plasma within 4 h. The limited stability is largely due to time-dependent generation or loss of labile factors, particulary

Table 6 Summary of key pre-analytical recommendations about storage conditions

Storage conditions	Store samples at room temperature (15–25 °C) until analysis.
	Perform whole blood assays <4 h after blood sampling and centrifugation <1 h.
	Extremes of temperature (e.g. both refrigerated or high) should be avoided.
	Store PPP at room temperature (15–25 °C) or at −80 °C until analysis.
	If the whole blood sample is centrifuged within 1 h of collection, the plasma can be left on top of the cells at room temperature up to 4 h prior to testing.
	Time from sampling to analysis depends on analyte: Samples for PT/INR have longer stability (24 h) at room temperature. Samples for aPTT should be performed using fresh plasma <4 h (<1 h in patients treated with unfractionated heparin). For platelet function assays, samples should rest at room temperature for at least 15 min before analysis. Testing should be completed <3–4 h of collection. For factors V and VIII analyses should be performed <3 h. Fibrinogen, protein C and antithrombin activity appear to remain relatively constant when stored at room temperature for up to 7 days. Protein S activity is unstable, with a statistically significant loss of activity at 8 h. VWF appears to be stable at room temperature for 48 h.

factor VIII and possibly factor V [83]. aPTT from patients receiving unfractionated heparin (UFH) therapy has shorter stability. For these samples, due to the variable heparin neutralization by platelet factor 4 (PF4), the delay before centrifugation should not exceed 1 h for a sample collected in citrate and 4 h in CTAD. If the whole blood sample is centrifuged within 1 h of collection, the plasma can be left on top of the cells at room temperature up to 4 h prior to testing [83]. This applies also to fibrinolysis parameters [35, 47, 52, 81, 83].

PT, aPTT and factor VIII tests from frozen samples cannot be performed [4]. Freezing has an inconstant and unpredictable effect on the results and may cause significant elevations of aPTT, but also PT [4, 84–86]. Poorly handled frozen material may also causes shortening of aPTT or PT [5]. If double centrifugation is not done when preparing a sample to be frozen this can lead to a lysis of residual platelets upon freezing of plasma sample and lead to shortened APTT results in heparinized patients [80].

Freezing leads to a marked decrease especially in FVIII activity [4, 87]. In case of a factor defect observed on a frozen sample, it is suggested to repeat the analysis on a fresh sample.

For platelet function assays, samples should rest at room temperature for at least 15 min before analysis. Testing should be completed within 3 to 4 h of collection [4, 5, 8, 15].

Stability of plasma samples for special coagulation assays (except FVIII, anti-FXa for UFH) is largely unknown. The shortest stability is observed for factors V and VIII. Analyses should be performed within 3 h.

For unknown reason, protein S is labile. It has been demonstrated that protein S activity is unstable, with a statistically significant loss of activity demonstrated at 8 h while fibrinogen, protein C and antithrombin activity appear to remain relatively constant when stored at room temperature for up to 7 days [83]. VWF appears to be stable at room temperature for 48 h [4].

Stability of the vitamin K-dependant factors has been reported to be 24 h at room temperature [4, 5, 83, 88]. For thrombin generation, direct plasma preparation is preferred to whole blood storage. When immediate analysis is not possible, plasma is most stable when incubated at room temperature, instead of 4 °C or 37 °C, most likely because of more activation and degradation of coagulation proteins at these temperatures [2].

For samples coming from external laboratories, it is important to check prior to analysis whether the aliquot external samples (fresh or frozen) really consist of citrated plasma. For specialized coagulation testing, most samples are sent as frozen samples, whilst samples for routine coagulation are more often sent as citrated blood (primary tube). Ideally, the primary tube should be received together with the aliquot tube [39]. It is not suggested to recentrifuge the aliquots coming from external laboratories.

c) long term plasma storage: Samples that cannot be tested within 4 h should be centrifuged and the plasma aliquot frozen [79] (Table 7).

For analyses that can be performed on frozen plasma, freezing should be fast (using rapid freezing technique like liquid nitrogen), and samples should be preferably stored at −70 °C (or below) rather than −20 °C. Plasma samples frozen at minus 20 °C remain stable for 2 weeks for most coagulation parameters [36, 49]. However, it is imperative that a frost-free freezer is not used [36, 44, 49, 83]. Plasma frozen at minus 80 °C remains stable for 6 – 18 months dependent on the parameter [47, 63, 64].

Prior to testing, frozen plasmas should be thawed rapidly at 37 °C (to prevent denaturing fibrinogen) and tested immediately. This usually takes at least 3–5 min for a 1–2 mL sample. The sample must be mixed gently to resuspend any cryoprecipitate [49].

The samples have to be thawed at least 5 min in a water bath at 37 °C and not at room temperature, on a bench or in a microwave oven. After thawing they should be gently stirred [2, 36]. After thawing, and for thrombin generation measurements, plasma is best analysed immediately [2]. Freeze-thawing may produce phospholipid rich membrane microvesicles from platelet damage which may then mask the presence of a lupus anti-coagulant [89].

If a pathological parameter is obtained on a frozen sample, this parameter is suggested to be re-tested on fresh plasma. Samples may not be re-frozen. Several aliquots (suggested volume of 500–1200 μL) should be prepared as a backup. Frozen aliquots should be transported on dry ice [36].

Table 7 Summary of key pre-analytical recommendations about freezing and thawing

Freezing and thawing	Do not perform PT, aPTT and factor VIII tests from frozen samples.
	Centrifuge samples that cannot be tested within 4 h and frozen the plasma aliquot.
	Use rapid freezing technique (liquid nitrogen).
	Store samples at −70 °C (or below) rather than −20 °C.
	Plasma samples frozen at minus 20 °C remain stable for 2 weeks.
	Plasma frozen at minus 80 °C remains stable for 6 – 18 months dependent on the parameter.
	Do not re-freeze samples (but prepare a sufficient number of aliquots).
	Thaw samples rapidly at 37 °C (to prevent denaturing fibrinogen) at least 5 min in a water bath at 37 °C and not at room temperature, on a bench or in a microwave oven. Test immediately.
	After thawing, mix the sample gently to resuspend any cryoprecipitate. Do not vortex or shake.
	Do not re-frozen samples.

Conclusion

Continuous monitoring and management of pre-analytical errors is crucial in order to improve the quality of the pre-analytical phase, which is essential for patient care. Standardization efforts are essential to control and prevent errors and to ensure the quality of exploration in haemostasis. They are also necessary for all clinical laboratories accredited by International Organization for Standardization (ISO) document 15189. The accurate standardization of the pre-analytical phase is of pivotal importance to achieve reliable results of coagulation tests.

Owing to the development of large laboratory networks and of decentralized phlebotomy services and analytical laboratories, standardized and unequivocal procedures and protocols are essential for sample collection, including patient preparation, specimen acquisition, handling and storage. These procedures are intended to prevent these problems and to protect against complications and patient mismanagement that could otherwise arise when specimens are not collected properly in order to achieve accurate and reliable coagulation measurements.

The effects of pre-analytical variables on the reliability and consistency of screening tests is often forgotten due to a lack of understanding and awareness. This can be improved by educating healthcare professionals who are involved in drawing blood for testing.

Acknowledgements
Not applicable.

Funding
Not applicable.

Authors' contributions
AM and FM performed the review of the literature and designed the manuscript. AM drafted the manuscript. All authors read and approved the final manuscript.

Competing interests
The authors declare that they have no competing interests.

Author details
[1]Université catholique de Louvain, CHU UCL Namur, Namur Thrombosis and Hemostasis Center (NTHC), NARILIS, Haematology Laboratory, B-5530 Yvoir, Belgium. [2]Maastricht University Medical Centre and Cardiovascular Research Institute (CARIM), Department of Internal Medicine, Maastricht, The Netherlands.

References

1. Guder WG. History of the preanalytical phase: a personal view. Biochem Med (Zagreb). 2014;24:25–30.
2. Loeffen R, Kleinegris MC, Loubele ST, Pluijmen PH, Fens D, van Oerle R, ten Cate H, Spronk HM. Preanalytic variables of thrombin generation: towards a standard procedure and validation of the method. J Thromb Haemost. 2012;10:2544–54.
3. Cornes M, van Dongen-Lases E, Grankvist K, Ibarz M, Kristensen G, Lippi G, Nybo M, Simundic AM, Working Group for Preanalytical Phase EFoCC, Laboratory M. Order of blood draw: Opinion Paper by the European Federation for Clinical Chemistry and Laboratory Medicine (EFLM) Working Group for the Preanalytical Phase (WG-PRE). Clin Chem Lab Med. 2016;55:27–31.
4. Guder WG, Narayanan S. Pre-Examination Procedures in Laboratory Diagnostics: Preanalytical Aspects and Their Impact on the Quality of Medical Laboratory Results. De Gruyter; 2015.
5. Kitchen S, Olson JD, Preston FE. Quality in Laboratory Hemostasis and Thrombosis. Bognor Regis: Wiley-Blackwell, 2nd Edition. 2013; 22–44.
6. van Dongen-Lases EC, Cornes MP, Grankvist K, Ibarz M, Kristensen GB, Lippi G, Nybo M, Simundic AM. Working group for preanalytical phase EFoCC, laboratory M. Patient identification and tube labelling - a call for harmonisation. Clin Chem Lab Med. 2016;54:1141–5.
7. Rodeghiero F, Tosetto A, Abshire T, Arnold DM, Coller B, James P, Neunert C, Lillicrap D, ISj VWF. Perinatal/pediatric hemostasis subcommittees working G. ISTH/SSC bleeding assessment tool: a standardized questionnaire and a proposal for a new bleeding score for inherited bleeding disorders. J Thromb Haemost. 2010;8:2063–5.
8. Harrison P, Mackie I, Mumford A, Briggs C, Liesner R, Winter M, Machin S. British committee for standards in H. Guidelines for the laboratory investigation of heritable disorders of platelet function. Br J Haematol. 2011;155:30–44.
9. Bonhomme F, Ajzenberg N, Schved JF, Molliex S, Samama CM, French A. Intensive care committee on evaluation of routine preoperative T, French society of a, intensive C. Pre-interventional haemostatic assessment: guidelines from the French society of anaesthesia and intensive care. Eur J Anaesthesiol. 2013;30:142–62.
10. Tosetto A, Castaman G, Rodeghiero F. Bleeders, bleeding rates, and bleeding score. J Thromb Haemost. 2013;11 Suppl 1:142–50.
11. Stepanian A, Biron-Andreani C. Primary hemostasis exploration. Ann Biol Clin (Paris). 2001;59:725–35.
12. Haute Autorité de Santé. Biologie des anomalies de l'hémostase. Service évaluation des actes professionnels. 2010. V n°5 du 20/10/10.
13. O'Donnell J, Laffan MA. The relationship between ABO histo-blood group, factor VIII and von Willebrand factor. Transfus Med. 2001;11:343–51.
14. Franchini M, Capra F, Targher G, Montagnana M, Lippi G. Relationship between ABO blood group and von Willebrand factor levels: from biology to clinical implications. Thromb J. 2007;5:14.
15. Cattaneo M, Cerletti C, Harrison P, Hayward CP, Kenny D, Nugent D, Nurden P, Rao AK, Schmaier AH, Watson SP, Lussana F, Pugliano MT, Michelson AD. Recommendations for the standardization of light transmission aggregometry: a consensus of the working party from the platelet physiology subcommittee of SSC/ISTH. J Thromb Haemost. 2013;11:1183–9.
16. Ozgonenel B, Rajpurkar M, Lusher JM. How do you treat bleeding disorders with desmopressin? Postgrad Med J. 2007;83:159–63.
17. Lipets EN, Ataullakhanov FI. Global assays of hemostasis in the diagnostics of hypercoagulation and evaluation of thrombosis risk. Thromb J. 2015;13:4.
18. Levine AB, Teppa J, McGough B, Cowchock FS. Evaluation of the prethrombotic state in pregnancy and in women using oral contraceptives. Contraception. 1996;53:255–7.
19. Brenner B. Haemostatic changes in pregnancy. Thromb Res. 2004;114:409–14.
20. Franchi F, Biguzzi E, Martinelli I, Bucciarelli P, Palmucci C, D'Agostino S, Peyvandi F. Normal reference ranges of antithrombin, protein C and protein S: effect of sex, age and hormonal status. Thromb Res. 2013;132:e152–7.
21. Sandset PM. Mechanisms of hormonal therapy related thrombosis. Thromb Res. 2013;131 Suppl 1:S4–7.
22. Raps M, Helmerhorst FM, Fleischer K, Dahm AE, Rosendaal FR, Rosing J, Reitsma P, Sandset PM, van Vliet HA. The effect of different hormonal contraceptives on plasma levels of free protein S and free TFPI. Thromb Haemost. 2013;109:606–13.
23. van Vliet HA, Bertina RM, Dahm AE, Rosendaal FR, Rosing J, Sandset PM, Helmerhorst FM. Different effects of oral contraceptives containing different progestogens on protein S and tissue factor pathway inhibitor. J Thromb Haemost. 2008;6:346–51.
24. Koenen RR, Christella M, Thomassen LG, Tans G, Rosing J, Hackeng TM. Effect of oral contraceptives on the anticoagulant activity of protein S in plasma. Thromb Haemost. 2005;93:853–9.
25. Armstrong E, Joutsi-Korhonen L, Lassila R. Interaction between clinic and laboratory. Thromb Res. 2011;127 Suppl 2:S2–4.
26. Centers for Disease Control and Prevention: http://www.cdc.gov. Accessed 17 Nov 2016.
27. Castaman G, Tosetto A, Goodeve A, Federici AB, Lethagen S, Budde U, Batlle J, Meyer D, Mazurier C, Goudemand J, Eikenboom J, Schneppenheim R, Ingerslev J, Habart D, Hill F, Peake I, Rodeghiero F. The impact of bleeding history, von Willebrand factor and PFA-100 ((R)) on the diagnosis of type 1 von Willebrand disease: results from the European study MCMDM-1VWD. Br J Haematol. 2010;151:245–51.
28. Tosetto A, Rodeghiero F, Castaman G, Goodeve A, Federici AB, Batlle J, Meyer D, Fressinaud E, Mazurier C, Goudemand J, Eikenboom J, Schneppenheim R, Budde U, Ingerslev J, Vorlova Z, Habart D, Holmberg L, Lethagen S, Pasi J, Hill F, Peake I. A quantitative analysis of bleeding symptoms in type 1 von willebrand disease: results from a multicenter European study (MCMDM-1 VWD). J Thromb Haemost. 2006;4:766–73.
29. Rodeghiero F, Castaman G, Tosetto A, Batlle J, Baudo F, Cappelletti A, Casana P, De Bosch N, Eikenboom JC, Federici AB, Lethagen S, Linari S, Srivastava A. The discriminant power of bleeding history for the diagnosis of type 1 von Willebrand disease: an international, multicenter study. J Thromb Haemost. 2005;3:2619–26.
30. Federici AB, Bucciarelli P, Castaman G, Mazzucconi MG, Morfini M, Rocino A, Schiavoni M, Peyvandi F, Rodeghiero F, Mannucci PM. The bleeding score predicts clinical outcomes and replacement therapy in adults with von Willebrand disease. Blood. 2014;123:4037–44.
31. O'Brien EC, Simon DN, Thomas LE, Hylek EM, Gersh BJ, Ansell JE, Kowey PR, Mahaffey KW, Chang P, Fonarow GC, Pencina MJ, Piccini JP, Peterson ED. The ORBIT bleeding score: a simple bedside score to assess bleeding risk in atrial fibrillation. Eur Heart J. 2015;36:3258–64.
32. Gresele P. Subcommittee on platelet physiology of the international society on T, Hemostasis Diagnosis of inherited platelet function disorders: guidance from the SSC of the ISTH. J Thromb Haemost. 2015;13:314–22.
33. Gresele P, Harrison P, Bury L, Falcinelli E, Gachet C, Hayward CP, Kenny D, Mezzano D, Mumford AD, Nugent D, Nurden AT, Orsini S, Cattaneo M. Diagnosis of suspected inherited platelet function disorders: results of a worldwide survey. J Thromb Haemost. 2014;12:1562–9.
34. Tosetto A, Castaman G, Plug I, Rodeghiero F, Eikenboom J. Prospective evaluation of the clinical utility of quantitative bleeding severity assessment in patients referred for hemostatic evaluation. J Thromb Haemost. 2011;9:1143–8.
35. Polack B, Schved JF, Boneu B. Groupe d'Etude sur l'Hemostase et la T. Preanalytical recommendations of the 'Groupe d'Etude sur l'Hemostase et la Thrombose' (GEHT) for venous blood testing in hemostasis laboratories. Haemostasis. 2001;31:61–8.
36. GFHT. (French Study Group on Hemostasis and Thrombosis). 2015. http://site.geht.org/site/Pratiques-Professionnelles/Documents-GEHT/Variables-Preanalytiques/Recommandations-Variables-preanalytiques_69_722.html. Accessed 3 Nov 2016.
37. Mullier F, Bailly N, Chatelain C, Chatelain B, Dogne JM. Pre-analytical issues in the measurement of circulating microparticles: current recommendations and pending questions. J Thromb Haemost. 2013;11:693–6.
38. Lima-Oliveira G, Salvagno GL, Lippi G, Danese E, Gelati M, Montagnana M, Picheth G, Guidi GC. Could light meal jeopardize laboratory coagulation tests? Biochem Med (Zagreb). 2014;24:343–9.
39. Rull G, Mohd-Zain ZN, Shiel J, Lundberg MH, Collier DJ, Johnston A, Warner TD, Corder R. Effects of high flavanol dark chocolate on cardiovascular function and platelet aggregation. Vascul Pharmacol. 2015;71:70–8.
40. O'Donnell J, Tuddenham EG, Manning R, Kemball-Cook G, Johnson D, Laffan M. High prevalence of elevated factor VIII levels in patients referred for thrombophilia screening: role of increased synthesis and relationship to the acute phase reaction. Thromb Haemost. 1997;77:825–8.
41. Lippi G, Salvagno GL, Montagnana M, Lima-Oliveira G, Guidi GC, Favaloro EJ. Quality standards for sample collection in coagulation testing. Semin Thromb Hemost. 2012;38:565–75.
42. Lee KW, Lip GY. Effects of lifestyle on hemostasis, fibrinolysis, and platelet reactivity: a systematic review. Arch Intern Med. 2003;163:2368–92.

43. Chen YW, Chen JK, Wang JS. Strenuous exercise promotes shear-induced thrombin generation by increasing the shedding of procoagulant microparticles from platelets. Thromb Haemost. 2010;104:293–301.
44. McCraw A, Hillarp A, Echenagucia M. Considerations in the laboratory assessment of haemostasis. Haemophilia. 2010;16 Suppl 5:74–8.
45. Lippi G, Becan-McBride K, Behulova D, Bowen RA, Church S, Delanghe J, Grankvist K, Kitchen S, Nybo M, Nauck M, Nikolac N, Palicka V, Plebani M, Sandberg S, Simundic AM. Preanalytical quality improvement: in quality we trust. Clin Chem Lab Med. 2013;51:229–41.
46. WHO Guidelines on Drawing Blood: Best Practices in Phlebotomy. Geneva; 2010. http://www.euro.who.int/__data/assets/pdf_file/0005/268790/WHO-guidelines-on-drawing-blood-best-practices-in-phlebotomy-Eng.pdf?ua=1.
47. CLSI GP41-A6 (replaces H03-A6). Procedures for the Collection of Diagnostic Blood Specimens by Venipuncture; Approved Standard—Sixth Edition. Vol. 27 No. 26.
48. Lima-Oliveira G, Lippi G, Salvagno GL, Montagnana M, Picheth G, Guidi GC. The effective reduction of tourniquet application time after minor modification of the CLSI H03-A6 blood collection procedure. Biochem Med (Zagreb). 2013;23:308–15.
49. Mackie I, Cooper P, Lawrie A, Kitchen S, Gray E, Laffan M, British Committee for Standards in H. Guidelines on the laboratory aspects of assays used in haemostasis and thrombosis. Int J Lab Hematol. 2013;35:1–13.
50. Riley RS, Tidwell AR, Williams D, Bode AP, Carr ME. Laboratory Evaluation of Hemostasis. http://www.pathology.vcu.edu/media/pathology/clinical/coag/LabHemostasis.pdf.
51. Lippi G, Ippolito L, Zobbi V, Sandei F, Favaloro EJ. Sample collection and platelet function testing: influence of vacuum or aspiration principle on PFA-100 test results. Blood Coagul Fibrinolysis. 2013;24:666–9.
52. Becton, Dickinson and Company (BD) Diagnostics : http://www.bd.com. Accessed 17 Nov 2016.
53. Lippi G, Salvagno GL, Adcock DM, Gelati M, Guidi GC, Favaloro EJ. Right or wrong sample received for coagulation testing? tentative algorithms for detection of an incorrect type of sample. Int J Lab Hematol. 2010;32:132–8.
54. Smock KJ, Crist RA, Hansen SJ, Rodgers GM, Lehman CM. Discard tubes are not necessary when drawing samples for specialized coagulation testing. Blood Coagul Fibrinolysis. 2010;21:279–82.
55. Raijmakers MT, Menting CH, Vader HL, van der Graaf F. Collection of blood specimens by venipuncture for plasma-based coagulation assays: necessity of a discard tube. Am J Clin Pathol. 2010;133:331–5.
56. Adcock DM, Kressin DC, Marlar RA. Minimum specimen volume requirements for routine coagulation testing: dependence on citrate concentration. Am J Clin Pathol. 1998;109:595–9.
57. CLSI H21-A5: Collection, Transport, and Processing of Blood Specimens for Testing Plasma-Based Coagulation Assays and Molecular Hemostasis Assays; Approved Guideline—Fifth Edition. Vol. 28 No. 5.
58. Ernst DJ, Ernst C. Phlebotomy tools of the trade: part 4: proper handling and storage of blood specimens. Home Healthc Nurse. 2003;21:266–70.
59. Arora S, Kolte S, Dhupia J. Hemolyzed samples should be processed for coagulation studies: the study of hemolysis effects on coagulation parameters. Ann Med Health Sci Res. 2014;4:233–7.
60. Favaloro EJ, Adcock Funk DM, Lippi G. Pre-analytical variables in coagulation testing associated with diagnostic errors in hemostasis. Lab Med. 2012;43:1–10.
61. Lippi G, Plebani M, Favaloro EJ. Interference in coagulation testing: focus on spurious hemolysis, icterus, and lipemia. Semin Thromb Hemost. 2013;39:258–66.
62. Lacroix R, Judicone C, Poncelet P, Robert S, Arnaud L, Sampol J, Dignat-George F. Impact of pre-analytical parameters on the measurement of circulating microparticles: towards standardization of protocol. J Thromb Haemost. 2012;10:437–46.
63. Lacroix R, Judicone C, Mooberry M, Boucekine M, Key NS, Dignat-George F, The ISSCW. Standardization of pre-analytical variables in plasma microparticle determination: results of the international society on thrombosis and haemostasis SSC collaborative workshop. J Thromb Haemost. 2013;11:1190–3.
64. Adcock Funk DM, Lippi G, Favaloro EJ. Quality standards for sample processing, transportation, and storage in hemostasis testing. Semin Thromb Hemost. 2012;38:576–85.
65. Bolliger D, Seeberger MD, Tanaka KA, Dell-Kuster S, Gregor M, Zenklusen U, Grapow M, Tsakiris DA, Filipovic M. Pre-analytical effects of pneumatic tube transport on impedance platelet aggregometry. Platelets. 2009;20:458–65.
66. Lance MD, Henskens YM. Effect of pneumatic tube transport on rotational thromboelastometry. Br J Anaesth. 2013;110:142.
67. Lance MD, Kuiper GJ, Sloep M, Spronk HM, van Oerle R, ten Cate H, Marcus MA, Henskens YM. The effects of pneumatic tube system transport on ROTEM analysis and contact activation assessed by thrombin generation test. Thromb Res. 2012;130:e147–50.
68. Lance MD, Marcus MA, van Oerle R, Theunissen HM, Henskens YM. Platelet concentrate transport in pneumatic tube systems–does it work? Vox Sang. 2012;103:79–82.
69. Daves M, Giacomuzzi K, Tagnin E, Jani E, Adcock Funk DM, Favaloro EJ, Lippi G. Influence of centrifuge brake on residual platelet count and routine coagulation tests in citrated plasma. Blood Coagul Fibrinolysis. 2014;25:292–5.
70. Nelson S, Pritt A, Marlar RA. Rapid preparation of plasma for 'Stat' coagulation testing. Arch Pathol Lab Med. 1994;118:175–6.
71. Pappas AA, Palmer SK, Meece D, Fink LM. Rapid preparation of plasma for coagulation testing. Arch Pathol Lab Med. 1991;115:816–7.
72. Lippi G, Franchini M, Montagnana M, Salvagno GL, Poli G, Guidi GC. Quality and reliability of routine coagulation testing: can we trust that sample? Blood Coagul Fibrinolysis. 2006;17:513–9.
73. Lippi G, Rossi R, Ippolito L, Zobbi V, Azzi D, Pipitone S, Favaloro EJ, Funk DM. Influence of residual platelet count on routine coagulation, factor VIII, and factor IX testing in postfreeze-thaw samples. Semin Thromb Hemost. 2013;39:834–9.
74. Lippi G, Salvagno GL, Montagnana M, Manzato F, Guidi GC. Influence of the centrifuge time of primary plasma tubes on routine coagulation testing. Blood Coagul Fibrinolysis. 2007;18:525–8.
75. Boudaoud L, Divaret G, Marie P, Bezeaud A. Rapid centrifugation for routine coagulation testing. Ann Biol Clin (Paris). 2006;64:315–7.
76. Sultan A. Five-minute preparation of platelet-poor plasma for routine coagulation testing. East Mediterr Health J. 2010;16:233–6.
77. Ageno W, Buller HR, Falanga A, Hacke W, Hendriks J, Lobban T, Merino J, Milojevic IS, Moya F, van der Worp HB, Randall G, Tsioufis K, Verhamme P, Camm AJ. Managing reversal of direct oral anticoagulants in emergency situations. Anticoagulation Education Task Force White Paper. Thromb Haemost. 2016;116:1003–10.
78. Pollack Jr CV, Reilly PA, Eikelboom J, Glund S, Verhamme P, Bernstein RA, Dubiel R, Huisman MV, Hylek EM, Kamphuisen PW, Kreuzer J, Levy JH, Sellke FW, Stangier J, Steiner T, Wang B, Kam CW, Weitz JI. Idarucizumab for dabigatran reversal. N Engl J Med. 2015;373:511–20.
79. Suchsland J, Friedrich N, Grotevendt A, Kallner A, Ludemann J, Nauck M, Petersmann A. Optimizing centrifugation of coagulation samples in laboratory automation. Clin Chem Lab Med. 2014;52:1187–91.
80. Mayo Medical Laboratories. Ensuring Specimen Integrity: Proper Processing and Handling of Specimens for Coagulation Testing. http://www.mayomedicallaboratories.com/articles/communique/2008/10update1.html.
81. Salvagno GL, Lippi G, Montagnana M, Franchini M, Poli G, Guidi GC. Influence of temperature and time before centrifugation of specimens for routine coagulation testing. Int J Lab Hematol. 2009;31:462–7.
82. Bohm M, Taschner S, Kretzschmar E, Gerlach R, Favaloro EJ, Scharrer I. Cold storage of citrated whole blood induces drastic time-dependent losses in factor VIII and von Willebrand factor: potential for misdiagnosis of haemophilia and von Willebrand disease. Blood Coagul Fibrinolysis. 2006;17:39–45.
83. Kottke-Marchant K, David B. Laboratory hematology practice. Wiley-Blackwell. 2012;31:416–7.
84. Zurcher M, Sulzer I, Barizzi G, Lammle B, Alberio L. Stability of coagulation assays performed in plasma from citrated whole blood transported at ambient temperature. Thromb Haemost. 2008;99:416–26.
85. Rao LV, Okorodudu AO, Petersen JR, Elghetany MT. Stability of prothrombin time and activated partial thromboplastin time tests under different storage conditions. Clin Chim Acta. 2000;300:13–21.
86. Alesci S, Borggrefe M, Dempfle CE. Effect of freezing method and storage at −20° C and −70° C on prothrombin time, aPTT and plasma fibrinogen levels. Thromb Res. 2009;124:121–6.
87. Bach J, Haubelt H, Hellstern P. Sources of variation in factor VIII, von Willebrand factor and fibrinogen measurements: implications for detecting deficiencies and increased plasma levels. Thromb Res. 2010;126:e188–95.
88. Marlar RA, Gausman JN. Laboratory testing issues for protein C, protein S, and antithrombin. Int J Lab Hematol. 2014;36:289–95.
89. A Practical Guide to Laboratory Haemostasis: http://www.practical-haemostasis.com/index.html. Accessed 17 Nov 2016.

6

New horizon in platelet function: with special reference to a recently-found molecule, CLEC-2

Yukio Ozaki[1*], Shogo Tamura[2,3] and Katsue Suzuki-Inoue[2]

From The 9th Congress of the Asian-Pacific Society on Thrombosis and Hemostasis
Taipei, Taiwan.

Abstract

Platelets play a key role in the pathophysiological processes of hemostasis and thrombus formation. However, platelet functions beyond thrombosis and hemostasis have been increasingly identified in recent years. A large body of evidence now exists which suggests that platelets also play a key role in inflammation, immunity, malignancy, and furthermore in organ development and regeneration, such as the liver.

We have recently identified CLEC-2 on the platelet membrane, which induces intracellular activation signals upon interaction of a snake venom, rhodocytin. Later we discovered that podoplanin, present in renal podocytes and lymphatic endothelial cells, both of which are not accessible to platelets in blood stream, is an endogenous ligand for CLEC-2. In accord with our expectation, platelet-specific CLEC-2 knockout mice have a phenotype of edema, lymphatic vessel dilatation, and the presence of blood cells in lymphatic vessels. It is suggested that lymphatic/blood vessel separation during the developmental stage is governed by cytokines released from platelets activated by the interaction between platelet CLEC-2 and podoplanin present on lymphatic endothelial cells.

Recombinant CLEC-2 bound to early atherosclerotic lesions and normal arterial walls, co-localizing with vascular smooth muscle cells (VSMCs). Flow cytometry and immunocytochemistry showed that recombinant CLEC-2, but not an anti-podoplanin antibody, bound to VSMCs, suggesting that CLEC-2 ligands other than podoplanin are present in VSMCs. Protein arrays and Biacore analysis were used to identify S100A13 as a CLEC-2 ligand in VSMCs. S100A13 was released upon oxidative stress, and expressed in the luminal area of atherosclerotic lesions.

Megakaryopoiesis is promoted through the CLEC-2/podoplanin interaction in the vicinity of arterioles, not sinusoids or lymphatic vessels. There exist podoplanin-expressing bone-marrow (BM) arteriolar stromal cells, tentatively termed as BM fibroblastic reticular cell (FRC)-like cells, and megakaryocyte colonies were co-localized with periarteriolar BM FRC-like cells in the BM. CLEC-2/podoplanin interaction induces BM FRC-like cells to secrete CCL5 to facilitate proplatelet formation. These observations indicate that a reciprocal interaction with between CLEC-2 on megakaryocytes and podoplanin on BM FRC-like cells contributes to the periarteriolar megakaryopoietic microenvironment in mouse BM.

Keywords: Platelets, Thrombosis, Beyond hemostasis, Immunity, CLEC-2, Lymphangiogeneis, Smooth muscle cells, Megakaryopoiesis

Abbreviations: CLEC-2, C-type lectin-like receptor 2; LEC, Lymphatic endothelial cell; VSMC, Vascular smooth muscle cell; HUVEC, Human umbilical vein-derived endothelial cell; TLR, Toll-like receptor; BM, Bone marrow; NET, Neutrophil extracellular trap; FRC, Fibroblastic reticular cell

* Correspondence: yozaki@fch.or.jp
[1]Fuefuki Central Hospital, 47-1 Yokkaichiba, Isawa, Fuefuki 406-0032, Yamanashi, Japan
Full list of author information is available at the end of the article

Background

Platelets play a key role in the pathophysiological processes of hemostasis and thrombus formation. However, platelet functions beyond thrombosis and hemostasis have been increasingly identified in recent years. This review reports on the newly identified platelet functions beyond hemostasis, especially with the reference to CLEC-2.

Introduction

In primitive organisms such as horseshoes crabs, except for red blood cells, there is only one additional type of blood cells, hemocytes, which is involved in bactericidal function, inflammation, immunity, and hemostasis. In more highly evolved creatures, there are five types of white blood cells and platelets which respectively take care of specific functions, and platelets have long been considered to be an expert in thrombosis and hemostasis but nothing else. However, as described above, platelets are now increasingly considered to play as liaison interactive effects between different cell types and tissues.

Platelets are the second most abundant cell type in the circulation after red blood cells. Platelets contain three types of cytoplasmic granules, including α-granules, dense granules and lysosome, which contain a large number of autocrine and paracrine substances. Recent reports demonstrate that intra-granular proteins are differentially released upon different stimulation, suggesting that platelets can provide specific substances to specific tissues in appropriate conditions. In addition to its vast number in circulation, its small size and its ability to form microparticles which trespass various tissues, allows the detection of small breaches in any space as well as in the circulation. Microparticles are small fragments of membranes shed by mechanisms often involving metalloproteases. While leukocytes and endothelial cells can also produce microparticles, the majority (70 to 90 %) of microparticles in the circulation is considered to come from activated platelets. Platelet-derived microparticles express adhesive molecules and they may also contain proinfmmatory molecules such as IL-1β which may communicate proinflammatory signals to extravascular tissues. Furthermore, platelet-derived microparticles are also known to contain microRNA, which, upon release from microparticles, may be transferred to other cell types, where they modulate inflammation and immunity, as well as in developmental biology and angiogenesis. Thus, platelets and their microparticles can be figuratively described as the best drug-delivery system in living things [1].

Discovery of CLEC-2

Rhodocytin, a snake venom obtained from the Malayan pit viper, *Calloselasma rhodostoma* activates platelets with a manner similar to collagen. Rhodocytin affinity chromatography and TOF-MASS spectrometry were utilized, and we identified a new class of platelet activation receptor, c-type lectin-like receptor 2 (CLEC-2) [2].

CLEC-2 belongs to the family of the non-classical C-type lectins. It contains one C-type lectin-like domain (CLTD) but lacking the consensus sequence for binding sugars and calcium. CLEC-2 assumes two forms, 32- and 40-kDaMW with varying degrees of glycosylation, in platelets. Its cytoplasmic tail contains a conserved YxxL sequence. The immunoreceptor tyrosine-based motif (ITAM) which plays an essential role of signal transduction in GPVI-related platelet activation has two tyrosine residues (tandem YxxL motif). In ITAM-related activation, both tyrosine residues undergo phosphorylation, and Syk with two SH2 domains which recognize phosphorylated tyrosine binds to this ITAM. In contrast, CLEC-2 has only a single cytoplasmic YxxL motif (hemITAM). However, we found that the intracellular signaling pathway elicited by CLEC-2-rhodocytin interaction is quite similar to that of GPVI (Fig. 1). Recent findings suggest that CLEC-2 exists as monomers and dimers at the resting state, and that when platelets are activated with CLEC-2 agonists, it assumes more profuse dimer formation or oligomerization, with resultant Syk interaction.

While CLEC-2 is expressed to a limited degree in liver sinusoidal endothelial cells, and liver Kupffer cells, CLEC-2 is abundantly and specifically expressed on platelets and megakaryocytes in humans . In mice, in addition to platelets, neutrophils and macrophages also express CLEC-2, and it appears to mediate phagocytosis and proinflammatory cytokine expression.

Lymphangiogenesis

Podoplanin was identified as an endogenous ligand for CLEC-2 [3]. Podoplanin is a sialo-glycoprotein, which is extensively O-glycosilated. It is highly expressed in renal podocytes, the name of which derives from, but it is also present in lung type I alveolar macrophages and lymphatic endothelial cells (LEC). In fact, it is often used as a marker for lymphatic vessels. It is also present on some types of tumor cells, and is responsible for tumor cell-induced platelet aggregation and tumor metastasis. A role for CLEC-2 in the developmental stage has been shown with CLEC-2 knockout mice with the phenotypes of blood-lymphatic vessel malseparation and edema [4, 5] (Fig. 2). Mice lacking signaling molecules such as Syk, PLCγ2, SLP-76, also manifest the similar phenotypes, and it is of interest that these signals are utilized by CLEC-2 for platelet activation. Knockout mice of podoplanin, the ligand for CLEC-2, also have blood lymphatic vessel malseparation and edema. One the other hand, mice lacking GPVI which also use the similar signaling pathway for platelet activation do not have this kind of phenotypes,

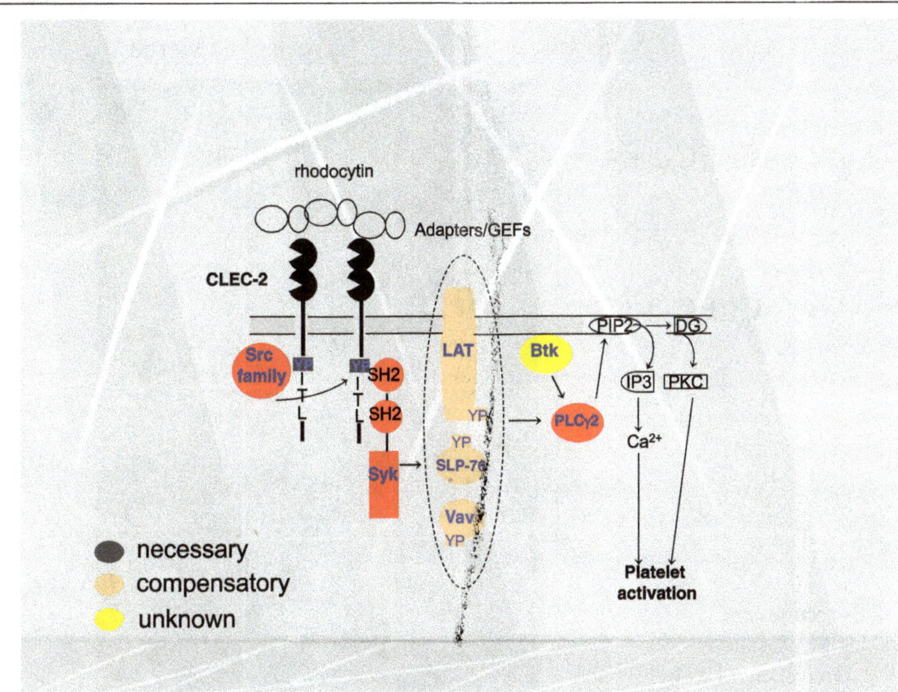

Fig. 1 Signal transduction pathway mediated through CLEC-2. Overall, the signal transduction pathway is strikingly similar to that of GPVI, involving a number of signaling molecules related to tyrosine kinases. Upon association with its agonists, CLEC-2 assumes multimerization, and Syk and Src family kinases mediates tyrosine phosphorylation of its hemITAM, which is followed by downstream signals culminating in PLCγ2 activation. Signaling molecules required for full activation of platelets are marked in *red*, those which are partially required are marked in *orange*, and those which can be spared are marked in *yellow*

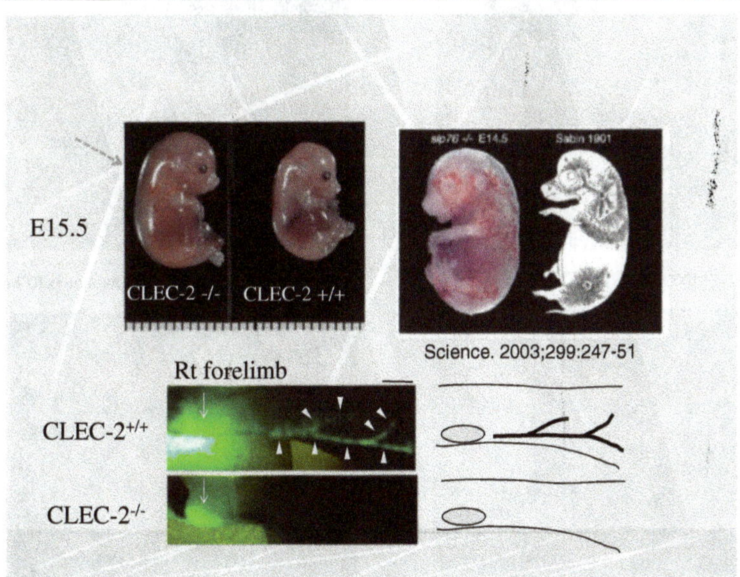

Fig. 2 CLEC-2 knockout mice have abnormal lymphatic vessels. CLEC-2 knockout mice (*upper left inlet*) are edematous with dilated vessels, the pattern of which is quite similar to the distribution of lymphatic vessels of porcine fetus (*upper right inlet*), which was reported previously elsewhere. We found that the injected dye does not run into lymphatic vessels of the CLEC-knockout, suggesting for the presence of lymphatic vessel malformation (*lower inlets*)

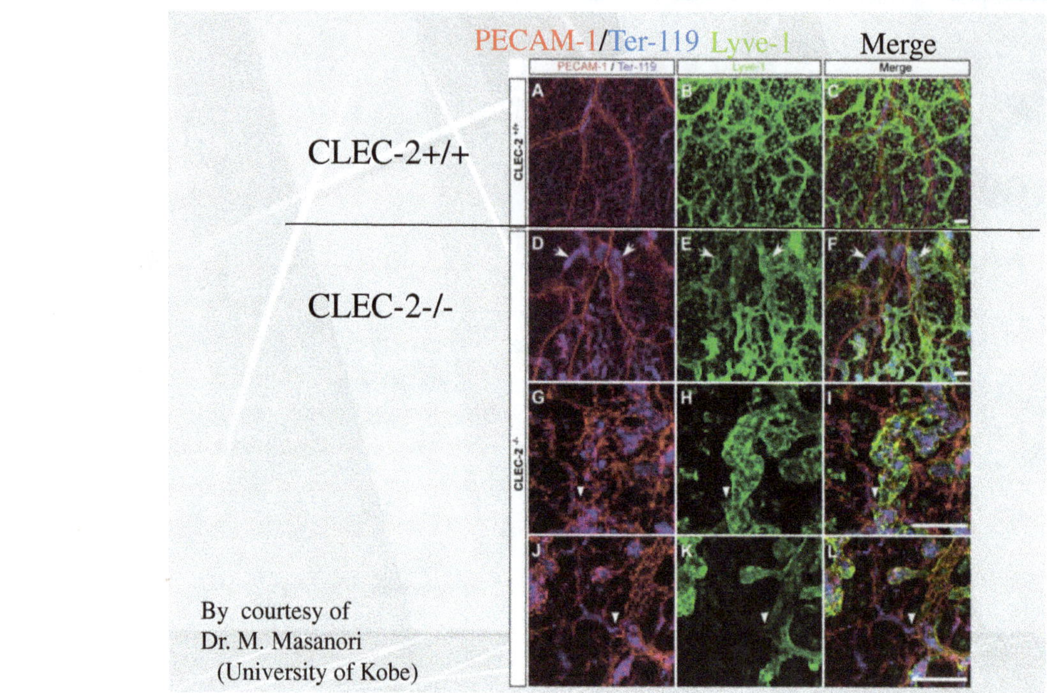

Fig. 3 CLEC-2-knockout mice have dilated, torturous lymphatic vessels. While blood vessels and lymphatic vessels are distinctly separated in wild-type, they were intermingled with each other with CLEC-2-knockout mice, and the lymphatic vessels are dilated and torturous. PECAM-1 stains blood vessels, and Lyve-1 stains lymphatic endothelial cells. At the sites indicated by *arrowheads*, blood vessels and lymphatic vessels appear to be connected

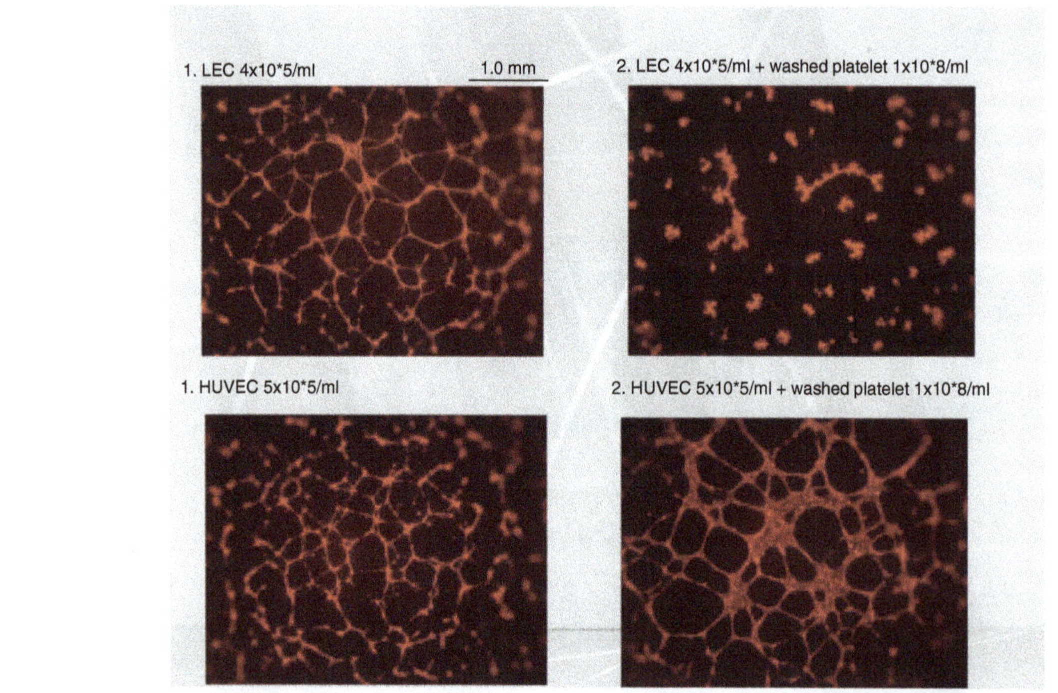

Fig. 4 The supernatant of activated platelets inhibited tube formation of lymphatic endothelial cells (LEC) but not that of human umbilical venous endothelial cells (HUVEC). The *upper left inlet* shows the pattern of LEC tube formation without platelets, and the *upper right inlet* shows that LEC tube formation is disturbed in the presence of washed platelets which express CLEC-2. On the other hand, tube formation of HUVEC (*lower left inlet*) is not affected in the presence of platelets (*lower right inlet*)

suggesting that podoplanin-CLEC-2-interaction play an essential role. Since LEC lack these signaling molecules, we assumed that platelet activation, elicited by the binding between CLEC-2 on the platelet membrane and podoplanin on the surface of LEC podoplanin, is required for normal separation of blood/lymphatic vessels in the developmental stage. However, since neutrophils and dendritic cells in mice also express CLEC-2, and these signaling molecules are also present in those cells, we sought to confirm this hypothesis by producing platelet-specific CLEC-2 knockout mice.

In line with our expectation, platelet-specific CLEC-2 knockout mice manifest edema, lymphatic vessel dilatation, and the leakage of blood cells in lymphatic vessels

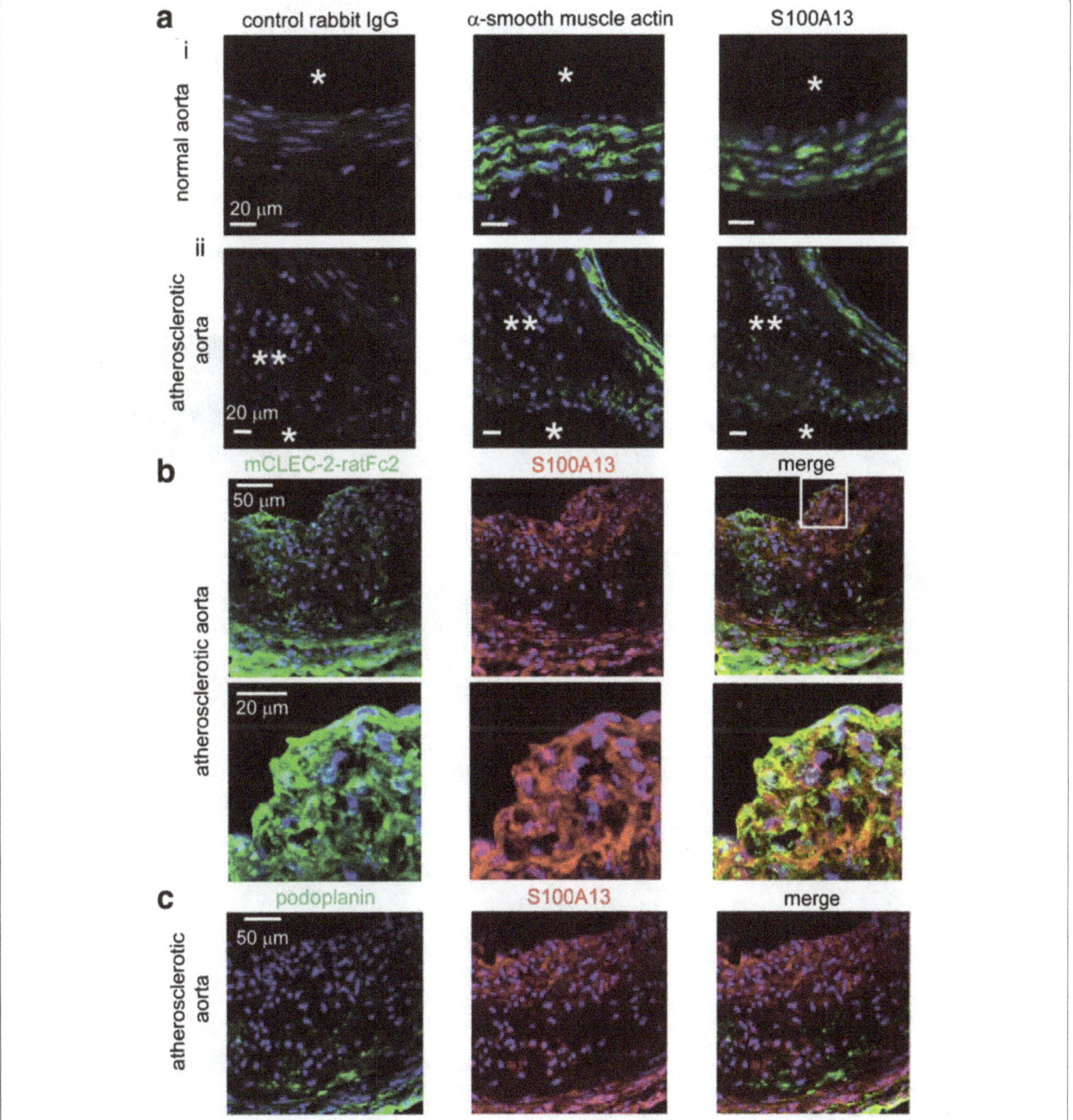

Fig. 5 S100A13 is present in the normal aorta, and its distribution coincides with that of smooth muscle cells. In figures **a**, the distribution patterns of smooth muscle actin is similar to that of S100A12. Figures **b** show that CLEC-2 binding is abundantly present in atherosclerotic aorta, but less so in the normal aorta, and the binding of CLEC-2 colocalizes with that of S100A13. Podoplanin which is a ligand for CLEC-2 is expressed in the atherosclerotic tissues. However, the distribution of podoplanin is distinct from that of S100A13 (figures **c**), suggesting that CLEC-2 binding in the normal and atherosclerotic aorta is attributed to its binding to S100A13, but not to podoplanin

[6] (Fig. 3). We have reached a conclusion that CLEC-2 expressed in platelets but not in other cells plays an important role in the normal separation of blood/lymphatic vessels. However, in contrast to pan-CLEC-2 deficient mice, the platelet-specific CLEC-2 mice, are not lethal at the stage of fetus or neonates, suggesting that CLEC-2 expressed in cells other than platelets are important somehow in maintaining life in the developmental stage.

There remains an interesting and important issue as to the mechanism by which the binding between podoplanin on the surface of LEC and CLEC-2 on the platelet surface regulates the lymphatic/blood vessel separation. Wild-type platelets with CLEC-2, but not CLEC-2 deficient platelets, inhibited LEC migration, proliferation and tube formation when co-incubated with LEC, and that granule contents released from activated platelets were responsible for this inhibitory effects. We found that cytokines belonging to the TGF-β superfamily play a role for this effect [6] (Fig. 4). Taken together, we suggest that the separation of lymphatic vessels from blood vessel during the developmental stage is regulated by cytokines released from platelets upon the interaction between CLEC-2 on the platelet membrane and podoplanin on lymphatic endothelial cells.

Thrombosis and hemostasis

We generated chimeric mice whose blood cells were derived from the liver cells of CLEC-2-knockout fetus, in order to evaluate the role of CLEC-2 in thrombosis and hemostasis, since CLEC-2-knockout mice were lethal at the fetus/birth stage. Platelets taken from CLEC-2(−) chimeric mice had normal functions such as platelet adhesion and spreading. However, multilayer formation of platelets under the flow system or in vivo thrombus formation was significantly suppressed, in comparison to wild-type mice [5]. Stable thrombus formation under high shear stress requires the expression of CLEC-2 in platelets [7]. Although podoplanin may be focally detected in

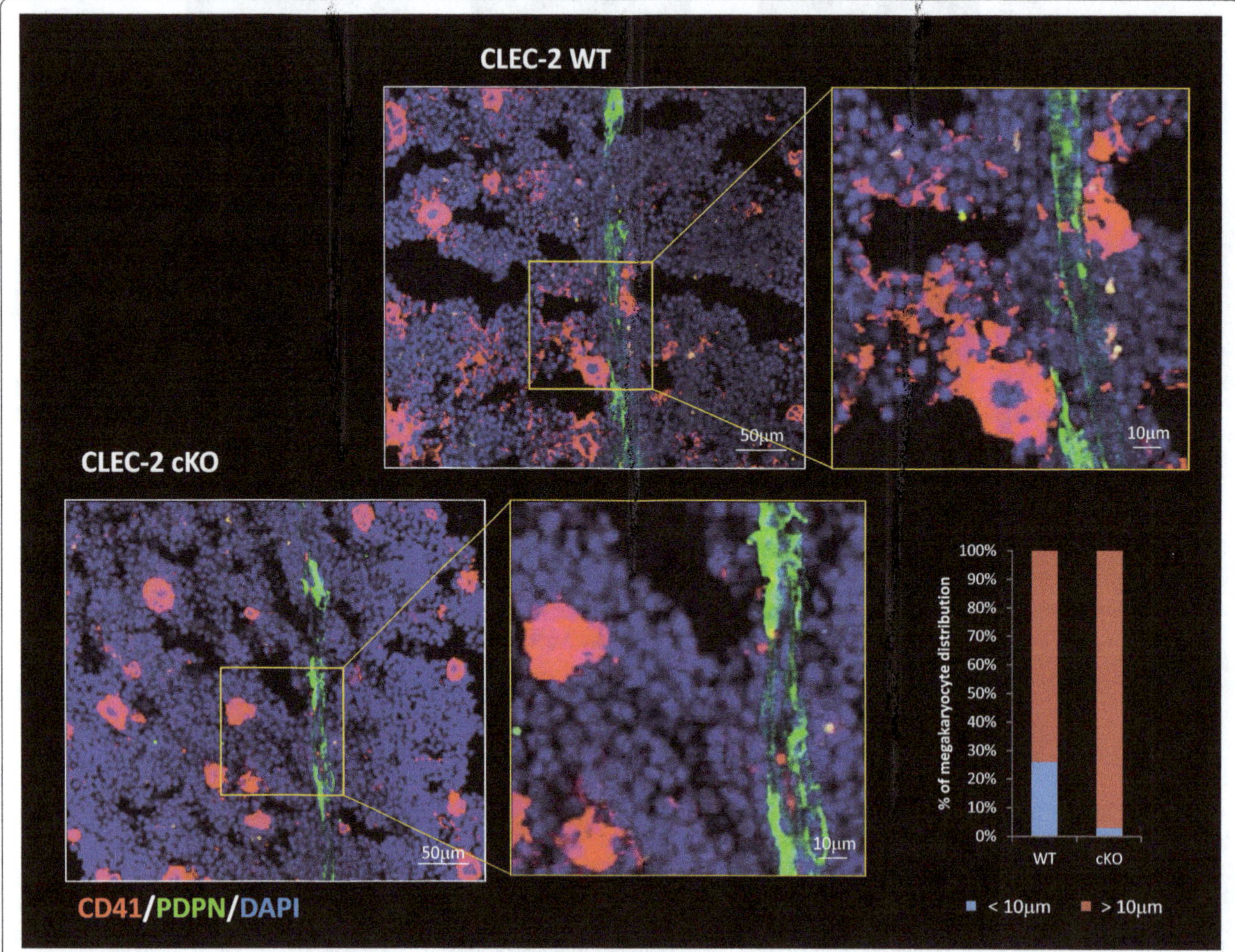

Fig. 6 CD41⁺ clusters were formed adjacent to the podoplanin⁺ stromal cells in the BM CD41⁺ clusters which represent megakaryocytes were observed, lying close to the podoplanin⁺ stromal cells lining vasculature in the bone marrow. However, this phenomenon is not present with CLEC-2 knockout mice. The *right inlet* shows the quantitative distribution of megakaryocytes within 10 μm of vasculature in wild-type mice vs. CLEC-2 knockout

advanced atherosclerotic lesions [8], it is not expressed in normal subendothelial matrix, suggesting that there should be some ligands other than podoplanin for CLEC-2. We next searched for CLEC-2 ligands in normal vessel walls. Recombinant CLEC-2 bound to early atherosclerotic lesions and normal arterial walls, whose localization coincided with vascular smooth muscle cells (VSMCs). Flow cytometric study and immunocytochemistry revealed that recombinant CLEC-2, but not an anti-podoplanin antibody, bound to VSMCs, suggesting that VSMCs express certain CLEC-2 ligands other than podoplanin. The time to occlusion in a FeCl3-induced animal thrombosis model was significantly prolonged in CLEC-2 knockout mice. Since our FeCl3-induced injury model causes laceration in the internal elastic lamina, we assume that the interaction between CLEC-2 and its ligands in VSMCs exposed by laceration induces thrombus formation. Using protein arrays and Biacore analysis, we identified S100A13 as a CLEC-2 ligand in VSMCs [9]. S100A13 was released upon oxidative stress, and expressed in the luminal area of atherosclerotic lesions. Its staining pattern is distinct from podoplanin, and unlike podoplain which is only expressed in atherosclerotic lesions, but not in normal vessels, S100A13 is present in the normal vasculature, and its expression is enhanced in the atherosclerotic lesions (Fig. 5). However, it appears that there is as-yet unidentified CLEC-2 ligand in VSMCs which potently activates platelets, since S100A13 remains to be relatively weak in platelet activation.

Previously, CLEC-2 was considered to play only a minor role in hemostasis, because CLEC-2 knockout resulted in no or only a moderate increase in bleeding time. However, a recent report on severely defective hemostasis in GPVI and CLEC-2 double knockout mice suggests that GPVI and CLEC-2 compensate for each other, preventing severe blood loss, that they serve together to play a key role in hemostasis [10]. In the closely related context, it is of note that GPVI and CLEC-2 with the shared signal transduction pathways such as Syk, SLP-76, and PLCγ2 play a critical role in maintaining vascular integrity during development and inflammation [11].

Role of platelets in liver regeneration

There is an increasing body evidence to suggest that platelets are involved in various stages of liver regeneration. They are not only involved in the early phase of liver generation, but platelet transfusion and thrombocytosis can enhance hepatocyte regeneration after liver injury. Recent studies have reported that platelets are recruited to the sinusoidal and Disse's space and probably due to direct contact with certain cell types such as stellate cells and sinusoidal endothelial cells, they release bioactive compounds which stimulate hepatocyte proliferation [12]. However, up to date, the molecules on the

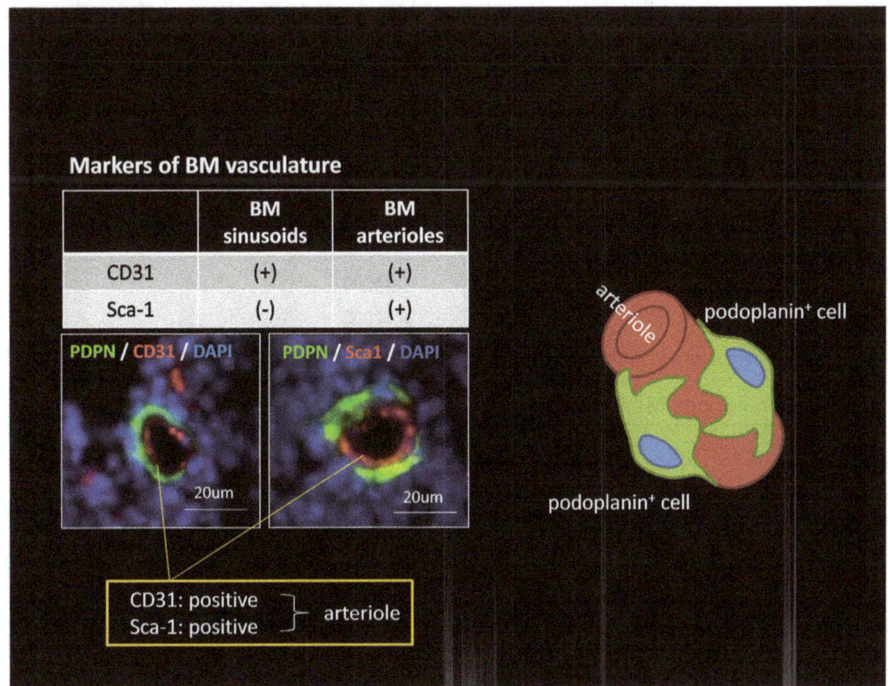

Fig. 7 BM arteriolar stromal cells are podoplanin-positive. There are three type of vessels in the bone marrow, arterioles, sinusoids and lymphatic vessels. Only the bone marrow (BM) arteriolar stromal cells (CD31- and Sca-1-positive) are podoplanin-positive, and these cells are tentatively termed as BM fibroblastic reticular cell (FRC)-like cells. BM-FRC-like cells surround arterioles as illustrated in the *right inlet*

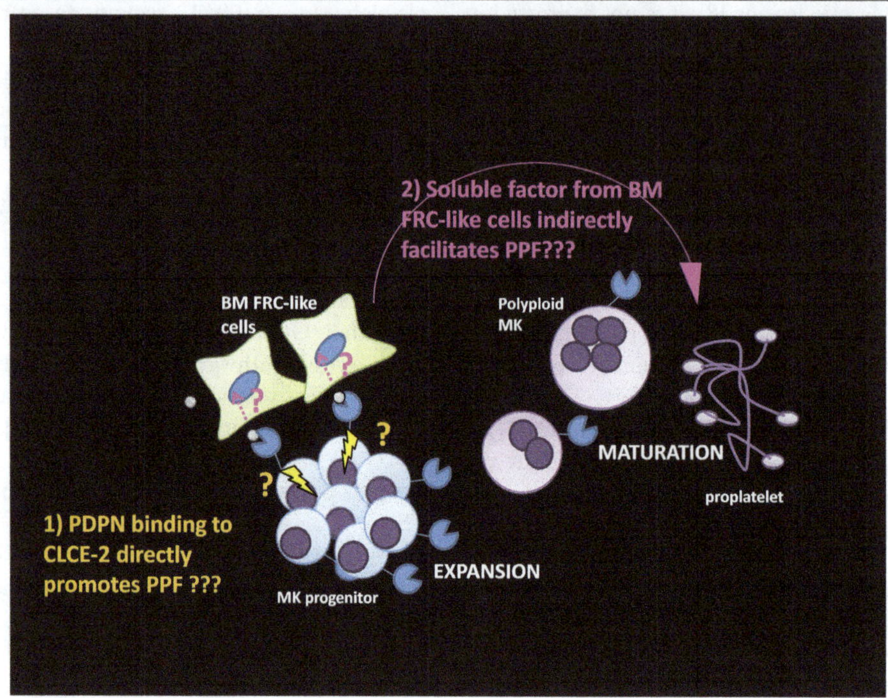

Fig. 8 Hitherto, we have found that podoplain/CLEC-2 interaction induces megakaryocyte expansion. We then asked whether podoplain/CLEC-2 interaction acts on megakaryocytes to induce proplatelet formation, or on BM FCR-like cells which then contributes to proplatelet formation. Two hypotheses are depicted in Fig. 8

platelet membranes which are involved in this process have not been identified.

We have recently found that hepatocyte proliferation is attenuated by clopidogrel, which inhibits platelet activation, and that liver regeneration is impaired with CLEC-2-knockout mice, suggesting that CLEC-2 on the platelet membrane is the key molecule which links with platelets and hepatocyte proliferation (manuscript being submitted).

Megakaryopoiesis and thrombopoiesis

Megakaryopoiesis encompasses the sequential differentiation of hematopoietic stem cells into megakaryocytes, followed by thrombopoiesis in which maturation of

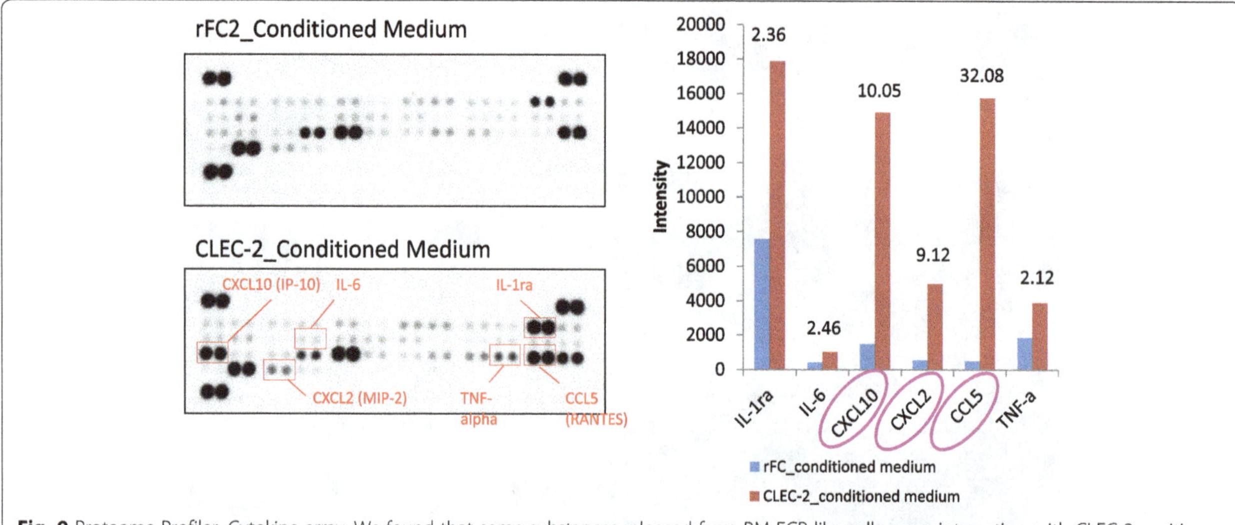

Fig. 9 Proteome Profiler_Cytokine array. We found that some substances released from BM FCR-like cells upon interaction with CLEC-2-positive megakaryocytes serve to induce proplatelet formation. By the use of proteome profile cytokine array, three cytokines were identified, CXCL10, CXCL2, andCCL5. CCL5 was identified to be the most potent molecule released from BM FCR-like cells to induce proplatelet formation in megakaryocytes

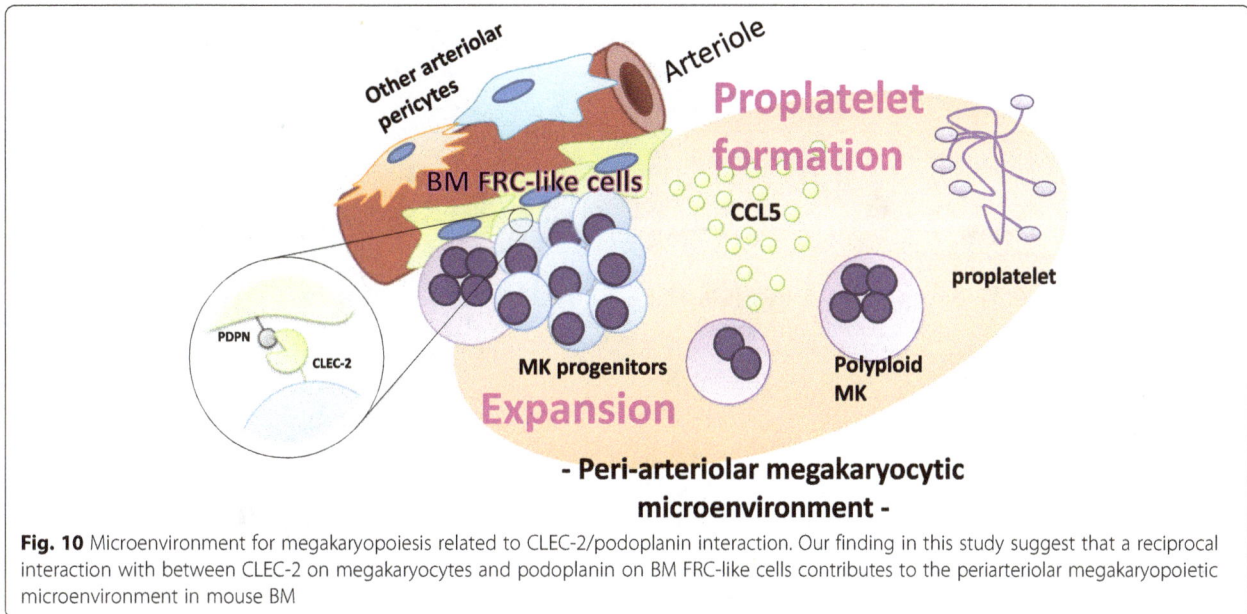

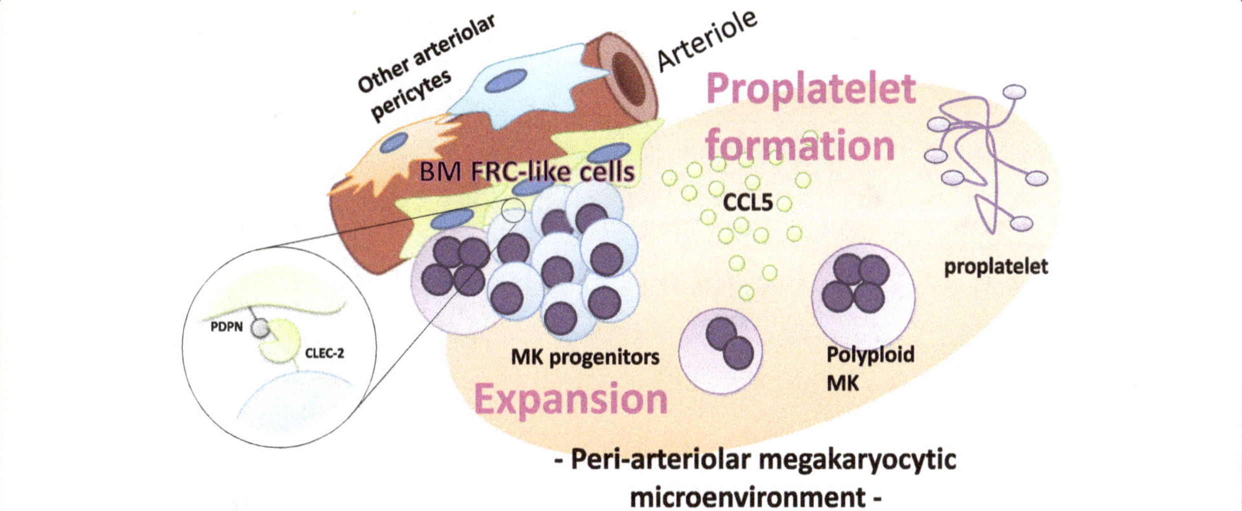

Fig. 10 Microenvironment for megakaryopoiesis related to CLEC-2/podoplanin interaction. Our finding in this study suggest that a reciprocal interaction with between CLEC-2 on megakaryocytes and podoplanin on BM FRC-like cells contributes to the periarteriolar megakaryopoietic microenvironment in mouse BM

megakaryocytes occurs with production of numerous platelets. CLEC-2 is expressed on platelets and megakaryocytes, and thrombocytopenia occurs with deletion of platelet/megakaryocyte CLEC-2 in mice. Megakaryopoiesis is promoted through the CLEC-2/podoplanin interaction in the vicinity of vessels, and we found that this occurs in the vicinity of arterioles, not sinusoids or lymphatic vessels (Fig. 6). We found that podoplanin-expressing stromal cells exit adjacent to BM arterioles, and tentatively termed these cells as BM fibroblastic reticular cell (FRC)-like cells (Fig. 7). There was a significant decrease in the number of immature megakaryocytes in platelet/megakaryocyte-specific CLEC-2 conditional knockout (cKO) mice. CLEC-2 WT megakaryocyte expansion was enhanced *in vitro* by the addition of recombinant podoplanin, but this did not occur with cKO megakaryocytes. Furthermore, megakaryocyte colonies appeared to nest adjacent to periarteriolar BM FRC-like cells in the BM. Co-culture of megakaryocytes with BM FRC-like cells maintained megakaryocyte expansion, which appeared to be dependent upon the CLEC-2/podoplanin interaction. We then asked whether podoplain/CLEC-2 interaction acts on megakaryocytes to induce proplatelet formation, or on BM FCR-like cells which then contributes to proplatelet formation, in addition to the megakaryocyte expansion (Fig. 8). We found that the CLEC-2/podoplanin interaction induces BM FRC-like cells to secrete CCL5 to facilitate proplatelet formation (Fig. 9). These observations suggest that a reciprocal interaction between CLEC-2 on megakaryocytes and podoplanin on BM FRC-like cells contributes to the megakaryopoietic microenvironment in the periarteriolar space in mouse BM [13] (Fig. 10).

Conclusions

There is an increasing body of evidence to suggest that platelets participate in various patho-physiological processes beyond those related to thrombosis and hemostasis, and that CLEC-2 on the platelet membrane by interacting with its ligands, podoplanin and others, contributes to a number of these processes.

Authors' contributions
ST performed the experiments related to megakaryopoiesis. KS analyzed and interpreted the entire data related to CLEC-2. YO gave advice to the project, and was a major contributor in writing this manuscript. All authors read and approved the final manuscript.

Competing interests
The authors declare that they have no competing interests.

Author details
[1]Fuefuki Central Hospital, 47-1 Yokkaichiba, Isawa, Fuefuki 406-0032, Yamanashi, Japan. [2]Department of Laboratory Medicine, University of Yamanashi, 1110 Shimokato, Chuo, Yamanashi 409-3898, Japan. [3]Department of Pathophysiological Laboratory Sciences, Nagoya University Graduate School of Medicine, 1-1-20, Oosachi Minami, Higashi, Nagoya 461-8673, Aichi, Japan.

References

1. McFadyen JD, Kaplan ZS. Platelets are not just for clots. Transfus Med Rev. 2015;26:110–9.
2. Suzuki-Inoue K, Fuller GL, Garcia A, Eble JA, Pohlmann S, Inoue O, et al. A novel Syk-dependent mechanism of platelet activation by the C-type lectin receptor CLEC-2. Blood. 2006;107:542–9.
3. Suzuki-Inoue K, Kato Y, Inoue O, Kaneko MK, Mishima K, Yatomi Y, et al. Involvement of the snake toxin receptor CLEC-2, in podoplanin-mediated platelet activation, by cancer cells. J Biol Chem. 2007;282:25993–6001.
4. Bertozzi CC, Schmaier AA, Mericko P, Hess PR, Zou Z, Chen M, et al. Platelets regulate lymphatic vascular development through CLEC-2-SLP-76 signaling. Blood. 2010;116:661–70.
5. Suzuki-Inoue K, Inoue O, Ding G, Nishimura S, Hokamura K, Eto K, et al. Essential in vivo roles of the C-type lectin receptor CLEC-2: embryonic/neonatal lethalilty of CLEC-2-deficient mice by blood/lymphatic misconnections and impaired thrombus formation of CLEC-2-deficient platelets. J Biol Chem. 2010;285:24494–507.
6. Osada M, Inoue O, Ding G, Shirai T, Ichise H, Hirayama K, et al. Platelet activation receptor CLEC-2 regulates blood/lymphatic vessel separation by inhibiting proliferation, migration, and tube-formation of lymphatic endothelial cells. J Biol Chem. 2012;287:22241–52.
7. May F, Hagedorn I, Pleines I, Bender M, Vogtle T, Eble J, et al. CLEC-2 is an essential platelet-activating receptor in hemostasis and thrombosis. Blood. 2009;114:3464–72.
8. Hatakeyama K, Kaneko MK, Kato Y, Ishikawa T, Nishihira K, Tsujimoto Y, et al. Podoplanin expression in advanced atherosclerotic lesions of human aortas. Thromb Res. 2012;129:e70–6.
9. Inoue O, Hokamura K, Shirai T, Osada M, Tsukiji N, Hatakeyama K, et al. Vascular smooth muscle cells stimulate platelets and facilitate thrombus formation through platelet CLEC-2: implications in atherothrombosis. PLoS One. 2015;10:e0139357. 1–28.
10. Bender M, May F, Lorenz V, Thielmann I, Hagedorn I, Finney BA, et al. Combined in vivo depletion of glycoprotein VI and C-type lectin-lie receptor 2 severely compromises hemostasis and abrogates arterial thrombosis in mice. Arterioscler Thromb Vasc Biol. 2013;33:926–34.
11. Lee RH, Bergmeier WW. Platelet immunoreceptor tyrosine-based activation motif (ITAM) and hemiITAM signaling and vascular integrity in inflammation and development. J Thromb Haemost. 2016;14:645–54.
12. Myer J, Lejmi E, Fontana P, Morel P, Gonelle-Gispert C, Buhler L. A focus on the role of platelets in liver regeneration: Do platelet-endothelia cell interactions initiate the regenerative process? J Hepatol. 2015;63:1263–71.
13. Tamura S, Suzuki-Inoue K, Tsukiji N, Shirai T, Sasaki T, Osada M, et al. Podoplanin-positive periarteriolar stromal cells promote megakaryocyte growth and proplatelet formation in mice by CLEC-2. Blood. 2016;127:1701–10.

7

Procoagulatory changes induced by head-up tilt test in patients with syncope: observational study

Viktor Hamrefors[1,2,3], Artur Fedorowski[1,4*†], Karin Strandberg[5], Richard Sutton[6] and Nazim Isma[1,7†]

Abstract

Background: Orthostatic hypercoagulability is proposed as a mechanism promoting cardiovascular and thromboembolic events after awakening and during prolonged orthostasis.

We evaluated early changes in coagulation biomarkers induced by tilt testing among patients investigated for suspected syncope, aiming to test the hypothesis that orthostatic challenge evokes procoagulatory changes to a different degree according to diagnosis.

Methods: One-hundred-and-seventy-eight consecutive patients (age, 51 ± 21 years; 46% men) were analysed. Blood samples were collected during supine rest and after 3 min of 70° head-up tilt test (HUT) for determination of fibrinogen, von Willebrand factor antigen (VWF:Ag) and activity (VWF:GP1bA), factor VIII (FVIII:C), lupus anticoagulant (LA1), functional APC-resistance, and activated prothrombin time (APTT) with and without activated protein C (C+/−). Analyses were stratified according to age, sex and diagnosis.

Results: After 3 min in the upright position, VWF:Ag (1.28 ± 0.55 vs. 1.22 ± 0.54; $p < 0.001$) and fibrinogen (2.84 ± 0.60 vs. 2.75 ± 0.60, $p < 0.001$) increased, whereas APTT/C+/− (75.1 ± 18.8 vs. 84.3 ± 19.6 s; $p < 0.001$, and 30.8 ± 3.7 vs. 32.1 ± 3.8 s; $p < 0.001$, respectively) and APC-resistance (2.42 ± 0.43 vs. 2.60 ± 0.41, $p < 0.001$) decreased compared with supine values. Significant changes in fibrinogen were restricted to women ($p < 0.001$) who also had lower LA1 during HUT ($p = 0.007$), indicating increased coagulability. Diagnosis vasovagal syncope was associated with less increase in VWF:Ag during HUT compared to other diagnoses (0.01 ± 0.16 vs. 0.09 ± 0.17; $p = 0.004$).

Conclusions: Procoagulatory changes in haemostatic plasma components are observed early during orthostasis in patients with history of syncope, irrespective of syncope aetiology. These findings may contribute to the understanding of orthostatic hypercoagulability and chronobiology of cardiovascular disease.

Keywords: Orthostatic stress, Hypercoagulability, Coagulation factors, Partial thromboplastin time, Fibrinogen, von Willebrand factor

Background

It has long been observed that major cardiovascular and thromboembolic events show higher incidence after awakening, which has been partly explained by increased platelet activity during morning hours [1–4]. In parallel, a phenomenon of "orthostatic hypercoagulability", i.e. increase in plasma procoagulants independent of postural volume shift and extravascular fluid escape, has been reported [5–7]. The prothrombotic changes during passive orthostasis were first detected in healthy volunteers without history of syncope, cardiovascular or thromboembolic disease. Similar changes in coagulation factors were induced by lower-body negative pressure in volunteers who developed vasovagal reflex but, interestingly, those who did not develop the reflex showed no significant alterations in coagulation factors [8]. Changes in the coagulation system have also been detected during vasovagal reflex activation: a study

* Correspondence: Artur.fedorowski@med.lu.se
†Equal contributors
[1]Department of Clinical Sciences Malmö, Lund University, SE 205-02 Malmö, Sweden
[4]Department of Cardiology, Skåne University Hospital, Inga Marie Nilssons gata 46, SE 205-02 Malmö, Sweden
Full list of author information is available at the end of the article

performed in subjects with von Willebrand disease has demonstrated increased antigen concentration of von Willebrand factor (VWF:Ag), VWF-Ristocetin-cofactor, and factor VIII activity (FVIII:C) after fainting prompted by fear of venepuncture [9]. In a previous study, we have observed that von Willebrand factor is increased in patients with orthostatic hypotension compared with other patients investigated for suspected syncope, irrespective of body position [10]. However, we have also noticed that both groups demonstrated procoagulatory changes during passive orthostasis evoked by head-up tilt test (HUT). In this study, we took the opportunity to analyse plasma samples collected at rest and during the early phase of HUT to assess how passive orthostasis impacts coagulation factors. We aimed to test the hypothesis that passive orthostasis during HUT would evoke procoagulatory changes and that these changes would differ according to HUT diagnosis.

Methods

Patients and inclusion/exclusion criteria

The present study was performed from November 2011 to October 2012 as a part of the ongoing Syncope Study of Unselected Population in Malmo (SYSTEMA) project, a single-centre observational study on syncope aetiology [11]. During this period, 233 consecutive patients underwent head-up tilt test (HUT) due to unexplained syncope and/or orthostatic intolerance. Patients were included if they accepted blood sampling during HUT (n = 183), and excluded if they were on current oral anti-coagulation therapy with warfarin (n = 5), leaving 178 patients that were eligible for the final inclusion. None of the included patients had a diagnosed bleeding disorder. All patients provided written informed consent and were included in further analyses. The Regional Ethical Review Board of Lund University approved the study protocol including blood sampling during tilt testing.

Head-up tilt test

Study participants were requested to take their regular medication and fast for 2 h before the test, although they were allowed to drink water. The examination was based on a specially designed HUT protocol, which included peripheral vein cannulation, supine rest for 15 min and HUT with optional nitroglycerine provocation after 20 min of passive HUT according to the Italian protocol [12]. Beat-to-beat blood pressure (BP) and ECG were continuously recorded using a Nexfin monitor (BMEYE, Amsterdam, The Netherlands) [13]. The detailed description of the examination protocol has been previously published [14]. The final HUT diagnoses were concordant with the current European Society of Cardiology guidelines [15].

Blood sampling

Blood was collected during supine rest before and after 3 min of 70° HUT (during passive phase, prior to optional nitroglycerine administration) in citrated tubes (BD Vacutainer®, 4,5 mL, 0,109 M sodium citrate). Samples were immediately centrifuged for 20 min at 2000 x g. Plasma was separated and immediately frozen at −70 °C.

Coagulation analyses

APTT was performed at the accredited hospital laboratory using a BCS-XP analyzer (Siemens Healthcare, Marburg, Germany) with the Actin FSL reagents (Siemens Healthcare, Marburg, Germany), with and without addition of activated protein C (reference interval in healthy individuals for test without activated protein C, 26–33 s). The analysis of plasma fibrinogen concentration was performed using the Dade Thrombin reagent on a Sysmex CS-5100 analyser (Siemens). The reference interval has been established locally as 2–4 g/L. The coagulation analyses below were performed on a BCS-XP instrument (Siemens). The original plasma-based activated protein C resistance (APC-resistance) test was performed with COATEST APC Resistance test (Chromogenix, Mölndal, Sweden). Reference interval was >2.1. The activity of von Willebrand factor (VWF:GP1bA) was analysed with an immunoassay based on an antibody against glycoprotein 1b (GP1b) and a GP1b construct that binds VWF in the sample (Innovance VWF:Ac; Siemens). Reference interval established locally was 0,5–2.0 kU/L. Antigen concentration of von Willebrand factor (VWF:Ag) was measured with a latex-enhanced immunoassays (Siemens). Reference interval was 0.6–2.7 kIU/L. Screening test for lupus anticoagulant (LA1) was performed with a clot-based assay: LA1 (Siemens). Reference interval was <42 s. Factor VIII activity assay (FVIII:C) was performed with a chromogenic substrate method (Coatest FVIII SP, Chromogenic). Reference interval was 0.5–2.0 kIU/L. Imprecision measured as a coefficient of variation was 2% for VWF:Ag (at 1.2 kIU/L), 3% for VWF:GP1bA (at 0.9 kIU/L), 4% for LA1: (at 40 s), 3% for FVIII: (at 0.8 and 1.5 kIU/L), and 2–4% for fibrinogen (at 1 g/L, 2%; at 3 g/L, 4%).

Statistical analyses

Independent samples Student's t-test was used to compare continuous variables between men and women whereas paired samples Student's t-test was used to compare changes in coagulation parameters measured in supine position and during HUT, respectively. Analyses regarding coagulation parameters were stratified according to sex and age (younger vs. older adults; 65 years). Changes in coagulation parameters during HUT according to diagnosis were specifically tested by comparing the changes in subjects with VVS versus all other diagnoses (including negative HUT) and comparing the changes in subjects with OH (classical + delayed form) versus all other diagnoses, using independent samples Student's t-test. Categorical variables were compared using Pearson's chi-square test. All analyses were performed using IBM SPSS Statistics version 23 (SPSS Inc., Chicago, IL, USA). All tests were two-sided whereby $p < 0.05$ was considered statistically significant.

Results

Patient characteristics stratified by gender are shown in Table 1. Men were older and had lower resting heart rate. Sixty-nine (38.8%) patients were diagnosed with vasovagal reflex syncope (VVS), whereas 49 (27.5%) patients met OH criteria. Further, 7 patients had carotid sinus syndrome, 7 postural orthostatic tachycardia syndrome, 9 initial OH, 5 psychogenic pseudosyncope and 17 (9.6%) underwent HUT without a definitive diagnosis (i.e. negative test). Table 2 shows data on measurements of coagulation markers in supine and after 3 min of HUT. All patients had a significantly increased level of VWF:Ag and fibrinogen after 3 min of HUT, whereas APC-resistance ratio and APTT were significantly decreased compared with resting supine values. There were no significant differences between supine and HUT regarding FVIII, VWF:GP1bA and LA1. All parameters were within the reference interval for healthy individuals. In gender-stratified analyses, only women had significantly increased fibrinogen and demonstrated a shorter LA1 time during HUT (see: Table 3). Stratification of study population by the age of 65 years showed similar distribution of changes in coagulation parameters (Table 4). A final diagnosis of VVS was associated with less increase in VWF:Ag during orthostasis (0.01 ± 0.16) compared to all other diagnoses (0.09 ± 0.17; $p = 0.004$). The changes in coagulation parameters were not different in patients diagnosed with OH compared with all other diagnoses ($p > 0.05$).

Table 1 Characteristics and risk factors in 178 consecutive patients with unexplained syncope, mean ± SD or n (%)

	All patients $n = 178$	Men $n = 81$ (46)	Women $n = 97$ (54)	*p*-value
Patient characteristics				
Age (years)	50.9 ± 20.9	56.0 ± 18.7	46.6 ± 21.8	0.003
BMI (kg/ m2)	25.6 ± 4.6	26.0 ± 3.6	25.3 ± 5.3	0.34
Systolic BP (mmHg)	131 ± 18.7	131 ± 17.1	132 ± 20.0	0.78
Diastolic BP (mmHg)	71 ± 8.0	71 ± 8.8	70 ± 7.6	0.44
Heart rate (bpm)	67.7 ± 11.7	65.4 ± 12.7	69.6 ± 10.6	0.016
Risk factors (%)				
Hypertension	28.8	35.0	23.7	0.10
Diabetes mellitus	6.7	8.6	5.2	0.36
History of MACE[a]	3.9	7.4	1.0	0.029
History of stroke	1.7	2.5	1.0	0.46
Present tobacco use	15.7	16.0	15.5	0.92

BMI, body mass index; BP, blood pressure; MACE[a] (=major coronary event) was defined as history of myocardial infarction, unstable angina, CABG, or PCI

Discussion

The present study illustrates the impact of passive orthostatic challenge on haemostatic plasma components in a series of unselected patients with a history of unexplained syncope. During early phase of head-up tilt test, fibrinogen, APTT, VWF:Ag, and APC-resistance demonstrated significant procoagulatory changes. Although relative changes in the assessed coagulation markers were small, indeed, within the test imprecision range for fibrinogen, the directionality of these changes consequently pointed at the increased coagulability on standing.

Fibrinogen, as acute-phase glycoprotein, may be elevated in any form of inflammation and is also involved in formation of blood clots not only through fibrinformation, but also through its effect on specific platelet receptors and blood viscosity. Higher levels of fibrinogen are associated with cardiovascular disease [16–19] and its degradation products accumulate in the atherosclerotic plaque [20]. Interestingly, fibrinogen increased most in women who also demonstrated procoagulatory LA1 changes. The exact mechanisms behind these gender-specific propensities are not known and were not the subject of this study, however, hormonal differences may be one of the possible explanations [21]. Thus, orthostatic procoagulatory changes in fibrinogen, LA1, and FVIII seem mainly to affect women who are at higher risk of thromboembolic events compared with men [22]. As thromboembolic events are more common in the morning hours [3], orthostatic increase in fibrinogen and FVIII may act as a facilitator of thrombus generation after awakening and assuming an upright position, in a relative dehydrated state after a night's rest.

Notably, APTT was reduced on orthostasis irrespective of the analysed subgroup. Shortening of APTT usually indicates increased activity of FVIII in association with inflammatory conditions [23]. As APTT involves both fibrinogen and FVIII, which first and foremost increased in women, it seems that other factors such as prothrombin, V, IX, X, XI, and XII may have undergone orthostatic changes too. Unfortunately, our test panel did not detect this. Shortening of APTT, although within the normal range, may have thromboembolic consequences, as indicated by a previous study [24]. We believe that shortened APTT indicates a hypercoagulable state, as was also shown in a study by Mina et al. [25]. This is supported by other clinical studies performed on patients with acute coronary events [26, 27].

Table 2 Coagulation markers in supine and after 3 min head-up tilt (HUT) in 178 patients with unexplained syncope, mean ± SD or n (%)

	All patients	*p*-value*	Men	Women	*p*-value¶
N (%)	178		81 (46)	97 (54)	
FVIII:C *supine* (kIE/L)	1.06 ± 0.38	0.43	1.07 ± 0.32	1.04 ± 0.41	0.56
FVIII:C *HUT* (kIE/L)	1.07 ± 0.36		1.07 ± 0.35	1.07 ± 0.36	0.98
VWF:Ag *supine* (kIE/L)	1.22 ± 0.54	<0.001	1.28 ± 0.56	1.17 ± 0.51	0.17
VWF:Ag *HUT* (kIE/L)	1.28 ± 0.55		1.33 ± 0.59	1.24 ± 0.52	0.31
VWF:GP1bA *supine* (kIE/L)	1.24 ± 0.55	0.20	1.30 ± 0.59	1.19 ± 0.52	0.19
VWF:GP1bA *HUT* (kIE/L)	1.26 ± 0.56		1.31 ± 0.64	1.23 ± 0.49	0.34
Fibrinogen *supine* (g/L)	2.75 ± 0.60	<0.001	2.67 ± 0.57	2.81 ± 0.62	0.11
Fibrinogen *HUT* (g/L)	2.84 ± 0.60		2.73 ± 0.59	2.93 ± 0.60	0.022
LA1 *supine* (sec)	31.2 ± 3.7	0.066	31.9 ± 3.50	30.7 ± 3.8	0.027
LA1 *HUT* (sec)	31.1 ± 4.7		32.0 ± 3.92	30.5 ± 5.2	0.030
APC-resistance *supine*	2.60 ± 0.41	<0.001	2.65 ± 0.39	2.57 ± 0.42	0.17
APC-resistance *HUT*	2.42 ± 0.43		2.49 ± 0.41	2.36 ± 0.44	0.044
APTT/C+ *supine* (sec)	84.3 ± 19.6	<0.001	85.8 ± 19.8	83.1 ± 19.5	0.36
APTT/C+ *HUT* (sec)	75.1 ± 18.8		77.4 ± 18.7	73.1 ± 18.7	0.13
APTT/C- *supine* (sec)	32.1 ± 3.8	<0.001	32.1 ± 4.1	32.1 ± 3.6	1.0
APTT/C- *HUT* (sec)	30.8 ± 3.7		30.8 ± 3.8	30.7 ± 3.7	0.83

*supine vs. HUT paired samples t-test; ¶ men vs. women independent samples t-test; FVIII, factor VIII; VWF:Ag, von Willebrand factor antigen; vVWF:GP1bA, von Willebrand factor GP1bA activity; LA1, lupus anticoagulant-screening; APC-resistance, activated protein C resistance; APTT, activated prothrombin time; C+/–, with/without activated protein C

Furthermore, we observed elevated levels of VWF during orthostasis. It has been reported that higher levels of VWF are associated with a 3-fold increased risk for severe coronary heart disease [28–30]. Our results are consistent with other studies, linking changes in VWF and FVIII to the vasovagal reflex, artificially induced orthostatic stress and presyncope [5, 6, 8]. The von Willebrand factor is the largest plasma protein and plays a key role in primary haemostasis as cofactor in platelet adhesion and platelet aggregation. This platelet adhesion is promoted by a platelet membrane receptor glycoprotein (GPIb –IX-V) when circulating VWF attaches to the sub-endothelium collagen and serves as a bridge between tissue and platelets [31].

Table 3 Gender-stratified changes in coagulation markers during head-up tilt among 178 patients with unexplained syncope

	Men	*p*-value*	Women	*p*-value*
N (%)	81 (46)		97 (54)	
Δ FVIII:C (kIE/L)	0.00 ± 0.16	0.64	0.02 ± 0.13	0.091
Δ VWF:Ag (kIE/L)	0.04 ± 0.18	0.030	0.07 ± 0.15	<0.001
Δ VWF:GP1bA (kIE/L)	0.01 ± 0.25	0.86	0.03 ± 0.18	0.067
Δ Fibrinogen (g/L)	0.06 ± 0.32	0.12	0.12 ± 0.22	<0.001
Δ LA1 (sec)	−0.13 ± 3.23	0.72	−0.56 ± 1.96	0.007
Δ APC-resistance	−0.16 ± 0.26	<0.001	−0.21 ± 0.26	<0.001
Δ APTT/C+ (sec)	−8.3 ± 13.7	<0.001	−9.9 ± 10.6	<0.001
Δ APTT/C- (sec)	−1.2 ± 2.4	<0.001	−1.4 ± 1.7	<0.001

*supine vs. HUT paired samples t-test; FVIII, factor VIII; VWF:Ag, von Willebrand factor antigen; vWF:GP1bA, von Willebrand factor GP1bA activity; LA1, lupus anticoagulant-screening; APC-resistance, activated protein C resistance; APTT, activated prothrombin time; C+/–, with/without activated protein C

Previous studies performed on healthy subjects have shown that platelet aggregability is increased in the morning, when the incidence of cardiovascular events such as myocardial infarct, sudden cardiac death and transient myocardial ischemia is higher [1, 32–35]. However, data on the changes in haemostatic plasma components in the same settings are very sparse and we believe that this study may contribute to the understanding of cardiovascular chronobiology. Our results confirm that changing from supine to upright body position induces activation of the coagulation system and promotes a hypercoagulable state during early orthostasis. The physiological role of orthostatic hypercoagulability may be to protect the body against increased bleeding risk during activities of daily life or be a result of higher hydrostatic pressure in the lower body, which will activate the endothelial response and release of coagulation factors.

The activation of haemostatic plasma components may support the hypothesis of tight cooperation between procoagulatory factors and platelets, and its impact on the development of cardiovascular events. Whether or not cardiovascular events such as myocardial infarct, sudden cardiac death, transient myocardial ischemia,

Table 4 Age-stratified changes in coagulation markers during head-up tilt among 178 patients with unexplained syncope

	Age < 65 years	*p*-value*	Age ≥ 65 years	*p*-value*
N (%)	119 (67)		59 (33)	
Δ FVIII:C (kIE/L)	0.02 ± 0.15	0.17	−0.01 ± 0.15	0.55
Δ VWF:Ag (kIE/L)	0.04 ± 0.15	0.006	0.10 ± 0.19	<0.001
Δ VWF:GP1bA (kIE/L)	0.02 ± 0.22	0.35	0.02 ± 0.19	0.37
Δ Fibrinogen (g/L)	0.10 ± 0.30	<0.001	0.07 ± 0.20	0.009
Δ LA1 (sec)	−0.40 ± 2.88	0.14	−0.31 ± 1.92	0.25
Δ APC-resistance	−0.16 ± 0.24	<0.001	−0.24 ± 0.28	<0.001
Δ APTT/C+ (sec)	−8.5 ± 12.2	<0.001	−10.6 ± 11.9	<0.001
Δ APTT/C- (sec)	−1.3 ± 2.1	<0.001	−1.3 ± 2.0	<0.001

*supine vs. HUT paired samples t-test; FVIII, factor VIII; VWF:Ag, von Willebrand factor antigen; vWF:GP1bA, von Willebrand factor GP1bA activity; LA1, lupus anticoagulant-screening; APC-resistance, activated protein C resistance; APTT, activated prothrombin time; C+/−, with/without activated protein C

and stroke during morning hours are promoted by synergic effects of both orthostatic hypercoagulability and increased platelet aggregability remains to be further explored.

Finally, patients diagnosed with vasovagal reflex syncope (VVS) demonstrated less pronounced changes in vWF:Ag than the rest of study population, whereas those with OH did not differ from non-OH patients. The former may be due to relatively younger age of VVS patients, although this study does not allow further speculations on the cause of this difference, whereas the latter implies that procoagulatory orthostatic changes are independent of BP fluctuations on standing.

Limitations

The conclusions of our study may be underpowered due to some important limitations (listed below). Thus, we would like to emphasize that the current study may be useful as a "proof of concept" for a larger and improved study design, in which these limitations could be overcome. No control group including healthy individuals was included and there were no measurements of coagulation parameters in subjects that did not undergo HUT. As the participants of the current study are part of the ongoing larger SYSTEMA project [11], no prospective sample size assessment was done, prior to the study. We were not able to measure specific markers of activated coagulation, such as thrombin-antithrombin-complex (TAT) or D-dimer, which would have been informative. Furthermore, since data on hereditary thrombophilia and levels or function of platelets were not registered, it was not feasible to separate possible contributions of these variables to hypercoagulability. Procoagulants were measured after 3 min of HUT only and we do not have data on how the prolonged standing might influence the assessed coagulation factors. However, determination of early orthostatic changes may have precluded the possible effects of intravascular volume escape observed during prolonged standing on the concentration of procoagulatory proteins. Also of relevance, even though the observed rise in coagulation markers is in direction during HUT, we cannot exclude a similar reaction if subjects were to be provoked by physical stress that did not involve orthostasis (such as on a supine ergometer bicycle). Finally, our study design and the fact that we did not measure potentially important coagulation proteases such as thrombin, factor Xa and tissue factor involved in atherosclerosis development, precludes us from drawing any conclusions on whether syncope induced hypercoagulability might also contribute to the development of atherosclerosis.

Conclusions

Procoagulatory changes in haemostatic plasma components can be observed during early phase of passive orthostatic challenge irrespective of syncope diagnosis. These findings may contribute to the understanding of orthostatic hypercoagulability and chronobiology of cardiovascular disease.

Abbreviations

APC-resistance: Activated protein C resistance; APTT: Activated partial thromboplastin time; FVIII:C: Factor VIII activity; HUT: Head-up tilt test; LA1: Lupus anticoagulant; OH: Orthostatic hypotension; VVS: Vasovagal syncope; VWF:Ag: Antigen concentration of von Willebrand factor; VWF:GP1bA: Activity of von Willebrand factor

Acknowledgments

Authors would like to thank Philippe Burri, Amna Ali, Elisabeth Persson and Shakila Modaber for their support and engagement during this study.

Funding

This study was supported by grants from the European Research Council (StG 282,225), Swedish Medical Research Council, the Swedish Heart and Lung Foundation, the Medical Faculty of Lund University, the Crafoord Foundation, the Ernhold Lundströms Research Foundation, the Hulda and Conrad Mossfelt Foundation, and the Anna Lisa and Sven-Erik Lundgrens Foundation.

Authors' contributions
AF preformed all the examinations. VH, AF and NI performed statistical analyses and drafted the manuscript. KS and RS, added specific sections of manuscript (coagulation analyses, interpretation of results, and discussion). All authors contributed equally to critical review of manuscript and final editing. AF supported the work by grants. All authors read and approved the final manuscript.

Competing interests
The authors declare that they have no competing interests.

Author details
[1]Department of Clinical Sciences Malmö, Lund University, SE 205-02 Malmö, Sweden. [2]Department of Internal Medicine, Skåne University Hospital, SE 205-02 Malmö, Sweden. [3]Department of Medical Imaging and Physiology, Skåne University Hospital, SE 205-02 Malmö, Sweden. [4]Department of Cardiology, Skåne University Hospital, Inga Marie Nilssons gata 46, SE 205-02 Malmö, Sweden. [5]Centre for Thrombosis and Haemostasis, Skåne University Hospital, SE 205-02 Malmö, Sweden. [6]National Heart and Lung Institute, Imperial College, Hammersmith Hospital Campus, Ducane Road, London W12 0NN, UK. [7]Department of Cardiology, Skåne University Hospital, SE 221-85 Lund, Sweden.

References

1. Tofler GH, Brezinski D, Schafer AI, Czeisler CA, Rutherford JD, Willich SN, et al. Concurrent morning increase in platelet aggregability and the risk of myocardial infarction and sudden cardiac death. N Engl J Med. 1987; 316(24):1514–8.
2. Goldberg RJ, Brady P, Muller JE, Chen ZY, de Groot M, Zonneveld P, et al. Time of onset of symptoms of acute myocardial infarction. Am J Cardiol. 1990;66(2):140–4.
3. Gallerani M, Manfredini R, Ricci L, Grandi E, Cappato R, Calo G, et al. Sudden death from pulmonary thromboembolism: chronobiological aspects. Eur Heart J. 1992;13(5):661–5.
4. Elliott WJ. Circadian variation in the timing of stroke onset: a meta-analysis. Stroke. 1998;29(5):992–6.
5. Masoud M, Sarig G, Brenner B, Jacob G. Orthostatic hypercoagulability: a novel physiological mechanism to activate the coagulation system. Hypertension. 2008;51(6):1545–51.
6. Masoud M, Sarig G, Brenner B, Jacob G. Hydration does not prevent orthostatic hypercoagulability. Thromb Haemost. 2010;103(2):284–90.
7. Cvirn G, Schlagenhauf A, Leschnik B, Koestenberger M, Roessler A, Jantscher A, et al. Coagulation changes during presyncope and recovery. PLoS One. 2012;7(8):e42221.
8. Kraemer M, Kuepper M, Nebe-vom Stein A, Sorgenfrei U, Diehl RR. The influence of vasovagal response on the coagulation system. Clin Auton Res. 2010;20(2):105–11.
9. Casonato A, Pontara E, Bertomoro A, Cattini MG, Soldera C, Girolami A. Fainting induces an acute increase in the concentration of plasma factor VIII and von Willebrand factor. Haematologica. 2003;88(6):688–93.
10. Isma N, Sutton R, Hillarp A, Strandberg K, Melander O, Fedorowski A. Higher levels of von Willebrand factor in patients with syncope due to orthostatic hypotension. J Hypertens. 2015;33(8):1594–601.
11. Fedorowski A, Burri P, Juul-Moller S, Melander O. A dedicated investigation unit improves management of syncopal attacks (syncope study of unselected population in Malmo–SYSTEMA I). Europace. 2010;12(9):1322–8.
12. Bartoletti A, Alboni P, Ammirati F, Brignole M, Del Rosso A, Foglia Manzillo G, Menozzi C, Raviele A, Sutton R. 'The Italian Protocol': a simplified head-up tilt testing potentiated with oral nitroglycerin to assess patients with unexplained syncope. Europace. 2000;2(4):339–42.
13. Eeftinck Schattenkerk DW, van Lieshout JJ, van den Meiracker AH, Wesseling KR, Blanc S, Wieling W, et al. Nexfin noninvasive continuous blood pressure validated against Riva-Rocci/Korotkoff. Am J Hypertens. 2009;22(4):378–83.
14. Nilsson D, Sutton R, Tas W, Burri P, Melander O, Fedorowski A. Orthostatic changes in Hemodynamics and cardiovascular biomarkers in Dysautonomic patients. PLoS One. 2015;10(6):e0128962.
15. Moya A, Sutton R, Ammirati F, Blanc JJ, Brignole M, Dahm JB, et al. Guidelines for the diagnosis and Management of Syncope (version 2009): the task force for the diagnosis and management of syncope of the European Society of Cardiology (ESC). Eur Heart J. 2009;30(21):2631–71.
16. Meade TW, Mellows S, Brozovic M, Miller GJ, Chakrabarti RR, North WR, et al. Haemostatic function and ischaemic heart disease: principal results of the Northwick Park heart study. Lancet. 1986;2(8506):533–7.
17. Kannel WB, Wolf PA, Castelli WP, D'Agostino RB. Fibrinogen and risk of cardiovascular disease. The Framingham study. JAMA. 1987;258(9):1183–6.
18. Yarnell JW, Baker IA, Sweetnam PM, Bainton D, O'Brien JR, Whitehead PJ, et al. Fibrinogen, viscosity, and white blood cell count are major risk factors for ischemic heart disease. The Caerphilly and speedwell collaborative heart disease studies. Circulation. 1991;83(3):836–44.
19. Stec JJ, Silbershatz H, Tofler GH, Matheney TH, Sutherland P, Lipinska I, et al. Association of fibrinogen with cardiovascular risk factors and cardiovascular disease in the Framingham offspring population. Circulation. 2000;102(14):1634–8.
20. Smith EB, Keen GA, Grant A, Stirk C. Fate of fibrinogen in human arterial intima. Arteriosclerosis. 1990;10(2):263–75.
21. Blomback M, Konkle BA, Manco-Johnson MJ, Bremme K, Hellgren M, Kaaja R. Issues ISSoWsH: Preanalytical conditions that affect coagulation testing, including hormonal status and therapy. J Thromb Haemost. 2007;5(4):855–8.
22. Group ECW. Venous thromboembolism in women: a specific reproductive health risk. Hum Reprod Update. 2013;19(5):471–82.
23. Ng VL. Prothrombin time and partial thromboplastin time assay considerations. Clin Lab Med. 2009;29(2):253–63.
24. Korte W, Clarke S, Lefkowitz JB. Short activated partial thromboplastin times are related to increased thrombin generation and an increased risk for thromboembolism. Am J Clin Pathol. 2000;113(1):123–7.
25. Mina A, Favaloro EJ, Mohammed S, Koutts J. A laboratory evaluation into the short activated partial thromboplastin time. Blood Coagul Fibrinolysis. 2010;21(2):152–7.
26. Pinelli A, Trivulzio S, Rossoni G. Activated partial thromboplastin time correlates with methoxyhydroxyphenylglycol in acute myocardial infarction patients: therapeutic implications for patients at cardiovascular risk. In Vivo. 2014;28(1):99–104.
27. Abdullah WZ, Moufak SK, Yusof Z, Mohamad MS, Kamarul IM. Shortened activated partial thromboplastin time, a hemostatic marker for hypercoagulable state during acute coronary event. Transl Res. 2010;155(6):315–9.
28. Whincup PH, Danesh J, Walker M, Lennon L, Thomson A, Appleby P, Rumley A, Lowe GD. von Willebrand factor and coronary heart disease: prospective study and meta-analysis. Eur Heart J. 2002;23(22):1764–70.
29. Willeit P, Thompson A, Aspelund T, Rumley A, Eiriksdottir G, Lowe G, et al. Hemostatic factors and risk of coronary heart disease in general populations: new prospective study and updated meta-analyses. PLoS One. 2013;8(2):e55175.
30. Morange PE, Simon C, Alessi MC, Luc G, Arveiler D, Ferrieres J, et al. Endothelial cell markers and the risk of coronary heart disease: the prospective epidemiological study of myocardial infarction (PRIME) study. Circulation. 2004;109(11):1343–8.
31. Berndt MC, Shen Y, Dopheide SM, Gardiner EE, Andrews RK. The vascular biology of the glycoprotein Ib-IX-V complex. Thromb Haemost. 2001;86(1):178–88.
32. Brezinski DA, Tofler GH, Muller JE, Pohjola-Sintonen S, Willich SN, Schafer AI, et al. Morning increase in platelet aggregability. Association with assumption of the upright posture. Circulation. 1988;78(1):35–40.
33. Willich SN, Tofler GH, Brezinski DA, Schafer AI, Muller JE, Michel T, et al. Platelet alpha 2 adrenoceptor characteristics during the morning increase in platelet aggregability. Eur Heart J. 1992;13(4):550–5.
34. Muller JE. Morning increase of onset of myocardial infarction. Implications concerning triggering events. Cardiology. 1989;76(2):96–104.
35. Muller JE. Circadian variation and triggering of acute coronary events. Am Heart J. 1999;137(4 Pt 2):S1–8.

8

CD163 macrophage and erythrocyte contents in aspirated deep vein thrombus are associated with the time after onset

Eiji Furukoji[1†], Toshihiro Gi[2†], Atsushi Yamashita[2*], Sayaka Moriguchi-Goto[3], Mio Kojima[2], Chihiro Sugita[4], Tatefumi Sakae[1], Yuichiro Sato[3], Toshinori Hirai[1] and Yujiro Asada[2]

Abstract

Background: Thrombolytic therapy is effective in selected patients with deep vein thrombosis (DVT). Therefore, identification of a marker that reflects the age of thrombus is of particular concern. This pilot study aimed to identify a marker that reflects the time after onset in human aspirated DVT.

Methods: We histologically and immunohistochemically analyzed 16 aspirated thrombi. The times from onset to aspiration ranged from 5 to 60 days (median of 13 days). Paraffin sections were stained with hematoxylin and eosin and antibodies for fibrin, glycophorin A, integrin α2bβ3, macrophage markers (CD68, CD163, and CD206), CD34, and smooth muscle actin (SMA).

Results: All thrombi were immunopositive for glycophorin A, fibrin, integrin α2bβ3, CD68, CD163, and CD206, and contained granulocytes. Almost all of the thrombi had small foci of CD34- or SMA-immunopositive areas. CD68- and CD163-immunopositive cell numbers were positively correlated with the time after onset, while the glycophorin A-immunopositive area was negatively correlated with the time after onset. In double immunohistochemistry, CD163-positive cells existed predominantly among the CD68-immunopositive macrophage population. CD163-positive macrophages were closely localized with glycophorin A, CD34, or SMA-positive cell-rich areas.

Conclusions: These findings indicate that CD163 macrophage and erythrocyte contents could be markers for evaluation of the age of thrombus in DVT. Additionally, CD163 macrophages might play a role in organization of the process of venous thrombus.

Keywords: CD163, Deep vein thrombus, Erythrocyte, Macrophage

Background

Venous thromboembolisms are a global health problem. The annual incidence of venous thromboembolism ranges from 0.75 to 2.69 per 1000 individuals in Western Europe, North America, Australia, and Argentina. This incidence has recently increased to between 2 and 7 per 1000 among those aged 70 years or older [1]. In a series of 140 cases of fatal pulmonary embolisms, the emboli originated in the iliac veins (4.5%), femoral veins (20.7%), and deep crural veins (74.8%) [2]. The pathological findings of venous thrombus vary with the time after onset. Pathological findings include platelet aggregation and fibrin formation with erythrocytes and neutrophils, lysis of cellular components, endothelial reactions and fibroblast proliferation, and replacement of thrombi with fibrous tissue and formation of recanalized vessels. Findings of deep vein thrombosis (DVT) have been obtained from pathological and forensic examinations, and are affected by degenerative changes at postmortem, therapeutic effects, and circulatory disturbance in the agonal stage.

* Correspondence: atsushi_yamashita@med.miyazaki-u.ac.jp
†Equal contributors
[2]Department of Pathology, Faculty of Medicine, University of Miyazaki, 5200 Kihara, Kiyotake, Miyazaki 889-1692, Japan
Full list of author information is available at the end of the article

Thrombolytic therapy can be more effective in selected patients with DVT compared with anticoagulant treatment alone [3, 4]. Addition of catheter-directed thrombolysis in conventional anticoagulant treatment for acute DVT reduces the risk of post-thrombotic syndrome by 14% at a 2-year follow-up and 28% at a 5-year follow up [5, 6]. Thrombolytic therapy results in a substantial increase in the risk of bleeding. Therefore, identification of a marker that reflects the age of thrombus is of particular concern. Alternatively activated macrophages are related to resolution of inflammation, tissue repair, and angiogenesis [7]. Therefore, we hypothesize that alternatively activated macrophages reflect the age of thrombus, as well as endothelial and fibroblastic proliferation.

Aspiration thrombectomy has been used to restore vascular patency alone and in conjunction with thrombolytic agents [8]. For treatment of acute DVT, aspiration thrombectomy with or without stenting is superior to anticoagulant therapy alone in terms of ensuring venous patency and improving clinical symptoms [9]. Technological advances have allowed evaluation the pathological changes in culprit thrombi in patients with DVT.

This pilot study aimed to determine the cellular and molecular components, and to identify a marker that reflects the time after onset in human aspirated DVT.

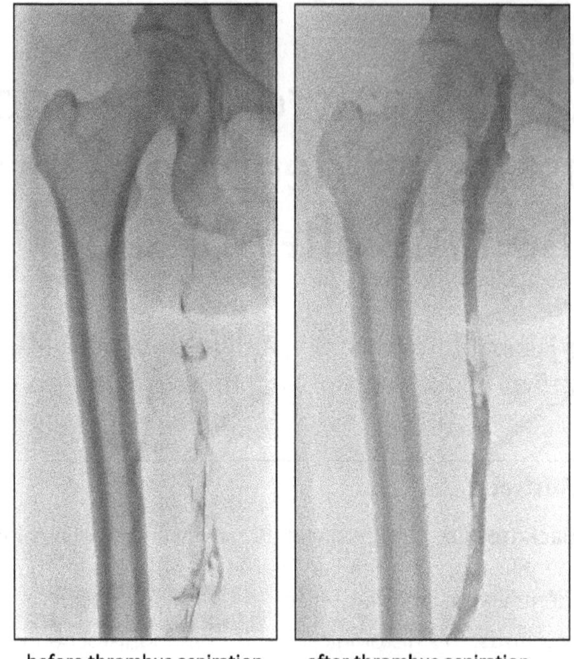

Fig. 1 Representative images of X-ray venography before and after thrombus aspiration. X-ray venography shows an extensive filling defect before thrombus aspiration along the femoral vein, and a considerable reduction in the defect after thrombus aspiration

Methods

Aspirated thrombi from patients with DVT

The ethics committee of the Miyazaki University approved the study protocol (approval no. 427). We obtained informed consent from the patients with DVT. Sixteen thrombi were obtained from 16 patients (8 men and 8 women; age range, 35–78 years) with DVT who were diagnosed based on clinical symptoms, laboratory data, and clinical imaging findings. The thrombi were mainly aspirated from the proximal portion of the thrombi with a guiding catheter (Guider Softip Guiding Catheter; Boston Scientific Japan, Tokyo, Japan). This catheter was placed from the popliteal vein to the iliac vein (10 cases), the leg vein to the inferior vena cava (5), and the subclavian vein to the superior vena cava (1). X-ray venography showed an extensive filling defect in the femoral vein before thrombus aspiration and reduction of the filling defect after thrombus aspiration (Fig. 1). An additional movie file shows this in more detail (see Additional file 1). We estimated the time of onset based on clinical symptoms and a medical interview. The times from onset to aspiration varied from 5 to 60 days, with a median of 13 days. The underlying diseases of the patients included the following: trauma and long-term immobilization ($n = 5$), idiopathic ($n = 3$), malignant tumor postoperatively ($n = 2$), chronic inflammatory disease ($n = 2$), Budd–Chiari syndrome ($n = 1$), chronic renal failure ($n = 1$), peripheral artery disease ($n = 1$), and gynecologic surgery ($n = 1$). Thirteen of 16 patients were intravenously administered heparin for 1 to 30 days, and six of 16 patients were intravenously administered thrombolytic agents for 1 to 12 days before thrombus aspiration.

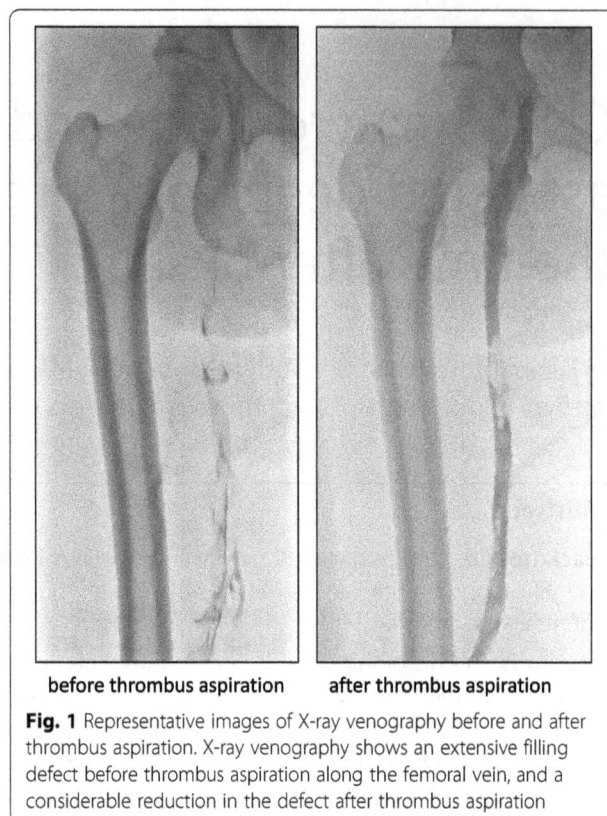

All aspirated thrombi were immediately fixed in 4% paraformaldehyde and embedded in paraffin for histological evaluation. Sections (4-μm thick) were stained with hematoxylin and eosin and morphologically assessed. Consecutive sections were immunohistochemically analyzed.

Immunohistochemistry

Consecutive 4-μm slices were immunohistochemically stained using antibodies against α-smooth muscle actin (SMA) (mouse monoclonal, clone 1A4; Dako, Glostrup, Denmark), CD34 (mouse monoclonal, QBEnd 10; Dako), CD68 (mouse monoclonal, clone PGM-1; Dako), CD163, a macrophage scavenger receptor (mouse monoclonal, clone 10D6; Leica Microsystems, Newcastle upon Tyne, UK), CD206, mannose receptor C type 1 (mouse monoclonal, clone 5C11; LifeSpan Biosciences, Inc., Seattle, WA, USA), fibrin (mouse monoclonal, clone T2G1; Accurate Chemical & Scientific Corp., Westbury, NY, USA), glycophorin A (mouse monoclonal, clone JC159; Dako), and platelet integrin α2bβ3 (sheep polyclonal; Affinity Biologicals Inc., Hamilton, CA, USA). The sections were stained with Envision (DAKO) or donkey anti-sheep IgG secondary antibody (Jackson ImmunoResearch, Baltimore, MA, USA). Horseradish peroxidase activity was visualized using 3, 3′-diaminobenzidine tetrahydrochloride. The immunostaining controls included non-immune mouse or sheep IgG instead of primary antibodies.

We performed double immunohistochemical staining for CD163 (rabbit polyclonal; DB Biotech, Kosice, Slovakia) and CD68 (Dako), CD163 (DB Biotech) and CD34 (Dako), CD163 (DB Biotech) and glycophorin A (Dako), and CD163 (DB Biotech) and SMA (Dako) using the MACH2 Double Stain kit (Biocare Medical, Concord, CA, USA).

Quantitative methods

The sizes of the thrombi were measured in sections under a microscope using the NIS-Element-D 3.2 image analysis software (Nikon, Tokyo, Japan). Areas that were immunopositive for CD34, fibrin, integrin α2bβ3, glycophorin A, and SMA were semiquantified using the Win Roof color image analysis software (Mitani, Fukui, Japan) (Fig. 2) [10]. These areas are expressed as the ratios of positively stained areas per thrombus area. The number of granulocytes without lytic change was counted in the five most cellular fields under a 20× objective lens, and is expressed as the number per mm^2. The immunopositive cell numbers for CD68, CD163, and CD206 in venous thrombi were counted in the five most heavily stained fields under a 20× objective lens. Cell density is expressed as the number of immunopositive cells per mm^2.

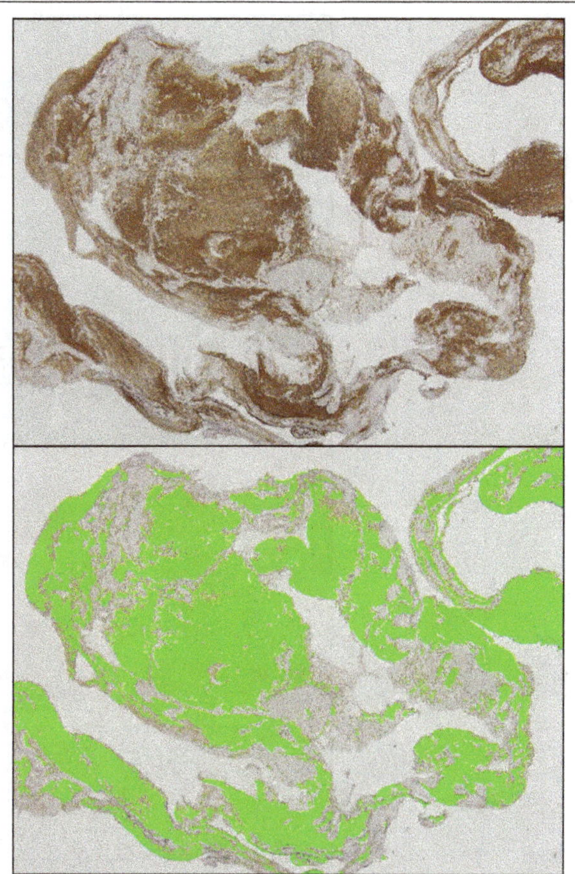

Fig. 2 Representative immunohistochemical image of glycophorin A and its color-extracted image in image analysis. Immunopositive areas were extracted using specific protocols based on the color parameters of hue, lightness, and saturation. The data are expressed as ratios (%) of the extracted light *green* areas in the areas of thrombus

Statistical analysis

All data are presented as medians and interquartile ranges. Differences between individual groups were tested using the Kruskal–Wallis test with Dunn's multiple comparison tests (GraphPad Prizm 6; GraphPad Software Inc., San Diego, CA, USA). The relationships between factors were evaluated using Spearman's rank correlation coefficients. Values of $P < 0.05$ were considered significant.

Results

Macro- and microscopic findings from aspirated venous thrombi

The aspirated thrombi were red or mixed red and white (Fig. 3a). The thrombi were composed of erythrocyte-rich areas, eosinophilic granular or fibrinous areas, and granulocytes or mononuclear leukocytes (Fig. 3b). Neutrophils were mainly accumulated at the border of erythrocyte-rich areas and eosinophilic granular or fibrinous areas (Fig. 3b). The thrombi showed various degrees of cell lytic change (Fig. 3c) and infiltration of macrophage-like cells in part (Fig. 3d). One half of the thrombi focally exhibited organizing reactions with infiltration of mononuclear leukocytes (Fig. 3e).

Immunohistochemical findings from aspirated thrombi

All venous thrombi were immunopositive for glycophorin A, platelet integrin α2bβ3, and fibrin (Fig. 4, Table 1). Among them, glycophorin A- ($p < 0.0001$) and fibrin-immunopositive areas ($p < 0.01$) were larger than those of the integrin α2bβ3-immunopositive area (Table 1). The thrombi had small foci of CD34- and SMA-immunopositive areas (Table 1). Flat CD34-positive cells covered the surface of thrombi and formed microvessels. CD34 and SMA-immunopositive areas were positively correlated ($r = 0.73$, $p < 0.01$). There were CD68- and CD163-immunopositive mononuclear cells and stellate cells in all thrombi. The numbers of CD68- ($p < 0.01$) and CD163-positive cells ($p < 0.0001$) were significantly greater than those of the CD206-positive cells (Table 1). Immunopositive areas and cell numbers

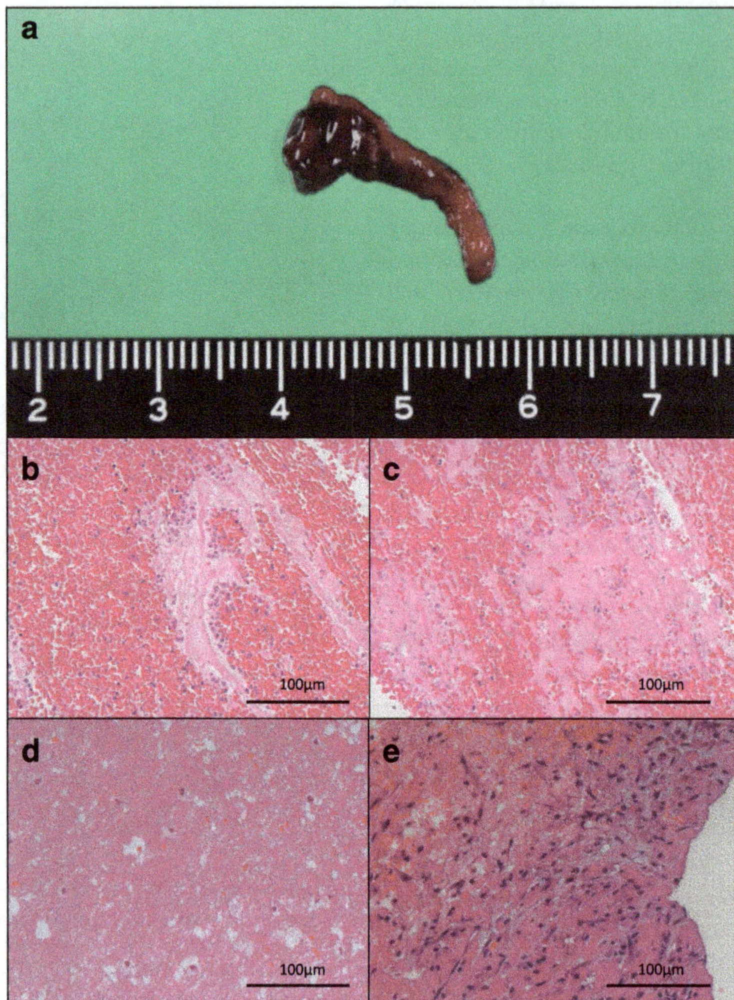

Fig. 3 Representative macro- and microscopic images of aspirated deep vein thrombi. **a**. Representative macroscopic image of an aspirated thrombus. The aspirated thrombus is *red* or *mixed red* and *white*. **b**. Representative image of a fresh thrombus composed of erythrocyte-rich areas, eosinophilic granular or fibrinous areas, and polymorphonuclear or mononuclear leukocytes. Neutrophils are mainly accumulated at the border of the erythrocyte-rich and eosinophilic areas (9 days after onset). **c**. Representative image of lytic changes, including the loss of cellular morphology, karyolysis, and karyorrhexis (9 days after onset). **d**. Representative image of macrophage-like cells (60 days after onset). **e**. Representative image of an organizing reaction showing fibroblastic/myofibroblastic proliferation, leukocytic infiltration, and matrix deposition (33 days after onset). Hematoxylin and eosin stain (**b**–**d**)

were not different in patients with ($n = 13$) or without heparin and/or thrombolytic therapy ($n = 3$).

Relationships between the time after onset and cellular and molecular parameters

Table 1 shows the relationships between the time after onset and cellular and molecular parameters. CD68- and CD163-immunopositive cell numbers were positively correlated with the time after onset, while the glycophorin A-immunopositive area was negatively correlated with the time after onset (Table 1, Fig. 5). There were no significant correlations of the time after onset with granulocyte number, CD34-immunopositive area, and SMA-immunopositive area.

Localization of CD163-positive cells in DVT

Double immunohistochemical staining showed colocalization of CD68- and CD163-positive cells, accumulation of CD163-positive cells in erythrocyte-rich areas, and phagocytosis of erythrocyte fragments. Oval or stellate CD163-positive cells were also accumulated in CD34- and SMA-immunopositive areas (Fig. 6).

Discussion

The present study showed that the majority of macrophages expressed CD163 in aspirated thrombi from patients with DVT and that CD163 macrophages were closely distributed in erythrocyte-, CD34-, and SMA-immunopositive cell-rich areas. Additionally, CD163

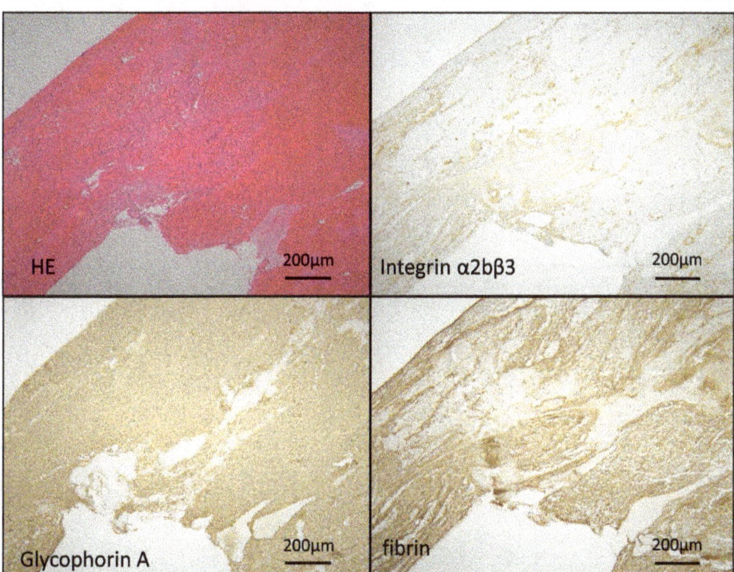

Fig. 4 Representative immunohistochemical images of an aspirated deep vein thrombus. The thrombus is stained with hematoxylin and eosin (HE) and antibodies for glycophorin A, integrin α2bβ3, and fibrin. The thrombus is rich in glycophorin A and fibrin

macrophage or erythrocyte contents were positively or negatively correlated with the time after onset.

The traditional view is that deep vein thrombi are composed of erythrocytes with a large amount of fibrin and relatively few platelets [11]. This view is based on hematoxylin and eosin staining. Takahashi et al. [12] immunohistochemically examined the attached portions of deep vein thrombi in autopsy cases of venous thromboembolism and found that fibrin and erythrocyte contents tended to exceed the platelet content. However, there were no significant differences among the contents in the thrombi. Fibrin, erythrocyte, and platelet contents were consistently present in aspirated thrombi, and the thrombi were rich in erythrocytes and fibrin. These findings support the traditional view. Our findings also suggested that thrombus content differed in the portion of DVT, because aspirated thrombi were mainly obtained from the proximal portion of the thrombi. Additionally, we identified a time-dependent change in erythrocyte content, but not fibrin and platelet contents, within 60 days after onset.

Table 1 Components of deep vein thrombi and their relationships with the time after onset

	Median (interquartile range)	Correlation coefficient	*p* value
fibrin (%)	31 (24–41)	−0.11	0.67
glycophorin A (%)	46 (34–49)	−0.76	<0.001
integrin α2bβ3 (%)	14 (8–18)	0.04	0.89
CD34 (%)	0.06 (0.02–0.29)	0.35	0.18
SMA (%)	0.01 (0.001–0.07)	0.23	0.38
Granulocytes (/mm^2)	204 (57–501)	−0.18	0.49
CD68 (/mm^2)	263 (122–460)	0.60	<0.05
CD163 (/mm^2)	308 (221–553)	0.64	<0.01
CD206 (/mm^2)	67 (30–92)	0.44	0.09

SMA smooth muscle actin
Data were analyzed using Spearman's rank correlation coefficient

Monocytes/macrophages are cellular components of venous thrombi. These cells appear around the edges of ligation-induced thrombi and become evenly distributed through the thrombi as resolution progresses in the rat [13]. Macrophage content time-dependently increases in experimental venous thrombi in the rat within 21 days [13] and peak at 7 days in mice [14] and 14 days in rabbits [15]. The positive relationship between macrophage content and the time after onset in aspirated thrombi is compatible with that of experimental studies. This relationship suggests that the thrombus resolution process is delayed in humans.

CD163 is a scavenger receptor for the hemoglobin–haptoglobin (HbHp) complex in macrophages. Several microenvironmental factors affect CD163 expression. Interleukin (IL)-6, IL-10, and glucocorticoids upregulate the expression of CD163 in monocytes/macrophages, while tumor necrosis factor-α, IL-1β, interferon-γ, lipopolysaccharide, IL-4, IL-13, oxidative stress, and hypoxia downregulate this expression [16]. High concentrations of HbHp complex also induce CD163 expression with an increase in secretion of IL-6 and IL-10 [17]. Hemoglobin that is released from lytic erythrocytes in venous thrombi is likely to enhance HbHp complex formation and upregulates CD163 expression in thrombus-associated macrophages. Previous studies have suggested

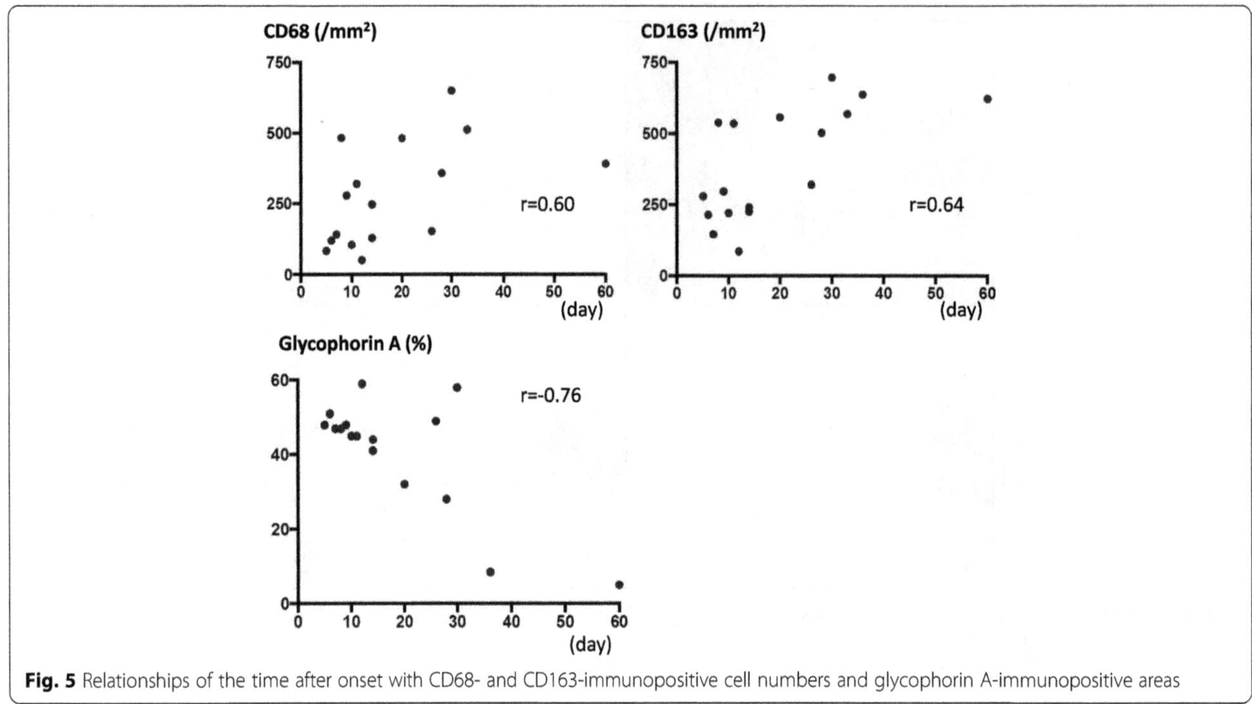

Fig. 5 Relationships of the time after onset with CD68- and CD163-immunopositive cell numbers and glycophorin A-immunopositive areas

a role for the binding of the HbHp complex to CD163 in anti-inflammatory responses of macrophages [18]. Macrophages in M2 or M2-like activation mode are related to resolution of inflammation, tissue repair, and remodeling via anti-inflammatory cytokine and angiogenic factor production, and extracellular matrix digestion and deposition [7]. Macrophages modulate the function and growth of human mesenchymal stem cells [19]. Therefore, interactions with endothelial cells, fibroblasts, and tissue stem cells could be important components of the role of macrophages in angiogenesis and tissue repair. CD163 macrophages are frequently localized to areas of interstitial fibrosis, collagen deposition, and accumulation of SMA-positive myofibroblastic cells in chronic kidney allograft injury [20]. The interactions between endothelial cells, myofibroblasts/SMCs, and CD163 macrophages are not fully understood. However, erythrophagocytosis and the nearby distribution of CD163 macrophages, endothelial cells, and myofibroblasts/ SMCs suggest that CD163 macrophages play a role in venous thrombus resolution/organization.

CD206 is known as a mannose receptor C type 1 that recognizes sugars on microorganisms and some endogenous glycoproteins. CD206 and CD163 are upregulated in human atherosclerotic lesions with intraplaque hemorrhages [21]. However, CD206 expression is not prominent in DVT. In contrast to CD163, CD206 is upregulated by IL-4 and IL-13 [7]. These results suggest that there are microenvironmental differences between thrombus organization and hemorrhagic, atherosclerotic plaques.

There are small foci of CD34- and SMA-immunopositive areas in nearly all thrombi. Experimental stasis-induced venous thrombi have shown that microvessels or myofibroblasts and/or SMCs appear at 5 and 7 days, respectively, and that these areas time-dependently increase [22]. Although we observed a positive relationship between CD34- and SMA-immunopositive areas, these positive areas did not significantly correlate with the time after onset. This discrepancy could be due to the dynamic process of human DVT and the small foci of CD34- and SMA-immunopositive areas (Table 1) of the aspirated thrombi in this study.

There are several biomarkers for diagnosis of DVT, active coagulation, and post-thrombotic syndrome. Because CD163 macrophage and erythrocyte contents were positively or negatively correlated with the time after onset in our study, soluble CD163 (sCD163) and some erythrocyte markers might predict acuity of DVT. CD163 is shed from the macrophage surface into the circulation as sCD163, and sCD163 levels increase during inflammation and macrophage activation [23]. Therefore, sCD163 could be a possible marker for evaluating thrombus organization in patients with DVT without inflammatory diseases. Suades et al. [24] reported higher erythrocyte (glycophorin A-positive)-derived microparticle levels in acute coronary syndrome compared with control subjects. Because the thrombus size in DVT is larger than coronary thrombus size, glycophorin A-positive microparticles could be a possible marker for the acute phase of DVT.

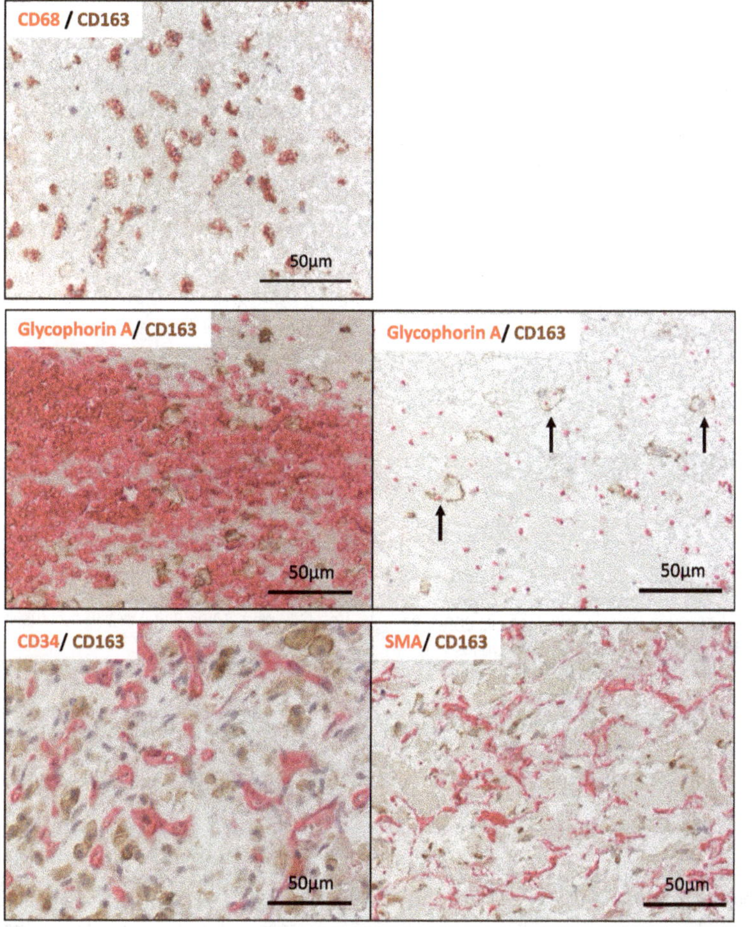

Fig. 6 Localization of CD163 in aspirated deep vein thrombi. Double immunohistochemical staining for CD68 and CD163 (upper panel), glycophorin A and CD163 (middle panels), and CD163 and CD34 or SMA (lower panels). Expression of CD163 is visualized as a *brown* stain. Expression of CD68, glycophorin A, CD34, and SMA are visualized as a *red* stain. Most of the CD163-immunopositive cells (*brown*) are immunopositive for CD68 (*red*) (upper panel). CD163-immunopositive cells in erythrocyte-rich areas and phagocytosis of erythrocyte fragments can be seen (arrows, middle panels). Oval or stellate CD163-immunopositive cells in CD34- and SMA-immunopositive organizing areas can be seen (lower panels)

This study has several limitations. We estimated the time of onset based on clinical symptoms and a medical interview. However, the onset of symptoms does not always indicate the onset of thrombus formation. This discrepancy might affect quantification of immunostaining results. Our findings from aspirated thrombi only represent a part of DVT. This could affect the value of the immunopositive area, especially with CD34 and SMA. In our study, histological samples did not provide information about the dynamic processes of thrombus formation and thrombolysis. Immunopositive areas and cell numbers were not different in patients with or without heparin and/or thrombolytic therapy, although we cannot deny β error due to the low power in each group. Although the sample number was small, the findings regarding aspirated thrombi from patients with DVT are important for better understanding the pathophysiology of DVT.

Conclusions

We histologically and immunohistochemically analyzed aspirated thrombi that were obtained from patients with DVT. Our study shows CD163- and glycophorin A-immunopositive areas are positively or negatively correlated with the time after onset. CD163 and erythrocyte contents and related products could be markers for evaluating the age of DVT. CD163 macrophages might play a role in the organization of DVT.

Abbreviations

DVT: Deep vein thrombosis; HbHp: Hemoglobin–haptoglobin; IL: Interleukin; SMA: Smooth muscle actin

Acknowledgements

We thank Ritsuko Sotomura and Kyoko Ohashi for excellent technical assistance.

Funding

This study was supported in part by Grants-in-Aid for Scientific Research in Japan (Nos. 25460440, 23390084, 16K08670, and 16H05163) from the Ministry of Education, Science, Sports and Culture of Japan, Clinical Research from Miyazaki University Hospital, Mitsui Life Welfare Foundation, SENSHIN Medical Research Foundation, Intramural Research Fund (25-4-3) for Cardiovascular Diseases of the National Cerebral and Cardiovascular Center, and the Bayer Scholarship for Cardiovascular Research.

Authors' contributions

EF, TG, AY, YS, TH, and YA designed and planned the study. EF, TG, SMG, MK, CS, and TS performed the experiments. EF, TG, AY, and YA contributed to writing of the manuscript. All authors read and approved the final manuscript.

Competing interests

The authors declare that they have no competing interests.

Author details

[1]Department of Radiology, Faculty of Medicine, University of Miyazaki, 5200 Kihara, Kiyotake, Miyazaki 889-1692, Japan. [2]Department of Pathology, Faculty of Medicine, University of Miyazaki, 5200 Kihara, Kiyotake, Miyazaki 889-1692, Japan. [3]Department of Diagnostic Pathology, Miyazaki University Hospital, University of Miyazaki, 5200 Kihara, Kiyotake, Miyazaki 889-1692, Japan. [4]Department of Biochemistry and Microbiology, Faculty of Pharmaceutical Sciences, Kyusyu University of Health and Welfare, 1714-1 Yoshinomachi, Nobeoka 882-0072, Japan.

References

1. Raskob GE, Angchaisuksiri P, Blanco AN, Büller H, Gallus A, Hunt BJ, et al. Thrombosis: a major contributor to global disease burden. Semin Thromb Hemost. 2014;40:724–35.
2. Fineschi V, Turillazzi E, Neri M, Pomara C, Riezzo I. Histological age determination of venous thrombosis: a neglected forensic task in fatal pulmonary thrombo-embolism. Forensic Sci Int. 2009;186:22–8.
3. Francis CW, Marder VJ. Fibrinolytic therapy for venous thrombosis. Prog Cardiovasc Dis. 1991;34:193–204.
4. Fiengo L, Bucci F, Khalil E, Salvati B. Original approach for thrombolytic therapy in patients with Ilio-femoral deep vein thrombosis: 2 years follow-up. Thromb J. 2015;13:40.
5. Enden T, Haig Y, Kløw NE, Slagsvold CE, Sandvik L, Ghanima W, et al. Long-term outcome after additional catheter-directed thrombolysis versus standard treatment for acute iliofemoral deep vein thrombosis (the CaVenT study): a randomised controlled trial. Lancet. 2012;379:31–8.
6. Haig Y, Enden T, Grøtta O, Kløw NE, Slagsvold CE, Ghanima W, Sandvik L, et al. Post-thrombotic syndrome after catheter-directed thrombolysis for deep vein thrombosis (CaVenT): 5-year follow-up results of an open-label, randomised controlled trial. Lancet Haematol. 2016;3:e64–71.
7. Mantovani A, Biswas SK, Galdiero MR, Sica A, Locati M. Macrophage plasticity and polarization in tissue repair and remodelling. J Pathol. 2013;229:176–85.
8. Kwon SH, Oh JH, Seo TS, Ahn HJ, Park HC. Percutaneous aspiration thrombectomy for the treatment of acute lower extremity deep vein thrombosis: is thrombolysis needed? Clin Radiol. 2009;64:484–90.
9. Cakir V, Gulcu A, Akay E, Capar AE, Gencpinar T, Kucuk B, et al. Use of percutaneous aspiration thrombectomy vs. anticoagulation therapy to treat acute iliofemoral venous thrombosis: 1-year follow-up results of a randomised, clinical trial. Cardiovasc Intervent Radiol. 2014;37:969–76.
10. Okuyama N, Matsuda S, Yamashita A, Moriguchi-Goto S, Sameshima N, Iwakiri T, et al. Human coronary thrombus formation is associated with degree of plaque disruption and expression of tissue factor and hexokinase II. Circ J. 2015;79:2430–8.
11. Stein PD, Evans H. An autopsy study of leg vein thrombosis. Circulation. 1967;35:671–81.
12. Takahashi M, Yamashita A, Moriguchi-Goto S, Marutsuka K, Sato Y, Yamamoto H, et al. Critical role of von Willebrand factor and platelet interaction in venous thromboembolism. Histol Histopathol. 2009;24:1391–8.
13. McGuinness CL, Humphries J, Waltham M, Burnand KG, Collins M, Smith A. Recruitment of labelled monocytes by experimental venous thrombi. Thromb Haemost. 2001;85:1018–24.
14. Nosaka M, Ishida Y, Kimura A, Kondo T. Time-dependent appearance of intrathrombus neutrophils and macrophages in a stasis-induced deep vein thrombosis model and its application to thrombus age determination. Int J Legal Med. 2009;123:235–40.
15. Kuroiwa Y, Yamashita A, Miyati T, Furukoji E, Takahashi M, Azuma T, et al. MR signal change in venous thrombus relates organizing process and thrombolytic response in rabbit. Magn Reson Imaging. 2011;29:975–84.
16. Kowal K, Silver R, Sławińska E, Bielecki M, Chyczewski L, Kowal-Bielecka O. CD163 and its role in inflammation. Folia Histochem Cytobiol. 2011;49:365–74.
17. Ugocsai P, Barlage S, Dada A, Schmitz G. Regulation of surface CD163 expression and cellular effects of receptor mediated hemoglobin-haptoglobin uptake on human monocytes and macrophages. Cytometry A. 2006;69:203–5.
18. Philippidis P, Mason JC, Evans BJ, Nadra I, Taylor KM, Haskard DO, et al. Hemoglobin scavenger receptor CD163 mediates interleukin-10 release and heme oxygenase-1 synthesis: antiinflammatory monocyte-macrophage responses in vitro, in resolving skin blisters in vivo, and after cardiopulmonary bypass surgery. Circ Res. 2004;94:119–26.
19. Freytes DO, Kang JW, Marcos-Campos I, Vunjak-Novakovic G. Macrophages modulate the viability and growth of human mesenchymal stem cells. J Cell Biochem. 2013;114:220–9.
20. Ikezumi Y, Suzuki T, Yamada T, Hasegawa H, Kaneko U, Hara M, et al. Alternatively activated macrophages in the pathogenesis of chronic kidney allograft injury. Pediatr Nephrol. 2015;30:1007–17.
21. Finn AV, Nakano M, Polavarapu R, Karmali V, Saeed O, Zhao X, et al. Hemoglobin directs macrophage differentiation and prevents foam cell formation in human atherosclerotic plaques. J Am Coll Cardiol. 2012;59:166–77.
22. Nosaka M, Ishida Y, Kimura A, Kondo T. Time-dependent organic changes of intravenous thrombi in stasis-induced deep vein thrombosis model and its application to thrombus age determination. Forensic Sci Int. 2010;195:143–7.
23. Møller HJ. Soluble CD163. Scand J Clin Lab Invest. 2012;72:1–13.
24. Suades R, Padró T, Vilahur G, Martin-Yuste V, Sabaté M, Sans-Roselló J, et al. Growing thrombi release increased levels of CD235a (+) microparticles and decreased levels of activated platelet-derived microparticles. Validation in ST-elevation myocardial infarction patients. J Thromb Haemost. 2015;13:1776–86.

9

Comparison of different laboratory tests in the evaluation of hemorrhagic risk of patients using rivaroxaban in the critical care setting: diagnostic accuracy study

Marjorie Paris Colombini[1*], Priscilla Bento Matos Cruz Derogis[1], Valdir Fernandes de Aranda[1], João Carlos de Campos Guerra[1], Nelson Hamerschlak[2] and Cristóvão Luis Pitangueiras Mangueira[1]

Abstract

Background: Rivaroxaban is a direct oral anticoagulant designed to dispense with the necessity of laboratory monitoring. However, monitoring rivaroxaban levels is necessary in certain clinical conditions, especially in the critical care setting.

Methods: This is a diagnostic accuracy study evaluating sensitivity and specificity of prothrombin time (PT), activated partial thromboplastin time (aPTT), and Dilute Russell viper venom time (dRVVT), to evaluate the hemorrhagic risk in patients taking rivaroxaban. The study used a convenience sample of 40 clinically stable patients using rivaroxaban to treat deep vein thrombosis or atrial fibrillation admitted in a private hospital in Brazil, compared to a group of 60 healthy controls. The samples from patients were collected two hours after the use of the medication (peak) and two hours before the next dose (trough).

Results: The correlation with the plasmatic concentration measured by anti-FXa assay was higher for PT and dRVVTS. The PT and aPTT tests presented higher specificity, while dRVVT was 100% sensible.

Conclusions: There was a strong correlation between the tests and the plasma concentration of the drug. Additionally, our results demonstrated the potential use of dRVVT as a screening test in the emergency room and the need of a second test to improve specificity.

Keywords: Anticoagulants, Direct oral anticoagulants, Rivaroxaban, Clinical laboratory techniques, Prothrombin time, Russell's viper venom time

Background

The traditional anticoagulant drugs that exist for the prevention and treatment of venous thromboembolism (VTE), prevention of cerebral vascular accident in patients with atrial fibrillation (AF), and secondary prevention in patients with acute coronary syndrome (ACS) require constant laboratory monitoring, which is sometimes burdensome and inconvenient for the patient. Rivaroxaban is a direct oral anticoagulant (DOAC) that dispenses with this type of control. It is an antithrombotic drug, that acts directly inhibiting activated factor X, impeding the generation of thrombin, and consequently preventing the formation of clots. It also has the advantage that it can be administered in a single daily dose [1].

Rivaroxaban has high bioavailability after oral administration, with a maximum peak of action at around 1.5 to 2 h after use (peak action), a mean half-life of between 5 and 9 h in young patients and 12 to 13 h in those aged over 75 years. It is eliminated in two ways: two thirds are metabolized by the liver (via CYP3A4 and CYP2J2)

* Correspondence: marjorie@einstein.br
[1]Department of Diagnostic and Preventive Medicine and Clinical Laboratory, Hospital Israelita Albert Einstein, São Paulo, Brazil
Full list of author information is available at the end of the article

without any circulating active metabolite identified, and one third is excreted unaltered in the urine [2, 3].

Although direct oral anticoagulants have been designed to dispense the necessity of laboratory monitoring, the literature has demonstrated that this monitoring is potentially useful in certain conditions [2, 4, 5].

So far, it is known that rivaroxaban can prolong the times in the conventional clotting tests used to evaluate the risk of hemorrhage, such as prothrombin time (PT), activated partial thromboplastin time (aPTT), and thrombin time (TT), but it has not yet been possible to establish a therapeutic window of clinical interest that can be linearly correlated with the plasma concentration of the drug for these tests. The only two specific tests available to date, and that present correlation with the plasma concentration of the drug, are anti-FXa assay (indirect method) [1, 4], and liquid chromatography/mass spectrometry (direct method).

More recently, some authors have considered PT [6, 7] and dilute Russell viper venom time (dRVVT) [8–11] as the most promising tests for this type of monitoring. dRVVT evaluates only the common laboratory coagulation pathway test (factors X, V, II and I) after activation of factor X by Russell viper venom, minimizing the possibility of interference of dysfunction of the other clotting factors. There are also two different types of reagents in terms of the concentration of phospholipid used: the screen test (lowest concentration of phospholipid, dRVVTS) and the confirm test (highest concentration, dRVVTC) to evidence the presence of lupus anticoagulant. Exner et al., suggested that dRVVT could possibly be used to detect and maybe determine the plasmatic concentration of many anticoagulants, including rivaroxaban [11]. Douxfils et al. state also that the "russell viper venom time test" allows a rapid estimation of the intensity of anticoagulation mediated by rivaroxaban, although the authors did not differentiate the drugs type [12].

Altman and Gonzalez published a study in which they proposed that Russell's viper venom is the most sensitive for identifying patients at risk of hemorrhage or exhibiting low anticoagulant effect, but they emphasize the need for other studies, to establish the sensitivity of other methods and identify cut-off values [8].

Objective

The primary objective of our work was to compare the sensitivity, specificity, positive predictive value (PPV) and negative predictive value (NPV) of PT, aPTT and dRVVT, in order to exclude qualitatively the plasma concentrations that are relevant in critical care. The secondary objective was to correlate PT, aPTT, dRVVT (screen and confirm) assays with plasmatic concentration of the drug measured by the anti-Xa methodology in the same patients.

Methods

Study design, setting and ethics

This is a diagnostic observational study, conducted at a private hospital in São Paulo, Brazil, with a convenience sample of stable patients using the drug rivaroxaban.

The Institutional Review Board approved the protocol in advance under CAAE number: 34661614.1.0000.0071. All the subjects signed an informed consent form to perform blood tests and to participate in the study.

Subjects

The subjects of this study are all patients consecutively admitted in the period of September 22, 2014 to December 21, 2015, in daily use of rivaroxaban at daily doses of 10, 15 or 20 mg daily (single dose), due to diagnosed thrombosis of the lower limbs, or those at risk of embolism due to atrial fibrillation. Patients with creatinine clearance lower than 15 mL/min or using rivaroxaban twice-daily regiment were excluded.

Plasma of 60 healthy controls without any known defects in the blood coagulation was used to estimate the normal range for the PT, aPTT and dRVVT screen and confirm assays.

Laboratorial analytical methods

The patients' blood samples were collected on two separate occasions: two hours after the use of the medication ("peak" moment) and two hours before the next dose ("trough" moment). The samples were collected according to the norms recognized by the Clinical Laboratory of the hospital, in test tubes containing 3.2% sodium citrate anticoagulant (Sarstedt, Newton, NC). Conventional PT tests were performed with the reagent STA Neoplastine CI Plus 10 and aPTT with STA Cephascreen 4 and processed on a Stago STA-R Evolution coagulation analyzer (Stago, Asnières-sur-Seine, France).

The Russell viper venom test was processed with the reagent STA Staclot DRVV (Screen and Confirm; Stago, Asnières-sur-Seine, France), at different phospholipid concentrations; one low, designated dRVVTS, and the other with a high concentration, designated dRVVTC.

The evaluation of anti-FXa assay was performed with the reagent STA-Liquid Anti-FXa with specific calibrator for rivaroxaban (Stago, Asnières-sur-Seine, France).

Definitions

In this study, the following definitions were used:

- ≤ 30 ng/mL as the plasma concentration cut-off defined as safe for invasive procedures [13, 14];

- ≤ 50 ng/mL as the plasma concentration indicating moderate risk cut-off defined by Lim et al. [15] and Levy et al. [16];
- ≤ 100 ng/mL as the concentration that may lead to thrombolysis in ischemic stroke [14, 17];
- sensitivity as the proportion of individuals with a higher plasma concentration than the threshold (30 ng/mL, 50 ng/mL or 100 ng/mL) and a test result above normality;
- specificity as the proportion of individuals with a plasma concentration lower than the threshold (30 ng/mL, 50 ng/mL or 100 ng/mL) and a test result within normality range;
- positive predictive value (PPV) as the proportion of individuals with a positive test result who actually present plasma concentrations higher than the threshold (30 ng/mL, 50 ng/mL or 100 ng/mL);
- negative predictive value (NPV) as the proportion of individuals with a negative test result who do really present plasma concentrations lower than the threshold (30 ng/mL, 50 ng/mL or 100 ng/mL);
- correlation grades: coefficients < 0.2 meaning very weak correlation; 0.2 to 0.39 as weak correlations; 0.40 to 0.59 as moderate; 0.60 to 0.79 strong correlation; > 0.80 very strong [18].

Statistical analysis

The plasmatic concentrations were described as means, standard deviation and 95% confidence intervals (CI). Spearman's correlations were calculated between the anti-FXa assay values (above the lower limit of quantitation, LOQ, 25 ng/mL) and the laboratory tests of interest. The results were illustrated using scatter plots. The analyses were performed with the software GraphPad Prism 5 (GraphPad Software, San Diego, CA), considering a level of significance of 0.05. The results from healthy subjects were analyzed using the EP Evaluator 11.1.0.26 (Data Innnovations, LLC) software program. EP Evaluator follows the recommendations of the CLSI C28-A (Clinical and Laboratory Standards Institute guideline) [19]. The normal ranges were expressed in the 90% CI. The diagnostic test evaluation was calculated using the free online MEDCALC easy-to-use statistical software. CI for sensitivity and specificity are "exact" Clopper-Pearson CI; and, for the predictive values, the standard logit CI given by Mercaldo et al. [20] were used.

Results

Study group

In the study period, 40 patients required the use of anticoagulation and were included and evaluated (Table 1).

Table 1 Patients' baseline data

Gender	n (%)
Female	20 (50)
Male	20 (50)
Rivaroxaban dosage	n (%)
10 mg/day	12 (30.0)
15 mg/day	19 (47.5)
20 mg/day	9 (22.5)
Age	
Average (standard deviation)	69 (21)
Minimum and maximum age	27–95

Plasmatic concentration

The plasmatic concentration calculated by anti-FXa assay were as expected in trough, mainly less than the LOQ (25 ng/mL), for all dosages. In peak time, the results were: 63.4 ± 61.0 ng/mL (mean ± standard deviation, SD, with 95% CI: 24.7–102.1) for 10 mg; 142.5 ± 93.2 ng/mL (CI: 97.6–187.4) for 15 mg, and 203.4 ± 85.6 ng/mL (CI: 137.6–269.2) for 20 mg.

Correlation between different methods with plasmatic concentration

All results of PT, dRVVT screen and confirm (Figs. 1, 2 and 3) presented a strong positive correlation with anti-FXa assay ($r \geq 0.60$). The correlation of aPTT (Fig. 4) was only moderate ($r = 0.53$).

Normal range

Table 2 shows the normal range calculated for TP, aPTT, dRVVs and dRVVc.

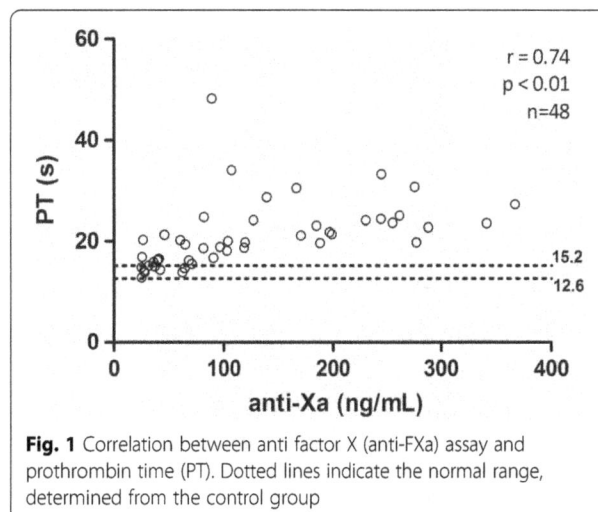

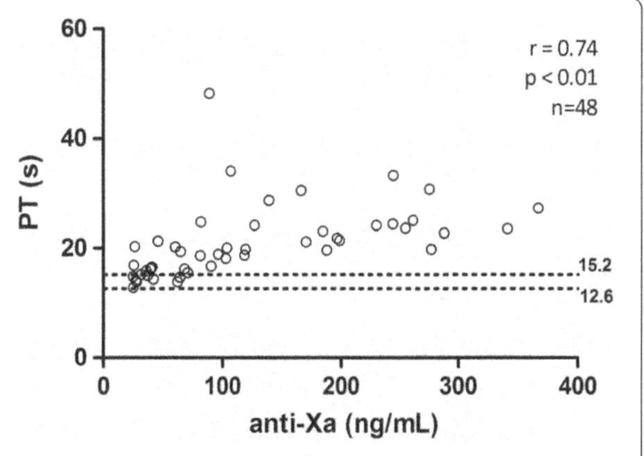

Fig. 1 Correlation between anti factor X (anti-FXa) assay and prothrombin time (PT). Dotted lines indicate the normal range, determined from the control group

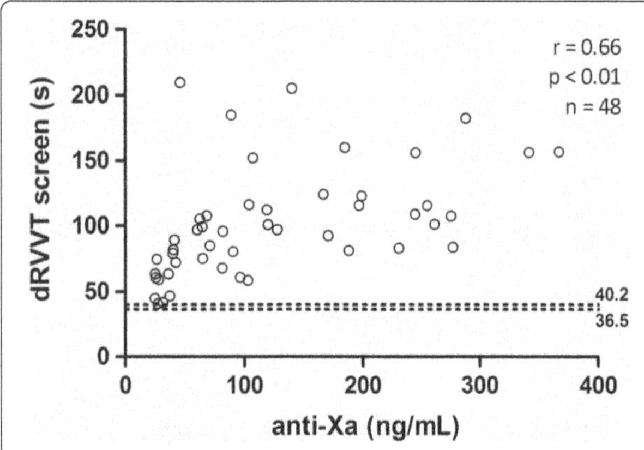

Fig. 2 Correlation between anti factor X (anti-FXa) and dilute Russell viper venom time (dRVVT) screen assays. Dotted lines indicate the normal range, determined from the control group

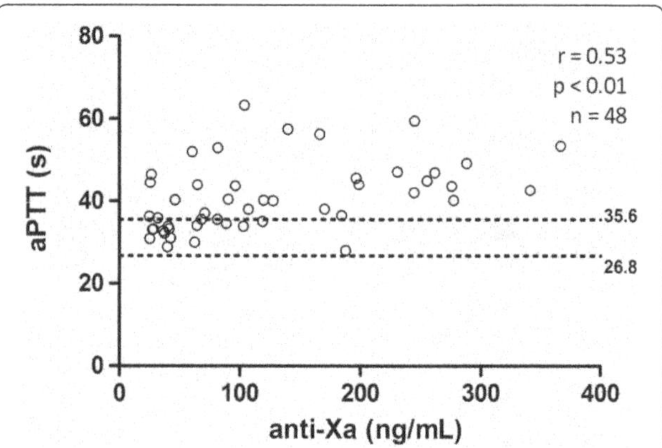

Fig. 4 Correlation between anti factor X (anti-FXa) assay and activated partial thromboplastin time (aPTT). Dotted lines indicate the normal range, determined from the control group

Sensitivity, specificity, PPV and NPV

Rivaroxaban concentration < 30 ng/mL was observed in 38/80 samples; < 50 ng/mL, in 46/80; and <100 ng/mL, in 57/80. Figs. 5, 6, 7, 8 and Tables 3, 4, 5 show the results dispersion and the performance of different tests according to different thresholds. It is possible to observe that, as the threshold increases, the TP and aPTT sensitivity also increases and specificity is reduced. dRVVs and dRVVc had the highest sensitivity regardless of the threshold adopted.

Discussion

Among the direct oral anticoagulants (DOACs), rivaroxaban has been widely used in medical practice, particularly because it dispenses with the necessity of laboratory control in the majority of patients [4, 5, 8]. However, in conditions where a laboratory evaluation is desirable, it has been demonstrated by many authors [1] that the test of choice, due to its high specificity, is the plasmatic concentration obtained by the chromogenic anti-FXa assay with specific calibrator for rivaroxaban.

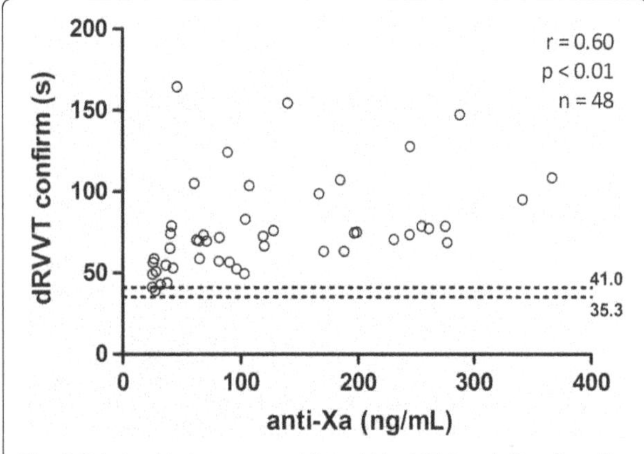

Fig. 3 Relationship between anti factor X (anti-FXa) and dilute Russell viper venom time (dRVVT) confirm assays. Dotted lines indicate the normal range, determined from the control group

According to Baglin et al. [21], three methodologies can be additionally used for rivaroxaban monitoring: activated partial thromboplastin time (aPTT), prothrombin time (PT) and plasmatic concentration determination. Recent data pointed dRVVT as an additional tool [8, 9].

Levy et al. [10] cited that is very important to know when the last dose of the direct oral anticoagulant was taken by the patient in order to determine whether the levels are likely to increase or fall over time. There are some situations, however, in that obtaining this information is impossible, and this happens frequently in the emergency setting [14]. Besides, some patients might metabolize anticoagulant drugs differently. Therefore, it is important to know the performance of the evaluation techniques that are available in the laboratory, so that a correct approach can be used in the emergency room. Because of that, this study sought to evaluate the correlation and performance of different tests regarding the plasmatic concentration of rivaroxaban.

The plasmatic concentrations measured by anti-FXa assay were comparable to Mueck et al. [22]. Our results also show that PT was most closely correlated to plasmatic concentration measured by anti-FXa assay, followed by dRVVTs, dRVVTc and aPTT. The PT and aPTT correlation to plasmatic concentration was strongly discussed by Francart et al. [23], depending on reagent type. Douxfils et al. studied the response of two PT reagents and correlated PT data to the plasma concentration measured by

Table 2 Normal range calculated using samples from 60 health volunteers

Tests	Lower limit (90% confidence interval)	Upper limit (90% confidence interval)
PT (seconds)	12.6 (12.37–12.85)	15.2 (14.96–15.44)
aPTT (seconds)	26.8 (26.1–27.5)	35.6 (34.7–36.6)
dRVVT screen (seconds)	36.5 (36.2–36.9)	40.2 (39.9–40.6)
dRVVT confirm (seconds)	35.3 (34.8–35.8)	41.0 (40.4–41.5)

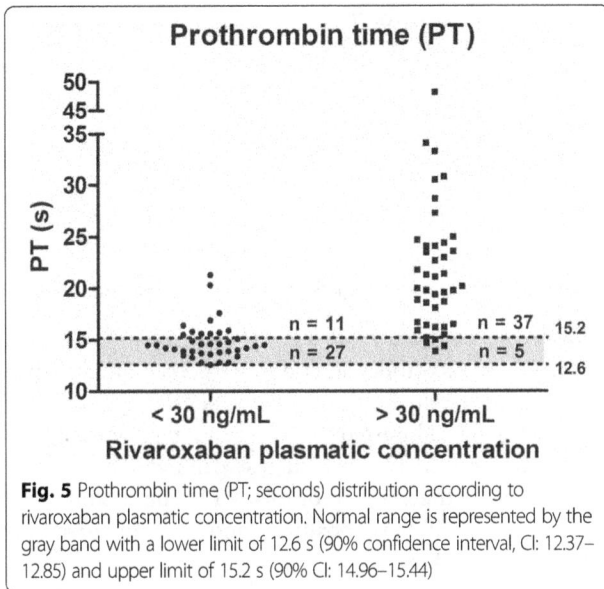

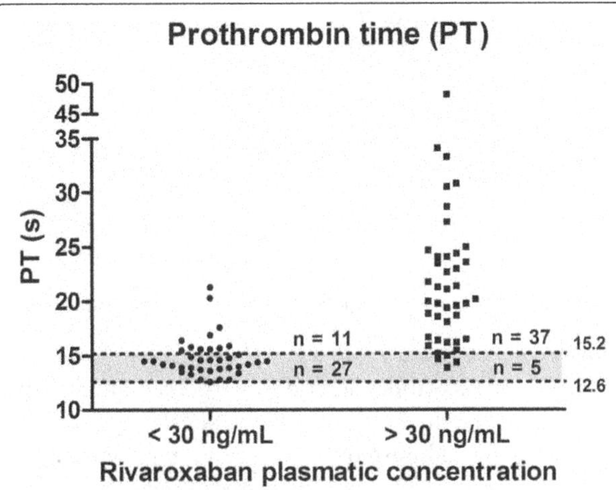

Fig. 5 Prothrombin time (PT; seconds) distribution according to rivaroxaban plasmatic concentration. Normal range is represented by the gray band with a lower limit of 12.6 s (90% confidence interval, CI: 12.37–12.85) and upper limit of 15.2 s (90% CI: 14.96–15.44)

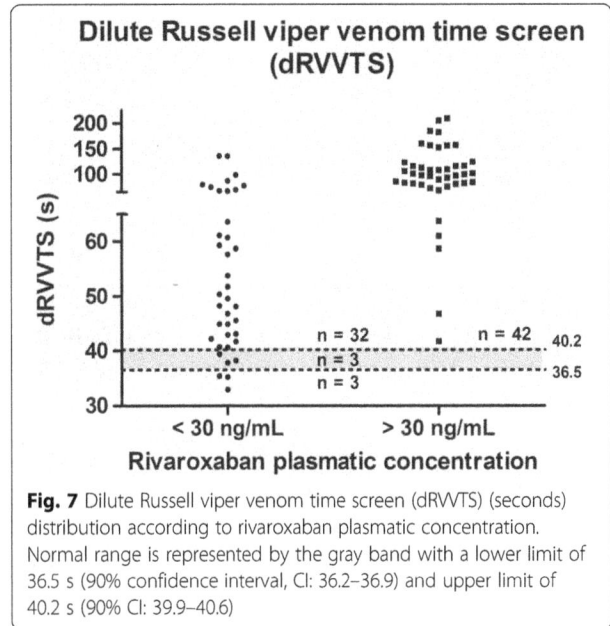

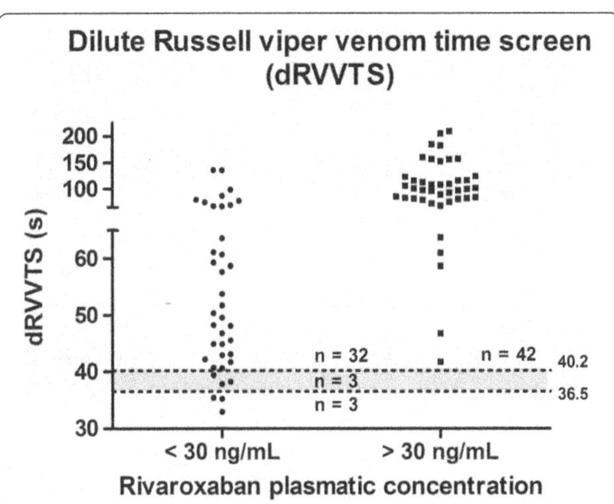

Fig. 7 Dilute Russell viper venom time screen (dRVVTS) (seconds) distribution according to rivaroxaban plasmatic concentration. Normal range is represented by the gray band with a lower limit of 36.5 s (90% confidence interval, CI: 36.2–36.9) and upper limit of 40.2 s (90% CI: 39.9–40.6)

HPLC-MS/MS. Correlation was found to be very strong (0.86) [9]. The differences between theirs and our results can be attributed to the characteristics of the patients evaluated, the reagents used and the methodology used in the plasmatic concentration measurement.

Gosselin et al. [10] correlated dRVVT to plasmatic concentration obtained by the direct method of liquid chromatography/mass spectrometry. They used the Siemens LA2 and Precision Biologics DRVVT reagents and presented a higher correlation coefficient (0.85 and 0.88, depending on the reagent). As for the PT and aPTT assays, the differences found can be attributed to the reagents, methods and even patients evaluated. In our study, if we isolate the results obtained with patients using 20 mg/day (n = 18), the correlation coefficient with anti-FXa assay would be 0.82.

Ebner et al. [14] recently described two thresholds of plasma concentration that are relevant in situations of emergency (30 and 100 ng/mL). Levy et al. [16] added the threshold of 50 ng/mL in cases of patients with severe bleeding. Lim et al., in 2016, described the same cut-off of 50 ng/mL for rivaroxaban, apixaban and dabigatran [15]. For this reason, the diagnostic test evaluation in our study was conducted using the three thresholds (< 30 ng/mL, < 50 ng/mL and <100 ng/mL).

Sensitivity and specificity of PT and aPTT were threshold-dependent. PT is indeed frequently described as

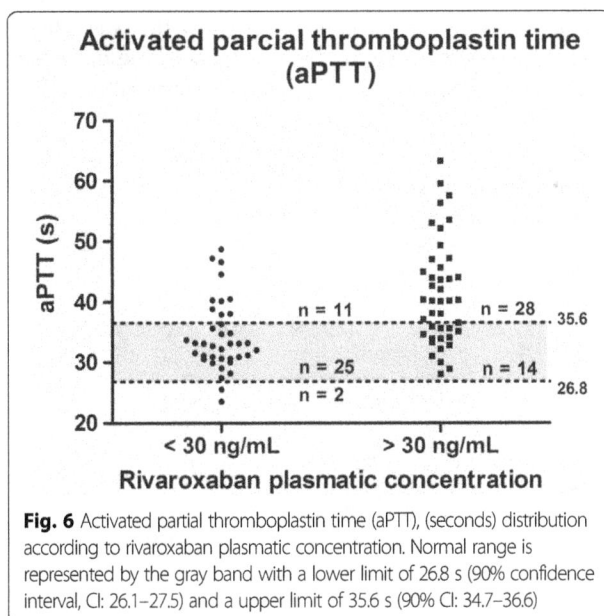

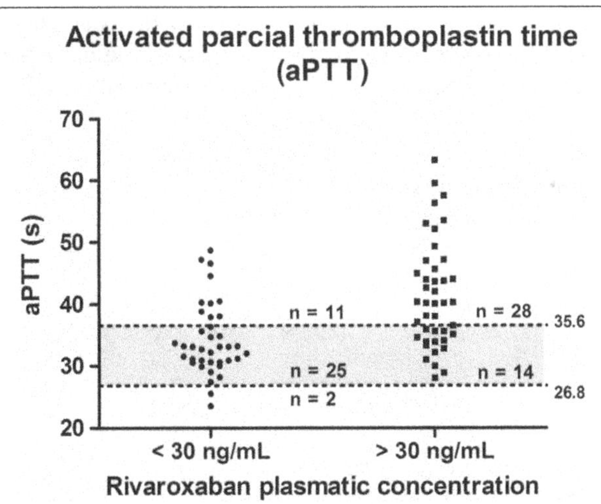

Fig. 6 Activated partial thromboplastin time (aPTT), (seconds) distribution according to rivaroxaban plasmatic concentration. Normal range is represented by the gray band with a lower limit of 26.8 s (90% confidence interval, CI: 26.1–27.5) and a upper limit of 35.6 s (90% CI: 34.7–36.6)

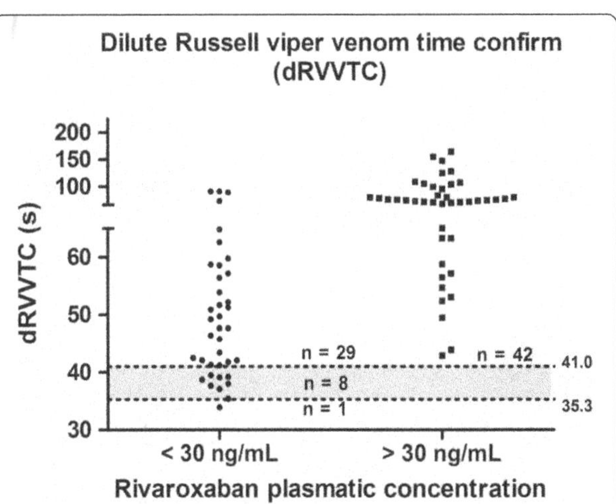

Fig. 8 Dilute Russell viper venom time confirm (dRVVTC) (seconds) distribution according to rivaroxaban plasmatic concentration. Normal range is represented by the gray band with a lower limit of 35.3 s (90% confidence interval, CI: 34.8–35.8) and upper limit of 41.0 s (90% CI: 40.4–41.5)

Table 3 Performance of four different tests for rivaroxaban monitoring (threshold: 30 ng/mL)

Test	Sensitivity (%, 95% CI)	Specificity (%, 95% CI)	PPV (%, 95% CI)	NPV (%, 95% CI)
PT	88 (74–96)	71 (54–85)	77 (67–85)	84 (70–93)
aPTT	67 (50–80)	71 (54–85)	72 (60–81)	66 (55–76)
dRVVs	100 (92–100)	16 (6–31)	57 (53–60)	100
dRVVc	100 (92–100)	24 (11–40)	59 (41–64)	100

PPV positive predictive value, *NPV* negative predictive value, *CI* confidence interval

an adequate test for rivaroxaban monitoring [4, 5, 24, 25]. Lim et al., in 2016, using the same reagent for PT assay, demonstrated a sensitivity and NPV above 90% for the cut-off of 50 ng/mL [15]. These results corroborate our findings. However, the observed differences in specificity and PPV can be attributed to the group studied. In addition to this influence, we believe that the differences in diagnostic accuracy related to aPTT may depend on the reagent used.

dRVVT screen and confirm tests presented maximum sensitivity and NPV, i.e., 100%, regardless of the threshold used. This would undoubtedly the safest test for exclusion of plasmatic concentration associated to hemorrhagic risk when the results are normal. The number of false positive results in relation to the total of exams for dRVVT screen and confirm varied from 32/80 to 51/80. These results are similar to the literature [7, 26].

Gosselin et al. [27], Exner et al. [11] described dRVVT as highly sensible for the presence of rivaroxaban. In fact, the authors described the application of dRVVT for many DOACs. Douxfils et al. [12] discussed also that dRVVT could be useful to assess pharmacodynamics of DOACs, with the advantage that it is a single test applied to different DOACs.

Gosselin et al. [27] describe that anticoagulants cause false results not only in coagulometric tests, as in the investigation of lupus anticoagulant, for example, but also in chromogenic tests. The interference of rivaroxaban on dRVVT was also described by other authors [26, 28, 29]. It is important to highlight that the sensitivity and specificity of a quantitative test are dependent on the cut-off value above or below which the test is positive [30].

Table 4 Performance of four different tests for rivaroxaban monitoring (threshold: 50 ng/mL)

Test	Sensitivity (%, 95% CI)	Specificity (%, 95% CI)	PPV (%, 95% CI)	NPV (%, 95% CI)
PT	94 (80–99)	65 (50–79)	67 (57–75)	94 (79–98)
aPTT	76 (59–89)	72 (57–84)	67 (55–77)	80 (69–89)
dRVVs	100 (90–100)	13 (5–26)	46 (43–49)	100
dRVVc	100 (90–100)	20 (9–34)	48 (44–51)	100

PPV positive predictive value, *NPV* negative predictive value, *CI* confidence interval

Table 5 Performance of four different tests for rivaroxaban monitoring (threshold: 100 ng/mL)

Test	Sensitivity (%, 95% CI)	Specificity (%, 95% CI)	PPV (%, 95% CI)	NPV (%, 95% CI)
PT	100 (85–100)	56 (42–69)	48 (41–55)	100
aPTT	100 (85–100)	67 (53–79)	55 (46–64)	100
dRVVs	100 (85–100)	11 (4–22)	31 (29–33)	100
dRVVc	100 (85–100)	16 (8–29)	32 (30–35)	100

PPV positive predictive value, *NPV* negative predictive value, *CI* confidence interval

Based on our results, we suggest that the patients with hemorrhagic risk (those with dRVVT screen and confirm tests above normality, that have sensitivity and low specificity) be submitted to a second test with higher diagnostic specificity (anti-Xa test calibrated with rivaroxaban or, in the absence of this, PT). This would allow the reduction of false positives and inadequate therapeutic interventions.

The potential limitations of this study must be considered, specially the reduced and highly homogeneous and clinically stable sample of patients, which might not be the case of other emergency settings. This must be considered in light of the fact that PPV and NPV are highly dependent on the disease prevalence.

Conclusions

In conclusion, our findings showed that there is a correlation between the tests studied and the plasma concentration of rivaroxaban, confirming the existing description in the literature. In addition, as shown by the sensitivity and specificity results, our study suggests the applicability of the tests evaluated in the screening of plasmatic concentration associated to hemorrhagic condition in patients using rivaroxaban. However, it is crucial that the laboratory informs the attending physician about the diagnostic limitations of this group of tests in the evaluation of patients using anticoagulants, using an appropriate and clear note in the lab results report. Additionally, our results show a cut-off dependent behavior of the tests that must be better investigated in future studies.

Abbreviations

ACS: Acute coronary syndrome; AF: Atrial fibrillation; anti-FXa: Anti factor X; aPTT: Activated partial thromboplastin time; C: Confirmatory; dRVVT: Dilute Russell viper venom time; PT: Prothrombin time; S: Screen; TT: Thrombin time; VTE: Venous thromboembolism

Acknowledgements

The authors thank Patricia Logullo for editorial assistance during manuscript preparation.

Funding

This study received no funding.

Authors' contributions
MPC, VFA, JCCG, NH and CLPM designed and coordinated the study. MPC, PBMCD analyzed and interpreted data and drafted the manuscript. MPC, VFA and JCCG carried out the assays, interpreted data and drafted the manuscript. PBMCD performed the statistical analysis. All authors read and approved the final manuscript.

Competing interests
The authors declare that they have no competing interests.

Author details
[1]Department of Diagnostic and Preventive Medicine and Clinical Laboratory, Hospital Israelita Albert Einstein, São Paulo, Brazil. [2]Department of Hematology, Hospital Israelita Albert Einstein, São Paulo, Brazil.

References

1. Tripodi A. The laboratory and the direct oral anticoagulants. Blood. 2013; 121(2):4032–5.
2. Leung LLK. Direct oral anticoagulants: Dosing and adverse effects. UpToDate. 2016. Available from: http://www.uptodate.com/contents/direct-oral-anticoagulants-dosing-and-adverse-effects?source=search_result&search=Direct+oral+anticoagulants&selectedTitle=1%7E131. Accessed in 2017 (May 15).
3. Kubitza D, Becka M, Mueck W, Zuehlsdorf M. The effect of extreme age, and gender, on the pharmacology and tolerability of rivaroxaban – an oral, direct factor FXa inhibitor. Blood. 2006;108:905. Available from: http://www.bloodjournal.org/content/108/11/905?sso-checked=true. Accessed in 2017 (May 15).
4. Tripodi A. The laboratory and the new oral anticoagulants. Clin Chem. 2013;59(2):353–62.
5. Baglin T, Hillarp A, Tripodi A, Elalamy I, Buller H, Ageno W. Measuring oral direct inhibitors (ODIs) of thrombin and factor Xa: a recommendation from the subcommittee on control of anticoagulation of the scientific and standardisation Committee of the International Society on thrombosis and haemostasis. J Thromb Haemost. 2013;11:756–760.
6. Tripodi A. Results expression for tests used to measure the anticoagulant effect of new oral anticoagulants. Thromb J. 2013;11(1):9.
7. Gosselin RC, Adcock DM. The laboratory's 2015 perspective on direct oral anticoagulant testing. J Thromb Haemost. 2016;14(5):886–93.
8. Altman R, Gonzalez CD. Simple and rapid assay for effect of the new oral anticoagulant (NOAC) rivaroxaban: preliminary results support further tests with all NOACs. Thromb J. 2014;12(1):7.
9. Douxfils J, Mani H, Minet V, Devalet B, Chatelain B, Dogné JM, et al. Non-VKA oral anticoagulants: accurate measurement of plasma drug concentration. Biomed Res Int. 2015;2015:345138.
10. Gosselin RC, Adcock Funk DM, Taylor JM, Francart SJ, Hawes EM, Friedman KD, et al. Comparison of anti-Xa and dilute Russell viper venom time assays in quantifying drug levels in patients on therapeutic doses of rivaroxaban. Arch Pathol Lab Med. 2014;138(12):1680–40.
11. Exner T, Ellwood L, Rubie J, Barancewicz A. Testing for new oral anticoagulants with LA-resistant Russells viper venom reagents. An in vitro study. Thromb Haemost. 2013;109(4):762–5.
12. Douxfils J, Chatelain B, Hjemdahl P, Devalet B, Sennesael AL, Wallemacq P, et al. Does the Russell viper venom time test provide a rapid estimation of the intensity of oral anticoagulation? A cohort study. Thromb Res. 2015;135(5):852–60.
13. Pernod G, Albaladejo P, Godier A, Samama CM, Susen S, Gruel Y, et al. Management of major bleeding complications and emergency surgery in patients on long-term treatment with direct oral anticoagulants, thrombin or factor-Xa inhibitors: proposals of the working group on perioperative haemostasis (GIHP) – march 2013. Arch Cardiovas Dis. 2013;106(6–7):382–93.
14. Ebner M, Birschmann I, Peter A, Spencer C, Härtig F, Kuhn J, et al. Point-of-care testing for emergency assessment of coagulation in patients treated with direct oral anticoagulants. Crit Care. 2017;21(1):32.
15. Li MS, Chapman K, Swanepoel P, Enjeti AK. Sensivity of routine coagulation assays to direct oral anticoagulants: patient samples versus commercial drug-specific calibrators. Pathology. 2016;48(7):712–9.
16. Levy JH, Ageno W, Chan NC, Crowther M, Verhamme P, Weitz JI. Subcommittee on control of anticoagulation. When and how to use antidotes for the reversal of direct oral anticoagulants: guidance from the SSC of the ISTH. J Thromb Haemost. 2016;14(3):623–7.
17. Steiner T, Böhm M, Dichgans M, Diener HC, Ell C, Endres M, et al. Recommendations for the emergency management of complications associated with the new direct oral anticoagulants (DOACs), apixaban, dabigatran and rivaroxaban. Clin Res Cardiol. 2013;102(6):399–412.
18. Evans JD. Straighforward statistics for the behavorial sciences. Califórnia: Brooks/Cole Publishing Company; 1996.
19. CLSI. Defining, establishing and verifying reference intervals in the clinical laboratory; approved guideline, third edition. CLSI document C28-A3. Wayne, PA: Clinical and Laboratory Standards Institute; 2008.
20. Mercaldo ND, Lau KF, Zhou XH. Confidence intervals for predictive values with an emphasis to case-control studies. Stat Med. 2007;26(10):2170–83.
21. Baglin T, Keeling D, Kitchen S. British Committee for Standards in haematology. Effects on routine coagulation screens and assessment of anticoagulant intensity in patients taking oral dabigatran or rivaroxaban: guidance from the British Committee for Standards in haematology. Br J Haematol. 2012;159(4):427–9.
22. Mueck W, Schwers S, Stampfuss J. Rivaroxaban and other novel oral anticoagulants: pharmacokinetics in healthy subjects, specific patient populations and relevance of coagulation monitoring. Thromb J. 2013;11(1):10.
23. Francart SJ, Hawes EM, Deal AM, Adcock DM, Gosselin R, Jeanneret C, et al. Performance of coagulation tests in patients on therapeutic doses of rivaroxaban a cross-sectional pharmacodynamic study based on peak and trough plasma levels. Thromb Haemost. 2014;111(6):1133–40.
24. Lippi G, Favaloro EJ. Recent guidelines and recommendations for laboratory assessment of the direct oral anticoagulants (DOACs): is there consensus? Clin Chem Lab Med. 2015;53(2):185–97.
25. Samuelson BT, Cuker A, Siegal DM, Crowther M, Garcia DA. Laboratory assessment of the anticoagulant activity of direct oral anticoagulants: a systematic Review. Chest. 2017;151(1):127–38.
26. Martinuzzo ME, Barrera LH, D'adamo MA, Otaso JC, Gimenez MI, Oyhamburu J. Frequent false-positive results of lupus anticoagulant tests in plasmas of patients receiving the new oral anticoagulants and enoxaparin. Int J Lab Hematol. 2014;36(2):144–50.
27. Gosselin R, Grant RP, Adcock DM. Comparison of the effect of the anti-Xa direct oral anticoagulants apixaban, edoxaban, and rivaroxaban on coagulation assays. Int J Lab Hematol. 2016;38(5):505–13.
28. Wong WH, Yip CY, Sum CL, Tan CW, Lee LH, Yap ES, et al. A practical guide to ordering and interpreting coagulation tests for patients on direct oral anticoagulants in Singapure. Ann Acad Med Singap. 2016;45(3):98–105.
29. van Os GM, de Laat B, Kamphuisen PW, Meijers JC, de Groot PG. Detection of lupus anticoagulant in the presence of rivaroxaban using Taipan snake venom time. J Thromb Haemost. 2011;9(8):1657–9.
30. Lalkhen AG, McCluskey A. Clinical tests: sensitivity and specificity. Contin Educ Anaesth Crit Care Pain. 2008;8(6):221-223. Available from: https://www.google.com.br/url?sa=t&rct=j&q=&esrc=s&source=web&cd=1&ved=0ahUKEwjVyYKvpfLTAhXEg5AKHQTiCRYQFggpMAA&url=http%3A%2F%2Fserene.me.uk%2Fhelpers%2Fsensitivity-specificity.pdf&usg=AFQjCNFKq268clQ1-Hi7t0SRB7ergjDvuw. Accessed in 2017 (May 15).

10

Non enzymatic upregulation of tissue factor expression by gamma-glutamyl transferase in human peripheral blood mononuclear cells

Valentina Scalise[1], Cristina Balia[1], Silvana Cianchetti[1], Tommaso Neri[1], Vittoria Carnicelli[1], Riccardo Zucchi[1], Maria Franzini[2], Alessandro Corti[2], Aldo Paolicchi[2], Alessandro Celi[1] and Roberto Pedrinelli[1*]

Abstract

Background: Besides maintaining intracellular glutathione stores, gamma-glutamyltransferase(GGT) generates reactive oxygen species and activates NFkB, a redox-sensitive transcription factor key in the induction of Tissue Factor (TF) gene expression, the principal initiator of the clotting cascade. Thus, GGT might be involved in TF-mediated coagulation processes, an assumption untested insofar.

Methods: Experiments were run with either equine, enzymatically active GGT or human recombinant (hr) GGT, a wheat germ-derived protein enzymatically inert because of missing post-translational glycosylation. TF Procoagulant Activity (PCA, one-stage clotting assay), TF antigen(ELISA) and TFmRNA(real-time PCR) were assessed in unpooled human peripheral blood mononuclear cell(PBMC) suspensions obtained from healthy donors through discontinuous Ficoll/Hystopaque density gradient.

Results: Equine GGT increased PCA, an effect insensitive to GGT inhibition by acivicin suggesting mechanisms independent of its enzymatic activity, a possibility confirmed by the maintained stimulation in response to hrGGT, an enzymatically inactive molecule. Endotoxin(LPS) contamination of GGT preparations was excluded by heat inactivation studies and direct determination(LAL method) of LPS concentrations <0.1 ng/mL practically devoid of procoagulant effect. Inhibition by anti-GGT antibodies corroborated that conclusion. Upregulation by hrGGT of TF antigen and mRNA and its downregulation by BAY-11-7082, a NFkB inhibitor, and N-acetyl-L-cysteine, an antioxidant, was consistent with a NFkB-driven, redox-sensitive transcriptional site of action.

Conclusions: GGT upregulates TF expression independent of its enzymatic activity, a cytokine-like behaviour mediated by NFκB activation, a mechanism contributing to promote acute thrombotic events, a possibility in need, however, of further evaluation.

Keywords: Gamma-glutamyltransferase, Tissue Factor, Cytokines, Oxidative Stress, NFkB

* Correspondence: roberto.pedrinelli@med.unipi.it
[1]Dipartimento di Patologia Chirurgica, Medica, Molecolare e dell'Area Critica, Università di Pisa, Pisa, Italy
Full list of author information is available at the end of the article

Background

Gamma-glutamyltransferase [GGT; (5-l-glutamyl)-peptide/amino acid 5-glutamyl transferase; EC 2.3.2.2], a member of the structural superfamily of the N-terminal nucleophilic hydrolases expressed by a wide number of cell types [1] including circulating monocytes [2, 3], hydrolyzes extracellular glutathione (GSH) to provide cysteine for its intracellular re-synthesis. Along with its pivotal role in that antioxidant biological process [1], however, GGT also generates reactive oxygen species (ROS) [4] and activates NFkB [5, 6], a redox-sensitive transcription factor [7] key in Tissue Factor (TF) gene expression [8], a major regulator of haemostasis and thrombosis [8, 9]. Therefore, deductive reasoning makes it plausible to hypothesize a cross-talk between GGT and TF, a possibility consistent with the highly consistent epidemiological association of circulating GGT levels with acute coronary events (see [10] for a review), a pathological process favoured by TF (see [11] for a review). The assumption, corroborated by recent reports of enzymatically active protein in human atheromatous plaques [12], requires, however, to document a mechanistic link between GGT and TF for which at the moment no evidence is available.

Aims

On the basis of that background, our aim was to evaluate the relationship between GGT and TF expression in human peripheral blood mononuclear cell (PBMC)s, a cell preparation capable of rapid TF induction in response to various proinflammatory stimuli [8].

Methods

Chemicals and standards

Unless stated otherwise, all reagents were from Sigma, Milano, Italy.

Cell isolation and culture

Human PBMC suspensions were obtained from unpooled buffy coats left over from blood bank draws taken from healthy donors with the approval of the local ethics committee of the Azienda Ospedaliero Universitaria Pisana, kept at room temperature and utilized within a maximum of 4 h from withdrawal. As detailed elsewhere [13], leukocytes were isolated from fresh buffy coats diluted 1:1 with sodium citrate 0.38 % in saline solution, mixed gently with 0.5 volume of 2 % Dextran T500 and left for 40 min for erythrocyte sedimentation. The leukocyte-rich supernatant was recovered and centrifuged for 10 min at 200xg. The pellet was resuspended in 30 mL of sodium citrate solution, layered over 15 mL of Ficoll-Hypaque and centrifuged for 30 min at 400xg at 20 °C. The PBMC-rich ring (3×10^6 cells/mL) was recovered, washed twice in sodium citrate 0.38 % and resuspended in polypropylene tubes in no glucose RPMI 1640 medium supplemented with 100 U/mL penicillin-streptomycin.

All reagents and solutions used for cell isolation and cultures were prepared with endotoxin-free water and glassware was rendered endotoxin-free by exposure to high temperature. Drugs were kept in stock solution and diluted in serum-free RPMI at the appropriate concentrations immediately before use. Cell viability, as assessed by dimethyl thiazolyl diphenyl tetrazolium (MTT), was verified (>85 % of viable cells) throughout all experimental phases.

The final PBMC preparations typically contain 25–35 % monocytes, negligible proportions of neutrophils (<5 %) and 65–75 % lymphocytes, a cell line with some but limited procoagulant potential [14]. Moreover, interferences from contaminating platelets [15] were excluded by absent procoagulant activity in clotting assays carried out in PBMC-free preparations as verified in pilot experiments, so that stimulated TF expression should be considered by and large a result of activated monocytes.

GGT

GGT experiments were carried out by using either equine, enzymatically active GGT purified according to already described procedures [16], or human recombinant(hr)GGT (Abnova, Taipei, Taiwan), a protein synthesized by wheat germ eukaryotic translational apparatuses in which lack of post-translational glycosylation forbids the generation of enzymatically active molecules [17, 18]. Confirming that assumption, GSH as measured by standard methods [19] was not cleaved by hrGGT in contrast with the hydrolysis induced by equine GGT, an effect this latter abolished by acivicin (10^{-4} M), a glutamate analogue with potent, non competitive GGT inhibiting properties [20], inactive on hrGGT (Fig. 1).

To exclude interferences from endotoxin (LPS) contamination [21], experiments were carried out with GGT preparations boiled for 30 min before their addition to PBMCs, a procedure expected to abrogate the biological effect of GGT but not the procoagulant power of heat-resistant LPS [21]. In the light of heat sensitivity of some LPS strains [22], endotoxin concentration was also measured in hrGGT-primed cultures by LAL (Limulus Amebocyte Lysate) chromogenic endpoint assay (Hycult Biotech, Uden, The Netherlands) [23] and the procoagulant effect of contaminant LPS levels was then tested in quiescent PBMCs. Finally, we assessed the effect of hrGGT-inhibition by an anti-GGT polyclonal antibody (Abnova, Taipei, Taiwan), 2.5 μg/mL, a concentration chosen according to preliminary concentration-response experiments (not shown), as compared with the appropriate isotype IgG control.

The role of NFkB was indirectly assessed by using BAY-11-7082 (10^{-5}M), a validated NFkB inhibitor [24],

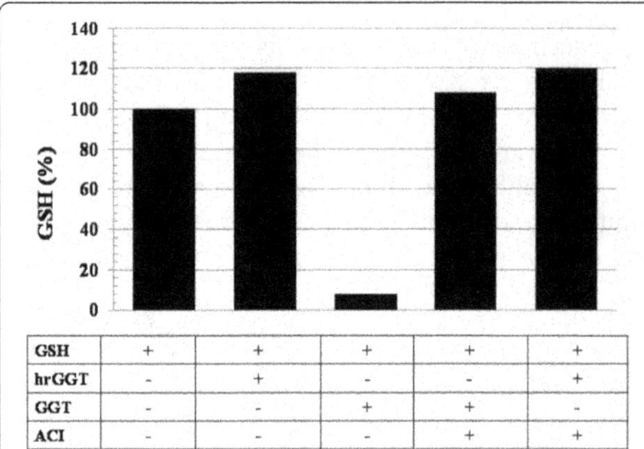

GSH	+	+	+	+	+
hrGGT	-	+	-	-	+
GGT	-	-	+	+	-
ACI	-	-	-	+	+

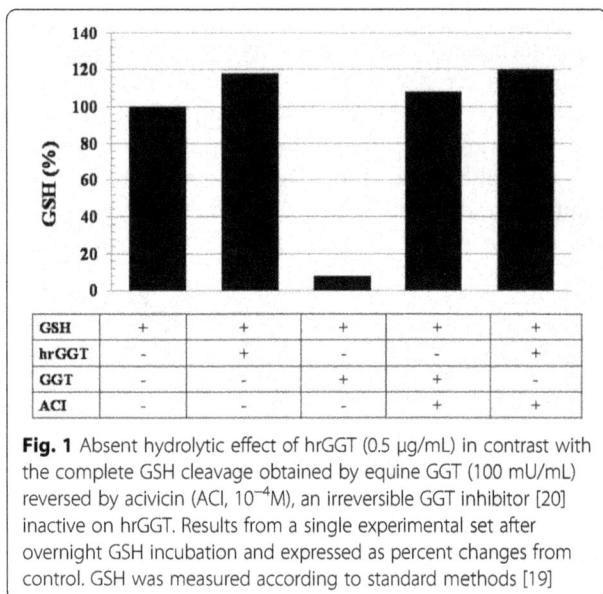

Fig. 1 Absent hydrolytic effect of hrGGT (0.5 μg/mL) in contrast with the complete GSH cleavage obtained by equine GGT (100 mU/mL) reversed by acivicin (ACI, 10^{-4}M), an irreversible GGT inhibitor [20] inactive on hrGGT. Results from a single experimental set after overnight GSH incubation and expressed as percent changes from control. GSH was measured according to standard methods [19]

as well as N-acetyl-L-cysteine (NAC, 10^{-3}M), an antioxidant with inhibitory effect on NFkB [25].

Experimental methods

TF Procoagulant Activity (PCA)

PCA was assessed by a one-stage clotting time test in PBMCs disrupted by three freeze–thaw cycles as reported previously [26]. Disrupted cells (100 μL) were mixed with 100 μL of normal human plasma at 37 °C, adding 100 μl of 25 mM $CaCl_2$ at 37 °C. Time to clot formation was recorded and values converted to arbitrary units (AU) by comparison with a standard human brain TF calibration curve covering clotting times from 20 to 600 s. The standard TF preparation was arbitrarily assigned a value of 1000 AU/mL and a representative conversion of clotting times to AU is as follows: 100 AU-21 s, 10 AU-40s, 1 AU-82 s, 0.1-187 s, 0.01 AU-375 s, 0.001 AU-600 s.

"Baseline" values were defined as clotting times above 375 s (0.01 AU) and refer to quiescent, non activated, untreated PBMCs. Experiments were run in triplicate and averaged.

TF antigen(ag)

Cells were disrupted by three repeated freeze–thaw cycles and debris pelleted by centrifugation at 100xg for 1 h at 4 °C and supernatants used for ELISA according to manufacturer's instructions (Imubind TF kit Sekisui Diagnostics, West Malling, United Kingdom). Within and between assay variability was 3.5 and 5.5 %, respectively.

TF mRNA

Total RNA was extracted from PBMCs using the RNeasy mini kit (Qiagen, Hilden, Germany). RNA concentration and purity were determined by optical density measurement via Nanodrop (Thermo Fisher Scientific, Wilmington, Delaware USA). A mixture of 0.5 ng total RNA per sample was retro-transcribed with random primer-oligodT into complementary DNA (cDNA) using the Quantitect Reverse Transcription Kit (Qiagen, Hilden, Germany). The retro-transcription cycle was performed at 25 °C for 5 min, 42 °C for 30 min and 95 °C for 3 min. RealTime-PCR was carried out in a iQ5 Real Time PCR System and SsoAdvanced Sybr Green Supermix (Bio-Rad Laboratories, Hercules, CA) was employed on the basis of the manufacturer's conditions: 95 °C, 30s; 40 cycles 95 °C, 5 s, 60 °C, 15 s;a final melting protocol with ramping from 65 °C to 95 °C with 0,5 °C increments of 5 s was performed. The primers sequence for RealTime-PCR were: TF, sense 5'-TTGGCAAGGACTT AATTTATACAC-3', antisense 5'-CTGTTCGGGAGGGA ATCAC-3'; GAPDH, sense: 5'-CCCTTCATTGACCTCA ACTACATG-3' and antisense: 5'-TGGGATTTCCATTGA TGACAAGC-3' (Invitrogen, Monza, Italy). All samples were analysed in duplicate and averaged. The relative expression of the target gene was normalized to the level of GAPDH in the same cDNA.

PCA and TFag were assayed after a 18 h incubation period while TFmRNA was evaluated after a 2 h interval. BAY 10–772, NAC and anti-GGT polyclonal antibody were added 30 min prior to GGT stimulation.

PCA, ELISA and Q-PCR results in each control and experimental group were all generated from suspensions containing equal number of cells (3×10^6 PBMCs/mL).

Statistics

Statistical differences were tested by Mann–Whitney test. Data were reported as means ± SD unless otherwise reported. A two-tailed p-level <0.05 was the threshold for statistical significance.

Results

GGT stimulates TF expression independent of its enzymatic properties

Equine GGT (100 mU/mL) stimulated TF PCA, an effect insensitive to GGT inhibition by acivicin (10^{-4}M) (Fig. 2). Incubation of the samples with an antihuman TF antibody (30 μg/mL; IgG, American Diagnostica) abolished more than 95 % of the PCA indicating its dependence upon TF (data not shown).

hrGGT, an enzymatically inactive protein induced a graded, concentration-dependent PCA stimulation without evidence of a plateau (Fig. 3, left panel). As a comparison, PCA in response to the peak hrGGT concentration (1.0 μg/mL) used in those studies was in the range obtained under identical experimental conditions by a well characterized procoagulant agonist such as LPS at a standard concentration of 0.1 μg/mL (from 0.01 ± 0.008 to 1.12 ± 0.2 AU) [13].

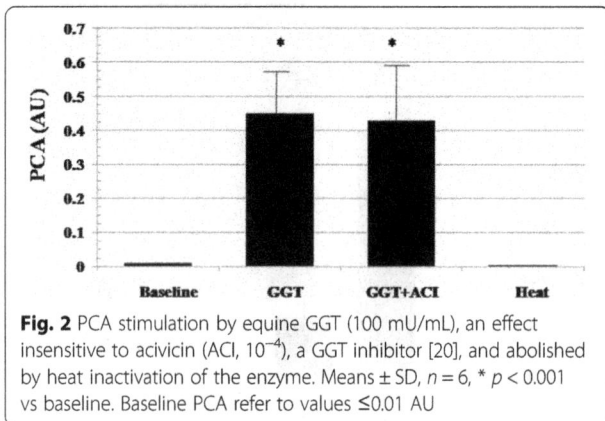

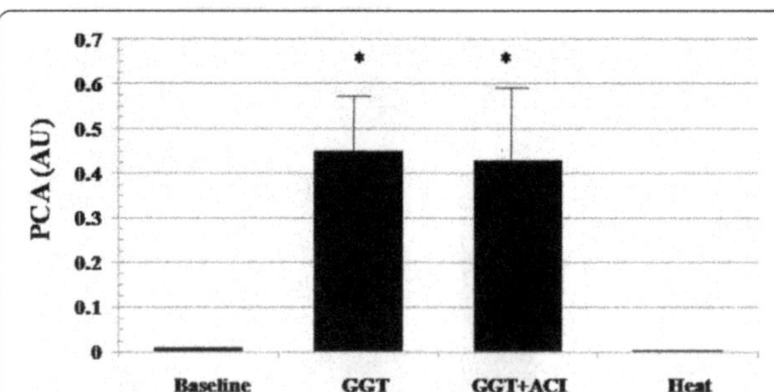

Fig. 2 PCA stimulation by equine GGT (100 mU/mL), an effect insensitive to acivicin (ACI, 10^{-4}), a GGT inhibitor [20], and abolished by heat inactivation of the enzyme. Means ± SD, $n = 6$, * $p < 0.001$ vs baseline. Baseline PCA refer to values ≤0.01 AU

Taking into account its equieffectiveness to natural GGT, 100 mU/mL, all further studies were carried out with hrGGT, 0.5 μg/mL, and the time course of its effect on PCA is reported in Fig. 3, right panel.

LPS contamination does not explain GGT-induced TF expression

Heat inactivation abrogated the effect of either natural GGT (Fig. 2) or hrGGT (data not shown).

LPS determination in hrGGT preparations averaged 0.07 ± 0.02 ng/mL (n = 4 replicates), a concentration that did not affect baseline PCA to a statistically significant extent quite in contrast with hrGGT (Fig. 4, left panel).

hrGGT-induced procoagulant responses were downregulated by an anti-GGT IgG polyclonal antibody (Fig. 4, right panel).

hrGGT induces TF transcription by activating NFkB and increasing ROS generation

hrGGT, 0.5 μg/mL, induced an increase in both TFag and mRNA (Fig. 5, left and right panel). BAY-11-7082 (10^{-5}M) inhibited both GGT-stimulated TF protein and activity (Fig. 6, left and right panel), an inhibitory effect on PCA shared by NAC (10^{-3}M, from 0.35 ± 0.07 to 0.09 ± 0.01, $p < 0.001$, $n = 7$).

Discussion

Discussion of the effects of GGT on TF expression needs some preliminary comments about endotoxin contamination, an important concern in the light of the frequent pollution by that bacterial product of cell cultures even if grown in carefully controlled experimental conditions [22]. However, three orders of considerations make that possibility unlikely. First, GGT-induced PCA was abrogated by heat, a procedure generally ineffective on heat-resistant LPS [21]. Secondly, LPS levels in our preparation were less than <0.1 ng/mL, a concentration with a minor, if any, procoagulant action and certainly far less than that of GGT, a behaviour excluding an important role for heat-sensitive LPS strains [22]. Thirdly, inhibition of TF activity by an anti-GGT antibody provided additional proof of the specificity of the procoagulant response to hrGGT.

Having this background in mind, the main and original outcome of this study was the demonstration of the procoagulant properties of GGT and their independence from the enzymatic action of the molecule. That latter, quite intriguing conclusion is based upon the insensitivity of natural GGT-stimulated PCA to acivicin, a highly specific GGT inhibitor [20] and, more importantly, by the maintained procoagulant effect of hrGGT, a wheat germ-derived protein devoid of enzymatic activity because of a missing post-translational glycosylation apparatus [17, 18], an assumption fully verified by our GSH hydrolysis experiments reported in Fig. 1. Thus, hrGGT induced a concentration-dependent procoagulant effect, increased TFag and upregulated mRNA, a behaviour this latter showing that GGT-induced TF gene transcription is an early event since our mRNA assays

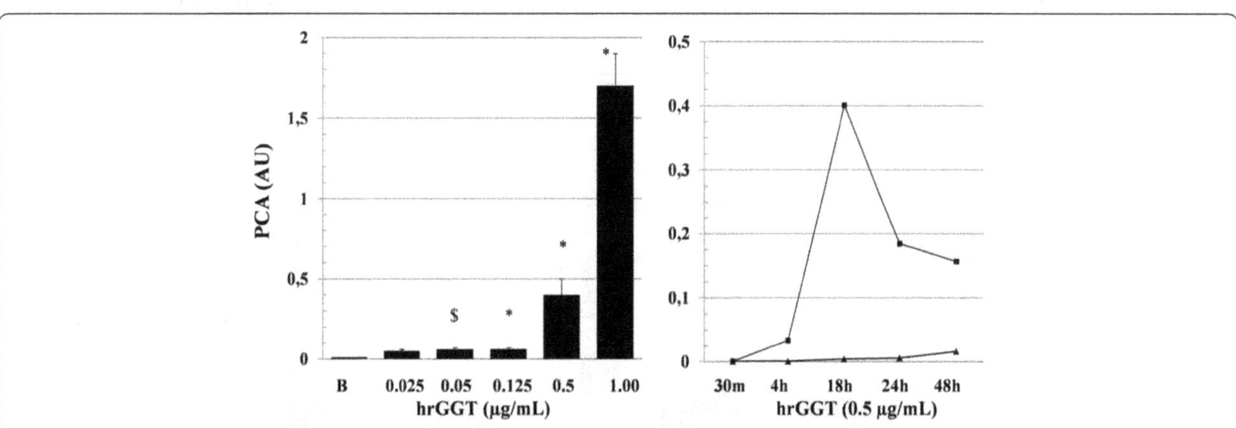

Fig. 3 *Left panel*: Concentration-dependent increase in PCA in response to hrGGT, an enzymatically inactive protein. Means ± SD, $n = 7$, \$ $p < 0.05$ and * $p < 0.001$ vs baseline (B). *Right panel*: Time course of PCA in PBMCs stimulated by hrGGT, 0.5 μg/mL (■), as compared to quiescent cell preparations (▲). Means, n = 4. Baseline PCA refer to values ≤0.01 AU

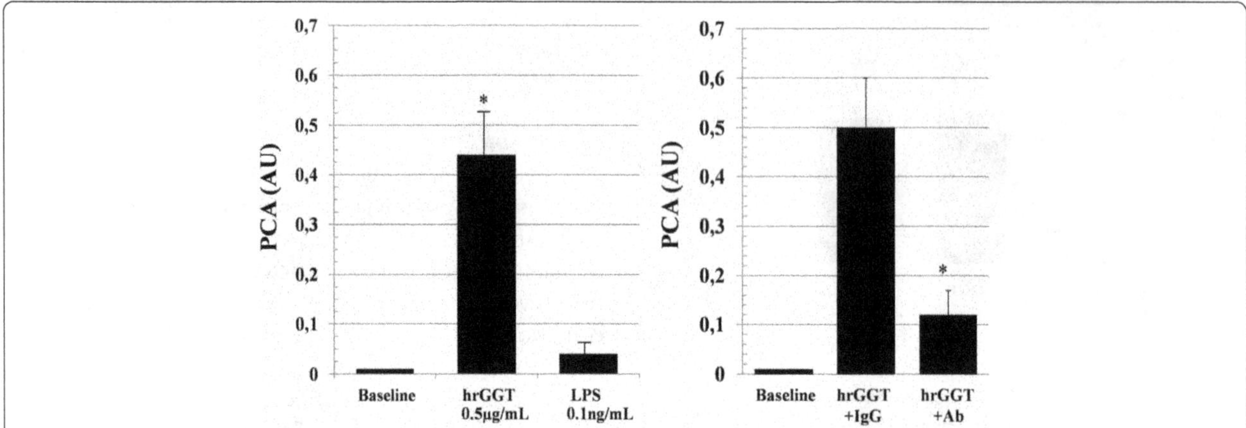

Fig. 4 *Left panel*: Procoagulant effect of LPS concentrations in the contaminant range (0.1 ng/mL) relative to baseline values and hrGGT-primed values. Means ± SD, $n = 3$, $^*p < 0.001$ vs LPS. *Right panel*: Inhibition of hrGGT(0.5 µg/mL)-stimulated PCA by a specific anti-hrGGT polyclonal IgG antibody (Ab, 2.5 µg/mL). Means ± SD, $n = 7$, $^*p < 0.001$ vs hrGGT+ IgG isotype control. Baseline PCA refer to values ≤0.01 AU

were obtained after only 2 h of exposure to the molecule, quite similar in this regard to the response induced by unrelated cytokines and inflammatory agonists (e.g. [27]). However, additional studies are needed to evaluate the pattern of GGT-induced gene expression over a longer time course and the reader should also be aware that our PCR procedure based upon the use of GAPDH as a single and quite variable reference gene may present some technical limitations [28, 29]. Moreover, GGT-induced TF gene transcription was likely located at the level of NFkB activation given the inhibitory effect of BAY-10-772, a pharmacological antagonist [24] of that crucial controller of redox stimuli converging upon TF gene [7, 8]. The conclusion was strengthened by the negative modulation of PCA exerted by NAC, a sulfhydryl-group donor that, by increasing the antioxidant thiol pool and scavenging the excess of intracellular ROS, downregulates NFkB [25]. Therefore, our data, besides constituting, to the best of our knowledge, the first demonstration of a direct TF procoagulant effect of GGT, also provide consistent, albeit admittedly indirect, evidence for increased ROS production and NFkB activation as the pathophysiological mechanism linking GGT to TF expression in PBMCs.

That GGT might induce ROS generation is a concept dating back to two decades ago or so when Glass and Stark showed oxidative damage of cell surface proteins and membrane lipids as a consequence of GSH cleavage by GGT inducing auto-oxidation of the sulfur via a Fenton reaction resulting in the iron–dependent production of oxygen radicals [30]. However, that mechanism, which requires an enzymatically functional GGT molecule, cannot evidently apply to our data. Rather, direct, non enzymatic TF stimulation is closely consonant with similar results obtained in evaluating the role of the GGT as a bone resorbing factor [31]. The data open obvious questions about the GGT-operated signal transduction pathways upstream NFkB activation including the mechanisms allowing membrane permeation of the exogenous protein and the interaction with its intracellular

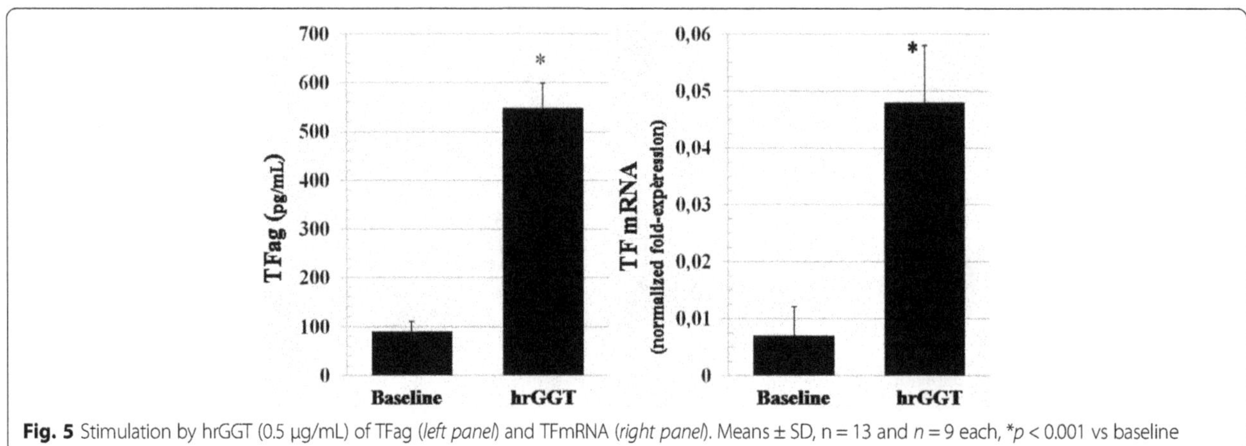

Fig. 5 Stimulation by hrGGT (0.5 µg/mL) of TFag (*left panel*) and TFmRNA (*right panel*). Means ± SD, n = 13 and $n = 9$ each, $^*p < 0.001$ vs baseline

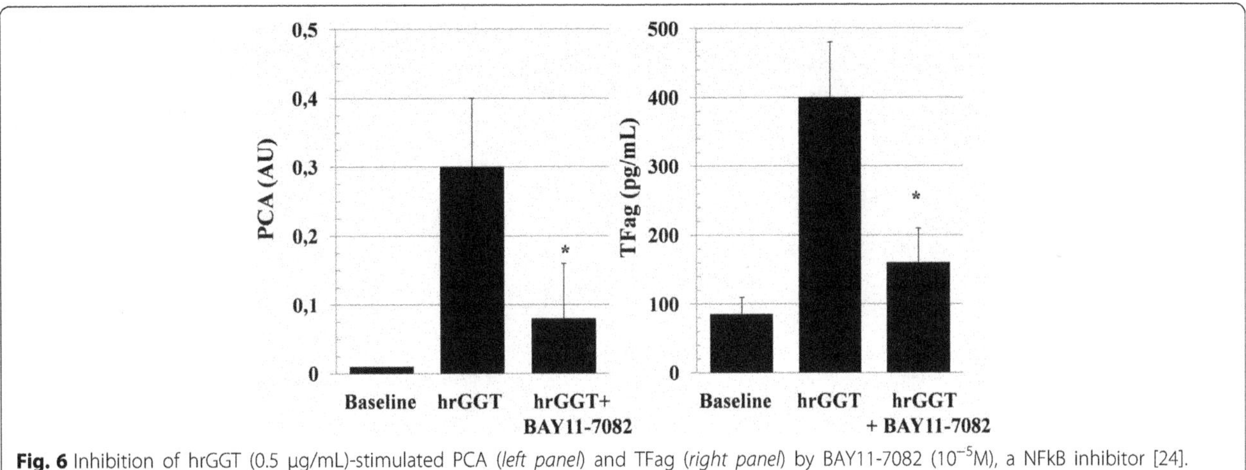

Fig. 6 Inhibition of hrGGT (0.5 μg/mL)-stimulated PCA (*left panel*) and TFag (*right panel*) by BAY11-7082 (10^{-5}M), a NFkB inhibitor [24]. Means ± SD, $n = 7$each, $*p < 0.001$ vs hrGGT. Baseline PCA refer to values ≤0.01 AU

targets. Although our results cannot answer this specific point, one might conjecture of a specific but insofar not identified GGT-receptor or lipid-driven endocytosis [32]. Perhaps, some role may play a chemokine-like CX3C motif contained in the GGT molecule [33] or exogenous GGT might mimick cytokine-like activities of GGT-related proteins produced by genes different from the GGT1 [34]. For example, the GGT2 gene located close to the GGT1 chromosomal region seems to encode for a full length, enzymatically inactive protein, not localized to the plasma membrane [35] and, according to some Authors, involved in redox modulation [36]. It might also be possible to envisage protein-protein interactions leading to the expression of other procoagulant cytokines. Additional unresolved questions to be addressed in future studies regard an understanding of how the enzymatic and non-enzymatic activity of GGT may complement each other as well as the role of circulating GGT levels in the activation of the TF procoagulant pathway.

The data reported in this study may have pathophysiological and clinical relevance. In fact, previous experiments have shown upregulated GGT transcription in response to NADPH oxidase-mediated ROS generation [37] as well as to agents endowed with TF-stimulating properties [8] such as Tumor Necrosis Factor(TNF)-alpha [38] and phorbol esters [39]. Moreover, monocytes, a cell line harbouring GGT [2, 3], have recently been shown to release a GGT fraction when exposed to LPS [40], a product of Gram-negative bacteria that initiates the pathogen-induced inflammatory response [41] of which activation of coagulation is a prominent component [9]. In that framework, thus, it is conceivable to hypothesize a vicious circle by which circulating or within-plaque [12, 40] GGT stimulates TF expression, and plaque-derived cytokines induce procoagulant GGT expression [38]. Both arms of this self-reverberating mechanism hinging around NFkB activation [42] may amplify the pro-thrombotic potential of vulnerable atheromatous plaques possibly in synergism with TF expressed by activated B- and T-lymphocytes [14, 43], a tempting but at the moment only speculative hypothesis worth being pursued in future studies.

Conclusions

Our data provide the first evidence of a procoagulant action of GGT, a result that adds to the long [8] and enlarging (e.g. [44, 45]) list of TF-inducing agents acting through NFkB activation. In showing the independence of that effect from its enzymatic activity, the data raise the issue of the proinflammatory and prothrombotic potential of GGT as a cytokine-like protein. However, further work is needed to understand more precisely the extent to which in-vitro data can be transferred to in-vivo conditions and the possible pathophysiological importance of this mechanism in cardiovascular risk modulation.

Abbreviations

ag: Antigen; AU: Arbitrary Units; $CaCl_2$: Calcium Chloride; DNA: Deoxyribonucleic acid; ELISA: Enzyme-linked immunosorbent assay; GAPDH: Glyceraldehyde-3-phosphate dehydrogenase; GGT: Gamma-glutamyltransferase; GSH: Glutathione; Hr: Human recombinant; Ig: Immunoglobulin; LAL: Limulus Amebocyte Lysate; LPS: Lipopolysaccharide; MTT: Dimethyl thiazolyl diphenyl tetrazolium; NAC: N-acetyl-L-cysteine; NADP: Nicotinamide adenine dinucleotide phosphate; NFkB: Nuclear factor kappa-light-chain-enhancer of activated B cells; PBMC: Peripheral Blood Mononuclear Cell; PCA: Procoagulant activity; PCR: Polymerase Chain Reaction; RNA: Deoxyribonucleic acid; ROS: Reactive Oxygen Species; RPMI: Roswell Park Memorial Institute; SD: Standard deviation; TF: Tissue Factor; TNF: Tumour Necrosis Factor

Acknowledgements

Not applicable.

Funding

Funding for the study was provided by grants from Università degli Studi di Pisa. All Authors are part of the teaching and research staff of the Università degli Studi di Pisa.

Authors' contributions

VS carried out the PCA studies; CB carried out the TF antigen experiments; VC carried out the PCR gene expression; AC & MF performed the statistical analysis, SC & TN drafted the manuscript; RZ, AC & AP participated in design of the study; RP conceived the study and coordinated the research team. All authors read and approved the final manuscript.

Competing interests

The authors declare that they have no competing interests.

Author details

[1]Dipartimento di Patologia Chirurgica, Medica, Molecolare e dell'Area Critica, Università di Pisa, Pisa, Italy. [2]Dipartimento di Ricerca Traslazionale e delle Nuove Tecnologie in Medicina e Chirurgia, Università di Pisa, Pisa, Italy.

References

1. Whitfield JB. Gamma glutamyl transferase. Crit Rev Clin Lab Sci. 2001;38:263–355.
2. Täger M, Ittenson A, Franke A, Frey A, Gassen HG, Ansorge S. Gamma-Glutamyl transpeptidase-cellular expression in populations of normal human mononuclear cells and patients suffering from leukemias. Ann Hematol. 1995;70:237–42.
3. Novogrodsky A, Tate SS, Meister A. Gamma-Glutamyl transpeptidase, a lymphoid cell-surface marker: relationship to blastogenesis, differentiation, and neoplasia. Proc Natl Acad Sci U S A. 1976;73:2414–8.
4. Paolicchi A, Dominici S, Pieri L, Maellaro E, Pompella A. Glutathione catabolism as a signaling mechanism. Biochem Pharmacol. 2002;64:1027–35.
5. Accaoui MJ, Enoiu M, Mergny M, Masson C, Dominici S, Wellman M, et al. Gamma-glutamyltranspeptidase-dependent glutathione catabolism results in activation of NF-kB. Biochem Biophys Res Commun. 2000;276:1062–7.
6. Dominici S, Visvikis A, Pieri L, Paolicchi A, Valentini MA, Comporti M, et al. Redox modulation of NF-kappaB nuclear translocation and DNA binding in metastatic melanoma. The role of endogenous and gamma-glutamyl transferase-dependent oxidative stress. Tumori. 2003;89:426–33.
7. Schreck R, Albermann K, Baeuerle PA. Nuclear factor kappa B: an oxidative stress-responsive transcription factor of eukaryotic cells (a review). Free Radic Res Commun. 1992;17:221–37.
8. Camerer E, Kolstø AB, Prydz H. Cell biology of tissue factor, the principal initiator of blood coagulation. Thromb Res. 1996;81:1–41.
9. Levi M, van der Poll T, Büller HR. Bidirectional relation between inflammation and coagulation. Circulation. 2004;109:2698–704.
10. Kunutsor SK, Apekey TA, Khan H. Liver enzymes and risk of cardiovascular disease in the general population: a meta-analysis of prospective cohort studies. Atherosclerosis. 2014;236:7–17.
11. Tatsumi K, Mackman N. Tissue factor and atherothrombosis. J Atheroscler Thromb. 2015;22:543–9.
12. Pucci A, Franzini M, Matteucci M, Ceragioli S, Marconi M, Ferrari M, et al. b-Gamma-glutamyltransferase activity in human vulnerable carotid plaques. Atherosclerosis. 2014;237:307–13.
13. Balia C, Petrini S, Scalise V, Neri T, Carnicelli V, Cianchetti S, et al. Compound 21, a selective angiotensin II type 2 receptor agonist, downregulates lipopolysaccharide-stimulated tissue factor expression in human peripheral blood mononuclear cells. Blood Coagul Fibrinolysis. 2014;25:501–6.
14. Mechiche H, Cornillet-Lefebvre P, Nguyen P. A subpopulation of human B lymphocytes can express a functional Tissue Factor in response to phorbol myristate acetate. Thromb Haemost. 2005;94:146–54.
15. Camera M, Brambilla M, Facchinetti L, Canzano P, Spirito R, Rossetti L, et al. Tissue factor and atherosclerosis: not only vessel wall-derived TF, but also platelet-associated TF. Thromb Res. 2012;129:279–84.
16. Franzini M, Bramanti E, Ottaviano V, Ghiri E, Scatena F, Barsacchi R, et al. A high performance gel filtration chromatography method for gamma-glutamyltransferase fraction analysis. Anal Biochem. 2008;374:1–6.
17. West MB, Segu ZM, Feasley CL, Kang P, Klouckova I, Li C, Novotny MV, et al. Analysis of site-specific glycosylation of renal and hepatic γ-glutamyl transpeptidase from normal human tissue. J Biol Chem. 2010;285:29511–24.
18. West MB, Wickham S, Quinalty LM, Pavlovicz RE, Li C, Hanigan MH. Autocatalytic cleavage of human gamma-glutamyl transpeptidase is highly dependent on N-glycosylation at asparagine 95. J Biol Chem. 2011;286:28876–88.
19. Baker MA, Cerniglia GJ, Zaman A. Microtiter plate assay for the measurement of glutathione and glutathione disulfide in large numbers of biological samples. Anal Biochem. 1990;190:360–5.
20. Smith TK, Ikeda Y, Fujii J, Taniguchi N, Meister A. Different sites of acivicin binding and inactivation of gamma-glutamyl transpeptidases. Proc Natl Acad Sci U S A. 1995;14(92):2360–4.
21. Majde JA. Endotoxin detection. Immunol Today. 1992;13:328–9.
22. Gao B, Tsan MF. Endotoxin contamination in recombinant human heat shock protein 70 (Hsp70) preparation is responsible for the induction of tumor necrosis factor alpha release by murine macrophages. J Biol Chem. 2003;278:174–9.
23. Lindsay GK, Roslansky PF, Novitsky TJ. Single-step, chromogenic Limulus amebocyte lysate assay for endotoxin. J Clin Microbiol. 1989;27:947–51.
24. García MG, Alaniz L, Lopes EC, Blanco G, Hajos SE, Alvarez E. Inhibition of NF-kappaB activity by BAY 11–7082 increases apoptosis in multidrug resistant leukemic T-cell lines. Leuk Res. 2005;29:1425–34.
25. Renard P, Zachary MD, Bougelet C, Mirault ME, Haegeman G, Remacle J, et al. Effects of antioxidant enzyme modulations on interleukin-1-induced nuclear factor kappa B activation. Biochem Pharmacol. 1997;53:149–60.
26. Celi A, Pellegrini G, Lorenzet R, De Blasi A, Ready N, Furie BC, et al. P-selectin induces the expression of tissue factor on monocytes. Proc Natl Acad Sci U S A. 1994;91:8767–71.
27. Mueller J, Rox JM, Madlener K, Poetzsch B. Quantitative tissue factor gene expression analysis in whole blood: development and evaluation of a real-time PCR platform. Clin Chem. 2004;50:245–7.
28. Bustin SA, Benes V, Garson JA, Hellemans J, Huggett J, Kubista M, et al. The MIQE guidelines: minimum information for publication of quantitative real-time PCR experiments. Clin Chem. 2009;55:611–22.
29. Dheda K, Huggett JF, Bustin SA, Johnson MA, Rook G, Zumla A. Validation of housekeeping genes for normalizing RNA expression in real-time PCR. Biotechniques. 2004;37:112–4. 116, 118–9.
30. Glass GA, Stark AA. Promotion of glutathione-gamma-glutamyl transpeptidase-dependent lipid peroxidation by copper and ceruloplasmin: the requirement for iron and the effects of antioxidants and antioxidant enzymes. Environ Mol Mutagen. 1997;29:73–80.
31. Niida S, Kawahara M, Ishizuka Y, Ikeda Y, Kondo T, Hibi T, et al. Gamma-glutamyltranspeptidase stimulates receptor activator of nuclear factor-kappaB ligand expression independent of its enzymatic activity and serves as a pathological bone-resorbing factor. J Biol Chem. 2004;279:5752–6.
32. Schubert T, Römer W. How synthetic membrane systems contribute to the understanding of lipid-driven endocytosis. Biochim Biophys Acta. 2015; 1853(11Pt B):2992–3005.
33. Kinlough CL, Poland PA, Bruns JB, Hughey RP. Gamma-glutamyltranspeptidase: disulfide bridges, propeptide cleavage, and activation in the endoplasmic reticulum. Methods Enzymol. 2005;401:426–49.
34. Heisterkamp N, Groffen J, Warburton D, Sneddon TP. The human gamma-glutamyltransferase gene family. Hum Genet. 2008;123:321–32.
35. West MB, Wickham S, Parks EE, Sherry DM, Hanigan MH. Human GGT2 does not autocleave into a functional enzyme: A cautionary tale for interpretation of microarray data on redox signaling. Antioxid Redox Signal. 2013;19:1877–88.
36. Moon DO, Kim BY, Jang JH, Kim MO, Jayasooriya RG, Kang CH, Choi YH, Moon SK, Kim WJ, Ahn JS, Kim GY. K-RAS transformation in prostate epithelial cell overcomes H2O2-induced apoptosis via upregulation of gamma-glutamyltransferase-2. Toxicol In Vitro. 2012;26:429–34.
37. Ravuri C, Svineng G, Pankiv S, Huseby NE. Endogenous production of reactive oxygen species by the NADPH oxidase complexes is a determinant of γ-glutamyltransferase expression. Free Radic Res. 2011;45:600–10.
38. Reuter S, Schnekenburger M, Cristofanon S, Buck I, Teiten MH, Daubeuf S, et al. Tumor necrosis factor alpha induces gamma-glutamyltransferase expression via nuclear factor-kappaB in cooperation with Sp1. Biochem Pharmacol. 2009;77:397–411.
39. Pandur S, Ravuri C, Moens U, Huseby NE. Combined incubation of colon carcinoma cells with phorbol ester and mitochondrial uncoupling agents results in synergic elevated reactive oxygen species levels and increased γ-glutamyltransferase expression. Mol Cell Biochem. 2014;388:149–56.

40. Belcastro E, Franzini M, Cianchetti S, Lorenzini E, Masotti S, Fierabracci V, Pucci A, et al. Monocytes/macrophages activation contributes to b-gamma-glutamyltransferase accumulation inside atherosclerotic plaques. J Transl Med. 2015;13:325. doi:10.1186/s12967-015-0687-6.
41. Beutler B, Hoebe K, Du X, Ulevitch RJ. How we detect microbes and respond to them: the Toll-like receptors and their transducers. J Leukoc Biol. 2003;74:479–85.
42. Ritchie ME. Nuclear Factor-kB is selectively and markedly activated in humans with unstable angina pectoris. Circulation. 1998;98:1707–13.
43. De Palma R, Cirillo P, Ciccarelli G, Barra G, Conte S, Pellegrino G, et al. Expression of functional tissue factor in activated T-lymphocytes in vitro and in vivo: A possible contribution of immunity to thrombosis? Int J Cardiol. 2016;218:188–95.
44. Napoleone E, Di Santo A, Amore C, Baccante G, di Febbo C, Porreca E, et al. Leptin induces tissue factor expression in human peripheral blood mononuclear cells: a possible link between obesity and cardiovascular risk? J Thromb Haemost. 2007;5:1462–8.
45. Calabrò P, Cirillo P, Limongelli G, Maddaloni V, Riegler L, Palmieri R, et al. Tissue factor is induced by resistin in human coronary artery endothelial cells by the NF-κB-dependent pathway. J Vasc Res. 2011;48:59–66.

11

Is it safe to withhold long-term anticoagulation therapy in patients with small pulmonary emboli diagnosed by SPECT scintigraphy?

R. Ghazvinian*, A. Gottsäter and J. Elf

Abstract

Background: The need for anticoagulation therapy (AC) in patients with subsegmental pulmonary embolism (SSPE) diagnosed by computed tomography of the pulmonary arteries (CTPA) has been questioned, as these patients run low risk for recurrent venous thromboembolism (VTE) during 3 months of follow-up. Whether this applies also to patients with small PE diagnosed with pulmonary scintigraphy has not yet been evaluated, however.

Methods: We therefore retrospectively evaluated 54 patients (mean age 62 ± 19 years, 36 [67 %] women) with small PE diagnosed by ventilation/perfusion singe photon emission computed tomography (V/P SPECT) who did not receive conventional long-term AC.

Results: More than half of our patients (36[67 %]) received less than 48 h of AC, 11 (20 %) patients were treated for 2–14 days, and 7 (13 %) for 15–30 days. The majority (28 [52 %]) of our patients had a non-low simplified pulmonary emboli severity index (S-PESI), and 7 (13 %) had malignancy. D-dimer was negative in 18 (33 %), positive in 10 (19 %), and not analyzed in 28 (52 %) patients. Phlebography of the lower extremities had been performed with negative result in one patient.

During 90 days of follow up no deaths or PE occurred. Seven patients were readmitted to hospital, whereof two (2/54 [4 %]) were diagnosed with deep venous thrombosis (DVT) necessitating AC therapy.

Conclusion: In conclusion, withholding longterm AC therapy in patients with SSPE diagnosed by V/P SPECT resulted in 4 % risk for recurrence of VTE during 90 days of follow up, and can therefore currently not be recommended.

Keywords: Withholding conventional AC therapy, V/P SPECT, Small PE, Subsegmental pulmonary embolism

Background

The annual incidence rates of deep venous thrombosis (DVT) and pulmonary embolism (PE) are approximately 0.5–1 per 1000 inhabitants [1]. The clinical presentation of PE extends from asymptomatic patients to shock states, but most patients (95 %) are normotensive and present with breathing difficulties or pleuritic pain [2]. The use of multiple-detector computed tomography pulmonary angiography (CTPA), has led to an increased number of diagnosed sub-segmental pulmonary emboli (SSPE), accounting for around 5–15 % of PE cases [3].

Albeit CTPA is considered the primary diagnostic tool for detection of PE and is available 24 h a day, 7 days a week, there are alternative methods [4]. Using planar ventilation-perfusion lung scan (V/Q scan), the majority of patients with suspected PE have non-diagnostic examinations [5]. Prospective management studies demonstrated that patients with low or intermediate probability V/Q scan, low pretest probability of PE, and negative compression ultrasonography can be safely managed without anticoagulation [6, 7]. Lung scintigraphy has been further developed, however. Modern ventilation/

* Correspondence: Raein.Ghazvinian@skane.se
Lund University, Division of Vascular Medicine, Skåne University Hospital, Ruth Lundskogs Gata 10, S-205 02 Malmö, Sweden

perfusion single photon emission computed tomography (V/P SPECT) and "holistic" interpretation criteria reduce the risk for non-diagnostic findings, and increases the sensitivity and specificity for diagnosis of PE [8]. With this technique PE can be classified as segmental or subsegmental and graded according to the percentage of the pulmonary vascular bed affected [8].

Some diagnostic challenges persist, however. Even though the use of multi-detector CTPA or V/P SPECT in combination with diagnostic algorithms as for example the Wells score [9] has increased the diagnostic accuracy of PE, the mortality of the disease has remained consistent [10–12]. This might indicate that many of the small SSPE treated after detection with CTPA may be of low clinical significance [4]. In fact, treatment of SSPE in patients with high bleeding risk, and low risk for recurrent venous thromboembolism (VTE) might perhaps even be contraindicated due to increased risk of bleeding and other treatment complications. Whether it is safe to withhold anticoagulant (AC) treatment in patients with SSPE diagnosed by CTPA and negative bilateral ultrasound of the legs is currently evaluated in an ongoing trial [13], but whether this approach is applicable to patients with small PE diagnosed by V/P SPECT has not yet been assessed.

In 898 patients diagnosed with PE by V/P SPECT, we previously reported risk of recurrence and bleeding in 307 patients with small PE undergoing home treatment with AC [14]. We now report a retrospective follow-up of patients with PE diagnosed by V/P SPECT in whom conventional long-term AC therapy for different reasons had been withheld.

Methods

All consecutive 898 patients with acute PE diagnosed by V/P SPECT between 2007 and 2011 at Lund University Hospital, Sweden were included in a prospective registry [14]. V SPECT had been performed after inhalation of aerosolized 99 m TC-Technegas to the lung in the supine position with acquisition lasting for 11 min, and P SPECT with a dual-head gamma camera in the supine position after i.v. administration of 50 MBq 99mTc-macroaggregated albumin. V SPECT illuminates ventilated areas and leaves areas with reduced/absent ventilation on the imaging screen, whereas P SPECT illuminates areas where blood flow is normal but leaves areas without perfusion on the imaging screen. PE was diagnosed and quantified by counting segments showing complete or relative mismatch between ventilation and perfusion defects [8].

After diagnosis, patients were clinically assessed according to a pre specified clinical algorithm [14]. Conventional long-term AC treatment defined as therapeutic doses of low molecular heparin or vitamin-K antagonist for at least three months according to current guidelines [1, 12] was withheld by the clinician if the V/P SPECT result was interpreted as falsely positive for technical reasons (non diagnostic for PE), if the perfusion defect was thought to represent an old and no longer clinically relevant embolization, or if the embolization was thought to be too clinically irrelevant to merit treatment. Withholding of long-term treatment also required that patients were hemodynamically stable, did not have clinical signs or symptoms of DVT, and that the extent of perfusion defects in the V/P SPECT images was less than ≤ 20 % of the pulmonary vascular bed. Based on these criteria, 54 patients (6 %, mean age 62 ± 19 years, 36 [67 %] women) did not receive conventional long-term AC therapy. AC treatment of shorter duration was, however, given to many of these patients during the diagnostic work-up as summarized in Table 1. Baseline data, clinical characteristics including retrospective calculation of sPESI score [15], additional imaging procedures, quantification of perfusion defects on V/P SPECT, d-dimer, and troponin T/ brain natriuretic peptide (NT-BNP) results were collected from patient files. Readmissions, recurrent VTE, and death during 90 days after the final dose of AC therapy were assessed by review of hospital records and imaging databases.

Results

Background data

Twenty (37 %) patients had a predisposing factor for VTE; active cancer, previous surgery, immobilization, pregnancy, contraceptive pill use, trauma or previous DVT (Table 1). Data on concomitant diseases, sPESI scores, and the number of auxiliary investigations such as D-dimer, compression ultrasound, contrast phlebography and CTPA are also shown in Table 1.

Follow-up

No deaths occurred during 90 days of follow up after the final dose of AC therapy. Seven patients (13 %) were readmitted to hospital, in 5 cases (9 %) for suspected VTE. One patient (2 %) underwent CTPA, without signs of PE. Four patients (7 %) underwent phlebography or ultrasound of the lower extremities, whereof two (2[4 %]) were diagnosed with DVT necessitating long-term AC therapy (Fig. 1).

One 71 year old man who had received AC for 24 h was readmitted 38 days after the final AC dose because of swelling of the left leg, and ultrasound showed DVT extending up to the external iliac vein provoked by plaster cast immobilization due to a tibial fracture. One 92 years old woman who had received AC for 20 days was readmitted 52 days after the final dose of AC therapy due to swelling of the right leg. Ultrasound showed DVT extending up to the common femoral vein.

Table 1 Baseline characteristics and duration of anticoagulant (AC) therapy in 54 patients with small pulmonary embolism diagnosed by ventilation/perfusion single photon emission computed tomography (V/P SPECT) who did not receive conventional long-term AC. N(%)

Predisposing factors for thrombosis n(%)	
Malignancy	7 (13)
Oral contraception	1 (2)
Surgery or immobilization	5 (9) (one with malignancy)
Trauma	1 (2)
Previous venous thromboembolism	4 (7)
Pregnancy	2 (4)
Concomitant diseases n(%)	
Congestive heart failure	18 (33)
Chronic obstructive pulmonary disease or asthma	9 (17)
Investigations n(%)	
D-dimer	28 (52), negative in total 18 (33)
NT-proBNP	9 (17), negative in total 8 (15)
Troponin T	28 (52), negative in total 24 (44)
Venous ultrasound or phlebography	1 (2), negative in total 1 (2)
CTPA	17 (31), positive in 6 (11)
Risk stratification n(%)	
sPESI score 0	12 (22)
sPESI score 1	28 (52)
sPESI score 2	11 (20)
sPESI score 3	2 (4)
sPESI score 4	1 (2)
Duration of anticoagulant therapy n(%)	
<48 hours	34 (63)
2–14 days	11 (20)
15–30 days	7 (13)
31–90 days	2 (4)

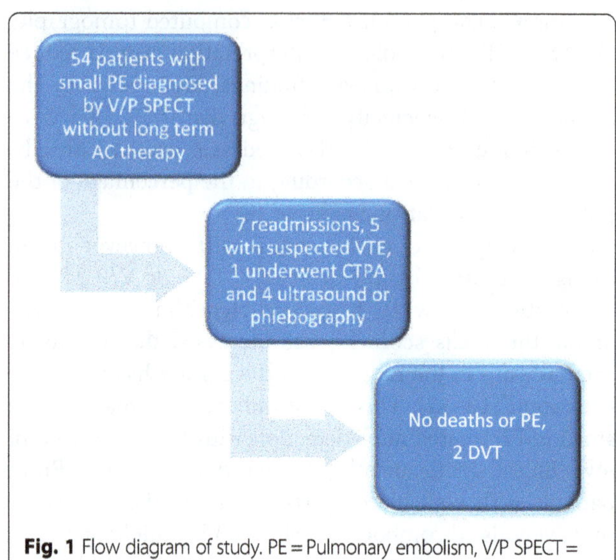

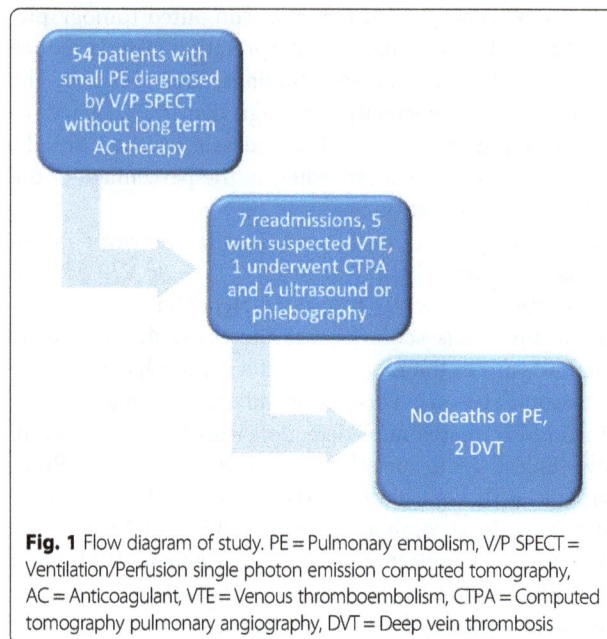

Fig. 1 Flow diagram of study. PE = Pulmonary embolism, V/P SPECT = Ventilation/Perfusion single photon emission computed tomography, AC = Anticoagulant, VTE = Venous thromboembolism, CTPA = Computed tomography pulmonary angiography, DVT = Deep vein thrombosis

Discussion

To our knowledge, this is the first retrospective study in which withholding of conventional long-term AC therapy has been clinically evaluated in patients with a diagnosis of small PE made by V/P SPECT. We report two cases of DVT during a follow up period of three months (4 %), but no PE or death. These figures are comparable higher than what has been reported when AC therapy has been withheld in SSPE patients diagnosed by CTPA. Goy et al retrospectively study reported no recurrences (0 %) among 30 patients but that treatment provoked major bleeding in 2/43 patients treated with AC [3]. Moreover, Carrier and coworkers summarized no recurrences in 60 patients with SSPE diagnosed with CTPA in combination with a negative compression ultrasonography [4], when reviewing data from four different reports [10, 16–18]. These low numbers must be compared with the results of den Exter et al who reported that 4/116 (3.5 %) patients with SSPE treated with AC had a recurrent VTE during 3 months follow up challenging the assumption that SSPE patients have a low risk profile and better clinical outcome compared to patients with more proximal PE [19].

In a cross-sectional survey on clinician's opinions on SSPE [20], it was shown that physicians are comfortable with withholding of therapy if the 3 month risk for recurrent VTE is <2 %. This means that our algorithm with a cutoff of <20 % extension of perfusion defects in the V/P SPECT images leads to a rate of VTE recurrence that would not be considered acceptable for the majority of clinicians. Whether the use of a lower limit of PE extension on V/P SPECT such as for example <5 % or <10 % would have resulted in a lower risk for recurrent DVT remains to be systematically investigated. The extension of the perfusion defects on V/P SPECT in our two patients later diagnosed with VTE was <10 %, and use of this cut-off would therefore not have resulted in any VTE diagnoses during follow-up in our material.

Whether a normal result on bilateral lower extremity ultrasonography should be requested before AC therapy is withheld in patients with confirmed small PE on V/P SPECT also needs to be further evaluated. Whereas this strategy has been used after SSPE diagnosis with CTPA [3] and is currently under further scientific evaluation [13], none of our two patients later diagnosed with DVT had undergone ultrasound or phlebography when the decision to abstain from long-term AC therapy was made.

Whether results of the s-PESI score [17] can be used to predict which patient with small PE that will develop VTE during follow-up is still unclear. Retrospectively calculated s-PESI scores differed in the two patients with VTE during follow-up in our study; zero in the male patient and three in the female patient. Our male patient had an elevated D-dimer which was thought to be caused by concomitant disease, whereas D-dimer was not assessed in the female patient. The combination of Wells score [9] and D-dimer in the diagnostic work-up of PE [1, 12] is only applicable in outpatients without too many comorbidities.

The results of our study underlines the importance of the ongoing prospective study [13] performed to evaluate the safety of withholding AC therapy in patients with SSPE. It is important to note, however, that the results of this trial will only be applicable in patients in whom PE is diagnosed by CTPA and in whom serial ultrasound of the lower extremities is negative. Our results indicate that the future study results cannot be extrapolated to patients with small PE diagnosed by V/P SPECT, at least not without routinely performing bilateral compression ultrasonography of the lower extremities.

The discrepancies in results between our and previous [3, 4, 10, 16–19] might also be caused by differences in the composition of the study populations. When relating our results to previously published data [10, 15–17, 21], our patients were of comparable age (62 years vs 65 and 56 years in the studies of Goy et al. [3] and den Exter et al [19]). The prevalence of malignancy was lower in our study (13 % vs 28 and 18 %) respectively, however. Furthermore, one third of our patients had congestive heart failure (CHF) and 17 % had chronic obstructive pulmonary disease (COPD), figures higher than the 9 % for both CHF and COPD reported by den Exter et al. [19].

Among patients with malignancies and PE, the risk for recurrent VTE is increased among those with symptomatic PE, compared to those with incidentally detected asymptomatic disease [20]. In our study, however, no VTE was detected during follow-up of the 7 patients with known malignancies.

The duration of AC treatment given during diagnostic work-up and initial hospital care is another important issue. In the majority (63 %) of our patients who received less than 48 h of AC therapy, one case of VTE occurred, whereas the other case of VTE was diagnosed in the group (13 %) of patients receiving 15-30 days of AC therapy. The risk of recurrence during the first three months is approximately 2 % [22], and the concept of generally prescribing one month of AC to patients diagnosed with small PE with V/P SPECT, thereby limiting the risk of bleeding, also needs to be further investigated.

The aim of our retrospective study was not to compare V/P SPECT with CTPA in diagnosis of small PE, but PE diagnosis made on V/P SPECT nevertheless had been reassessed with CTPA in 31 % of patients, and was confirmed in a third of these. This reflects that the clinical decision to withhold long term AC therapy was made in three different situations after a positive V/P SPECT; when the result was believed to be non diagnostic, when the perfusion defect was thought to represent a no longer clinically relevant embolization, and when the embolization was thought to be clinically irrelevant. The reason to perform CTPA is most evident in the first of these three scenarios, and in 11 of our patients the PE diagnosis was dropped after a negative CTPA. In the 6 patients in whom long-term AC therapy was withheld in spite of positive results on both V/P SPECT and CTPA, therapy was withheld by the clinician for the third of the above reasons.

A recent paper comparing diagnostic performance between CTPA and V/P SPECT reported that these modalities were equivalent with respect to receiver operating curves (ROC) analysis, with areas under curve (AUC) of 0.99 (95 % CI 0.96–1.00) and 0.98 (95 % CI 0.94–1.00) for V/P SPECT and CTPA, respectively [23].

The main study limitation is of course that we conducted a retrospective clinical follow-up, and not a randomized prospective study. Furthermore, as the decision to withhold conventional long-term AC therapy was made on different ground, our patient material is heterogeneous. Nevertheless, we think that it represents practice in an often occurring difficult clinical situation.

Conclusions

Withholding of conventional long term AC therapy in patients diagnosed with small PE with V/P SPECT was associated with a 4 % risk of VTE diagnosis during 3 months of follow-up. This would not be considered acceptable for the majority of clinicians, and the concept can at the present stage therefore not be recommended.

Abbreviations

AC, anticoagulation; AUC, area under curve; CHF, chronic heart failure; COPD, chronic obstructive pulmonary disease; CTPA, computed tomography pulmonary arteries; DVT, deep vein thrombosis; PE, pulmonary embolism; ROC, reciever operating curves; S-PESI, simplified pulmonary emboli severity index; SSPE, subsegmental pulmonary embolism; V/P SPECT, ventilation/perfusion single photon emission computed tomography; V/Q scan, ventilation-perfusion lungscintigraphy; VTE, venous thromboembolism.

Acknowledgement

None.

Funding

No funding was obtained for this article.

Authors' contributions

RG and JE contributed to the study concept and design, and acquisition of the data. RG, AG, and JE all contributed to data analysis and interpretation, and drafting and critical revision of the manuscript. Statistical analysis was performed by RG.

Competing interests

The authors state that they have no conflicts of interests.

References

1. Torbicki A, Perrier A, Konstantinides S, Agnelli G, Galiè N, Pruszczyk P, Bengel F, Brady AJ, Ferreira D, Janssens U, Klepetko W, Mayer E, Remy-Jardin M, Bassand JP. Guidelines on the diagnosis and management of acute pulmonary embolism: the Task Force for the Diagnosis and Management of Acute Pulmonary Embolism of the European Society of Cardiology (ESC). Eur Heart J. 2008;29(18):2276–315.
2. Kasper W, Konstantinides S, Geibel A, Olschewski M, Heinrich F, Grosser KD, Rauber K, Iversen S, Redecker M, Kienast J. Management strategies and determinants of outcome in acute major pulmonary embolism: results of a multicenter registry. J Am Coll Cardiol. 1997;30(5):1165–71.
3. Goy J, Lee J, Levine O, Charudhry S, Crowther M. Sub-segmental pulmonary embolism in three academic teaching hospitals: a review of management and outcomes. J Thromb Haemost. 2015;13:214–8.
4. Carrier M, Righini M, Le Gal G. Symptomatic subsegmental pulmonary embolism: what is the next step? J Thromb Haemost. 2012;10:1486–90.
5. Stein PD, Henry JW. Prevalence of acute pulmonary embolism in central and subsegmental pulmonary arteries and relation to probability interpretation of ventilation/perfusion lung scans. Chest. 1997;111:1246–8.
6. Perrier A, Bounameaux H, Morabia A, de Moerloose P, Slosman D, Didier D, P-f U, Junod A. Diagnosis of pulmonary embolism by a decinsion analysis-based strategy including clinical probability, D-dimer levels, and ultrasonography: a management study. Arch Intern Med. 1996;156:531–6.
7. Salaun PY, Couturaud F, Le Duc-Pennec A, Lacut K, Le Roux PY, Guillo P, Pennec PY, Cornily JC, Leroyer C, Gal G. Noninvasive diagnosis of pulmonary embolism. Chest. 2011;139:1294–8.
8. Bajc M, Neilly JB, Miniati M, Scheumichen C, Meignan M, Jonson B. EANM guidelines for ventilation/perfusion scintigraphy : Part 1. Pulmonary imaging with ventilation/perfusion single photon emission tomography. Eur J Nucl Med Mol Imaging. 2009;36:1356–70.
9. Wells PS, Anderson DR, Rodger M, Stiell I, Dreyer JF, Barnes D, Forgie M, Kovacs G, Ward J, Kovacs MJ. Excluding pulmonary embolism at the bedside without diagnostic imaging: management of patients with suspected pulmonary embolism presenting to the emergency department using a simple clinical model and d-dimer. Ann Intern Med. 2001;135:98–107.
10. Pena E, Kimton M, Dennie C, Peterson R, Le Gal G, Carrier M. Difference in interpretation of computed tomography pulmonary angiography diagnosis of subsegmental thrombosis in patients with suspected pulmonary embolism. J Thromb Haemost. 2012;10:496–8.
11. Wiener R, Schwartz LM, Woloshin S. Time trends in pulmonary embolism in the United States: evidence of overdiagnosis. Arch Intern Med. 2011;171:831–7.
12. Kearon C, Akl EA, Comerota AJ, Prandoni P, Bounameaux H, Goldhaber SZ, Nelson ME, Wells PS, Gould MK, Dentali F, Crowther M, Kahn SR. Antithrombotic therapy for VTE disease: antithrombotic therapy and prevention of thrombosis, 9thed: American college of chest physicians evidence-based clinical practice guidelines. Chest. 2012;141:419S–94.
13. A study to evaluate the safety of withholding anticoagulation in patients with subsegmental PE who have a negative serial bilateral lower extremity ultrasound (SSPE). https://clinicaltrials.gov/ct2/show/NCT01455818. Accessed at Aug 13, 2014.
14. Elf J, Jögi J, Bajc M. Home treatment of patients with small to medium sized acute pulmonary embolism. J Thromb Thrombolysis. 2015;39:166–72.
15. Masotti L, Panigada G, Landini G, Pieralli F, Corradi F, Lenti S, Migliacci R, Arrigucci S, Frullini A, Bertieri MC, Tatini S, Fortini A, Cascinelli I, Mumoli N, Giuntoli S, De Palma A, Crescenzo V, Piacentini M, Tintori G, Dainelli A, Levantino G, Fabiani P, Risaliti F, Mastriforti R, Voglino M, Carli V, Meini S. Simplified PESI score and sex difference in prognosis of acute pulmonary embolism: a brief report from a real life study. J Thromb Thrombolysis. 2015; 9:1–7.
16. Donato AA, Scheirer JJ, Atwell MS, Gramp J, Duszak Jr R. Clinical outcomes in patients with suspected acute pulmonary embolism and negative helical computed tomographic results in whom anticoagulant was withheld. Arch Intern Med. 2003;163(17):2033–8.
17. Eyer BA, Goodman LR, Washington L. Clinicians' response to radiologists' reports of isolated subsegmental pulmonary embolism or inconclusive interpretation of pulmonary embolism using MDCT. AJR Am J Roentgenol. 2005;184(2):623–8.
18. Carrier M, Kimpton M, Le Gal G, Kahn SR, Kovacs MJ, Wells PS, Anderson DR, Rodger MA. The management of a sub-segmental pulmonary embolism: a cross-sectional survey of Canadian thrombosis physicians. J Thromb Haemost. 2011;9:1412–5.
19. den Exter PL, Van Es J, Klok AF, Kroft LJ, Kruip MJHA, Kamphuisen PW, Büller, Huisman MV. Risk profile and clinical outcome of symptomatic subsegmental acute pulmonary embolism. Blood. 2013;122(7):1144–9.
20. den Exter PL, Hooijer J, Dekkers OM, Huisman MV. Risk of recurrent venous thromboembolism and mortality in patients with cancer incidentally diagnosed with pulmonary embolism: a comparison with symptomatic patients. J Clin Oncol. 2011;29:2405–9.
21. Le Gal G, Righini M, Parent F, van Strijen M, Couturaud F. Diagnosis and management of subsegmental pulmonary embolism. J Thromb Haemost. 2006;4:724–31.
22. Prins MH, Lensing AW, Bauersachs R, van Bellen B, Bounameaux H, Brighton TA, Cohen AT, Davidson BL, Decousus H, Raskob GE, Berkowitz SD, Wells PS. Oral rivaroxaban versus standard therapy for the treatment of symptomatic venous thromboembolism: a pooled analysis of the EINSTEIN-DVT and PE randomized studies. Thromb J. 2013;11:21.
23. Phillips JJ, Straiton J, Staff RT. Planar and SPECT ventilation/perfusion imaging and computed tomography for the diagnosis of pulmonary embolism: a systematic review and meta-analysis of the literature, and cost and dose comparison. Eur J Radiol. 2015;84(7):1392–400.

12

Identification of novel mutations in congenital afibrinogenemia patients and molecular modeling of missense mutations in Pakistani population

Arshi Naz[1*], Arijit Biswas[2,6], Tehmina Nafees Khan[1,7], Anne Goodeve[3,8], Nisar Ahmed[4], Nazish Saqlain[4], Shariq Ahmed[1,7], Ikram Din Ujjan[5], Tahir S Shamsi[1,7] and Johannes Oldenburg[2,9]

Abstract

Background: Congenital afibrinogenemia (OMIM #202400) is a rare coagulation disorder that was first described in 1920. It is transmitted as an autosomal recessive trait that is characterized by absent levels of fibrinogen (factor I) in plasma. Consanguinity in Pakistan and its neighboring countries has resulted in a higher number of cases of congenital fibrinogen deficiency in their respective populations. This study focused on the detection of mutations in fibrinogen genes using DNA sequencing and molecular modeling of missense mutations in all three genes [Fibrinogen gene alpha (FGA), beta (FGB) and gamma (FGG)] in Pakistani patients.

Methods: This descriptive and cross sectional study was conducted in Karachi and Lahore and fully complied with the Declaration of Helsinki. Patients with fibrinogen deficiency were screened for mutations in the Fibrinogen alpha (*FGA*), beta (*FGB*) and gamma (*FGG*) genes by direct sequencing. Molecular modeling was performed to predict the putative structure functional impact of the missense mutations identified in this study.

Results: Ten patients had mutations in *FGA* followed by three mutations in *FGB* and three mutations in *FGG*, respectively. Twelve of these mutations were novel. The missense mutations were predicted to result in a loss of stability because they break ordered regions and cause clashes in the hydrophobic core of the protein.

Conclusions: Congenital afibrinogenemia is a rapidly growing problem in regions where consanguinity is frequently practiced. This study illustrates that mutations in *FGA* are relatively more common in Pakistani patients and molecular modeling of the missense mutations has shown damaging protein structures which has profounding effect on phenotypic bleeding manifestations in these patients.

Keywords: Afibrinogenemia, Molecular modeling, *FGA* gene, Consanguinity, Inherited bleeding disorder

Background

Hemostasis is the normal physiological response that prevents blood loss following vascular injury. It is dependent on an intricate series of events involving platelets and specific coagulation factors. Inherited bleeding disorders can be grouped into abnormalities of primary and secondary hemostasis. Fibrinogen (Factor I) deficiency can originate from congenital or acquired causes. Congenital afibrinogenemia (*OMIM #202400*) is a rare coagulation disorder that was first described in 1920 [1]. It is as a recessive autosomal inherited trait characterized by the absence of fibrinogen (factor I) in plasma [2]. The disease has a worldwide prevalence of 1–2 per million in the general population [3]. Fibrinogen is a 340 KDa hexameric protein of hepatic origin with multiple functions including roles in platelet aggregation and platelet plug formation and is an acute phase reactant [4]. It is secreted as zymogen similar to all other clotting factors and needs to be activated prior to its participation in the coagulation cascade. It consist of

* Correspondence: labarshi@yahoo.com; labarshi2013@gmail.com
[1]National Institute of Blood Diseases and Bone Marrow Transplantation, Karachi University of Bonn, ST 2/A, Block-17, Gulshan-e-Iqbal KDA scheme, 24, Karachi, Pakistan
Full list of author information is available at the end of the article

three pairs (Aα, Bβ and Gγ) of polypeptide chains [5] encoded by three genes (*FGA, FGB and FGG*) clustered in a region of approximately 50 kb on chromosome 4q28-q31 [6, 7]. The normal plasma levels of fibrinogen are 4 g/l [8, 9] and its half-life is approximately 100 h/4 days [10]. The main role of fibrinogen in hemostasis is to strengthen the platelet plug by converting into its polymeric insoluble form called fibrin by thrombin [11]. The fibrin meshwork traps red blood cells and platelets to form a plug which stops bleeding from site of injury. The absence of fibrinogen may result in excessive blood loss after a trauma. Moreover spontaneous bleeding events can occur. Fibrinogen defects are classified as quantitative (Hypofibrinogenemia and Afibrinogenemia, depending upon the partial or complete absence of fibrinogen) or qualitative (Dysfibrinogenemia and Hypodysfibrinogenemia) [12]. The most common symptom associated with fibrinogen deficiency is umbilical stump bleeding with other secondary bleeding manifestations including epistaxis, gum bleeding, cutaneous bleeding, muscle hematoma and haemarthrosis [13].

Congenital fibrinogen deficiency is considered as rare coagulation disorder but its incidence is growing higher in those regions where consanguineous partnerships are common [14, 15]. Pakistan is the country with high ratio of consanguinity resulting in increasing numbers of rare inherited bleeding disorders including congenital afibrinogenemia. Our focus was to identify the mutations, assess the possible structure functional impact of affected protein by using molecular modeling/silico analysis tools. In addition to this, the study also encompasses the insight for possible mutational spectrum in frequently involved fibrinogen gene which may contribute for future prenatal diagnosis of carriers of these defects in Pakistani population.

Methods

Patient inclusion and exclusion criteria

This study, involving human subjects, was performed according to the Declaration of Helsinki, 1975, revised in 2000, and was approved by the relevant institutional Ethical Committee. Patients with congenital afibrinogenemia i.e. absent or undetectable levels of fibrinogen antigen (0–0.1 g/dl) and it activity in plasma were selected for this study. These low levels excluded acquired causes of fibrinogen deficiency, such as liver disease and consumptive coagulopathies, leukemia or other factor deficiencies. Patients from across Pakistan were recruited from centers including Karachi (Sindh) and Lahore (Punjab). A written informed consent was taken from patients and guardians incase of minor. Sampling was performed independent of sex or age. A comprehensive questionnaire was completed containing information about the patient's demographics and disease symptoms. A diagnosis was made on the basis of history and quantitative analysis. All subjects were registered at Hemophilia Society of Pakistan. Samples from all centers were collected and initially processed and saved at the National Institute of Blood Diseases (NIBD) for coagulation profile, biochemistry tests including liver profile and viral markers. DNA sequencing was performed in NIBD genome department, Karachi.

Sample collection and lab assays

Blood samples from patients were collected in 3.2% sodium citrate for coagulation profile in serum (RST) for biochemistry analysis, including liver profile and viral profile, (HBsAg, Anti HCV and HIV) and in K_2EDTA for complete blood count and DNA extraction for amplification and sequencing. All sampling was performed with supportive infusion of cryoprecipitate to avoid bleeding. Platelet-poor plasma was collected by centrifugation of citrate tubes at 4000×g for 10 min and coagulation profile was performed, including PT, APTT and fibrinogen assay, using the Clauss method. Liver function tests (direct and indirect bilirubin, ALT, AST and alkaline phosphatase) and viral markers (HBsAg, anti HCV and HIV) were performed to exclude any acquired cause of afibrinogenemia.

Genetic analysis was performed after isolation of genomic DNA using standard protocols, exons and intron-exon junctions of the fibrinogen genes were amplified by polymerase chain reaction [16] and sequenced [17] as previously described.

Pathogenecity scoring

Pathogenecity scoring was done by five prediction tools to predict the possible structure functional impact of affected protein in identified novel missense mutations. The prediction software tool Poly-phen2 (polymorphism phenotyping v2), (http://genetics.bwh.havard.edu/pph2/ accessed on 20th April 2015) was used to assess the possible impact of substitution on structure and function in human SNPs (Single nucleotide polymorphism). MUPRO (predictions of protein stability changes upon mutations), (http://mupro.proteomics.ics.uci.edu/ accessed on 20th April 2015) utilizes an SVM (support vector machines) model to predict the changes in stability as a result of single-site mutations, primarily from sequential information, and optionally provided structural information. The result only predicts whether the alteration in single amino acid will lead to destabilization or not. MUPRO predictions are reported with the confidence score (C score). A positive score indicates higher stability whereas a negative score shows the mutation decreases the protein stability (http://mupro.proteomics.ics.uci.edu/ accessed on 20th April 2015). SNP&GO (Single nucleotide polymorphism and GO terms, http://snps.biofold.org/snps-and-go

accessed on 20th April 2015). SIFT (Sorting Intolerant from Tolerant, http://sift.jcvi.org accessed 20th April 2015) are algorithms which predict whether an amino acid substitution will affect protein function based on sequence homology and the physical properties of amino acids. A SIFT score of less than 0.05 is predicted to be deleterious. A substitution with a score greater than or equal to 0.05 is predicted to be tolerated (http://www.exeterlaboratory.com/molecular-genetics/). Provean (http://provean.jcvi.org/about.php) accessed on 27th January 2015) has the default threshold of −2.5 that means if the score of a variant is equal or below this threshold then the mutation is said to be deleterious and if the threshold is above −2.5, the score of variant is said to have neutral effects. Protein accession numbers were provided by Uniprot (Universal Protein Resource, http://www.uniprot.org/) and wild type color fasta sequence was first accessed (http://pga.gs.washington.edu/data/fga/fga.Colorfasta.html) on 27th January 2015 and later on 20th April 2015.

Structural analysis of novel missense mutations using molecular modeling

Among the six reported novel missense mutations from this study, four mutations were located in an area of the alpha chain that has no resolved crystal/NMR-based structure (Nuclear magnetic Resonance). Thus, to assess the putative structural effect of these mutations, we modeled this region on the ITASSER (Iterative Threading ASSEmbly Refinement) threading modeling server (http://zhanglab.ccmb.med.umich.edu/I-TASSER/; accessed on 12th November 2014). The model for this region was then joined to the remaining beta chain for which the structure has already been determined and submitted in the protein structure database (PDB file ID: 3GHG; 2.9 Å resolution). Model joining was performed by replacing the last two amino acid residues common to the model and the crystal structure (PDB file ID: 3GHG; chain A) (PDB: Protein Data Base, ID: Identity, 3ghg is a 4-character unique identifier of every entry in the Protein Data Bank) downloaded from the protein structure database (http://rcsb.org/pdb/home/home.do;) accessed 20th November 2014) to maintain the dihedral angles for the full model at the point of joining the same. The complete model was refined by a short solvated simulation lasting 500 ps as described in Krieger et al., 2004 (Force field: Yamber3, periodic boundary conditions, temperature: 298 K, water density: 0.997 g/L, pH: 7.4). The local neighborhood of the wild type residue corresponding to the reported mutation was investigated to establish a logical hypothesis for the effect of the mutation. An additional one missense mutations (p.Trp432Arg) in the beta chain lies on the structurally resolved region of the PDB file 3GHG; chain B). Similarly the local molecular environment for this wild-type residue was also inspected. All structural analysis and image rendering were performed with YASARA (Yet Another Scientific Artificial Reality Application) version 12.8.6 (www.yasara.org/).

Results

Mutations were identified in all 13 patients. The major bulk of identified mutations is present in *FGA* gene which tends to be the most frequently occurring mutation site in our study population. Ten patients who have mutations in *FGA* gene are individual unrelated probands.

Mutations in *FGB* gene are less frequent as compared to *FGA*.

In *FGA* gene, eight mutations were identified as novel and the remaining two were reported mutations. Eight novel mutations include five missense, one nonsense and two frameshift mutations including homozygous and a compound heterozygous frameshift mutation. The two nonsense mutations in *FGA* are reported in literature. There is one more mutation with reported status in proband (C3). This patient had compound heterozygous mutation with frameshift as novel mutation and nonsense as reported.

We identified three mutations in *FGB* including one novel missense mutation (C9) and two homozygous nonsense mutations reported in siblings.

The *FGG* gene mutations are the rarest of all three fibrinogen genes. We detected three novel mutations including two similar nonsense mutations in siblings and one frameshift mutation in unrelated proband in different exons of *FGG* gene (Table 1).

All patients had markedly absent fibrinogen levels (0 g/l) and prolonged PT >120 s and APTT >180 s (Table 2).

Structural analysis of novel missense mutations using molecular modeling

A) alpha chain missense mutations

All four novel missense mutations from the α-chain reported in this study were present in a region (residues 220–860) of the α-chain, which had no resolved/known crystal structure. The region surrounding the reported mutations (residues 300–400) was relatively poorly conserved with most of it missing from some fibrinogen homologues.

Among the mutated residues, p.Pro302 was present in all homologues, which contained this part. The p.Ser325 residue was also conserved in all homologues with the exception of *Musmusculus,* where it was substituted by an Asn. The two Thr residues, p.Thr302 and p.Thr331, were relatively variable and substituted by Ser or Asp in a few homologues. Only in the homologue from *Canis lupus familiaris* was one of the Thr residues (p.Thr302) observed to be substituted by an Ala residue, which has been reported as a mutated residue for both Thr

Table 1 Genotypic expression of mutations in fibrinogen gene (*FGA, FGB & FGG*)

IP #	Gene	Exon	Mutation	Amino Acid change	Zygosity	Mutation type	Reported/Novel
C1	***FGA***	1	c.24C > A	p.Cys8[a]	Homozygous	Nonsense	Ref [23] €
C2		2	c.143_144 del AA	p.Lys(AAA)48Arg fs9[a]	Compound Heterozygous	Frame shift	Novel mutation
C3		5	c.846delG	p.Gln282Thr fsx83[a]	Compound Heterozygous	Frame shift	Novel mutation
		4	c.385C > T	p.Arg129[a]	Homozygous	Nonsense	Ref [24] €
C4		4	c.385 C > T	p.Arg129[a]	Homozygous	Nonsense	Ref [24] €
C5		5	c.598C > T	p.Gln183[a]	Homozygous	Nonsense	Novel mutation
C6		5	c.904C > G	p.Pro302Ala	Homozygous	Missense	Novel mutation
C7		5	c.913A > G	p.Thr 305 Ala	Homozygous	Missense	Novel mutation
C8		5	c.992A > G	p.Thr331Ala	Homozygous	Missense	Novel mutation
C9		5	c.992A > G	p.Thr331Ala	Homozygous	Missense	Novel mutation
C10		5	c.974A > G	p.Ser325Gly	Homozygous	Missense	Novel mutation
C11A	***FGB***	2	c.141 > T	p.Arg47[a]	Homozygous	Nonsense	Ref [25] €
C11B		2	c.141C > T	p.Arg47[a]	Homozygous	Nonsense	Ref [25] €
C9		8	c.1294 T > A	p.Trp 432Arg	Homozygous	Missense	Novel mutation
C12	***FGG***	2	c.120_126dupTTCTTCA	TTCTTCA	Homozygous	Frame shift	Novel mutation
C13A		4	c.361A > T	p.Lys121[a]	Homozygous	Nonsense	Novel mutation
C13B		4	c.361A > T	Lys121[a]	Homozygous	Nonsense	Novel mutation

Identified novel and reported mutations in three genes of fibrinogen. The letter A and B with patient code designate the sibling status. € (reported mutation,) c (complimentary deoxyribonucleic acid), A (adenine), T (thymine), C (cytosine), G (guanine), Lys (lysine), Arg (arginine), Tyr (tyrosine), Pro (proline), Trp (tryptophan), Thr (threonine), Gln (glycine), Cys = cystine, fs = frame shift, [a] stop codon number, *FGA* (fibrinogen Aα-chain gene), *FGB* (fibrinogen Bβ-chain gene), *FGG* (fibrinogen Gγ-chain gene

Table 2 Assessment of coagulation markers and bleeding scores with consanguinity/ethnicity

IP#	Fibrinogen Level (g/l)	Thrombin Time (Sec)	Prothrombin Time (Sec)	Activated partial thromboplastin Time (aPTT)(Sec)	Bleeding Score	Consanguinity	Interfamilial Relation	Ethnic Origin
C1	0.01	23	>120	>180	20	positive	Unrelated	Urdu Speaking
C2	0.02	24	>120	>180	21	positive	Unrelated	Punjabi
C3	0	33	>120	>180	22	positive	Unrelated	Punjabi
C4	0.1	24	>120	>180	17	positive	Unrelated	Urdu Speaking
C5	0.02	31	>120	>180	20	positive	Unrelated	Sindhi
C6	0.01	25	>120	>180	20	positive	Unrelated	Urdu speaking
C7	0.02	29	>120	>180	22	positive	Unrelated	Sindhi
C8	0.0	30	>120	>180	20	positive	Unrelated	Sindhi
C9	0.0	32	>120	>180	22	positive	Unrelated	Punjabi
C10	0.01	25	>120	>180	16	positive	Unrelated	Punjabi
C11A	0.02	28	>120	>180	18	positive	**	Punjabi
C11B	0.01	24	>120	>180	16	positive		Punjabi
C12	0.0	30	>120	>180	21	positive	Unrelated	Punjabi
C13	0.01	24	>120	>180	20	positive	Unrelated	Punjabi
C14	0.0	26	>120	>180	21	positive	Unrelated	Punjabi
C15A	0.02	24	>120	>180	20	positive	**	Punjabi
C15B	0.01	25	>120	>180	21	positive		Punjabi

Shows the individual test values of PT, aPTT and fibrinogen (Claus Method), consanguinity and the relationship status. Bleeding score calculated, Tosetto et al. [26]. ** Siblings, *NA* not available, *s* (seconds). The fibrinogen levels in all patients were found to be equal to or lower than 0.1 g/l (Normal Range 2-4 g/dl), PT more than 120 s (Normal Range 9–11 s) aPTT more than 180 s (Normal Range 24–27 s) and prolonged thrombin time (normal range 10–13 s). Ethnicity explains the frequency of majorly affected, thickly populated and largest province of Pakistan (Punjab) residues in our study. Modeling of this region showed that this region could be split into two central cores, each of which is organized as a beta sheet surrounded by flexible coils (Fig. 1). The two cores are connected by a central long helix. The first core, apart from being surrounded by flexible coils, also contains a few short helices. Three of the four reported mutated residues were located on these short helices with the exception that p.Ser325 is located on a short loop connecting one of the short helices to the central core. The residues p.Pro302, p.Thr305 and p.Thr331 are partially buried, with the p.Pro302 and p.Thr305 side chains oriented toward the central core beta sheets. The residues p.Pro302 and p.Thr305 participate in intra-helical hydrogen bonds with each other and with p.Ser399 and p.Arg308, respectively. The residue p.Thr331 lies at the edge of a short helix and also participates in intra-helical hydrogen bonding (p.Gly327). Interestingly, within the fold on which all four of these mutations reside, lysine residue p.Lys322 is known to be cross-linked to ∝ – 2 antiplasmin proteins and a glutamine residue, p.Gln347, which participates in inter-chain cross-links during clot formation.

B) Beta chain missense mutations

The one novel missense mutations (p.Trp432Arg) reported in the chain occurs in a highly conserved region. (Fig. 2).

The residues are completely conserved in homologues that have been used for the present alignment. The p.Trp432 residue lies completely in the densely packed hydrophobic core of the C-terminal region of chain. This densely packed hydrophobic core consists of a number of other aromatic acids, which are in close proximity to p.Trp432 (p.His400 and p.His438, p.Trp433 and p.Tyr434). The p.Trp432 residue hydrogen bond contacts with p.Tyr434 and p.Ser406.

Pathogenecity score

Pathogenecity scoring of six novel missense mutations identified in *FGA* and *FGB* was done on five different pathogenicity scoring software (Table 3). Out of five missense mutations of *FGA*, two mutations were found to have damaging effect and decreased protein stability calculated by two different softwares (MUPRO and Provean). Other software didn't show the deleterious effect for the same two mutations identified in two unrelated proband. In *FGB* gene the missense mutation was found to be damaging or deleterious and showed decreased structure stability. The damaging effect and lack of protein stability in structure may lead to the bleeding manifestations in patients which can vary from mild to severe bleeding.

Discussion

Fibrinogen deficiency is a rare inherited bleeding disorder that is characterized by two subtypes of either reduced or completely absent levels of fibrinogen in the blood [18]. *FGA* is documented as the most affected gene in literature [19, 20]. We have found the larger chunk of mutations in *FGA* gene in our set of data. A total of 169 mutations in fibrinogen are reported on the Human Gene Mutation Database (http://www.hgmd.cf.ac.uk/ac/index.php) date accessed August 12, 2014). Consanguinity involving

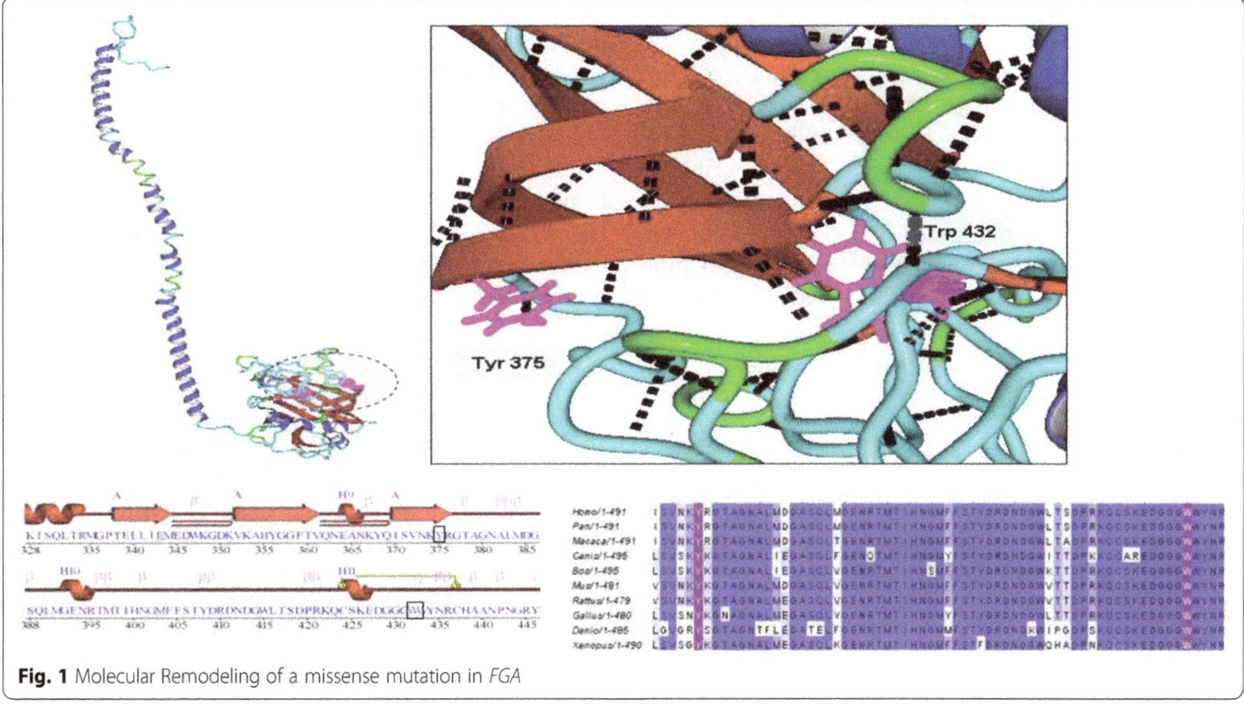

Fig. 1 Molecular Remodeling of a missense mutation in *FGA*

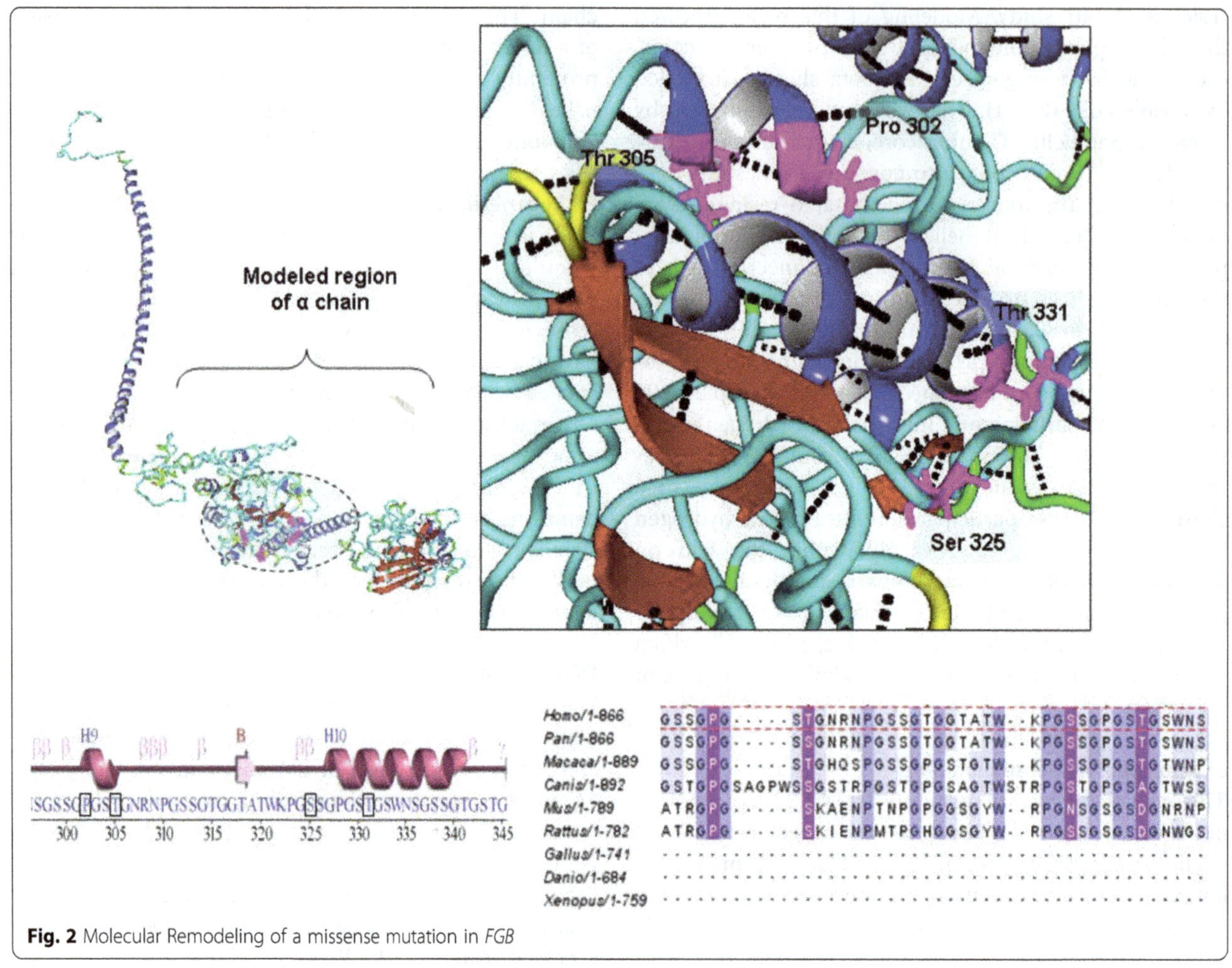

Fig. 2 Molecular Remodeling of a missense mutation in *FGB*

first and second cousin marriages is accelerating the spread of disease in areas such as Pakistan, Iran, the Middle East, China and the far Middle East, including Turkey, in societies where consanguinity is frequent. The spectrum of causative mutations for afibrinogenemia is interesting as *FGA* appears to stand out from the two other fibrinogen genes [21]. The predominant inheritance pattern was homozygous with a high proportion of nonsense mutations followed by missense mutations in our study results. A frame shift mutation (p.Glu262AspfsX158) in FGA exon 5 reported in one study is predicted as truncated polypeptide. It is associated with exceptionally long stretch of abnormal residues in homozygous patient with congenital afibrinogenemia [22]. Frameshift mutation (p.Gln282Thr fsx83*) and (p. Lys (AAA) 48Arg fs9*) are the novel compound heterozygous mutations which have manifested deletions along with frameshift defects. The

Table 3 Pathogenicity score of missense mutations

Missense Mutations	Polyphen- 2		Provean		MUpro		SNP&GO		Sift	
	Score	prediction	Score	prediction	SVM score	Protein structure stability	Score	Prediction	Score	Prediction
p.Pro302Ala	0.028	Benign	−4.257	Deleterious	−0.797	Decrease stability	(0.4)	Neutral	0.00	Benign
p.Thr 305 Ala	0.00	Benign	−0.387	Neutral	0.134	Increase stability	(0.05)	Neutral	0.00	Benign
p.Thr331Ala	0.025	Benign	−1.100	Neutral	0.122	Increase stability	(0.03)	Neutral	0.00	Benign
p.Thr331Ala	0.025	Benign	−1.100	Neutral	0.122	Increase stability	(0.03)	Neutral	0.00	Benign
p.Ser325Gly	0.014	Benign	−2.331	Neutral	−0.063	Decrease stability	(0.1)	Neutral	0.00	Benign
p.Trp 432Arg	1.00	Damaging	−12.18	Deleterious	−0.411	Decrease stability	(0.8)	Disease	Na	Na

Pathogenecity of missense mutations was calculated by five different softwares to check for the protein structure stability and deleterious effects. *Na* not available

bleeding phenotype is severe as these mutations worsen the symptoms due to combined effect of compound mutation and truncation of polypeptide chain.

Three missense mutations (Pro302Ala, Thr305Ala and Thr331Ala) in the alpha chain reside on short helices surrounding a central beta sheet core. All these mutations are non-conservative in nature, i.e., the Pro302Ala substitution results in the replacement of a rigid imino group with a smaller, more flexible residue, and the Thr305Ala and Thr302Ala substitutions result in the replacement of polar side chains by smaller but hydrophobic side chains. In addition, the introduction of alanine in these regions will most likely disrupt some of the intra-helical hydrogen bonds, thereby breaking the helical structure surrounding the central core. Because these short helices provide order and stability around an otherwise disordered coiled-coil region, their disruption might result in a loss of stability for this region and the alpha chain. The third mutation in this chain, Ser325Gly, is also non-conservative, i.e., it results in the substitution of a polar residue to a very small and flexible Gly residue. Because the wild-type residue already lies on the flexible loop, the introduction of a small residue will make this region more disordered and therefore unstable. Moreover, because all four missense mutations belong to a fold of the alpha chain that might be interacting with Factor XIII (this fold also contains the Lys and Gln residues that participate in interchain cross linking and cross linking to alpha 2- antiplasmin), conformational changes induced by these mutations on this fold might interfere with the interaction of fibrinogen alpha chain with Factor XIII. The one beta chain missense mutation resides on a highly conserved region of the beta chain, most likely because many of the residues of this region contribute to the stability of its densely packed hydrophobic core. The p.Trp432Arg substitution occurs in the middle of the hydrophobic core. The introduction of a large polar, positively charged residue instead of a hydrophobic aromatic one would destabilize the hydrophobic core of this region. Thus, the mutation affects the stability of the beta chain by disrupting its C-terminal hydrophobic core.

Conclusions

Rare inherited bleeding disorder specifically congenital afibrinogenemia has a growing incidence especially in regions like Pakistan where consanguinity factor is strongly present. Our study is purely based on Pakistani patients of congenital afibrinogenemia. It has shown the frequently affected gene *FGA* in our set of patients. We have documented the pathogenicity scores for missense mutations as a description for protein molecule stability and functional defects. We have also performed molecular modeling to see the structural defects and damages and their impact on the clinical manifestation of patients. In this way the genotype well correlated with phenotype of these patients.

Abbreviations

Ala: Alanine; ALT: Alanine transaminase; Anti-HCV: Anti hepatitis C antibodies; aPTT: Activated partial thromboplastin time; Arg: Arginine; Asn: Asparagine; AST: Aspartate transaminase; C score: Confidence score; EDTA: Ethylenediaminetetraacetic acid; FGA: Fibrinogen gene alpha; FGB: Fibrinogen gene beta; FGG: Fibrinogen gene gamma; HBsAG: Hepatitis B surface antigen; HIV: Human immunodeficiency virus; ITASSER: Iterative threading assembly refinement; KDa: Kilo daltons; Poly-phen2: Polymorphism phenotyping v2; Pro: Proline; Provean: Protein variation effect analyzer; PT: Prothrombin time; SIFT: Sorting intolerant from tolerant; SNP: Single nucleotide polymorphism; SNP&GO: Single nucleotide polymorphism and GO terms; SVM: Support vector machine; Trp: Tryptophan; TT: Thrombin time; UniProt: Universal protein resource; YASARA: Yet another scientific artificial reality application

Acknowledgements

We thank all the patients and their families who participated in this study. We acknowledge Marguerite Neerman-Arbez (Professor, Department of Genetic Medicine and Development University Medical Centre) Switzerland for generously providing primer sequences and help with validation of the results. We would also like to acknowledge the contribution of Dr. Philipe de Moerloose (Hôpitaux Universitaires de Genève HUG) for their unconditional support in establishing the technique. We would like to thank Dr.Shahla Tariq and Dr. Ayisha Imran from Chughtai's Lab, Lahore for their contribution in providing samples for this study.

Funding

This entire project had been funded by Novo Nordisk Hemophilia Foundation (NNHF) as PK-4 funding. All expenditures inclusive of collection of samples till their processing and sequencing were carried out under the PK-4 funding. The processing of all samples from CBC, DNA extraction, PCR and Direct sequencing was conducted in our institution under PK4 project.

We sent extracted DNAs of four samples to University of Geneva, Switzerland, for sequencing and validated their results and interpretations in our institution as well and the entire portion of molecular modeling was done in Bonn, Germany. The manuscript writing, Study design and interpretation of the data were completely independent of the role of funding body and done without any monetary expenditure.

Consent

All participant/guardians in case of minors has given their consent by signing the consent forms in English and local language after proper explanation of the procedure and purpose.

Authors' contributions

AN designed and supervised the research.

AB reviewed the data, performed molecular remodeling and edited the text.

TNK wrote the paper and analyzed the samples.

AG reviewed the paper, edited the text and contributed to the mutation nomenclature and other necessary changes in the text.

NA provides samples from the Children's Hospital Lahore.

NS Helped in making diagnosis and sample collection from the Children's Hospital Lahore.

SA DNA extraction, PCR and gene sequencing of samples. Result analyses.

IDU reviewed paper.

TSS project approval and secured funding for this study.

JO Supported in establishing the technique and validation of results along with data review. All authors read and approved the final manuscript

Competing interests
The authors declare that they have no competing interests.

Author details
[1]National Institute of Blood Diseases and Bone Marrow Transplantation, Karachi University of Bonn, ST 2/A, Block-17, Gulshan-e-Iqbal KDA scheme, 24, Karachi, Pakistan. [2]Institute of Experimental Hematology and Transfusion Medicine, Bonn, Germany. [3]University of Shieffield, Shiefield, United Kingdom. [4]Children's Hospital, Resident, Paediatric hematology, Main Ferozpur Road, Lahore, Pakistan. [5]Liaquat university of medical and health sciences, Jamshoro, Pakistan. [6]Institute of Experimental Hematology and Transfusion Medicine, AG, FXIII Room No. 2.308 Sigmund Freud Street-25, 53127 Bonn, Germany. [7]National Institute of blood diseases and bone marrow transplantation, ST 2/A, Block-17, Gulshan-e-Iqbal KDA scheme, 24, Karachi, Pakistan. [8]Clinical Scientist and Professor of Molecular Medicine, Sheffield Diagnostic Genetics Service, Sheffield Children's NHS Foundation Trust, Western Bank, Sheffield S10 2TH, UK. [9]Institute of Experimental Hematology and Transfusion Medicine, Sigmund Freud Street-25, 53127 Bonn, Germany.

References

1. Peyvandi F, Haertel S, Knaub S, Mannucci P. Incidence of bleeding symptoms in 100 patients with inherited afibrinogenemia or hypofibrinogenemia. Journal of Thrombosis and Haemostasis. 2006;4:1634–7.
2. Acharya S, Dimichele D. Rare inherited disorders of fibrinogen. Haemophilia. 2008;14:1151–8.
3. Neerman-Arbez M, De Moerloose P, Bridel C, Honsberger A, Sconborner A, Rossier C, Peerlinck K, Claeyssens S, Di Michele D, D'oiron R, Dreyfus M, Laubriat-Bianchin M, Dieval J, Antonarakis SE, Morris MA. Mutations in the fibrinogen Aa gene account for the majority of cases of congenital afibrinogenemia. Blood. 2000;96:149–52.
4. Janciauskiene S, Welte T, Mahadev R. Acute Phase Proteins: Structure and Function Relationship. Acute Phase Proteins - Regulation and Functions of Acute Phase Proteins. 2011;.
5. Neerman-Arbez M, De Moerloose P, Honsberger A, Parlier G, Arnuti B, Biron C, Borg J, Eber S, Meili E, Peter-Salonen K, Ripoll L, Vervel C, d'Oiron R, Staeger P, Antonarakis SE, Morris MA. Molecular analysis of the fibrinogen gene cluster in 16 patients with congenital afibrinogenemia: novel truncating mutations in the FGA and FGG genes. Human genetics. 2001; 108:237–40.
6. Anwar M, Iqbal H, Gul M, Saeed N, Ayyub M. Congenital afibrinogenemia: report of three cases. Journal of Thrombosis and Haemostasis. 2005;3:407–9.
7. Neerman-Arbez M, De Moerloose P. Mutations in the fibrinogen gene cluster accounting for congenital afibrinogenemia: an update and report of 10 novel mutations. Human Mutation. 2007;28:540–53.
8. Asselta R, Duga S, Tenchini M. The molecular basis of quantitative fibrinogen disorders. Journal of Thrombosis and Haemostasis. 2006;4:2115–29.
9. Grieninger G, Lu X, Cao Y, Fu Y, Kudryk BJ, Galanakis DK, Hertzberg KM. Fib420, the novel fibrinogen subclass: newborn levels are higher than adult. Blood. 1997;90:2609–14.
10. Fang Y, DAI B, WANG X, FU Q, Dai J, Xie F, CAI X, WANG H, WANG Z. Identification of three FGA mutations in two Chinese families with congenital afibrinogenaemia. Haemophilia. 2006;12:615–20.
11. Asselta R, Duga S, Simonic T, Malcovati M, Santagostino E, Giangr EP, Mannucci P, Tenchini M. Afibrinogenemia: first identification of a splicing mutation in the fibrinogen gamma chain gene leading to a major gamma chain truncation. Blood. 2000;96:2496–500.
12. Casini A, Neerman-Arbez M, Ariëns R, de Moerloose P. Dysfibrinogenemia: from molecular anomalies to clinical manifestations and management. Journal of Thrombosis and Haemostasis. 2015;13(6):909–19.
13. Asselta R, Spena S, Duga S, Peyv IF, Malcovati M, Mannucci P, Tenchini M. Analysis of Iranian patients allowed the identification of the first truncating mutation in the fibrinogen Bbeta-chain gene causing afibrinogenemia. Haematologica. 2002;87:855–9.
14. Wu S, Wang Z, Dong N, Bai X, Ruan C. A novel nonsense mutation in the FGA gene in a Chinese family with congenital afibrinogenaemia. Blood coagulation & fibrinolysis. 2005;16(3):221–6.
15. Sumitha E, Jayandharan G, Arora N, Abraham A, David S, Devi GS, Shenbagapriya P, Nair SC, George B, Mathews V, Chandy M, Viswabandya A, Srivastava A. Molecular basis of quantitative fibrinogen disorders in 27 patients from India. Haemophilia. 2013;19:611–8.
16. Tyrrell DAJ. Polymerase Chain Reaction. BMJ. 1997;314(7073):5–5.
17. Sanger Sequencing Method | Thermo Fisher Scientific [Internet]. Thermofisher.com. 2017 [cited 2 Febuary 2017]. Available from: https://www.thermofisher.com/pk/en/home/lifescience/sequencing/sanger-sequencing/sanger_sequencing_method.html
18. Korte W, Poon M, Iorio A, Makris M. Thrombosis in Inherited Fibrinogen Disorders. Transfusion Medicine and Hemotherapy. 2017;44(2):70–6.
19. Neerman-Arbez M. Prenatal diagnosis for congenital afibrinogenemia caused by a novel nonsense mutation in the FGB gene in a Palestinian family. Blood. 2003;101(9):3492–4.
20. VU D, NEERMAN-ARBEZ M. Molecular mechanisms accounting for fibrinogen deficiency: from large deletions to intracellular retention of misfolded proteins. Journal of Thrombosis and Haemostasis. 2007;5:125–31.
21. Robert-Ebadi H, De Moerloose P, El Khorassani M, El Khattab M, Neerman-Arbez M. A novel frameshift mutation in FGA accounting for congenital afibrinogenemia predicted to encode an aberrant peptide terminating 158 amino acids downstream. Blood Coagulation & Fibrinolysis. 2009;20(5):385–7.
22. Levrat E, Aboukhamis I, de Moerloose P, Farho J, Chamaa S, Reber G, et al. A novel frameshift mutation in FGA (c.1846 del A) leading to congenital afibrinogenemia in a consanguineous Syrian family. Blood Coagulation & Fibrinolysis. 2011;22(2):148–50.
23. Asselta R, Platè M, Robusto M, Borhany M, Guella I, Soldà G, et al. Clinical and molecular characterisation of 21 patients affected by quantitative fibrinogen deficiency. Thrombosis and Haemostasis. 2014;113(3):567–76.
24. Palermo P, Barbados B, Asselta R, Duga S, Tenchini M. The molecular basis of quantitative fibrinogen disorders. Journal of Thrombosis and Haemostasis. 2006;4:2115–29.
25. Sheen C, Brennan S, Jabado N, George P. Fibrinogen Montreal: a novel missense mutation (A alpha D496N) associated with hypofibrinogenemia. Thrombosis and haemostasis. 2006;96:231–2.
26. Tosetto A, Rodeghiero F, Castaman G, Goodeve A, Federici A, Batlle J, Meyer D, Fressinaud E, Mazurier C, Goudemand J, Eikenboom J, Schneppenheim R, Budde U, Ingerslev J, Vorlova Z, Habart D, Holmberg L, Lethagen S, Pasi J, Hill F, Peake I. A quantitative analysis of bleeding symptoms in type 1 von Willebrand disease: results from a multicenter European study (MCMDM-1 VWD). J Thromb Haemost. 2006;4:766–73.

13

Pathways for outpatient management of venous thromboembolism

Robin Condliffe

Abstract

It has become widely recognised that outpatient treatment may be suitable for many patients with venous thromboembolism. In addition, non-vitamin K antagonist oral anticoagulants that have been approved over the last few years have the potential to be an integral component of the outpatient care pathway, owing to their oral route of administration, lack of requirement for routine anticoagulation monitoring and simple dosing regimens.

A robust pathway for outpatient care is also vital; one such pathway has been developed at Sheffield Teaching Hospitals in the UK. This paper describes the pathway and the arguments in its favour as an example of best practice and value offered to patients with venous thromboembolism.

The pathway has two branches (one for deep vein thrombosis and one for pulmonary embolism), each with the same five-step process for outpatient treatment. Both begin from the point that the patient presents (in the Emergency Department, Thrombosis Clinic or general practitioner's office), followed by diagnosis, risk stratification, treatment choice and, finally, follow-up.

The advantages of these pathways are that they offer clear, evidence-based guidance for the identification, diagnosis and treatment of patients who can safely be treated in the outpatient setting, and provide a detailed, stepwise process that can be easily adapted to suit the needs of other institutions. The approach is likely to result in both healthcare and economic benefits, including increased patient satisfaction and shorter hospital stays.

Keywords: Deep vein thrombosis, Oral anticoagulant, Patient pathway, Pulmonary embolism, Venous thromboembolism

Background

Historically, patients diagnosed with deep vein thrombosis (DVT) and pulmonary embolism (PE) have been treated as inpatients owing to the potential for serious complications, including death. In recent years it has been recognised that many patients with acute DVT may be safely treated in the outpatient setting. Furthermore, it is possible to identify patients with acute PE who are at low risk of deterioration and may also be suitable for ambulatory management or early discharge [1–4].

Appropriate outpatient management of DVT and PE may be beneficial to patients and the healthcare system alike. Potential benefits include improvements in patient satisfaction and reduced healthcare costs associated with a shorter hospital stay. Limited data are available to compare these outcomes and further research is needed [5]. Non-vitamin K antagonist (VKA) oral anticoagulant (NOAC) therapy may provide benefits for patient management in ambulatory care compared with low molecular weight heparin (LMWH) overlapping with, and followed by, a VKA [6]. NOAC therapy involves oral administration, no routine coagulation monitoring requirements, a single-drug approach (with rivaroxaban and apixaban) and fewer follow-up appointments [6].

One potential disadvantage of ambulatory care is that opportunities for follow-up, patient education and communication between primary and secondary care may be lost if a patient is discharged from hospital without an adequate protocol in place. Healthcare professionals (HCPs) at Sheffield Teaching Hospitals have developed a patient pathway for venous thromboembolism (VTE) management to improve the transition of patients from hospital to home. This pathway has proved effective in ensuring adequate follow-up and communication between all HCPs involved. The development of such a

Correspondence: Robin.Condliffe@sth.nhs.uk
Pulmonary Vascular Disease Unit, Sheffield Teaching Hospitals NHS Foundation Trust, Sheffield, UK

pathway can also help streamline processes and clinical decision-making, improving efficiency and ensuring consistent high-quality care. This article presents the Sheffield VTE management pathways for DVT and PE as examples of best practice, demonstrating their value in VTE management, and discusses the benefits of NOAC use in ambulatory care.

Venous thromboembolism management

In the UK, the management of DVT varies widely. A recent UK audit reported a lack of coordinated services in this area and called for standardised and consistent protocols [7]. The Sheffield pathway is an evidence-based pathway, developed by the whole VTE management team, in which low-risk patients may be treated in an ambulatory care setting, while patients at higher risk are admitted to hospital. This approach also reduces the associated burden on healthcare resources and patients' time. A treatment pathway also provides clarity in an area with a large choice of diagnostic tools, an increasing number of treatment options and various forms of presentation (e.g. provoked or unprovoked, mild, moderate or severe symptoms). In the past, many hospitals had an uncoordinated VTE management strategy with a range of diagnostic assessment, treatment, and patient follow-up pathways, depending on which department the patient presented to [8, 9]. Optimal VTE management includes rapid assessment, diagnosis and treatment; patient information and support; and follow-up. Follow-up allows clinical improvement to be confirmed, chronic complications to be monitored and an optimal anticoagulation approach to be planned.

The Sheffield venous thromboembolism management pathway: deep vein thrombosis

Typically, a patient may enter the Sheffield DVT pathway in one of three ways. A patient may: 1) present directly to the Emergency Department and be transferred to the Thrombosis Clinic (open during working hours); 2) visit their general practitioner and be referred to the Thrombosis Clinic/Emergency Department; or 3) present as an inpatient (e.g. in the instance of a post-operative venous thromboembolic event). These three entry levels involve contact with several hospital HCPs, including nurses, VTE specialist nurses, junior doctors, pharmacists and consultants (collectively, the multidisciplinary team [MDT]). The type of VTE diagnosed and the patient's medical history determine which members of the MDT are involved in each individual patient pathway, including longer-term follow-up.

Step 1: Patient presentation

When a patient presents with suspected DVT, a general medical history and physical examination will be conducted; if DVT is considered likely, the patient will enter the DVT pathway (Fig. 1). If a specialist nurse in the Thrombosis Clinic is not available, an Emergency Department physician will assess the patient.

Step 2: Diagnosis in the thrombosis clinic (or by emergency department physician)

The validated two-level DVT Wells' score indicates whether a DVT is likely or unlikely based on the patients clinical signs, symptoms and through exclusion of other causes [10]. A score of ≥2 indicates that DVT is likely; a score of ≤1 indicates that DVT is unlikely (Table 1) [10]. The likelihood of DVT can be further determined by a blood test for D-dimer, a degradation product of a blood clot. D-dimer levels are typically elevated in patients with an acute VTE [11]. However, a negative D-dimer result is more clinically important in order to 'rule out' DVT, because a positive result can arise in conditions other than DVT [11].

If DVT is considered a likely diagnosis, the patient will be sent for an ultrasound scan, preferably on the same day. If the ultrasound scan is scheduled for the following day or after a weekend, immediate anticoagulation with a LMWH injection is administered.

Step 3: Risk stratification

At the point of diagnosis, and when considering DVT treatment options, each patient must be assessed for complications and frailty. This may determine the treatment type, level of observation required and whether treatment can be safely administered at home. Most DVT cases can be managed safely at home, but for certain patients, for example if the event is post-operative or if the patient is at high risk of falling, a hospital stay may be required. Certain patients with proximal iliofemoral DVT may be candidates for catheter-directed thrombolysis. Risk of bleeding events within the first 3–6 months of

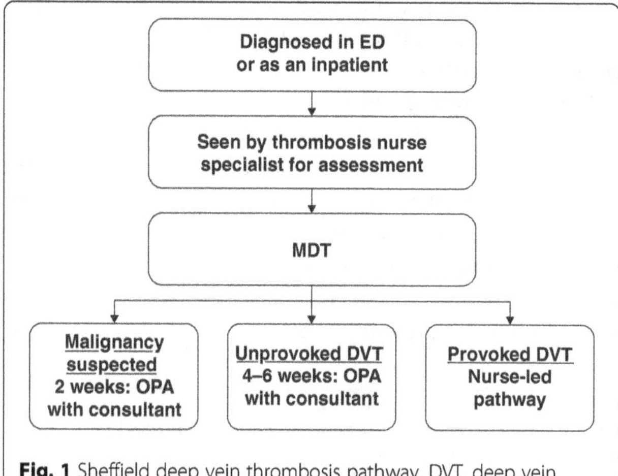

Fig. 1 Sheffield deep vein thrombosis pathway. DVT, deep vein thrombosis; ED, Emergency Department; MDT, multidisciplinary team; OPA, outpatient appointment

Table 1 Deep vein thrombosis Wells' score [10]

Criteria	Points
Active cancer	+1
Paralysis, paresis or recent plaster cast of the lower limb	+1
Bedridden for 3+ days or major surgery within 12 weeks	+1
Pain/tenderness along deep vein system	+1
Swollen leg	+1
Calf swelling >3 cm more than asymptomatic leg	+1
Pitting oedema in symptomatic leg only	+1
Collateral superficial veins	+1
History of DVT	+1
Alternative cause is considered at least as likely as DVT	−2
Outcome:	
DVT unlikely:	Score ≤1 (consider trauma, cellulitis)
DVT likely:	Score ≥2

DVT deep vein thrombosis

anticoagulation may be assessed using the HAS-BLED (Hypertension, Abnormal renal and liver function, Stroke, Bleeding, Labile international normalised ratios, Elderly, Drugs or alcohol) [12] or the RIETE (based on recent major bleeding, creatinine >1.2 mg/mL, anaemia, cancer, clinically overt PE and age >75 years) risk scores [13]. The HAS-BLED score was derived from patients receiving anticoagulation for atrial fibrillation. The utility of these studies in assessing early risk of bleeding is limited.

Step 4: Treatment strategy

In Sheffield, until recently, the majority of patients diagnosed with DVT were treated initially with LMWH while warfarin therapy was commenced. Patients receiving warfarin require routine coagulation monitoring to ensure that they stay within the therapeutic range, evaluated with the international normalised ratio [14]. Several other choices of anticoagulation are now available in Europe, with the NOACs apixaban, dabigatran, edoxaban and rivaroxaban approved for the treatment of acute DVT and PE [15–18]. These therapies do not require routine coagulation monitoring and have all been shown to be non-inferior to warfarin in terms of VTE recurrence [19–22].

To improve clinician familiarity and hence patient safety, we have elected to use a single NOAC for the initial treatment of VTE. In the Sheffield DVT pathway the majority of DVT cases are managed using rivaroxaban if patients have a creatinine clearance ≥30 mL/min, unless contraindicated. This oral, single-drug approach – 15 mg twice daily for the first 21 days and then 20 mg once daily for longer-term treatment – is a simple regimen that facilitates the majority of patients being treated at home [15]. Other NOACs are considered after initial anticoagulation on a case-by-case basis.

Step 5: Follow-up

An outpatient appointment with the thrombosis nurse at the Thrombosis Clinic is arranged for all patients undergoing outpatient management, approximately 21 days after the initial DVT event. This aligns with when the rivaroxaban dose, if rivaroxaban is the prescribed drug, is changed to 20 mg once daily. The patient is provided with education about their anticoagulation therapy, including the importance of adherence to treatment, warning signs for bleeding, symptoms of recurrent VTE and when to contact a HCP. The patient is also provided with a contact number for the Thrombosis Clinic if they need to access more information.

For patients with an unprovoked DVT, in which the cause of DVT is unclear, an outpatient appointment with a consultant haematologist is arranged to discuss long-term therapy. In patients for whom malignancy is suspected, an outpatient appointment is booked within 2 weeks of initial presentation to discuss options for further investigations or scans. Thrombophilia testing may also be arranged in selected patients. The initial treatment duration with rivaroxaban is 3 months, and longer-term treatment is discussed when appropriate.

The Sheffield venous thromboembolism management pathway: pulmonary embolism

Step 1: Patient presentation

Patients may present with symptoms indicative of an acute PE either to their general practitioner (leading to referral to the Emergency Department) or directly to the Emergency Department, where they enter into the PE pathway (Fig. 2).

Step 2: Diagnosis in the thrombosis clinic (or by emergency department physician)

The two-level Wells' PE score is used to determine whether PE is a likely or unlikely diagnosis [23]. The Wells' PE score – both the full and simplified versions – has been validated for use in clinical settings [24, 25]. The score includes clinical signs and symptoms of DVT, PE as the most likely diagnosis, heart rate >100 bpm, recent immobilisation or surgery, previous VTE, haemoptysis and active or previous malignancy (Table 2) [23]. If the simplified Wells' score suggests that PE is likely, the patient proceeds to diagnostic imaging, most commonly computed tomography pulmonary angiogram, with ventilation/perfusion single-photon emission computed

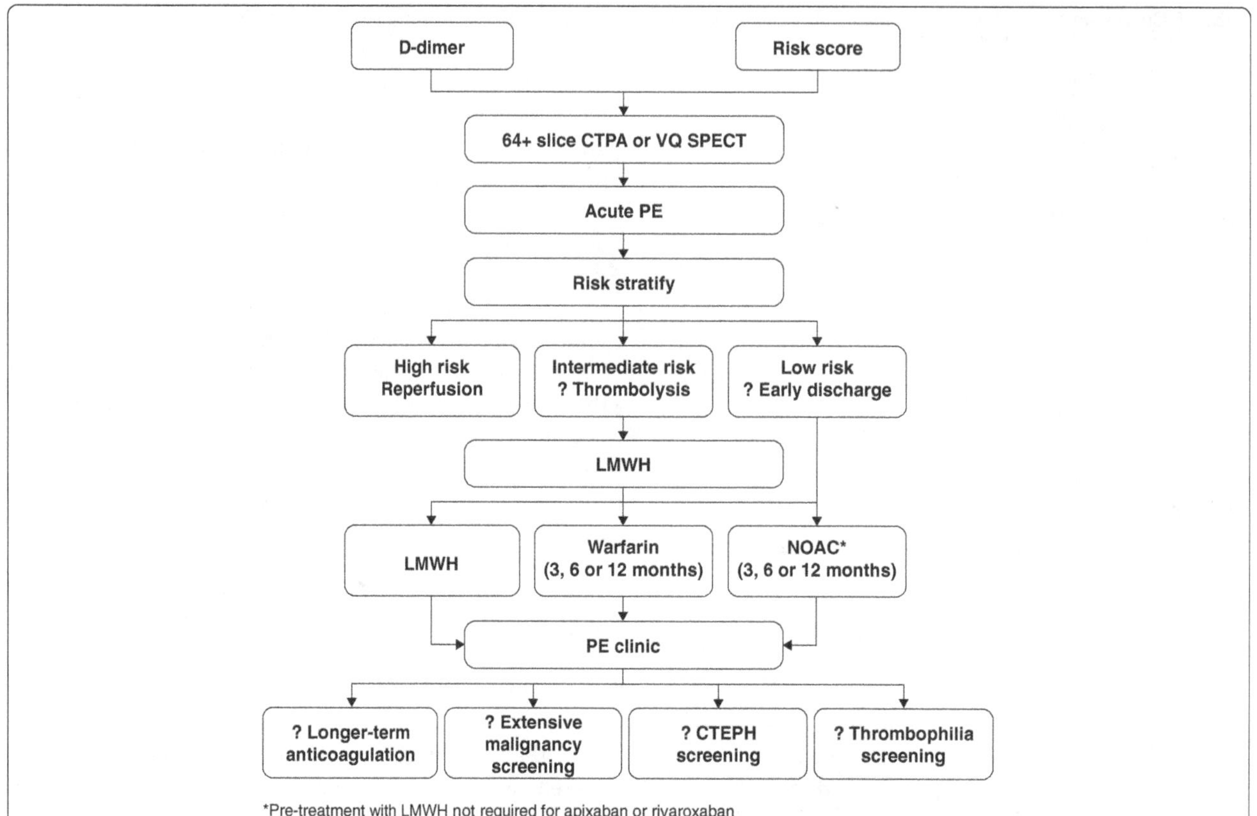

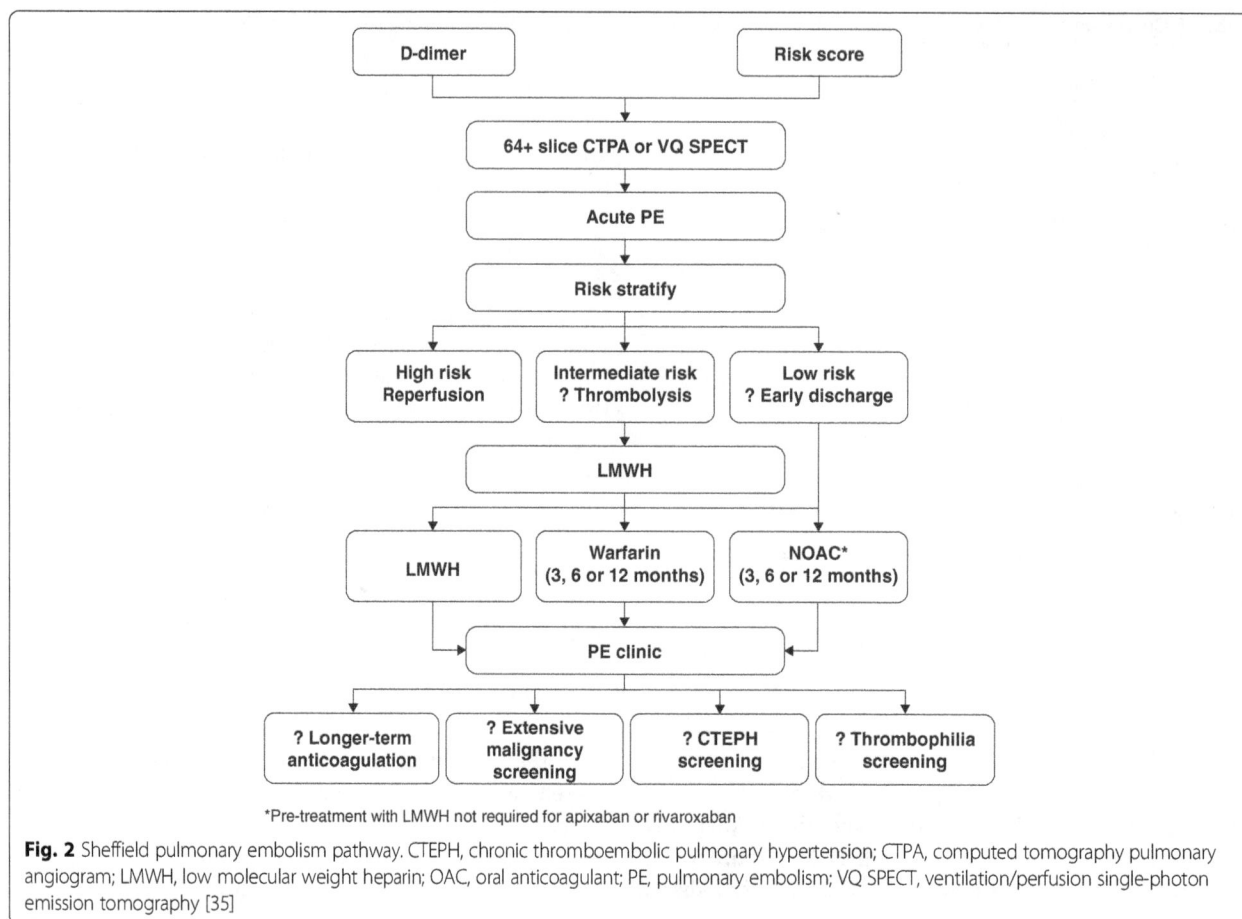

Fig. 2 Sheffield pulmonary embolism pathway. CTEPH, chronic thromboembolic pulmonary hypertension; CTPA, computed tomography pulmonary angiogram; LMWH, low molecular weight heparin; OAC, oral anticoagulant; PE, pulmonary embolism; VQ SPECT, ventilation/perfusion single-photon emission tomography [35]

Table 2 Simplified pulmonary embolism Wells' score [23, 25]

Clinical feature	Original score	Simplified score
Clinical signs and symptoms of DVT (minimum of leg swelling and pain with palpation of the deep veins)	3	1
An alternative diagnosis is less likely than PE	3	1
Heart rate ≥100 beats per minute	1.5	1
Immobilisation (for >3 days) or surgery in the previous 4 weeks	1.5	1
Previous DVT/PE	1.5	1
Haemoptysis	1	1
Active cancer	1	1
Outcome		
PE unlikely:	Score ≤4	Score 0 or 1
PE likely:	Score >4	Score ≥2

DVT deep vein thrombosis, *PE* pulmonary embolism

tomography being reserved for patients with significant renal dysfunction, contrast allergy or pregnancy. If the simplified Wells' score suggests that PE is unlikely, D-dimer levels are used to identify patients in whom diagnostic imaging is not required. Although withholding of anticoagulation in patients with levels below an age-adjusted D-dimer threshold (age in years × 10) was demonstrated to be associated with a very low risk of subsequent VTE, these data have not been validated in other populations [26]. Therefore, the current approach is to use a standard threshold of <500 ng/mL to exclude acute PE in patients with a simplified Wells' score of ≤4 [1].

Step 3: Risk stratification

Following diagnosis of acute PE, patients undergo risk assessment for early deterioration. Patients with low blood pressure (<90/60 mmHg) and/or signs of clinical shock (high-risk patients) should be considered for immediate reperfusion therapy, most commonly with systemic thrombolysis [1]. Non-high-risk patients may be further categorised into intermediate- and low-risk groups based on a combination of risk score and markers of right ventricular dysfunction and ischaemia [1].

The PESI and the sPESI are the two most validated clinical–physiological risk scoring systems (Table 3). Patients with a PESI class I–II or sPESI score of 0 are considered low risk (<3% risk of deterioration) and may be considered for outpatient management [1]. Aujesky et al. performed the largest randomised controlled trial of outpatient PE management to date and demonstrated that patients with PESI class I or II, who also did not meet certain exclusion criteria (Table 3), were not put at increased risk by early discharge [2]. If markers of right ventricular dysfunction or ischaemia (e.g. N-terminal of the prohormone brain natriuretic peptide or high-sensitivity troponin) are also negative, the risk of early PE-related deterioration is <1% [27, 28]. It is unclear whether these additional biomarkers should be a mandatory addition to the PESI or sPESI for identifying patients who can be considered for discharge. Although these additional tests may improve safety, this may be at the expense of the number of patients who would qualify for outpatient management. The HESTIA criteria provide an alternative approach to risk stratification, incorporating several clinical, practical and social issues (Table 4) [3]. The HESTIA study showed that the absence of any of these criteria could safely identify patients for outpatient management of PE [3]. On closer inspection, the HESTIA criteria are actually very similar to the exclusion criteria employed in the study by Aujesky et al. [2] (Table 4). Because the PESI and sPESI currently have more data supporting their use in risk stratification across the whole spectrum of patients with acute PE, the current protocol therefore incorporates PESI scoring in all patients diagnosed with acute PE (Fig. 3). The majority of social and practical exclusion criteria used by Aujesky et al. [2] have been incorporated. Currently, patients in our centre are also required to have a normal-sized RV on CTPA to fulfil criteria for outpatient management. It is possible that the criteria may become less conservative in the future in light of recent data and changing guidelines. For example, the HESTIA investigators observed that the presence of RV dilatation did not increase risk related to outpatient management, assuming that no HESTIA criteria were met [3].

Patients without hypotension but with PESI class III–V or sPESI class >0 are at intermediate risk of early deterioration and require hospital admission. Patients in this group who have both radiological evidence of right ventricular dysfunction (from CTPA or echocardiography, if performed) and elevated plasma biomarkers (BNP, NT-proBNP or troponin) are at intermediate-high risk of deterioration; this group require especially close monitoring and consideration for reperfusion therapy if there is evidence of further deterioration [1]. Other features, such as

Table 3 PESI and sPESI scores [33, 34]

Prediction factors	PESI	sPESI
Age >80 years	Age in years	1
Male gender	+10	-
Cancer	+30	1
Heart failure	+10	1[a]
Chronic lung disease	+10	
Pulse ≥110 beats/minute	+20	1
Systolic blood pressure <100 mmHg	+30	1
Respiratory rate ≥30 breaths/minute	+20	-
Temperature <36 °C	+20	-
Altered mental status	+60	-
Arterial oxyhaemoglobin saturation <90%	+20	1
Outcome		
Low risk:	Class I: ≤65 Class II: 66–85	PESI = 0
Intermediate risk:	Class III: 86–105	
High risk:	Class IV: 106–125 Class V: >125	PESI = ≥1

PESI Pulmonary Embolism Severity Index, *sPESI* simplified Pulmonary Embolism Severity Index
[a]Single combined category of chronic cardiopulmonary disease

Table 4 Comparison of HESTIA criteria and exclusion criteria used by Aujesky et al. [2, 3]

HESTIA criteria: Zondag [3]	Exclusion criteria: Aujesky [2]
Is the patient haemodynamically unstable?	SBP <100 mmHg
Is thrombolysis or embolectomy necessary?	
>24 h oxygen to maintain sats >90%	Oxygen saturation <90%
Active bleeding or high risk of bleeding	Active bleeding High risk of bleeding (stroke within the preceding 10 days, GI bleed within the last 14 days or platelet count <75,000/mm^3)
PE diagnosed on anticoagulation?	Therapeutic anticoagulation (INR ≥2.0) at diagnosis
Severe pain needing IV pain medication for >24 h	Chest pain needing opiates
Medical or social reason for treatment in hospital (infection, malignancy, no support system)	Barriers to treatment adherence or follow-up
CrCl <30 mL/min	Severe renal failure (CrCl <30 mL/min)
Severe liver impairment	
Documented history of HIT	HIT
Is the patient pregnant?	
	Obesity (weight >150 kg)

CrCl creatinine clearance, *GI* gastrointestinal, *HIT* heparin-induced thrombocytopenia, *INR* international normalised ratio, *IV* intravenous, *PE* pulmonary embolism, *SBP* systolic blood pressure

the presence of DVT on compression ultrasonography [29] or elevated lactate levels [30], may be useful in further refining identification of intermediate-to-high risk patients at particular risk of deterioration.

Step 4: Treatment strategy

Patients at high risk of early deterioration should undergo reperfusion therapy, most commonly with systemic thrombolysis, although catheter-directed therapy and surgical embolectomy will sometimes be necessary if there are significant contraindications to systemic thrombolysis. Patients at low or intermediate risk of deterioration are candidates for either LMWH/VKA, or a NOAC. We would generally treat patients at intermediate-high risk – in whom subsequent thrombolysis may potentially be necessary – with LMWH and a VKA. Patients at low risk of deterioration are considered for outpatient management. Although currently published studies regarding outpatient management of acute PE have utilised LMWH and VKA, the practical benefits of NOACs (especially the NOACs rivaroxaban and apixaban, which do not require pre-treatment with LMWH) make them an attractive method of anticoagulation in patients undergoing outpatient management. This role of rivaroxaban in outpatient PE management is currently being investigated in more detail in the multicentre HoT-PE study [31]. In intermediate-risk patients who are admitted, reassessment of PESI or sPESI score after 48 h may identify patients now suitable for early discharge and outpatient management [1].

Step 5: Follow-up

If patients undergo outpatient management, they are reviewed within 48 h by the VTE nurse specialist. The patient's clinical state is assessed to ensure no clinical deterioration. Results of initial malignancy screening are reviewed, including a focused history and examination, review of blood results and urinalysis. Dependent on the results of these tests, further tests may be arranged. The current anticoagulation method is reviewed and a plan for ongoing anticoagulation is made in conjunction with the patient. If the patient is treated with rivaroxaban, a second appointment is made for approximately 21 days after diagnosis which coincides with the change in dosing from 15 mg twice daily to 20 mg once daily.

Education and counselling are important components of patient care. At the time of PE diagnosis, an individual treatment plan will be provided and treatment options will be discussed. Later, outpatient appointments help to ensure patients understand the reasons behind why a PE occurred, the recommended treatment and why treatment adherence is important. It is also an opportunity for the patient to be fully reassured and for any questions or concerns to be discussed.

In Sheffield, we review patients at approximately 3 months following their acute PE at a consultant-led, combined respiratory-haematology clinic. The patient's initial history and radiological investigations are reviewed to confirm the diagnosis, the nature of the event (i.e. provoked or unprovoked) and to assess the likelihood of chronic complications. A proportion of patients with ongoing, new breathlessness will undergo further investigation (often a combination of echocardiography, nuclear perfusion scanning and/or computed tomography pulmonary angiogram) to assess for the presence of chronic thromboembolic pulmonary hypertension. Plans regarding ongoing anticoagulation management are then made. Longer-term anticoagulation is considered following unprovoked events, whereas anticoagulation can often be stopped after 3 months following strongly provoked clots. In selected patients thrombophilia testing may be indicated, while D-dimer level testing after withdrawing anticoagulation may further refine estimates of the risk of recurrence in selected patients with partially provoked events [32].

Conclusion

The Sheffield VTE management pathways for DVT and PE are examples of best practice within the UK. These pathways facilitate the smooth transition of patients from hospital to home, while maintaining regular patient follow-up. VTE management for many patients with distal DVT, proximal DVT or low-risk PE can be safely carried out as part of ambulatory care, particularly with the involvement of specialist anticoagulation nurses and the use of NOACs. Use of a pathway similar to the Sheffield VTE pathway may reduce the burden on secondary care and the length of hospital stays. Patient satisfaction may also increase with same-day diagnosis, shorter hospital stay, fewer injections, and follow-up in the same thrombosis service.

Abbreviations

CTEPH: Chronic thromboembolic pulmonary hypertension; CTPA: Computed tomography pulmonary angiogram; DVT: Deep vein thrombosis; HAS-BLED: Hypertension Abnormal renal and liver function, Stroke, Bleeding, Labile international normalised ratio, Elderly, Drugs or alcohol; HCP: Healthcare professional; HoT-PE: Home treatment of pulmonary embolism; LMWH: Low molecular weight heparin; MDT: Multidisciplinary team; NOAC: Non-vitamin K antagonist oral anticoagulant; OAC: Oral anticoagulant; OPA: Outpatient appointment; PE: Pulmonary embolism; PESI: Pulmonary Embolism Severity Index; sPESI: Simplified Pulmonary Embolism Severity Index; VKA: Vitamin K antagonist; VQ SPECT: Ventilation/perfusion single-photon emission tomography; VTE: Venous thromboembolism

Acknowledgement

The author would like to acknowledge Susan Croft, Tim Devey, Charlie Elliot, Rodney Hughes, Judith Hurdman, David Kiely, Joost VanVeen and Rhona Maclean for their extensive work in the development of the VTE pathways used within our trust. The author would also like to acknowledge Claudia Wiedemann, who provided editorial support with funding from Bayer Pharma AG.

Funding

Not applicable.

Authors' contributions
Not applicable.

Competing interests
R. Condliffe has received honoraria payments from Bayer for lecturing and advisory boards and from Daiichi Sankyo for advisory boards.

References

1. Konstantinides SV, Torbicki A, Agnelli G, Danchin N, Fitzmaurice D, Galiè N, et al. 2014 ESC guidelines on the diagnosis and management of acute pulmonary embolism. Eur Heart J. 2014;35:3033–69.
2. Aujesky D, Roy PM, Verschuren F, Righini M, Osterwalder J, Egloff M, et al. Outpatient versus inpatient treatment for patients with acute pulmonary embolism: an international, open-label, randomised, non-inferiority trial. Lancet. 2011;378:41–8.
3. Zondag W, Mos IC, Creemers-Schild D, Hoogerbrugge AD, Dekkers OM, Dolsma J, et al. Outpatient treatment in patients with acute pulmonary embolism: the Hestia Study. J Thromb Haemost. 2011;9:1500–7.
4. Condliffe R, Elliot CA, Hughes RJ, Hurdman J, Maclean RM, Sabroe I, et al. Management dilemmas in acute pulmonary embolism. Thorax. 2014;69:174–80.
5. Yoo HH, Queluz TH, El Dib R. Outpatient versus inpatient treatment for acute pulmonary embolism. Cochrane Database Syst Rev. 2014;11:CD010019.
6. Robertson L, Kesteven P, McCaslin JE. Oral direct thrombin inhibitors or oral factor Xa inhibitors for the treatment of deep vein thrombosis. Cochrane Database Syst Rev. 2015;6:CD010956.
7. Khanbhai M, Hansrani V, Burke J, Ghosh J, McCollum C. The early management of DVT in the North West of England: a nation-wide problem? Thromb Res. 2015;136:76–86.
8. House of Commons Health Committee. The Prevention of Venous Thromboembolism in Hospitalised Patients; Second Report of Session 2004–05. http://www.publications.parliament.uk/pa/cm200405/cmselect/cmhealth/99/99.pdf. Accessed 5 July 2016.
9. National Institute for Health and Care Excellence. Venous thromboembolism: reducing the risk for patients in hospital. 1. Recommendations. http://www.nice.org.uk/guidance/cg92/chapter/1-recommendations. Accessed 5 July 2016.
10. Wells PS, Anderson DR, Rodger M, Forgie M, Kearon C, Dreyer J, et al. Evaluation of D-dimer in the diagnosis of suspected deep-vein thrombosis. N Engl J Med. 2003;349:1227–35.
11. Wells PS, Owen C, Doucette S, Fergusson D, Tran H. Does this patient have deep vein thrombosis? JAMA. 2006;295:199–207.
12. Pisters R, Lane DA, Nieuwlaat R, de Vos CB, Crijns HJ, Lip GYH. A novel user-friendly score (HAS-BLED) to assess 1-year risk of major bleeding in patients with atrial fibrillation: the Euro Heart Survey. Chest. 2010;138:1093–100.
13. Ruíz-Giménez N, Suárez C, González R, Nieto JA, Todolí JA, Samperiz ÁL, et al. Predictive variables for major bleeding events in patients presenting with documented acute venous thromboembolism. Findings from the RIETE Registry. Thromb Haemost. 2008;100:26–31.
14. Weitz JI. Anticoagulation therapy in 2015: where we are and where we are going. J Thromb Thrombolysis. 2015;39:264–72.
15. Bayer Pharma AG. Xarelto® (rivaroxaban) Summary of Product Characteristics. 2016. http://www.ema.europa.eu/docs/en_GB/document_library/EPAR_-_Product_Information/human/000944/WC500057108.pdf. Accessed 21 Sep 2016.
16. Bristol-Myers Squibb, Pfizer. Eliquis® (apixaban) Summary of Product Characteristics. 2016. http://www.ema.europa.eu/docs/en_GB/document_library/EPAR_-_Product_Information/human/002148/WC500107728.pdf. Accessed 21 Sept 2016.
17. Boehringer Ingelheim International GH. Pradaxa® (dabigatran etexilate) Summary of Product Characteristics. 2016. http://www.ema.europa.eu/docs/en_GB/document_library/EPAR_-_Product_Information/human/000829/WC500041059.pdf. Accessed 21 Sep 2016.
18. Daiichi Sankyo Europe GH. Lixiana® (edoxaban) Summary of Product Characteristics. 2016. http://www.ema.europa.eu/docs/en_GB/document_library/EPAR_-_Product_Information/human/002629/WC500189045.pdf. Accessed 10 Jun 2016.
19. Agnelli G, Buller HR, Cohen A, Curto M, Gallus AS, Johnson M, et al. Oral apixaban for the treatment of acute venous thromboembolism. N Engl J Med. 2013;369:799–808.
20. Schulman S, Kearon C, Kakkar AK, Mismetti P, Schellong S, Eriksson H, et al. Dabigatran versus warfarin in the treatment of acute venous thromboembolism. N Engl J Med. 2009;361:2342–52.
21. The Hokusai-VTE Investigators. Edoxaban versus warfarin for the treatment of symptomatic venous thromboembolism. N Engl J Med. 2013;369:1406–15.
22. The EINSTEIN Investigators. Oral rivaroxaban for symptomatic venous thromboembolism. N Engl J Med. 2010;363:2499–510.
23. Wells PS, Anderson DR, Rodger M, Stiell I, Dreyer JF, Barnes D, et al. Excluding pulmonary embolism at the bedside without diagnostic imaging: management of patients with suspected pulmonary embolism presenting to the emergency department by using a simple clinical model and D-dimer. Ann Intern Med. 2001;135:98–107.
24. Wells PS, Anderson DR, Rodger M, Ginsberg JS, Kearon C, Gent M, et al. Derivation of a simple clinical model to categorize patients probability of pulmonary embolism: increasing the models utility with the SimpliRED D-dimer. Thromb Haemost. 2000;83:416–20.
25. Gibson NS, Sohne M, Kruip MJ, Tick LW, Gerdes VE, Bossuyt PM, et al. Further validation and simplification of the Wells clinical decision rule in pulmonary embolism. Thromb Haemost. 2008;99:229–34.
26. Righini M, van Es J, den Exter PL, Roy PM, Verschuren F, Ghuysen A, et al. Age-adjusted D-dimer cutoff levels to rule out pulmonary embolism: the ADJUST-PE study. JAMA. 2014;311:1117–24.
27. Lankeit M, Jimenez D, Kostrubiec M, Dellas C, Hasenfuss G, Pruszczyk P, et al. Predictive value of the high-sensitivity troponin T assay and the simplified Pulmonary Embolism Severity Index in hemodynamically stable patients with acute pulmonary embolism: a prospective validation study. Circulation. 2011;124:2716–24.
28. Jimenez D, Kopecna D, Tapson V, Briese B, Schreiber D, Lobo JL, et al. Derivation and validation of multimarker prognostication for normotensive patients with acute symptomatic pulmonary embolism. Am J Respir Crit Care Med. 2014;189:718–26.
29. Jiménez D, Aujesky D, Díaz G, Monreal M, Otero R, Martí D, et al. Prognostic significance of deep vein thrombosis in patients presenting with acute symptomatic pulmonary embolism. Am J Respir Crit Care Med. 2010;181:983–91.
30. Vanni S, Jimenez D, Nazerian P, Morello F, Parisi M, Daghini E, et al. Short-term clinical outcome of normotensive patients with acute PE and high plasma lactate. Thorax. 2015;70:333–8.
31. Barco S, Lankeit M, Binder H, Schellong S, Christ M, Beyer-Westendorf J, et al. Home treatment of patients with low-risk pulmonary embolism with the oral factor Xa inhibitor rivaroxaban. Rationale and design of the HoT-PE Trial. Thromb Haemost. 2016;116:191–7.
32. Palareti G, Cosmi B, Legnani C, Antonucci E, De Micheli V, Ghirarduzzi A, et al. D-dimer to guide the duration of anticoagulation in patients with venous thromboembolism: a management study. Blood. 2014;124:196–203.
33. Aujesky D, Perrier A, Roy PM, Stone RA, Cornuz J, Meyer G, et al. Validation of a clinical prognostic model to identify low-risk patients with pulmonary embolism. J Intern Med. 2007;261:597–604.
34. Jiménez D, Aujesky D, Moores L, Gómez V, Lobo JL, Uresandi F, et al. Simplification of the Pulmonary Embolism Severity Index for prognostication in patients with acute symptomatic pulmonary embolism. Arch Intern Med. 2010;170:1383–9.
35. Quadery R, Elliot CA, Hurdman J, Kiely DG, Maclean RM, Sabroe I, et al. Management of acute pulmonary embolism. Br J Hosp Med. 2015;76:C150–5.

14

Platelets and platelet adhesion molecules: novel mechanisms of thrombosis and anti-thrombotic therapies

Xiaohong Ruby Xu[1,2,3], Naadiya Carrim[2,4], Miguel Antonio Dias Neves[2], Thomas McKeown[2], Tyler W. Stratton[2], Rodrigo Matos Pinto Coelho[2], Xi Lei[2], Pingguo Chen[2,4], Jianhua Xu[5], Xiangrong Dai[6,7], Benjamin Xiaoyi Li[6,7,8] and Heyu Ni[1,2,4,5,9*]

From The 9th Congress of the Asian-Pacific Society on Thrombosis and Hemostasis
Taipei, Taiwan.

Abstract

Platelets are central mediators of thrombosis and hemostasis. At the site of vascular injury, platelet accumulation (i.e. adhesion and aggregation) constitutes the first wave of hemostasis. Blood coagulation, initiated by the coagulation cascades, is the second wave of thrombin generation and enhance phosphatidylserine exposure, can markedly potentiate cell-based thrombin generation and enhance blood coagulation. Recently, deposition of plasma fibronectin and other proteins onto the injured vessel wall has been identified as a new "protein wave of hemostasis" that occurs prior to platelet accumulation (i.e. the classical first wave of hemostasis). These three waves of hemostasis, in the event of atherosclerotic plaque rupture, may turn pathogenic, and cause uncontrolled vessel occlusion and thrombotic disorders (e.g. heart attack and stroke). Current anti-platelet therapies have significantly reduced cardiovascular mortality, however, on-treatment thrombotic events, thrombocytopenia, and bleeding complications are still major concerns that continue to motivate innovation and drive therapeutic advances. Emerging evidence has brought platelet adhesion molecules back into the spotlight as targets for the development of novel anti-thrombotic agents. These potential antiplatelet targets mainly include the platelet receptors glycoprotein (GP) Ib-IX-V complex, β3 integrins (αIIb subunit and PSI domain of β3 subunit) and GPVI. Numerous efforts have been made aiming to balance the efficacy of inhibiting thrombosis without compromising hemostasis. This mini-review will update the mechanisms of thrombosis and the current state of antiplatelet therapies, and will focus on platelet adhesion molecules and the novel anti-thrombotic therapies that target them.

Keywords: αIIbβ3, Anfibatide, GPIbα, GPVI, Hemostasis, Integrins, P-selectin, Stroke, Thrombosis

Abbreviations: ADP, Adenosine diphosphate; GLP-1R, Glucagon-like peptide 1 receptor; GP, Glycoprotein; ITAM, Immunoreceptor tyrosine-based activation motif; ITP, Idiopathic thrombocytopenic purpura; LLR, Leucine-rich repeat; PAR, Protease-activated receptor; PCI, Percutaneous coronary intervention; PDI, Protein disulphide isomerase; PSI, Plexin-semaphorin-integrin; TIA, Transient ischemic attack; TTP, Thrombotic thrombocytopenic purpura; VWF, von Willebrand factor

* Correspondence: nih@smh.ca
[1]Department of Laboratory Medicine and Pathobiology, University of Toronto, Toronto, ON, Canada
[2]Department of Laboratory Medicine, Keenan Research Centre for Biomedical Science, St. Michael's Hospital, Toronto, ON, Canada
Full list of author information is available at the end of the article

Background

Platelet adhesion, activation and aggregation are critical events in hemostasis and thrombosis [1–3]. Platelet adhesion molecules, αIIbβ3 integrin and the glycoprotein (GP) Ib-IX-V, are essential for these processes [4–6]. Other adhesion molecules, such as P-selectin, GPVI and cadherins, are also involved [7–10]. The important roles of adhesion molecules in normal hemostasis have been well demonstrated in bleeding disorders, for example, Glanzmann thrombasthenia (β3 integrin deficiency) [11] and Bernard-Soulier syndrome (GPIb-IX-V complex deficiency) [12]. However, under pathological conditions, excessive platelet function may lead to thrombotic diseases, such as myocardial infarction and ischemic stroke, which cause far more deaths each year than cancer or respiratory diseases [1, 2, 13–15]. Therefore, antiplatelet agents are vital for the treatment of thrombosis [16]. For over a decade, dual antiplatelet therapy with clopidogrel and aspirin has been considered a key treatment of patients with acute coronary syndrome [17, 18]. Nonetheless, some patients undergoing this combination therapy continue to suffer from recurrent thrombotic events, likely a result of platelet activation and aggregation occurring independently of ADP or thromboxane A2 receptor-mediated signalling pathways [17]. Thus, attenuating platelet adhesion appears to be a desirable strategy in effectively controlling pathological thrombosis [18]. Further understanding of the interactions between platelet adhesion molecules and their binding partners is therefore crucial in developing novel anti-thrombotic therapies. This review briefly summarizes the current knowledge of thrombosis and antiplatelet therapies, introduces a number of major platelet adhesion molecules, and highlights some recent advances in the new mechanisms of thrombosis, and anti-thrombotic therapies that are in clinical trials (unless otherwise indicated). There are several excellent available reviews regarding antiplatelet therapies, such as ADP antagonists (e.g. P2Y12 inhibitors), thromboxane antagonists and PAR-1/4 inhibitors [17, 18]. This mini-review will mainly focus on the therapeutic developments targeting platelet adhesion molecules.

Review

Arterial thrombosis and current state of antiplatelet therapies

Arterial thrombosis at the site of atherosclerotic plaque rupture may lead to uncontrolled vessel occlusion, resulting in life-threatening consequences (e.g. unstable angina, myocardial infarction and ischemic stroke) [1, 2, 13]. During plaque rupture, subendothelial matrix proteins, like collagen, von Willebrand factor (VWF), fibrinogen, fibronectin and laminin are exposed to circulation, leading to the rapid response of platelets [6]. Inappropriate platelet adhesion, activation and aggregation promote excessive platelet plug formation. Activated platelets can also provide negatively-charged surfaces that harbor coagulation factors and markedly potentiate cell-based thrombin generation and blood coagulation [1, 2, 19, 20]. The evolving concept of the "protein wave of hemostasis" indicates a potential role of platelet-released plasma fibronectin in thrombosis and hemostasis [21, 22]. Thus, platelets are key mediators of atherothrombosis, which are actively involved in all three waves of thrombus formation: protein wave, platelet accumulation, and blood coagulation [21, 23].

Current FDA-approved antiplatelet therapies (Fig. 1) mainly aim to (i) inhibit thromboxane A2 synthesis, which inhibits platelet activation (e.g. aspirin and triflusal); (ii) antagonize the function of platelet P2Y12 receptors, (e.g. clopidogrel, prasugrel, and ticagrelor); (iii) inhibit platelet integrin αIIbβ3 activity, which inhibits platelet aggregation, (e.g. abciximab, eptifibatide, and tirofiban); (iv) inhibit phosphodiesterase, which increases platelet cAMP/cGMP levels (e.g. dipyridamole and cilostazol) [24]. These antiplatelet drugs have significantly reduced cardiovascular deaths. However, limitations of current therapies, such as weak/poor inhibition of platelet function, excessive bleeding, thrombocytopenia and unexpected platelet activation are concerns that drive therapeutic advances [18, 25, 26]. In 2014, the FDA approved Vorapaxar, a novel antagonist of the thrombin receptor protease-activated receptor 1 (PAR1), which reduces the risk of heart attack and stroke in patients with atherosclerosis or peripheral arterial disease [27, 28]. However, Vorapaxar must not be used in patients who have histories of stroke, transient ischemic attack (TIA) or intracranial hemorrhage, since it increases the risk of intracranial bleeding [28, 29].

Platelet adhesion molecules in hemostasis and thrombosis: novel mechanisms and therapeutic opportunities

Platelet adhesion molecules are proteins/receptors on the platelet surface that interact with other cells or the extracellular matrix, including the integrin family (e.g. α2β1, α5β1, α6β1, αLβ2, αIIbβ3, and αvβ3) [4, 30, 31], the immunoglobulin superfamily (e.g. GPVI, FcγRIIA, ICAM-2, PECAM-1, JAMs and Cadherin 6), the leucine-rich repeat family (LRR; e.g. GPIb-IX-V complex), and the C-type lectin receptor family (e.g. P-selectin and CLEC-2), etc. [32–34]. Recent evidence has shown that platelet adhesion molecules play key roles in a variety of pathophysiological processes [23], such as hemostasis and thrombosis [4, 33], immune responses [35, 36], inflammation [35–37], atherosclerosis [38–40], lymphatic vessel development [41–44], angiogenesis [45–47], miscarriage [48, 49], and tumor metastasis [50–52]. Platelets

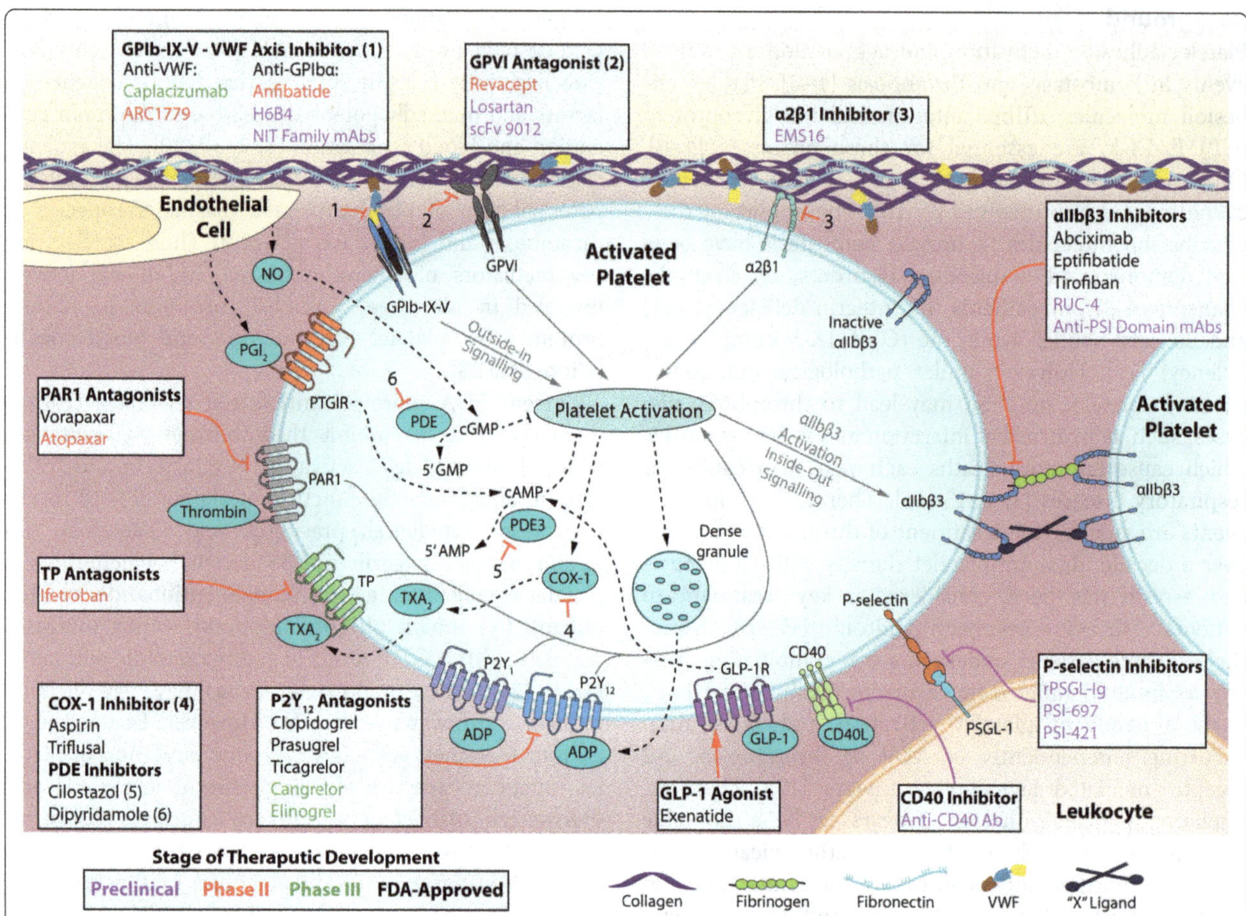

Fig. 1 Current and novel antiplatelet therapies. Platelet adhesion to an injury site at a vessel wall is mediated by the exposure and binding of subendothelial matrix proteins (e.g. collagen, VWF, fibrinogen, and fibronectin) to glycoprotein (GP) receptors on the platelet surface. VWF binding to the GPIb-IX-V complex, collagen binding to platelet GPVI and integrin α2β1 receptors trigger a signal transduction process resulting in the local release of platelet activation agonists, such as thromboxane A2 and ADP. These agonists along with thrombin produced from coagulation cascades and activated platelets, bind to platelet surface bound G-coupled receptors inducing further platelet activation. Activation of platelet integrin αIIbβ3 induces platelet aggregation mediated by fibrinogen/VWF or the yet undetermined "X" ligands. Leukocyte-platelet adhesion can be driven by the interaction between platelet surface P-selectin and its counter-receptor PSGL-1 situated upon the leukocyte surface. Inhibition of platelet activation is mainly mediated by the PDE/PDE3 regulated degradation and PGI_2, NO and GLP-1R regulated activation of cGMP or cAMP. Direct and indirect antithrombotic therapeutics are tabulated in the light colored boxes within the figure. The actions of antithrombotic therapies are depicted using *red* arrows, and some indirect antithrombotic agents (such as anti-atherosclerotic agents) are represented with *purple* arrows. Therapeutics, to name a few, listed in *black*, *green*, *red* and *purple* correspond to FDA-approved, phase III, phase II or preclinical development status, respectively. Numbered inhibitory arrows represent the actions of the correspondingly numbered therapies. Some other anti-platelet agents are not included, more information can be found in references 17, 18 and other publications. *Abbreviations*: *COX-1* cyclooxygenase 1 *GLP-1* glucagon-like peptide 1, *GLP-1R* glucagon-like peptide 1 receptor, *PAR* protease-activated receptor, *PDE* phosphodiesterase, *PSGL-1* P-selectin glycoprotein ligand 1, *TP* thromboxane prostanoid receptor, TXA_2 thromboxane A2; *VWF* von Willebrand factor

are versatile cells and the mechanisms of their diverse functions have emerged as hot research topics [23]. This review mainly focuses on their roles in thrombosis and as novel anti-thrombotic targets (Fig. 1).

The GPIb-IX-V complex: emerging targets of antiplatelet therapy

New insights into the GPIb-IX-V complex Platelet GPIb-IX-V complex (LRR family protein) has approximately 50,000 copies/platelet. It is composed of one GPIbα subunit disulfide-linked to two molecules of GPIbβ, and non-covalently linked with GPIX and GPV in a 2:4:2:1 ratio [53]. GPIb-IX-V is a key platelet receptor in initiating platelet translocation and adhesion to the vessel wall during vascular injury, especially under high shear stress (e.g. in small or stenosed arteries) [54, 55]. Platelet translocation onto the subendothelium is mediated by the binding of GPIbα to the immobilized VWF, a multimeric adhesive protein secreted from activated endothelial cells and platelets. The crystal structure of the GPIbα N-terminal ligand-binding domain and the VWF A1 domain gives useful information regarding their interaction [56].

This interaction induces intracellular signalling events that can activate integrins, leading to platelet stable adhesion and subsequent platelet aggregation. Interestingly, platelet-derived VWF was recently shown not essential for hemostasis and thrombosis, but instead fosters thrombo-inflammatory diseases such as ischemic stroke in mice via a GPIb-dependent mechanism [57]. This suggests that targeting GPIbα-VWF may be a promising anti-thrombotic strategy, particularly in thrombo-inflammatory conditions.

Furthermore, GPIb-IX-V complex has a high affinity for thrombin [58, 59]. Two thrombin binding sites on GPIbα LRR C-terminal flank region have been revealed [58]. Consequently, thrombin can activate platelets via GPIbα in two ways [60]: accelerating the cleavage of PAR-1 and platelet activation [61], or direct signaling via GPIbα, particularly after cleaving GPV, which is generally considered a "brake" in GPIb-IX-V activation [62, 63]. It is currently unknown but it is reasonable to consider that targeting both VWF and thrombin binding sites of GPIbα might provide additional benefits in effectively controlling thrombosis.

GPIbα can also interact with multiple other ligands, leading to platelet activation (e.g. thrombospondin [64] and P-selectin), pro-coagulant activity (e.g. factors XI [65], XII [66], VIIa [67] and kininogen [68]), inflammatory responses (e.g. P-selectin [69, 70], $\alpha_M\beta_2$ [71]), arterial remodeling [72] and others. Recently, the antibody-GPIbα interaction in immune thrombocytopenia has been highlighted. Some anti-GPIbα antibodies cause platelet activation and desialylation (removal of sugars), followed by the clearance of desialylated platelets via Ashwell-Morell receptors on hepatocytes [73, 74].

Developing novel antiplatelet agents against GPIbα

Given the critical roles of GPIbα or GPIbα-VWF interactions in platelet adhesion, particularly under stenosis high-shear conditions, they are attractive targets in attenuating thrombosis [54, 75, 76]. Currently, two such agents are in active clinical trials. ALX-0081 (Caplacizumab), an anti-VWF humanized single-variable-domain immunoglobulin (Nanobody), binds to the A1 domains of VWF with high affinity [77]. The phase I and II clinical trials of ALX-0081 in patients with stable angina undergoing percutaneous coronary intervention (PCI) or high risk PCI patients have shown a promising antiplatelet effects, and a relatively safe profile [77, 78]. The phase III clinical trials will investigate its effects on acquired thrombotic thrombocytopenic purpura (TTP) [79–81]. ARC1779, an anti-VWF aptamer, was previously reported as an encouraging agent; however, the clinical trial of ARC1779 was prematurely terminated [82]. These VWF inhibitors may be useful candidates for TTP treatment.

A direct anti-GPIbα drug, Anfibatide, is purified from the snake venom of *Agkistrodon acutus* [83, 84]. Notably, Anfibatide inhibits both VWF and α-thrombin binding to GPIbα, representing a more potent anti-thrombotic effect [85]. In experimental models, Anfibatide inhibited platelet adhesion, aggregation and thrombus formation, without increasing bleeding time [83]. The phase II human clinical trials have also shown the promise of Anfibatide being utilized as a novel antiplatelet agent in cardiovascular diseases without significantly affecting hemostasis in patients with non-ST segment elevation myocardial infarction (unpublished data) [85]. Additionally, anti-GPIbα antibody displayed a strong protective effect in the mouse stroke models without inducing significant intracranial bleeding [86–88]. Anfibatide has also been shown as a candidate to treat ischemic stroke in experimental models [89] (the same may hold true for anti-VWF therapy) and deserves further investigation. There are some other preclinical agents targeting GPIbα that are under investigation, such as h6B4-Fab [90], GPG-290 [91], and anti-GPIbα NIT family monoclonal antibodies [92]. The generation of these novel antagonists is reaching the forefront of treatment against heart attack and stroke, although the efficacy and safety of these drugs remain to be further established or evaluated in human clinical trials. Notably, there are currently no clinically available direct GPIbα antagonists.

GPVI: a potential anti-thrombotic target

GPVI (immunoglobulin superfamily protein) is exclusively expressed on platelets and megakaryocytes. It is associated with the Fc receptor γ-chain, which contains an immunoreceptor tyrosine-based activation motif (ITAM). Cross-linking by ligands, such as collagen, leads to ITAM-dependent signalling, and platelet activation. A possible anti-thrombotic benefit of targeting PI3-kinase/Akt pathway on ITAM receptors was suggested [93]. Fibrin has also been identified as a new GPVI ligand [94]. The GPVI ectodomain interacts with immobilized fibrin, which amplifies thrombin generation, and promotes thrombus stabilization [94, 95].

The role of platelet GPVI in the pathogenesis of ischemic stroke has been gradually acknowledged [96–98]. Notably, platelet adhesion/activation can enhance infarct growth by promoting an inflammatory response [88, 99, 100]. GPVI-mediated platelet activation can lead to the release of interleukin-1α that drives cerebrovascular inflammation [100]. GPVI may be thus a potential antiplatelet target [97, 101, 102]. In animal models, anti-GPVI protected against thrombosis, ischemia-reperfusion injury [103] and stroke [104]. In phase I clinical trials, Revacept (the humanized Fc fusion protein of the GPVI ectodomain), inhibited collagen-induced human platelet aggregation [105]. Phase II trials of Revacept in patients with carotid artery stenosis, TIA, or stroke are ongoing [106]. The efficacy and safety of Revacept in these patients will be further determined. Some other GPVI targeted agents that are under preclinical development, such as Losartan [107] and scFv9012 [108], have been shown to inhibit the binding of GPVI to collagen.

Platelet integrin receptors

Integrins are heterodimeric transmembrane receptors, which are involved in cell-cell and cell-matrix interactions [30]. There are six different integrins on platelet surfaces: α2β1, α5β1, α6β1, αLβ2, αIIbβ3, and αvβ3. Platelet integrin αIIbβ3 is the dominant integrin expressed on platelets. Given the critical roles of αIIbβ3 integrin in mediating platelet aggregation, αIIbβ3 antagonists have been widely used for nearly two decades.

Integrin αIIbβ3 as anti-thrombotic targets: lessons and opportunities Approximately 17 % of total platelet surface proteins are αIIbβ3 integrin, which contains both αIIb and β3 subunits [4]. Platelet "outside-in" signals are induced following platelet adhesion and platelet activation (e.g. GPIbα-VWF, GPVI/α2β1-collagen, $P2Y_{12}$-ADP, PARs-thrombin), resulting in an increased Ca^{2+} influx and ultimately "inside-out" signaling. These "inside-out" signals further drive the conformational changes of αIIbβ3, from a low to high affinity state for binding to its ligands (e.g. fibrinogen/fibrin, VWF, fibronectin, thrombospondin, vitronectin and unidentified "X" ligands) [109–112].

Fibrinogen, a major prothrombotic ligand of αIIbβ3, has been documented to be required for platelet aggregation for over 50 years. However, platelet aggregation still occurs in the absence of fibrinogen and VWF, although in the absence of αIIbβ3, aggregation is abolished [5, 8, 21, 113–116]. The discovery of "fibrinogen-independent platelet aggregation" demonstrates that unidentified αIIbβ3 ligands also mediate platelet aggregation [5, 8, 21, 113, 116], and have the potential to be novel anti-thrombotic targets. Interestingly, some ligands (e.g. plasma fibronectin, vitronectin) may block prothrombotic ligand (e.g. fibrinogen)-αIIbβ3 interactions and attenuate thrombosis [21, 117].

Three FDA-approved αIIbβ3 antagonists are available: Abciximab (ReoPro), Eptifibatide (Integrilin) and Tirofiban (Aggrastat) [118–120]. Abciximab is a fragmented antibody that binds close to the ligand binding-pocket on αIIbβ3. Eptifibatide, isolated from snake venom, binds via a KGD sequence and is a competitive inhibitor for fibrinogen-αIIbβ3, whilst tirofiban is a small molecule RGD inhibitor. Currently, αIIbβ3 antagonists are used in patients undergoing PCI and significantly decrease the incidence of myocardial infarction and death [121]. However, these antagonists can induce further conformational changes in the β3 subunit that may have negative consequences, such as exposing previously hidden epitopes, and causing platelet activation [122]. αIIbβ3 antagonists are also associated with intracranial hemorrhage in patients with acute ischemic stroke [123]. Therefore, a safer and more specific on-target drug is required to provide better patient care. Recently, a novel αIIbβ3 antagonist, RUC-4 (a more potent and more soluble congener of RUC-2 that disrupts Mg^{2+} binding to the metal ion-dependent adhesion site of αIIbβ3), is suggested for prehospital therapy of myocardial infarction in animal models, without significantly priming the receptor to bind fibrinogen [124]. However, the possibility of increased bleeding with therapeutic doses of RUC-4 remains to be evaluated [124].

The plexin-semaphorin-integrin (PSI) domain, located near the N-terminus of the β3 subunit, is highly conserved across the integrin family in different species, and contains seven cysteine residues which have been implicated in regulating β2 integrin activation [125, 126]. Previous studies described a role for cysteine-derived thiol/disulfide groups in the conformational switches of the β3 integrin [127–130]. Disulfide bond remodeling is mediated primarily by thiol isomerase enzymatic activity, which is derived from active CXXC thioredoxin motifs and plays a role in the activation of αIIbβ3 [131]. Our group has recently identified that integrin PSI domain has endogenous thiol isomerase function and could be a novel target for anti-thrombotic therapy (unpublished data) [132]. We found that both CXXC motifs of β3 integrin PSI domain are required to maintain the optimal enzyme function, since mutations to one or both of the CXXC motifs decrease or abolish their protein disulphide isomerase (PDI)-like activity. We developed anti-PSI monoclonal antibodies and found that these antibodies cross-reacted with β3 PSI domains of human and other species and specifically inhibited the PDI-like activity, integrin activation and reduced PAC-1 binding to β3 integrin. Importantly, anti-PSI abrogated murine and human platelet aggregation in vitro and thrombus growth ex vivo and in vivo in both small and large vessels without significantly affecting bleeding time or platelet count. Thus, integrin PSI domain contains endogenous PDI activity and is a key regulator of integrin activation that can be a new target for therapy.

Interestingly, targeting activated platelets αIIbβ3 has been considered into the development of novel fibrinolytic drugs, which may allow effective thrombolysis and thromboprophylaxis [14, 133]. For example, scFvSCE5 (a single-chain urokinase plasminogen activator fused to a small recombinant antibody that binds activated αIIbβ3) directly targets thrombi and exerts an effective thrombolysis [133]. A chimeric platelet-targeted urokinase prodrug (composed of a single-chain version of the variable region of an anti-αIIbβ3 mAb and a thrombin-activatable, low-molecular-weight pro-uPA) selectively targets new thrombus formation [134].

Other platelet integrins: α2β1, α6β1 and α5β1 Other integrin receptors may also be considered as novel anti-thrombotic targets [16, 135]. Platelet α2β1 promotes stable platelet adhesion to collagen and may be a viable option, since overexpression of α2β1 in humans increases atherothrombotic risk, but lower level of α2β1 does not enhance bleeding risk [16]. Experimental evidence shows that α2β1 inhibitors (e.g. snake venom EMS-16) reduced pathological thrombus formation in vivo [136–138]. Platelet α6β1, the main receptor for laminin, plays a role in platelet adhesion/activation and arterial thrombosis, and may also be a new target [135]. Platelet α5β1, the major receptor for fibronectin, plays a supplementary role in platelet adhesion [139], but evidence is lacking regarding the anti-thrombotic benefits of antagonizing α5β1.

Other novel anti-thrombotic candidates: Glucagon-like peptide 1 receptor, P-selectin, CD40/CD40L, and Toll-like receptors

Strategies to target other platelet receptors beyond adhesive proteins have also been developed, such as P2Y12, PAR1, TP, $5HT_{2A}$ antagonists [17, 140]. Interestingly, some chronic diseases, such as diabetes mellitus and atherosclerosis, are associated with arterial thrombosis [23, 141]. Recently, our group identified that a functional Glucagon-like peptide 1 receptor (GLP-1R) is expressed on human megakaryocytes and platelets [142]. Importantly, GLP-1R agonists (e.g. Exenatide), likely through increasing the intracellular cAMP levels, inhibit platelet function and thrombus formation [142]. This study provides important insights into why diabetic patients who are receiving GLP-1-targeted therapies have a reduced number of cardiovascular events [142, 143]. In addition, given the cross-talks between platelets and immune systems, thrombosis also intensively communicates with the inflammatory pathway [23]. Some anti-inflammatory/anti-atherosclerotic agents may therefore also indirectly inhibit thrombosis, especially in deep vein thrombosis [144]. For example, antagonists of P-selectin/PSGL-1, such as rPSGL-Ig [145], PSI-697 [146], PSI-421 [147], inhibit platelet-mediated leukocyte attachment and recruitment of procoagulant microparticles, and may represent a safe therapeutic intervention in accelerating thrombolysis [148]. Antagonists of CD40/CD40L [149], such as CD40 antibody, reduce atherosclerotic burden in a murine model [150]. In addition, as the important roles of Toll-like receptors in atherosclerosis are gradually recognized [151, 152], they may also be potential targets for the treatment of atherothrombosis.

Conclusions

Arterial thrombotic events, such as myocardial infarction and ischemic stroke, and venous thromboembolism, are three leading causes of morbidity and mortality worldwide [153]. Platelets play a central role in the pathogenesis of atherothrombosis, and contribute profoundly to the pathology of venous thrombosis [23]. Platelet adhesion molecules, act as the contacts between platelets and other cells or extracellular matrix proteins and, to a great extent, may determine the reactivity of platelets and thus are attractive anti-thrombotic targets (Fig. 1) [23]. Although evidence-based antiplatelet therapy has markedly improved patient care, on-treatment events and bleeding are still major concerns [17, 148].

Optimization of the use of currently available therapies, and improvements to the understanding of individual differences in response to anti-platelet treatments are still the most cost-effective treatment strategies [17, 148]. Additionally, improved understanding of the mechanisms of platelet accumulation has been critical for further developing novel antiplatelet therapies, such as the PAR1 antagonist Vorapaxar (recently approved by the FDA), GPIbα/VWF antagonists (e.g. ALX-0081 and Anfibatide; undergoing clinical trials), and GPVI antagonist (e.g. Revacept; undergoing clinical trials) (See section II. A-C). Another cost-effective strategy may be to repurpose already-established drugs by discovering novel mechanisms of action in anti-thrombotic diseases, such as the recently-identified GLP-1R agonist, Exenatide, an anti-diabetic drug that has potential anti-thrombotic effects [142, 154]. Future studies in the areas of atherothrombosis, inflammation, metabolic syndrome, diabetes, lipid metabolism and cancer-related thrombotic diseases in the next few years should advance our knowledge and the application of these and other new anti-platelet agents. Of note, clinical trials provide important evidence regarding the safety and efficacy of the treatments. However, difficulties such as narrow eligibility criteria, low enrollment of patients and the necessity to test the new drugs on top of the current dual antiplatelet therapy (e.g. aspirin and clopidogrel), may add complexity to the development of new drugs and also deserve our attention.

Acknowledgements

The authors would like to thank Dr. Richard O. Hynes, Dr. Zaverio M. Ruggeri, Dr. Denisa D. Wagner, and Dr. John Freedman for their long-term support for these research projects.

Funding

This work was supported by the Canadian Institutes of Health Research (MOP 119540, MOP 97918, and MOP 119551), Heart and Stroke Foundation of Canada (Ontario), Equipment Funds from Canada Foundation for Innovation, St. Michael's Hospital, and Canadian Blood Services; and research Funds from CCOA Therapeutics Inc and Lee's Pharmaceutical Holdings limited. X. R. X is a recipient of China National Scholarship award, Meredith & Malcolm Silver Scholarship in Cardiovascular Studies of Department of Laboratory Medicine and Pathobiology, and the Heart and Stroke/Richard Lewar Centre of Excellence Studentship award, University of Toronto. N.C. is a recipient of the Canadian Blood Services Postdoctoral Fellowship.

Authors' contributions

XRX and NC drafted the manuscript. MADN drew the figure. TM, TWS and RMPC contributed to preparation of the manuscript. XL, XD and BXL contributed to the original findings on the phase II human clinical trials of Anfibatide. PC and JX contributed to the original findings and further development of anti-PSI monoclonal antibodies. HN is the principal investigator who defined the topic and revised the manuscript. All of authors read, commented and approved the final manuscript.

Competing interests

J. X. is supported by the CCOA Therapeutics Inc. X. D. and B.X.L. are supported by the Lee's Pharmaceutical Holdings limited. Some of the research fund of the projects is supported by CCOA Therapeutics and Lee's Pharmaceutical Holdings limited. Canadian Blood Services have held the patents on the anti-GPIb NIT family monoclonal antibodies and anti-PSI monoclonal antibodies.

Author details

[1]Department of Laboratory Medicine and Pathobiology, University of Toronto, Toronto, ON, Canada. [2]Department of Laboratory Medicine, Keenan Research Centre for Biomedical Science, St. Michael's Hospital, Toronto, ON, Canada. [3]Guangdong Provincial Hospital of Chinese Medicine, Guangzhou University of Chinese Medicine, Guangzhou, Guangdong, People's Republic of China. [4]Canadian Blood Services, Toronto, ON, Canada. [5]CCOA Therapeutics Inc, Toronto, ON, Canada. [6]Lee's Pharmaceutical holdings limited, Shatin, Hong Kong, China. [7]Zhaoke Pharmaceutical co. limited, Hefei, Anhui, China. [8]Hong Kong University of Science and technology, Hong Kong, China. [9]Department of Medicine and Department of Physiology, University of Toronto, Toronto, ON, Canada.

References

1. Ruggeri ZM. Platelets in atherothrombosis. Nat Med. 2002;8:1227–34.
2. Mackman N. Triggers, targets and treatments for thrombosis. Nature. 2008;451:914–8.
3. Xu XR, Gallant RC, Ni H. Platelets, immune-mediated thrombocytopenias, and fetal hemorrhage. Thromb Res. 2016;141 Suppl 2:S76–9.
4. Ni H, Freedman J. Platelets in hemostasis and thrombosis: role of integrins and their ligands. Transfus Apher Sci. 2003;28:257–64.
5. Yang H, Reheman A, Chen P, Zhu G, Hynes RO, Freedman J, et al. Fibrinogen and von Willebrand factor-independent platelet aggregation in vitro and in vivo. J Thromb Haemost. 2006;4:2230–7.
6. Wang Y, Gallant RC, Ni H. Extracellular matrix proteins in the regulation of thrombus formation. Curr Opin Hematol. 2016;23:280–7.
7. Moroi M, Jung SM, Okuma M, Shinmyozu K. A patient with platelets deficient in glycoprotein VI that lack both collagen-induced aggregation and adhesion. J Clin Invest. 1989;84:1440–5.
8. Dunne E, Spring CM, Reheman A, Jin W, Berndt MC, Newman DK, et al. Cadherin 6 has a functional role in platelet aggregation and thrombus formation. Arterioscler Thromb Vasc Biol. 2012;32:1724–31.
9. Palabrica T, Lobb R, Furie BC, Aronovitz M, Benjamin C, Hsu YM, et al. Leukocyte accumulation promoting fibrin deposition is mediated in vivo by P-selectin on adherent platelets. Nature. 1992;359:848–51.
10. Yang H, Lang S, Zhai Z, Li L, Kahr WH, Chen P, et al. Fibrinogen is required for maintenance of platelet intracellular and cell-surface P-selectin expression. Blood. 2009;114:425–36.
11. Nurden AT. Platelet membrane glycoproteins: a historical review. Semin Thromb Hemost. 2014;40:577–84.
12. Lopez JA, Andrews RK, Afshar-Kharghan V, Berndt MC. Bernard-Soulier syndrome. Blood. 1998;91:4397–418.
13. Jackson SP. Arterial thrombosis–insidious, unpredictable and deadly. Nat Med. 2011;17:1423–36.
14. Reheman A, Xu X, Reddy EC, Ni H. Targeting activated platelets and fibrinolysis: hitting two birds with one stone. Circ Res. 2014;114:1070–3.
15. Writing Group Members, Mozaffarian D, Benjamin EJ, Go AS, Arnett DK, Blaha MJ, et al. Heart disease and stroke statistics-2016 update: a report from the American Heart Association. Circulation. 2016;133:e38–60.
16. Michelson AD. Antiplatelet therapies for the treatment of cardiovascular disease. Nat Rev Drug Discov. 2010;9:154–69.
17. Franchi F, Angiolillo DJ. Novel antiplatelet agents in acute coronary syndrome. Nat Rev Cardiol. 2015;12:30–47.
18. Gachet C. Antiplatelet drugs: which targets for which treatments? J Thromb Haemost. 2015;13 Suppl 1:S313–22.
19. Hou Y, Carrim N, Wang Y, Gallant RC, Marshall A, Ni H. Platelets in hemostasis and thrombosis: novel mechanisms of fibrinogen-independent platelet aggregation and fibronectin-mediated protein wave of hemostasis. J Biomed Res. 2015;29:437–44.
20. Wang H, Bang KW, Blanchette VS, Nurden AT, Rand ML. Phosphatidylserine exposure, microparticle formation and mitochondrial depolarisation in Glanzmann thrombasthenia platelets. Thromb Haemost. 2014;111:1184–6.
21. Wang Y, Reheman A, Spring CM, Kalantari J, Marshall AH, Wolberg AS, et al. Plasma fibronectin supports hemostasis and regulates thrombosis. J Clin Invest. 2014;124:4281–93.
22. Wang Y, Ni H. Fibronectin maintains the balance between hemostasis and thrombosis. Cell Mol Life Sci. 2016;73(17):3265–77. doi:10.1007/s00018-016-2225-y.
23. Xu XR, Zhang D, Oswald BE, Carrim N, Wang X, Hou Y, et al. Platelets are versatile cells: New discoveries in hemostasis, thrombosis, immune responses, tumor metastasis and beyond. Crit Rev Clin Lab Sci. 2016. Published online:1–69. doi: 10.1080/10408363.2016.1200008.
24. Metharom P, Berndt MC, Baker RI, Andrews RK. Current state and novel approaches of antiplatelet therapy. Arterioscler Thromb Vasc Biol. 2015;35:1327–38.
25. Michelson AD. Advances in antiplatelet therapy. Hematology Am Soc Hematol Educ Program. 2011;2011:62–9.
26. Jackson SP, Schoenwaelder SM. Antiplatelet therapy: in search of the 'magic bullet'. Nat Rev Drug Discov. 2003;2:775–89.
27. Morrow DA, Braunwald E, Bonaca MP, Ameriso SF, Dalby AJ, Fish MP, et al. Vorapaxar in the secondary prevention of atherothrombotic events. N Engl J Med. 2012;366:1404–13.
28. Adminstration USFaD. Drug Trials Snapshot Zontivity (vorapaxar). 2014. http://www.fda.gov/Drugs/InformationOnDrugs/ucm423935.htm. Accessed 15 June 2016.
29. ClinicalTrials.gov. 2011. https://clinicaltrials.gov/ct2/show/NCT00527943?term=Vorapaxar&rank=5. Accessed 15 June 2016.
30. Hynes RO. Integrins: bidirectional, allosteric signaling machines. Cell. 2002;110:673–87.
31. Mou Y, Ni H, Wilkins JA. The selective inhibition of beta 1 and beta 7 integrin-mediated lymphocyte adhesion by bacitracin. J Immunol. 1998;161:6323–9.
32. Clemetson KJ, Clemetson JM. Platelet receptors. In: Michelson AD, editor. Platelets. 3rd ed. Amsterdam: Academic Press/Elsevier; 2013. p. 169–94.
33. Varga-Szabo D, Pleines I, Nieswandt B. Cell adhesion mechanisms in platelets. Arterioscler Thromb Vasc Biol. 2008;28:403–12.
34. Tamura S, Suzuki-Inoue K, Tsukiji N, Shirai T, Sasaki T, Osada M, et al. Podoplanin-positive periarteriolar stromal cells promote megakaryocyte growth and proplatelet formation in mice by CLEC-2. Blood. 2016;127:1701–10.
35. Li C, Li J, Li Y, Lang S, Yougbare I, Zhu G, et al. Crosstalk between platelets and the immune system: old systems with new discoveries. Adv Hematol. 2012;2012:384685.
36. Semple JW, Italiano Jr JE, Freedman J. Platelets and the immune continuum. Nat Rev Immunol. 2011;11:264–74.

37. Wagner DD, Burger PC. Platelets in inflammation and thrombosis. Arterioscler Thromb Vasc Biol. 2003;23:2131–7.
38. Siegel-Axel D, Daub K, Seizer P, Lindemann S, Gawaz M. Platelet lipoprotein interplay: trigger of foam cell formation and driver of atherosclerosis. Cardiovasc Res. 2008;78:8–17.
39. Lindemann S, Kramer B, Seizer P, Gawaz M. Platelets, inflammation and atherosclerosis. J Thromb Haemost. 2007;5 Suppl 1:203–11.
40. Murphy AJ, Bijl N, Yvan-Charvet L, Welch CB, Bhagwat N, Reheman A, et al. Cholesterol efflux in megakaryocyte progenitors suppresses platelet production and thrombocytosis. Nat Med. 2013;19:586–94.
41. Hess PR, Rawnsley DR, Jakus Z, Yang Y, Sweet DT, Fu J, et al. Platelets mediate lymphovenous hemostasis to maintain blood-lymphatic separation throughout life. J Clin Invest. 2014;124:273–84.
42. Navarro-Nunez L, Langan SA, Nash GB, Watson SP. The physiological and pathophysiological roles of platelet CLEC-2. Thromb Haemost. 2013;109:991–8.
43. Osada M, Inoue O, Ding G, Shirai T, Ichise H, Hirayama K, et al. Platelet activation receptor CLEC-2 regulates blood/lymphatic vessel separation by inhibiting proliferation, migration, and tube formation of lymphatic endothelial cells. J Biol Chem. 2012;287:22241–52.
44. Herzog BH, Fu J, Wilson SJ, Hess PR, Sen A, McDaniel JM, et al. Podoplanin maintains high endothelial venule integrity by interacting with platelet CLEC-2. Nature. 2013;502:105–9.
45. Italiano Jr JE, Richardson JL, Patel-Hett S, Battinelli E, Zaslavsky A, Short S, et al. Angiogenesis is regulated by a novel mechanism: pro- and antiangiogenic proteins are organized into separate platelet alpha granules and differentially released. Blood. 2008;111:1227–33.
46. Chatterjee M, Huang Z, Zhang W, Jiang L, Hultenby K, Zhu L, et al. Distinct platelet packaging, release, and surface expression of proangiogenic and antiangiogenic factors on different platelet stimuli. Blood. 2011;117:3907–11.
47. Yougbare I, Lang S, Yang H, Chen P, Zhao X, Tai WS, et al. Maternal anti-platelet beta3 integrins impair angiogenesis and cause intracranial hemorrhage. J Clin Invest. 2015;125:1545–56.
48. Li C, Piran S, Chen P, Lang S, Zarpellon A, Jin JW, et al. The maternal immune response to fetal platelet GPIbalpha causes frequent miscarriage in mice that can be prevented by intravenous IgG and anti-FcRn therapies. J Clin Invest. 2011;121:4537–47.
49. Yougbare I, Wei-She T, Zdravic D, Chen P, Zhu G, Leong-Poi H, et al. Natural killer cells contribute to pathophysiology of placenta leading to miscarriage in fetal and neonatal alloimmune thrombocytopenia. Blood. 2015;126:2254.
50. Labelle M, Hynes RO. The initial hours of metastasis: the importance of cooperative host-tumor cell interactions during hematogenous dissemination. Cancer Discov. 2012;2:1091–9.
51. Labelle M, Begum S, Hynes RO. Platelets guide the formation of early metastatic niches. Proc Natl Acad Sci U S A. 2014;111:E3053–61.
52. Franco AT, Corken A, Ware J. Platelets at the interface of thrombosis, inflammation, and cancer. Blood. 2015;126:582–8.
53. Luo SZ, Mo X, Afshar-Kharghan V, Srinivasan S, Lopez JA, Li R. Glycoprotein Ibalpha forms disulfide bonds with 2 glycoprotein Ibbeta subunits in the resting platelet. Blood. 2007;109:603–9.
54. Jackson SP. The growing complexity of platelet aggregation. Blood. 2007;109:5087–95.
55. Ruggeri ZM, Mendolicchio GL. Adhesion mechanisms in platelet function. Circ Res. 2007;100:1673–85.
56. Huizinga EG, Tsuji S, Romijn RA, Schiphorst ME, de Groot PG, Sixma JJ, et al. Structures of glycoprotein Ibalpha and its complex with von Willebrand factor A1 domain. Science. 2002;297:1176–9.
57. Verhenne S, Denorme F, Libbrecht S, Vandenbulcke A, Pareyn I, Deckmyn H, et al. Platelet-derived VWF is not essential for normal thrombosis and hemostasis but fosters ischemic stroke injury in mice. Blood. 2015;126:1715–22.
58. Dumas JJ, Kumar R, Seehra J, Somers WS, Mosyak L. Crystal structure of the GpIbalpha-thrombin complex essential for platelet aggregation. Science. 2003;301:222–6.
59. Celikel R, McClintock RA, Roberts JR, Mendolicchio GL, Ware J, Varughese KI, et al. Modulation of alpha-thrombin function by distinct interactions with platelet glycoprotein Ibalpha. Science. 2003;301:218–21.
60. Andrews RK, Berndt MC. The GPIb-IX-V Complex. In: Michelson AD, editor. Platelets. 3rd ed. Amsterdam: Academic Press/Elsevier; 2013. p. 195–213.
61. De Candia E, Hall SW, Rutella S, Landolfi R, Andrews RK, De Cristofaro R. Binding of thrombin to glycoprotein Ib accelerates the hydrolysis of Par-1 on intact platelets. J Biol Chem. 2001;276:4692–8.
62. Ramakrishnan V, DeGuzman F, Bao M, Hall SW, Leung LL, Phillips DR. A thrombin receptor function for platelet glycoprotein Ib-IX unmasked by cleavage of glycoprotein V. Proc Natl Acad Sci U S A. 2001;98:1823–8.
63. Ni H, Ramakrishnan V, Ruggeri ZM, Papalia JM, Phillips DR, Wagner DD. Increased thrombogenesis and embolus formation in mice lacking glycoprotein V. Blood. 2001;98:368–73.
64. Jurk K, Clemetson KJ, de Groot PG, Brodde MF, Steiner M, Savion N, et al. Thrombospondin-1 mediates platelet adhesion at high shear via glycoprotein Ib (GPIb): an alternative/backup mechanism to von Willebrand factor. FASEB J. 2003;17:1490–2.
65. Baglia FA, Badellino KO, Li CQ, Lopez JA, Walsh PN. Factor XI binding to the platelet glycoprotein Ib-IX-V complex promotes factor XI activation by thrombin. J Biol Chem. 2002;277:1662–8.
66. Bradford HN, Pixley RA, Colman RW. Human factor XII binding to the glycoprotein Ib-IX-V complex inhibits thrombin-induced platelet aggregation. J Biol Chem. 2000;275:22756–63.
67. Weeterings C, de Groot PG, Adelmeijer J, Lisman T. The glycoprotein Ib-IX-V complex contributes to tissue factor-independent thrombin generation by recombinant factor VIIa on the activated platelet surface. Blood. 2008;112:3227–33.
68. Chavakis T, Santoso S, Clemetson KJ, Sachs UJ, Isordia-Salas I, Pixley RA, et al. High molecular weight kininogen regulates platelet-leukocyte interactions by bridging Mac-1 and glycoprotein Ib. J Biol Chem. 2003;278:45375–81.
69. Romo GM, Dong JF, Schade AJ, Gardiner EE, Kansas GS, Li CQ, et al. The glycoprotein Ib-IX-V complex is a platelet counterreceptor for P-selectin. J Exp Med. 1999;190:803–14.
70. Kaplan ZS, Zarpellon A, Alwis I, Yuan Y, McFadyen J, Ghasemzadeh M, et al. Thrombin-dependent intravascular leukocyte trafficking regulated by fibrin and the platelet receptors GPIb and PAR4. Nat Commun. 2015;6:7835.
71. Simon DI, Chen Z, Xu H, Li CQ, Dong J, McIntire LV, et al. Platelet glycoprotein ibalpha is a counterreceptor for the leukocyte integrin Mac-1 (CD11b/CD18). J Exp Med. 2000;192:193–204.
72. Chandraratne S, von Bruehl ML, Pagel JI, Stark K, Kleinert E, Konrad I, et al. Critical role of platelet glycoprotein ibalpha in arterial remodeling. Arterioscler Thromb Vasc Biol. 2015;35:589–97.
73. Li J, van der Wal DE, Zhu G, Xu M, Yougbare I, Ma L, et al. Desialylation is a mechanism of Fc-independent platelet clearance and a therapeutic target in immune thrombocytopenia. Nat Commun. 2015;6:7737.
74. Li J, Callum JL, Lin Y, Zhou Y, Zhu G, Ni H. Severe platelet desialylation in a patient with glycoprotein Ib/IX antibody-mediated immune thrombocytopenia and fatal pulmonary hemorrhage. Haematologica. 2014;99:e61–3.
75. Gresele P, Momi S. Inhibitors of the interaction between von Willebrand factor and platelet GPIb/IX/V. Handb Exp Pharmacol. 2012;(210):287–309.
76. Ulrichts H, Silence K, Schoolmeester A, de Jaegere P, Rossenu S, Roodt J, et al. Antithrombotic drug candidate ALX-0081 shows superior preclinical efficacy and safety compared with currently marketed antiplatelet drugs. Blood. 2011;118:757–65.
77. Bartunek J, Barbato E, Heyndrickx G, Vanderheyden M, Wijns W, Holz JB. Novel antiplatelet agents: ALX-0081, a Nanobody directed towards von Willebrand factor. J Cardiovasc Transl Res. 2013;6:355–63.
78. Muller O, Bartunek J, Hamilos M, Berza CT, Mangiacapra F, Ntalianis A, et al. von Willebrand factor inhibition improves endothelial function in patients with stable angina. J Cardiovasc Transl Res. 2013;6:364–70.
79. Peyvandi F, Scully M, Kremer Hovinga JA, Cataland S, Knobl P, Wu H, et al. Caplacizumab for acquired thrombotic thrombocytopenic purpura. N Engl J Med. 2016;374:511–22.
80. Lammle B. Thrombotic microangiopathy: caplacizumab accelerates resolution of acute acquired TTP. Nat Rev Nephrol. 2016;12:259–60.
81. Von VA. Willebrand factor–a new target for TTP treatment? N Engl J Med. 2016;374:583–5.
82. Blombery P, Scully M. Management of thrombotic thrombocytopenic purpura: current perspectives. J Blood Med. 2014;5:15–23.
83. Lei X, Reheman A, Hou Y, Zhou H, Wang Y, Marshall AH, et al. Anfibatide, a novel GPIb complex antagonist, inhibits platelet adhesion and thrombus formation in vitro and in vivo in murine models of thrombosis. Thromb Haemost. 2014;111:279–89.
84. Hou Y, Li BX, Dai X, Yang Z, Qian F, Zhang G, et al. The first in vitro and in vivo assessment of anfibatide, a novel glycoprotein ib antagonist, in mice and in a phase i human clinical trial. Blood. 2013;122:577.

85. Li B, Dai X, Yang Z, Qian F, Zhang G, Xu Z, et al. First ex vivo and in vivo assessment of anfibatide, a novel glycoprotein Ib-IV-V complex antagonist, in healthy human volunteers in phase I clinical trial. J Thromb Haemost. 2013;11 Suppl 2:23.
86. Nieswandt B, Kleinschnitz C, Stoll G. Ischaemic stroke: a thrombo-inflammatory disease? J Physiol. 2011;589:4115–23.
87. Stoll G, Kleinschnitz C, Nieswandt B. Molecular mechanisms of thrombus formation in ischemic stroke: novel insights and targets for treatment. Blood. 2008;112:3555–62.
88. Kleinschnitz C, Pozgajova M, Pham M, Bendszus M, Nieswandt B, Stoll G. Targeting platelets in acute experimental stroke: impact of glycoprotein Ib, VI, and IIb/IIIa blockade on infarct size, functional outcome, and intracranial bleeding. Circulation. 2007;115:2323–30.
89. Li TT, Fan ML, Hou SX, Li XY, Barry DM, Jin H, Luo SY, Kong F, Lau LF, Dai XR, Zhang GH, Zhou LL. A novel snake venomderived GPIb antagonist, anfibatide, protects mice from acute experimental ischaemic stroke and reperfusion injury. Br J Pharmacol.
90. Fontayne A, Meiring M, Lamprecht S, Roodt J, Demarsin E, Barbeaux P, et al. The humanized anti-glycoprotein Ib monoclonal antibody h6B4-Fab is a potent and safe antithrombotic in a high shear arterial thrombosis model in baboons. Thromb Haemost. 2008;100:670–7.
91. Hennan JK, Swillo RE, Morgan GA, Leik CE, Brooks JM, Shaw GD, et al. Pharmacologic inhibition of platelet vWF-GPIb alpha interaction prevents coronary artery thrombosis. Thromb Haemost. 2006;95:469–75.
92. Ni H, Zhu G. Novel monoclonal antibodies against platelet GPIb-alpha: potential anti-thrombotic drugs and research reagents for study of thrombosis and hemostasis. 2012. US8323652.
93. Moroi AJ, Watson SP. Impact of the PI3-kinase/Akt pathway on ITAM and hemITAM receptors: haemostasis, platelet activation and antithrombotic therapy. Biochem Pharmacol. 2015;94:186–94.
94. Alshehri OM, Hughes CE, Montague S, Watson SK, Frampton J, Bender M, et al. Fibrin activates GPVI in human and mouse platelets. Blood. 2015;126:1601–8.
95. Mammadova-Bach E, Ollivier V, Loyau S, Schaff M, Dumont B, Favier R, et al. Platelet glycoprotein VI binds to polymerized fibrin and promotes thrombin generation. Blood. 2015;126:683–91.
96. Bigalke B, Stellos K, Geisler T, Kremmer E, Seizer P, May AE, et al. Expression of platelet glycoprotein VI is associated with transient ischemic attack and stroke. Eur J Neurol. 2010;17:111–7.
97. Induruwa I, Jung SM, Warburton EA. Beyond antiplatelets: the role of glycoprotein VI in ischemic stroke. Int J Stroke. 2016. doi:10.1177/1747493016654532.
98. Al-Tamimi M, Gardiner EE, Thom JY, Shen Y, Cooper MN, Hankey GJ, et al. Soluble glycoprotein VI is raised in the plasma of patients with acute ischemic stroke. Stroke. 2011;42:498–500.
99. Stoll G, Kleinschnitz C, Nieswandt B. Combating innate inflammation: a new paradigm for acute treatment of stroke? Ann N Y Acad Sci. 2010;1207:149–54.
100. Thornton P, McColl BW, Greenhalgh A, Denes A, Allan SM, Rothwell NJ. Platelet interleukin-1alpha drives cerebrovascular inflammation. Blood. 2010; 115:3632–9.
101. Stegner D, Haining EJ, Nieswandt B. Targeting glycoprotein VI and the immunoreceptor tyrosine-based activation motif signaling pathway. Arterioscler Thromb Vasc Biol. 2014;34:1615–20.
102. Dutting S, Bender M, Nieswandt B. Platelet GPVI: a target for antithrombotic therapy?! Trends Pharmacol Sci. 2012;33:583–90.
103. Pachel C, Mathes D, Arias-Loza AP, Heitzmann W, Nordbeck P, Deppermann C, et al. Inhibition of platelet GPVI protects against myocardial ischemia-reperfusion injury. Arterioscler Thromb Vasc Biol. 2016;36:629–35.
104. Goebel S, Li Z, Vogelmann J, Holthoff HP, Degen H, Hermann DM, et al. The GPVI-Fc fusion protein Revacept improves cerebral infarct volume and functional outcome in stroke. PLoS One. 2013;8:e66960.
105. Ungerer M, Rosport K, Bultmann A, Piechatzek R, Uhland K, Schlieper P, et al. Novel antiplatelet drug revacept (Dimeric Glycoprotein VI-Fc) specifically and efficiently inhibited collagen-induced platelet aggregation without affecting general hemostasis in humans. Circulation. 2011;123:1891–9.
106. ClinicalTrials.gov. 2015. https://clinicaltrials.gov/ct2/show/NCT01645306?term=Revacept&rank=1. Accessed 15 June 2016.
107. Ono K, Ueda H, Yoshizawa Y, Akazawa D, Tanimura R, Shimada I, et al. Structural basis for platelet antiaggregation by angiotensin II type 1 receptor antagonist losartan (DuP-753) via glycoprotein VI. J Med Chem. 2010;53:2087–93.
108. Muzard J, Bouabdelli M, Zahid M, Ollivier V, Lacapere JJ, Jandrot-Perrus M, et al. Design and humanization of a murine scFv that blocks human platelet glycoprotein VI in vitro. FEBS J. 2009;276:4207–22.
109. Takagi J, Petre BM, Walz T, Springer TA. Global conformational rearrangements in integrin extracellular domains in outside-in and inside-out signaling. Cell. 2002;110:599–611.
110. Li R, Mitra N, Gratkowski H, Vilaire G, Litvinov R, Nagasami C, et al. Activation of integrin alphaIIbbeta3 by modulation of transmembrane helix associations. Science. 2003;300:795–8.
111. Vinogradova O, Vaynberg J, Kong X, Haas TA, Plow EF, Qin J. Membrane-mediated structural transitions at the cytoplasmic face during integrin activation. Proc Natl Acad Sci U S A. 2004;101:4094–9.
112. Vinogradova O, Velyvis A, Velyviene A, Hu B, Haas T, Plow E, et al. A structural mechanism of integrin alpha(IIb)beta(3) "inside-out" activation as regulated by its cytoplasmic face. Cell. 2002;110:587–97.
113. Ni H, Denis CV, Subbarao S, Degen JL, Sato TN, Hynes RO, et al. Persistence of platelet thrombus formation in arterioles of mice lacking both von Willebrand factor and fibrinogen. J Clin Invest. 2000;106:385–92.
114. Law DA, DeGuzman FR, Heiser P, Ministri-Madrid K, Killeen N, Phillips DR. Integrin cytoplasmic tyrosine motif is required for outside-in alphaIIbbeta3 signalling and platelet function. Nature. 1999;401:808–11.
115. Hodivala-Dilke KM, McHugh KP, Tsakiris DA, Rayburn H, Crowley D, Ullman-Cullere M, et al. Beta3-integrin-deficient mice are a model for Glanzmann thrombasthenia showing placental defects and reduced survival. J Clin Invest. 1999;103:229–38.
116. Reheman A, Yang H, Zhu G, Jin W, He F, Spring CM, et al. Plasma fibronectin depletion enhances platelet aggregation and thrombus formation in mice lacking fibrinogen and von Willebrand factor. Blood. 2009;113:1809–17.
117. Reheman A, Gross P, Yang H, Chen P, Allen D, Leytin V, et al. Vitronectin stabilizes thrombi and vessel occlusion but plays a dual role in platelet aggregation. J Thromb Haemost. 2005;3:875–83.
118. Topol EJ, Byzova TV, Plow EF. Platelet GPIIb-IIIa blockers. Lancet. 1999;353:227–31.
119. Phillips DR, Scarborough RM. Clinical pharmacology of eptifibatide. Am J Cardiol. 1997;80:11B–20B.
120. Egbertson MS, Chang CT, Duggan ME, Gould RJ, Halczenko W, Hartman GD, et al. Non-peptide fibrinogen receptor antagonists. 2. Optimization of a tyrosine template as a mimic for Arg-Gly-Asp. J Med Chem. 1994;37:2537–51.
121. Schneider DJ. Anti-platelet therapy: glycoprotein IIb-IIIa antagonists. Br J Clin Pharmacol. 2011;72:672–82.
122. Coller BS. alphaIIbbeta3: structure and function. J Thromb Haemost. 2015;13 Suppl 1:S17–25.
123. Ciccone A, Motto C, Abraha I, Cozzolino F, Santilli I. Glycoprotein IIb-IIIa inhibitors for acute ischaemic stroke. Cochrane Database Syst Rev. 2014;3:CD005208.
124. Li J, Vootukuri S, Shang Y, Negri A, Jiang JK, Nedelman M, et al. RUC-4: a novel alphaIIbbeta3 antagonist for prehospital therapy of myocardial infarction. Arterioscler Thromb Vasc Biol. 2014;34:2321–9.
125. Xiong JP, Stehle T, Goodman SL, Arnaout MA. A novel adaptation of the integrin PSI domain revealed from its crystal structure. J Biol Chem. 2004;279:40252–4.
126. Zang Q, Springer TA. Amino acid residues in the PSI domain and cysteine-rich repeats of the integrin beta2 subunit that restrain activation of the integrin alpha(X)beta(2). J Biol Chem. 2001;276:6922–9.
127. Ni H, Li A, Simonsen N, Wilkins JA. Integrin activation by dithiothreitol or Mn2+ induces a ligand-occupied conformation and exposure of a novel NH2-terminal regulatory site on the beta1 integrin chain. J Biol Chem. 1998; 273:7981–7.
128. Yan B, Smith JW. A redox site involved in integrin activation. J Biol Chem. 2000;275:39964–72.
129. Essex DW, Li M. Redox control of platelet aggregation. Biochemistry. 2003; 42:129–36.
130. Manickam N, Ahmad SS, Essex DW. Vicinal thiols are required for activation of the alphaIIbbeta3 platelet integrin. J Thromb Haemost. 2011;9:1207–15.
131. Wang L, Wu Y, Zhou J, Ahmad SS, Mutus B, Garbi N, et al. Platelet-derived ERp57 mediates platelet incorporation into a growing thrombus by regulation of the alphaIIbbeta3 integrin. Blood. 2013;122:3642–50.
132. Carrim N, Zhu G, Reddy E, Xu M, Xu X, Wang Y, et al. Integrin PSI domain has endogenous thiol isomerase function and is a novel target for anti-thrombotic therapy. J Thromb Haemost. 2015;13(Supplement S2):60.

133. Wang X, Palasubramaniam J, Gkanatsas Y, Hohmann JD, Westein E, Kanojia R, et al. Towards effective and safe thrombolysis and thromboprophylaxis: preclinical testing of a novel antibody-targeted recombinant plasminogen activator directed against activated platelets. Circ Res. 2014;114:1083–93.
134. Fuentes RE, Zaitsev S, Ahn HS, Hayes V, Kowalska M, Lambert MP, et al. A chimeric platelet-targeted urokinase prodrug selectively blocks new thrombus formation. J Clin Invest. 2016;126:483–94.
135. Schaff M, Tang C, Maurer E, Bourdon C, Receveur N, Eckly A, et al. Integrin alpha6beta1 is the main receptor for vascular laminins and plays a role in platelet adhesion, activation, and arterial thrombosis. Circulation. 2013;128:541–52.
136. Miller MW, Basra S, Kulp DW, Billings PC, Choi S, Beavers MP, et al. Small-molecule inhibitors of integrin alpha2beta1 that prevent pathological thrombus formation via an allosteric mechanism. Proc Natl Acad Sci U S A. 2009;106:719–24.
137. Marcinkiewicz C, Lobb RR, Marcinkiewicz MM, Daniel JL, Smith JB, Dangelmaier C, et al. Isolation and characterization of EMS16, a C-lectin type protein from Echis multisquamatus venom, a potent and selective inhibitor of the alpha2beta1 integrin. Biochemistry. 2000;39:9859–67.
138. Arlinghaus FT, Momic T, Ammar NA, Shai E, Spectre G, Varon D, et al. Identification of alpha2beta1 integrin inhibitor VP-i with anti-platelet properties in the venom of Vipera palaestinae. Toxicon. 2013;64:96–105.
139. Piotrowicz RS, Orchekowski RP, Nugent DJ, Yamada KY, Kunicki TJ. Glycoprotein Ic-IIa functions as an activation-independent fibronectin receptor on human platelets. J Cell Biol. 1988;106:1359–64.
140. Przyklenk K, Frelinger 3rd AL, Linden MD, Whittaker P, Li Y, Barnard MR, et al. Targeted inhibition of the serotonin 5HT2A receptor improves coronary patency in an in vivo model of recurrent thrombosis. J Thromb Haemost. 2010;8:331–40.
141. Ni H. The platelet "sugar high" in diabetes. Blood. 2012;119:5949–51.
142. Cameron-Vendrig A, Reheman A, Siraj MA, Xu XR, Wang Y, Lei X, et al. Glucagon-like peptide 1 receptor activation attenuates platelet aggregation and thrombosis. Diabetes. 2016;65:1714–23.
143. Monami M, Dicembrini I, Nardini C, Fiordelli I, Mannucci E. Effects of glucagon-like peptide-1 receptor agonists on cardiovascular risk: a meta-analysis of randomized clinical trials. Diabetes Obes Metab. 2014;16:38–47.
144. Martinod K, Wagner DD. Thrombosis: tangled up in NETs. Blood. 2014;123:2768–76.
145. Kumar A, Villani MP, Patel UK, Keith Jr JC, Schaub RG. Recombinant soluble form of PSGL-1 accelerates thrombolysis and prevents reocclusion in a porcine model. Circulation. 1999;99:1363–9.
146. Bedard PW, Clerin V, Sushkova N, Tchernychev B, Antrilli T, Resmini C, et al. Characterization of the novel P-selectin inhibitor PSI-697 [2-(4-chlorobenzyl)-3-hydroxy-7,8,9,10-tetrahydrobenzo[h] quinoline-4-carboxylic acid] in vitro and in rodent models of vascular inflammation and thrombosis. J Pharmacol Exp Ther. 2008;324:497–506.
147. Meier TR, Myers Jr DD, Wrobleski SK, Zajkowski PJ, Hawley AE, Bedard PW, et al. Prophylactic P-selectin inhibition with PSI-421 promotes resolution of venous thrombosis without anticoagulation. Thromb Haemost. 2008;99:343–51.
148. Kolandaivelu K, Bhatt DL. Novel antiplatelet therapies. In: Michelson AD, editor. Platelets. 3rd ed. Amsterdam: Academic Press/Elsevier; 2013. p. 1185–213.
149. Conde ID, Kleiman NS. Soluble CD40 ligand in acute coronary syndromes. N Engl J Med. 2003;348:2575–7.
150. Schonbeck U, Libby P. CD40 signaling and plaque instability. Circ Res. 2001; 89:1092–103.
151. Lin J, Kakkar V, Lu X. Essential roles of toll-like receptors in atherosclerosis. Curr Med Chem. 2016;23:431–54.
152. Hovland A, Jonasson L, Garred P, Yndestad A, Aukrust P, Lappegard KT, et al. The complement system and toll-like receptors as integrated players in the pathophysiology of atherosclerosis. Atherosclerosis. 2015;241:480–94.
153. Beckman MG, Hooper WC, Critchley SE, Ortel TL. Venous thromboembolism: a public health concern. Am J Prev Med. 2010;38:S495–501.
154. Husain M, Aameron-Vendrig A, Ni H. Methods for inhibiting platelet aggregation using glp-1 receptor agonists. Google Patents; 2014. WO2014066992.

15

Perioperative management of patients on direct oral anticoagulants

Virginie Dubois[1†], Anne-Sophie Dincq[1,2†], Jonathan Douxfils[2,3], Brigitte Ickx[4], Charles-Marc Samama[5], Jean-Michel Dogné[2,3], Maximilien Gourdin[1,2], Bernard Chatelain[2,6], François Mullier[2,6†] and Sarah Lessire[1,2*†]

Abstract

Direct oral anticoagulants (DOACs) have been licensed worldwide for several years for various indications. Each year, 10–15% of patients on oral anticoagulants will undergo an invasive procedure and expert groups have issued several guidelines on perioperative management in such situations. The perioperative guidelines have undergone numerous updates as clinical experience of emergency management has increased and perioperative studies including measurement of residual anticoagulant levels have been published. The high inter-patient variability of DOAC plasma levels has challenged the traditional recommendation that perioperative DOAC interruption should be based only on the elimination half-life of DOACs, especially before invasive procedures carrying a high risk of bleeding. Furthermore, recent publications have highlighted the potential danger of heparin bridging use when DOACs are stopped before an invasive procedure.

As antidotes are progressively becoming available to manage severe bleeding or urgent procedures in patients on DOACs, accurate laboratory tests have become the standard to guide their administration and their actions need to be well understood by clinicians.

This review aims to provide a systematic approach to managing patients on DOACs, based on recent updates of various perioperative guidance, and highlighting the advantages and limits of recommendations based on pharmacokinetic properties and laboratory tests.

Keywords: Anticoagulants, Perioperative period, Invasive procedures, Spinal anesthesia, Emergency care, Blood coagulation test

Background

The number of patients receiving treatment with direct oral anticoagulants (DOACs) is increasing, as clinical trials have demonstrated non-inferiority or superiority in terms of prevention and treatment of thrombo-embolic events [1–11] compared with vitamin K antagonists (VKAs).

Rapid onset and offset of action, short half-life and predictable anticoagulant effects without the need for routine monitoring were the key strengths on which these anticoagulants have been marketed. However, the perioperative management and monitoring of DOACs has proved to be challenging, especially as antidotes were not available immediately following their introduction.

Several expert guidelines [12–14] were developed as soon as DOACs became available to help physicians manage these drugs. More recently, sub-group analyses of the phase III trials as well as results of recent clinical studies [15, 16] have influenced further guidelines [17–19]. Nowadays, around 10–15% of patients on DOACs will have to interrupt their anticoagulant before an invasive procedure every year [20, 21]. Furthermore, antidotes are gradually being licensed [22, 23]. This review aims to summarize current guidance on the perioperative management of DOACs to reflect published research. The literature search was performed in PubMed using the following keywords: perioperative, anticoagulant, dabigatran, rivaroxaban, edoxaban and apixaban. Only publications in English were considered.

* Correspondence: sarah.lessire@uclouvain.be

†Equal contributors

1Université catholique de Louvain, CHU UCL Namur, Department of Anesthesiology, Yvoir, Belgium

2Namur Thrombosis and Hemostasis Center (NTHC), NAmur Research Institute of LIfe Sciences (NARILIS), Namur, Belgium

Full list of author information is available at the end of the article

INDICATIONS FOR DOACs

Dabigatran (a direct anti-IIa inhibitor), rivaroxaban and apixaban (two direct anti-Xa inhibitors) are licensed in the European Union for the prevention of venous thromboembolism (VTE) after orthopedic surgery (hip and knee arthroplasties), for the prevention of thromboembolic events due to non-valvular atrial fibrillation (NVAF), and in the treatment or secondary prophylaxis of VTE [24–26]. Rivaroxaban is also licensed in the European Union for the prevention of atherothrombotic events after acute coronary syndrome with elevated cardiac biomarkers.

Edoxaban is a direct anti-Xa inhibitor that has recently been licensed in the European Union for the prevention of thromboembolic events due to NVAF and the treatment or secondary prophylaxis of venous thromboembolism only [27].

These anticoagulants are given at fixed doses and do not require repetitive coagulation monitoring in the routine follow-up of patients. Table 1 summarizes the pharmacokinetic properties of DOACs. Clinical features such as advanced age, decreased creatinine clearance (CrCl) and some drug-drug interactions are indications for using lower DOAC doses in patients at risk of having supra-therapeutic anticoagulant levels at normal doses [24–27].

PERIOPERATIVE MANAGEMENT OF DOACs

Recent publications strongly recommend the development of institutional guidelines and hospital policies for the perioperative management of DOACs [17, 18]. A checklist including all aspects of the particular procedure and the patient characteristics that may increase the risks of bleeding or thrombosis should be available to guide the perioperative use of DOACs.

Table 2 shows items to consider in a perioperative checklist.

The thrombo-embolic risk of the patient

CHADS2 or CHA2DS2-VASc score

The CHADS2 score and the CHA2DS2-VASc score are used to predict AF-related thromboembolic risk in the absence of anticoagulation and to determine anticoagulant therapy [28, 29]. The CHA2DS2-VASc score has shown better discrimination of patients at truly low risk of thrombo-embolism (TE) [30]. Patients with chronic AF have twice the risk of postoperative stroke than patients without AF [31]. Currently, these scores are proposed to identify patients with AF at high TE risk in a perioperative setting, when they have more than 4 individual risk factors for stroke [19, 32, 33]. However, only the individual risk factors from the CHADS2 stroke risk index were assessed in stratifying the risk of postoperative stroke and not the global value of both scores. Therefore the utility of the CHADS2 and CHA2DS2-VASc scores to predict perioperative stroke needs to be prospectively validated [34].

Table 1 Pharmacokinetic properties of direct oral anticoagulants

	Dabigatran	Rivaroxaban	Apixaban	Edoxaban
Target	Factor IIa	Factor Xa	Factor Xa	Factor Xa
Prodrug	Yes	No	No	No
Tmax (h)	1.0–3.0	2.0–4.0	3.0–4.0	1.0–2.0
Half-life (h)	12-17 h	5–9: healthy individuals 11–13: elderly	8–15: healthy individuals	10–14
Bioavailability	3–7% pH sensitive	For 2.5 mg and 10 mg: 80–100% (fasting or fed) For 15-20 mg: 66%: (fasting) almost 100% (fed)	± 50%	62%
Metabolism	Conjugation	CYP-dependent and independent mechanism	CYP-dependent mechanism (25%)	CYP-dependent (<5%) and independent mechanism (<10%)
Active metabolites	Yes - acylglucuronides	No	No	Yes (<15%)
Elimination of absorbed dose	80% renal	33% unchanged via the kidney	27% renal	50% renal
	20% bile (glucuronide conjugation)	66% metabolized in the liver into inactive metabolites then eliminated via the kidney or the colon in an approximate 50% ratio	73% through the liver, the residue is excreted by the hepatobiliary route	50% metabolism and biliary/intestinal excretion
CYP substrate	No	CYP3A4, CYP2J2	CYP3A4	CYP3A4 (<5%)
P-gp substrate	DE: Yes	Yes	Yes	Yes
BRCP substrate	No	Yes	Yes	No

Tmax: time to reach peak concentration; CYP3A4: cytochrome P450 isozyme 3A4;
P-gp: P-glycoprotein; BRCP: Breast cancer resistance protein

Table 2 Items of the perioperative checklist

THE PERIOPERATIVE CHECKLIST
➢ The thrombo-embolic risk of the patient
➢ The bleeding risk of the patient
➢ Timing of stopping DOAC before an invasive procedure: • The bleeding risk of the invasive procedure • The elimination half-life of the DOAC used depending on the patient's ° renal function, liver function, and co-medication
➢ Specific considerations for some invasive procedures: ° Neuraxial anesthesia ° Atrial fibrillation ablation
➢ When should bridging therapy with heparin be suggested?
➢ Resuming a DOAC after an invasive procedure or surgery

Apart from these scores, patients with a recent history of stroke or transient ischemic attack (within 3 months) are considered as high TE risk. The 9th edition of the American College of Chest Physicians (ACCP) guidelines on perioperative management of antithrombotic therapy go further and suggest considering at high TE risk:

- Patients with AF and a prior stroke or transient ischemic attack (occurring >3 months before the planned surgery).
- Patients with a CHADS2 score < 5 having prior thromboembolism during temporary interruption of oral anticoagulants [32, 33].

Timing of last thrombo-embolic event

For patients with VTE, thrombosis, thrombus propagation and embolization can occur up to 12 months after diagnosis and initiation of the treatment. The ACCP guidelines consider that during interruption of anticoagulant treatment, the risk of recurrence of VTE is a high risk if the last acute VTE occurred less than 3 months ago, an intermediate risk if VTE occurred between 3 and 12 months ago, and a low risk if the last VTE occurred at least 12 months ago. The authors recommend taking individual patient factors into consideration, such as patients with remote (> 12 months ago), but severe VTE associated with pulmonary hypertension. These patients may be perceived as high risk though they would be classified as low risk [32].

Regarding patients with a VTE event <3 months, procedures requiring DOAC discontinuation during this time interval must be discussed with a multidisciplinary team to assess the urgency of the procedure. The procedure should be postponed if possible, and if not, a bridging therapy with heparin should be discussed due to the high case fatality of recurrent VTE during the initial 3 months (11.3% (CI, 8.0% to 15.2%)) [35]. Caution is advised in patients with initial symptomatic pulmonary embolism (PE) as they have a higher risk of recurrent VTE than those with initial deep vein thrombosis (DVT) without PE, and as they are at higher risk of recurrent symptomatic PE [36], with a case-fatality of 26.4% (95% CI, 16.7%–38.1%) [37].

Other risk factors

Patients with active cancer receiving chronic anticoagulation are prone to thrombosis and bleeding complications. Tafur et al. showed that patients with active cancer in whom anticoagulation (warfarin) was temporarily interrupted for an invasive procedure had significantly higher 3-month rates of VTE, major bleeds and death. These outcomes were observed only for those cancer patients receiving anticoagulant therapy for prior VTE events, not for patients on long-term anticoagulation for AF or mechanical heart valves (MHV) where the cancer status did not affect either thromboembolic or major bleeding outcomes [38].

Kaatz et al. showed that the 30-day postoperative incidence of stroke supports the premise that the perioperative milieu is prothrombotic [39]. Prolonged bed rest in healthy volunteers does not induce a hypercoagulability state [40], however this is not generalizable to the perioperative context and caution should be advised if prolonged immobilization is required post-surgery.

The ACCP guidelines consider certain types of surgery to be associated with an increased risk for stroke or other thromboembolism (eg, cardiac valve replacement, carotid endarterectomy, and major vascular surgery) [32].

The bleeding risk of the patient

The use of specific scores can help to assess the risk of major bleeding in patients with oral anticoagulant treatment. As these scores have never been validated in the perioperative setting to guide anticoagulant management, there is a real need to develop a bleeding risk score dedicated to surgical patients.

Different scores have been evaluated such as the **HAS-BLED score** [41], the **ORBIT bleeding risk score** [42] and the novel **biomarker-based ABC– bleeding risk score**. The last score performed better in predicting major bleeding in patients with atrial fibrillation than the HAS-BLED and ORBIT scores, but is probably more difficult to use in practice [43].

A high bleeding risk score should generally not suggest that oral anticoagulants are stopped, but modifiable bleeding risk factors should be identified and treated [44].

Time of stopping DOACs before an invasive procedure

Two main characteristics influence the timing for the last DOAC administration before an invasive procedure: the bleeding risk of the procedure and the elimination half-life of the DOAC.

The bleeding risk of invasive procedures

Invasive procedures should be classified as low or high bleeding risk. Various classifications of procedural bleeding risks have been published [19, 33, 45, 46].

Each institution should have a detailed list of the bleeding risks of all the invasive procedures that are performed there such as that presented in Table 3.

There is sufficient evidence that some procedures may be performed on patients receiving anticoagulant therapy (i.e. procedures with minimal risk), as for example superficial skin surgeries, parietal surgery, cataract surgery, and minor dental procedures [47]. It is suggested that the morning dose of anticoagulant should be omitted on the day of the procedure to avoid peak concentrations during the procedures [19].

Pacemaker or cardioverter-defibrillator devices can be implanted safely without stopping VKAs, but more evidence is needed about DOACs [48, 49]. The BRUISE CONTROL-2 trial, which is currently recruiting, aims to show that performing device surgery without interruption of the DOAC will result in a reduced rate of clinically significant hematoma [48].

The elimination half-life of the DOAC

The elimination half-life of DOACs can be increased by decreased renal function (dabigatran > > edoxaban > rivaroxaban and apixaban), severe liver insufficiency (rivaroxaban and apixaban > edoxaban > dabigatran) and co-medications.

a. ***Renal function***

The creatinine clearance (CrCl) must be calculated by the Cockcroft - Gault equation, as the Modified Diet in Renal Disease (MDRD) equation overestimates renal function at lower levels. Renal function should be systematically checked when underlying conditions might affect it [17].

b. ***Liver function***

None of the perioperative proposals recommend altering DOAC pre-procedural administration in cases of liver insufficiency. However, moderate to severe, chronic liver disease can increase rivaroxaban plasma concentrations. Therefore, liver function should be regularly rechecked in chronic or acute liver impairment.

c. ***Other risk factors***

Older age, extreme low body weight (<50 kg) and co-medication with important drug-drug interaction should also be researched as they can increase the half-life of DOACs or anticoagulant concentrations.

Drugs that strongly inhibit CYP3A4 and P-glycoprotein (P-gp) increase bleeding risks due to increased anticoagulation concentrations [50–52]. Anti-platelet agents, anti-inflammatory drugs, selective or non-selective serotonin re-uptake inhibitors and all anticoagulants are medications that, while not directly affecting DOAC metabolism or transport, increase the bleeding risk when co-administrated with DOACs. Despite drug-drug interactions that frequently occur in patients treated with NVAF [53], only a few perioperative proposals recommend an extra delay before surgery in such cases [18].

Table 4 summarizes recent guidance from various expert groups.

Specific consideration for some invasive procedures

Neuraxial anesthesia

Two multicenter studies have published findings on residual perioperative DOAC concentrations. Both concluded that 48 h without treatment might not guarantee the absence of residual anticoagulant effect at the time of the

Table 3 Examples of bleeding risk stratification for invasive procedures

Minimal risk of bleeding or feasible with on-therapy levels of direct oral anticoagulants[a]	Low to moderate risk of bleeding	High risk of bleeding
Tooth extraction: 1 to 3 teeth Periodontology Simple endoscopy without biopsy Superficial surgery (e.g. abscess incision or minor dermatologic procedures (small superficial excision) Cataract procedure Double J stent insertion	Endoscopy with simple biopsy Prostate or bladder biopsy Coronary angiography Simple abdominal hernia repair Anal surgery Gynecologic surgery: simple total laparoscopic hysterectomy Orthopedic surgery: hand surgery, arthroscopy Pace-maker or cardioverter-defibrillator implantation[b]	Neuraxial anesthesia Intracranial surgery Thoracic surgery Cardiac surgery Complex abdominal or gynecological cancer surgery Major orthopedic surgery Ear/Nose/Throat complex cancer surgery or specific surgery requiring good hemostasis (e.g. cochlear implant or thyroid surgery) Liver and kidney biopsy Transurethral prostate or bladder resection Extracorporeal shockwave lithotripsy Infected pace maker lead extraction (increased risk of cardiac tamponade) Robotic surgery

[a]We suggest realizing these procedures at trough levels of direct oral anticoagulants (e.g. avoiding the intake the morning of the procedure)
[b]Awaiting results of BRUISECONTROL-2 trial (NCT01675076) to decide whether device procedures can be safely realized on direct oral anticoagulants

Table 4 Summary of recent propositions for perioperative management of DOACs

DOAC			Dabigatran		Rivaroxaban - Apixaban		Edoxaban	
Bleeding risk of invasive procedure			LOW Bleeding risk	HIGH Bleeding risk	LOW Bleeding risk	HIGH Bleeding risk	LOW Bleeding risk	HIGH Bleeding risk
GIHP (Groupe d'Intérêt en Hémostase Péri-opératoire)	Preoperative interruption *No bridging (except patients with high risk of TE)*	CrCl ≥50 ml/min	Last dose ≥ 24 h before surgery	Last dose 4 days before surgery	Last dose ≥ 24 h before surgery	Last dose 3 days before surgery	Last dose ≥ 24 h before surgery	Last dose 3 days before surgery
		CrCl >30 ml/min		Last dose 5 days before surgery				
		For very high risk procedure (neuraxial anaesthesia)	Last dose 5 days before surgery					
	Resumption after invasive procedure or surgery		LOW Bleeding Risk: Resume minimum 6 h after invasive procedure or surgery HIGH Bleeding Risk: Prophylactic dose of LMWH, UFH or fondaparinux minimum 6 h after invasive procedure or surgery if venous thromboprophylaxis is indicated Therapeutic dose of DOACs when hemostasis is controlled (24-72 h) For neuraxial anesthesia with indwelling catheter: Resumption with LMWH or UFH until indwelling catheter is out					
Heidbuchel et al.	Preoperative interruption *No bridging*	CrCl ≥80 ml/min	≥ 24 h	≥ 48 h	≥ 24 h	≥ 48 h	≥ 24 h	≥ 48 h
		CrCl 50–80 ml/min	≥ 36 h	≥ 72 h	≥ 24 h	≥ 48 h	≥ 24 h	≥ 48 h
		CrCl 30–50 ml/min	≥ 48 h	≥ 96 h	≥ 24 h	≥ 48 h	≥ 24 h	≥ 48 h
		CrCl 15–30 ml/min	Not indicated	Not indicated	≥ 36 h	≥ 48 h	≥ 36 h	≥ 48 h
		CrCl <15 ml/min	No official indication for use					
	Resumption after invasive procedure or surgery		LOW Bleeding Risk: • DOACs 6-8 h HIGH Bleeding Risk: • Low TE risk ➔ resume DOACs 48-72 h after procedure • High TE risk ➔ prophylactic or intermediate dose of LMWH 6-8 h after procedure, resume DOACs when hemostasis is controlled (48-72 h)					
Spyropoulos et al.	Preoperative interruption *No bridging*	CrCl >50 mL/min	Last dose 2 days before surgery	Last dose 3 days before surgery	Last dose 2 days before surgery	Last dose 3 days before surgery	Last dose 2 days before surgery	Last dose 3 days before surgery
		CrCl 30–50 mL/min	Last dose 3 days before surgery	Last dose 4–5 days before surgery	Last dose 2 days before surgery	Last dose 3 days before surgery		
		CrCl 15–29 mL/min			Depends on patient and procedural factors	Depends on patient and procedural factors		

Table 4 Summary of recent propositions for perioperative management of DOACs *(Continued)*

	Resumption after invasive procedure or surgery	LOW Bleeding Risk: • DOACs 24 h HIGH Bleeding Risk: • Low TE risk ➔ resume DOACs 48-72 h after procedure • High TE risk ➔ consider a reduced dose of dabigatran (75 mg twice daily), rivaroxaban (10 mg once daily) or apixaban (2,5 mg twice daily) on the evening after surgery and on the following day (first postoperative day) after surgery.

CrCl: creatinine clearance, LMWH: low molecular weight heparin, UFH: unfractionated heparin, TE: thrombo-embolic

procedure in around 15% of patients and suggested that the period of stopping a DOAC before very high bleeding risk procedures requiring complete hemostatic function such as neuraxial anesthesia or intracranial surgery should be prolonged [16, 54].

Such findings are important as some expert groups have classified these procedures as having a similar risk of bleeding as other conventional high-risk procedures and recommend a minimum 48 h of stopping DOAC treatment in patients with normal CrCl (>80 ml/min) for dabigatran and with moderate to normal CrCl (CrCl >30 ml/min) in patients on rivaroxaban, apixaban or edoxaban [45].

Yet, procedures such as neuraxial anesthesia must be considered as major bleeding risk interventions that require complete hemostatic function. The overall incidences of neuraxial hematoma in patients receiving an epidural or spinal anesthesia are estimated to be 1/220,000 and 1/320,000 patients, respectively [55]. In the presence of risk factors such as multiple attempts, spinal abnormalities, inherited or acquired coagulopathies, and heparin administration, the bleeding risk can be increased by up to two orders of magnitude (e.g. 1/3600 in the study published by Moen et al. including female patients undergoing knee arthroplasty) [55–58].

Rosencher et al. [59] and Gogarten et al. [60] advise an interruption of two half-lives before neuraxial anesthesia, but firstly this recommendation is based only on the prophylactic dosage and secondly it does not take into account the huge inter and intra-individual variability of DOAC plasma concentrations [61].

Recent guidelines published by the American Society of Regional Anesthesia (ASRA) [62] recommend an interval of 5 half-lives to allow complete elimination between stopping oral anticoagulants and carrying out medium or high-risk pain procedures [62]. Due to the variability in DOAC metabolism and elimination, this interval corresponds to 4–5 days for dabigatran, and 3 days for rivaroxaban and apixaban [57, 63]. Similarly in a very cautious approach, the GIHP proposed 5 days of DOAC interruption before neuraxial anesthesia [19].

Douketis et al. commented recently on the latest ASRA guidance. With the high inter-individual variability of DOAC plasma concentration [15, 61], they warned that estimating the elimination half-life of DOACs using the glomerular filtration rate is not sufficient to determine the required stoppage period before neuraxial anesthesia. They suggested that the ideal timing of stopping DOAC treatment should be based on residual plasma concentration measured in the perioperative setting. Benzon et al. replied that further research projects implementing DOAC perioperative measurements need to be conducted to provide sufficient high quality evidence to guide perioperative DOAC interruption. For perioperative research purposes, the use of adapted specific laboratory tests to estimate low plasma concentration of DOACs need to be used and will be discussed in a later chapter.

Atrial fibrillation ablation

Catheter ablation (CA) for atrial fibrillation performed by venous femoral puncture is a common procedure performed worldwide. However, this procedure can cause potentially life threatening bleeding complications such as cardiac tamponade, and also carries a specific TE risk. For periprocedural anticoagulation, undergoing CA with uninterrupted warfarin became a standard as it was associated with fewer periprocedural strokes and minor bleeding complications than low molecular weight heparin (LMWH) [64]. For uninterrupted DOACs (rivaroxaban, dabigatran and apixaban), research evidence tends to the same conclusions as with uninterrupted warfarin [65–69]. However, there is an important variability in the definition of uninterrupted DOACs in the literature. For example, uninterrupted dabigatran can be defined as a last dose on the evening before CA [66] or in the morning of the procedure [70]. Studies should use a standard protocol for uninterrupted DOACs to allow comparison between results.

Unfractionated heparin (UFH) is given during the procedure for left-sided ablation as a prophylactic measure to prevent clot formation. Activated clotting time (ACT) is used to measure UFH anticoagulation during the procedure. However, several ex-vivo and in-vitro studies have shown that ACT can be influenced by concomitant DOAC in the plasma. Indeed, some studies report that it takes more time [70] and higher doses of UFH to reach the target ACT (300–400 s) than in patients undergoing CA with uninterrupted warfarin or acenocoumarol [70–72]. Other studies report that DOACs influence ACT baseline, according to the variable sensitivity of ACT to each DOAC and to the specific instrument used to measure ACT [73]. Further studies are needed to validate the safety and the relevance of the target ACT (300–400 s) with UFH during the procedure with uninterrupted DOACs.

When should bridging therapy with heparin be suggested?

The administration of LMWH after stopping oral anticoagulants was initially recommended to avoid a perioperative gap with insufficient anticoagulation.

The recommendations of the European Society of Anaesthesiology (ESA) published in 2013 [74] suggested that bridging therapy with heparins could be used when DOAC had a long preoperative interruption (5 days before surgery) in patients at high TE risk (for dabigatran, it considered patients with normal to mildly impaired renal function only) (grade 2C). Their categorization of patients at high risk of TE differed from the one proposed in the ACCP guidelines, as the ESA included patients with AF and CHADS2 score > 2.

Since the latter recommendations, several studies have failed to support the benefit of heparin bridging in reducing perioperative TE at DOAC arrest.

Schulman et al. published the first prospective trial of dabigatran perioperative management, without heparin bridging, except in postoperative situations where patients were fasting or when an indwelling neuraxial catheter was in place. They included 541 patients in two years and recorded only one transient ischemic attack (0.2%; 95% CI, 0–0.5). They concluded that bridging was not necessary for a standardized arrest of dabigatran in a perioperative context. However, the majority of invasive procedures had a low bleeding risk and most patients undergoing high bleeding risk procedures had a dabigatran interruption of only 48 h, which seems insufficient for procedures like neuraxial anesthesia [21, 75–78].

Several observational studies from clinical trials or national registries have shown a higher bleeding risk without reduction of TE with the use of heparin bridging in patients taking DOACs or warfarin [79]. However, in most studies heparin bridging and anticoagulant arrest were not standardized. Furthermore, the invasive procedures had mainly low to moderate bleeding risks and patients at high TE risks were again underrepresented in these trials. Therefore the ongoing PAUSE trial (NCT02228798) which aims to recruit 3300 patients on DOACs in a perioperative setting following a standardized protocol without heparin bridging and with residual DOAC concentration measurements on the day of the invasive procedure, may be able to recruit sufficient high-TE risk patients to strengthen the conclusions of the previous trials. The estimated study completion date is December 2018.

DOACs have a shorter elimination half-life than most VKAs and therefore heparin bridging has no clinical benefit in patients with a short period of perioperative DOAC interruption. The situation might be different for patients with high TE risk and prolonged DOAC arrest (> 72–96 h), e.g. before a neuraxial anesthesia. For prolonged arrest of DOAC, when the risk of TE outweighs the risk of bleeding, patients should benefit from a multidisciplinary management to decide if heparin bridging should be prescribed in order to reduce the perioperative gap without anticoagulant. The use of heparin bridging (LMWH or UFH) requires a clear protocol that should be readily available in each institution. For example, the dose and regimen of LMWH must be adapted according to the patient's clinical characteristics (e.g. weight and renal function) including the risk of bleeding [80]. Furthermore, both are parenteral anticoagulants which may cause heparin-induced thrombocytopenia and osteoporosis. The use of UFH requires hospitalization to monitor the anticoagulant level, but it has the advantage of being eliminated independently of the patient's renal function [81]. Indeed, a recent survey demonstrated that despite the evidence that bridging with heparin should be greatly reduced in clinical practice and reserved for particularly high TE settings, many physicians involved in perioperative management still continue to bridge patients with heparin at DOAC arrest without a standardized protocol [19, 33, 45, 46].

Resuming a DOAC after an invasive procedure or surgery

Advice about DOAC resumption after high bleeding-risk procedures is similar in the different expert guidelines: all recommend that therapeutic doses of DOACs should be deferred for 24–72 h [19, 45, 46]. If necessary, the use of a stepwise approach of bridging therapy with a prophylactic dose of heparin can be considered for patients at high TE risks [33]. Spyropoulos et al. instead propose a reduced dose of dabigatran (75 mg twice daily), rivaroxaban (10 mg once daily) or apixaban (2.5 mg twice daily) on the evening after surgery and on the day after surgery (first postoperative day). They recommend bridging therapy with heparins only in patients who cannot tolerate oral medications [19]. If patients are at high TE risks and hemostasis is not achieved, mechanical VTE prophylaxis should be considered. The GIHP suggest a bridge with heparin by the time an indwelling catheter is in place after neuraxial anesthesia [59].

For prophylactic DOAC resumption in a postoperative context, Rosencher et al. suggest that after neuraxial catheter withdrawal, the anticoagulant can be administered at *"8 hours minus its time to peak concentration (Tmax)"* (which varies from 1 to 4 h in DOACs). They suggest that it takes about 8 h for an initial platelet plug to solidify into a stable clot which will remain intact after administration of anticoagulants [59]. The presence of bleeding during needle puncture or catheter placement should further delay anticoagulant therapy post surgery for 24 h [62].

For pain procedures, the recent ASRA guidelines suggest that the first dose of DOAC can be administrated after an interval of 24 h, unless there is a high risk of VTE. A 12-h interval can be considered in some circumstances, depending on the physician's judgement [82].

For low bleeding-risk surgery, some experts recommend restarting DOACs 6–8 h after the end of surgery. Spyropoulos et al. recommend waiting 24 h before resuming the full dose of DOAC.

Table 4 describes the main propositions about DOAC resumption in the peri-procedural setting.

Planning safe resumption of DOAC treatment is essential as premature re-initiation of heparin therapy (within 24 h of a procedure) is an avoidable independent predictor of major bleeding [83, 84].

Doac laboratory testing

DOACs were initially marketed with the advantage of not requiring routine laboratory testing. However, use in frail or obese patients [22], as well as the management of emergencies in patients on DOACs necessitated the development of specific coagulation assays able to answer specific clinical questions accurately.

In the perioperative setting, the 2 main needs are: 1) to exclude clinically relevant concentrations of DOACs before a procedure carrying a high risk of bleeding (e.g. when DOAC interruption has been wrongly assessed or when emergencies require thrombolysis) and 2) to exclude supra-therapeutic plasma concentrations before urgent interventions. In addition, specific plasma levels have been suggested to warrant the administration of DOAC antidotes (i.e. 50 ng/ml for a patient with serious bleeding and 30 ng/ml in patients requiring urgent surgery that cannot be delayed and carries a high risk of bleeding) [85].

Reagents used for routine global assays such as activated partial thromboplastin time (aPTT) for dabigatran and prothrombin time (PT) for direct anti-Xa anticoagulants (rivaroxaban > edoxaban> > apixaban) are not sufficiently accurate to exclude clinically relevant plasma concentrations of DOACs [86–88]. However, both global assays can provide a qualitative assessment of DOACs in the on-therapy range, but their performances depend strongly on the reagent used and for apixaban, even high therapeutic levels may not be detected with PT [89, 90]. In contrast, the thrombin time is very sensitive to the presence of dabigatran and a normal TT excludes this [90]. However, slightly elevated TT does not assess accurately the residual effect of dabigatran due to lack of standardization. Furthermore, the sensitivity of various thrombin reagents can give different TT measurements for the same dabigatran plasma concentration [91–95].

Routine tests are not specific to DOAC and can be prolonged in many situations (e.g. trauma-induced coagulopathy) outside the intake of DOACs. This may lead to incorrect estimation of DOAC anticoagulant level.

For accurate estimation of DOAC plasma concentrations, laboratories must use specific assays with the appropriate methods for the expected DOAC plasma level. The choice of method will depend on the question the clinician needs to answer.

Some specific coagulation assays have adapted calibrators and methods for low plasma DOAC concentrations and these should therefore be used to assess levels <50 ng/ml [95]. These tests can provide accurate estimation in the perioperative setting when clinically relevant DOAC concentrations need to be excluded or when the estimation of DOAC plasma concentrations will guide antidote administration [23].

Importantly, laboratory scientists and clinicians should collaborate to establish an institutional protocol on when and how to test patients on DOACs to highlight what information is needed, to propose the appropriate tests and to provide the correct interpretation of results.

In addition, laboratories need to be informed about any clinical aspects of the patient that might influence the results (e.g. heparin bridging) so they can use the most appropriate test available or to adapt estimates of DOAC plasma concentrations and their significance.

Recently, experts highlighted the urgent need to make accurate, specific coagulation assays widely available [96] and the need for further research to improve the turn-around time of such tests (ideally less than 20 min) to speed up emergency management of patients on DOACs.

Other options to rapidly screen for the presence of DOACs

When a patient is unconscious and the clinical history is not available, the presence of dabigatran can be excluded if the TT is normal or its presence suspected if the TT is elevated. However, there is no routine assay with similar sensitivity for anti-Xa DOACs (rivaroxaban, apixaban and edoxaban), and therefore some authors reported the use of UFH or LMWH-calibrated heparin assays to screen the presence (or absence) of significant levels of a FXa DOAC. Indeed, LMWH- or UFH-calibrated methods can exclude significant levels of anti-Xa DOACs (< 30 ng/ml) and most coagulation analyzers can run the heparin assays. Furthermore, FDA-approved heparin calibrators and controls are commercially available, which is not the case for anti-Xa DOACs [97–100].

Although heparin assays are not specific and cannot distinguish between heparins and anti-Xa DOACs, their use could assist clinicians in emergency situations where the clinical history is not available (i.e. excluding anti-Xa activity in an unconscious patient who may benefit from thrombolysis).

One promising global assay that could be implemented easily on all coagulometers is the dilute Russell's Viper Venom Time (dRVV-T). Recent data suggest that this test could provide a rapid estimation of the intensity of anticoagulation with all DOACs without any specific calibrators, and the test can identify sub-therapeutic plasma levels. However, further studies are needed to confirm its clinical utility, as it is currently less widely available than the TT or the anti-Xa chromogenic assays [101].

Point of care monitoring and other global assays

Point-of-care (POC) monitoring and other global assays (e.g. thrombin generation assay (TGA), prothrombinase induced clotting time (PiCT), thromboelastography (TEG), thromboelastometry (TEM), and activated clotting time

(ACT)) have been tested for various DOACs. They can be useful to assess the efficacy of reversal agents. However, they are costly, lack standardization, are insufficiently studied and are not available in routine clinical practice [22, 23, 102]. In addition, they are often not sensitive enough to exclude clinically relevant concentrations of DOACs in the perioperative setting. Their use should therefore be restricted to specific clinical contexts.

Management of emergencies

Most episodes of bleeding in patients treated with DOACs can be managed with supportive measures and natural clearance of the drug.

A rapid assessment of the patient's anticoagulation level helps to determine the contribution of the anticoagulant to the bleeding, the need for a reversal strategy and to plan the best timing if an invasive procedure is required [102].

If emergencies require an invasive procedure that can be postponed, the timing for the procedure should be determined from the bleeding risk of the procedure and the residual anticoagulant level of DOACs. The GIHP suggest that a residual DOAC plasma concentration < 30 ng/ml should be reached before undertaking high bleeding risk surgery [102, 103]. A level > 400 ng/ml suggests a high risk of uncontrollable hemorrhage [22].

Recent ISTH guidance for the administration of DOAC antidotes [104] is partly based on DOAC plasma concentration. Experts consider that a threshold ≥50 ng/ml warrants the administration of an antidote in cases of serious bleeding. For urgent invasive procedures carrying a high risk of bleeding, the threshold is ≥30 ng/ml. If specific coagulation assays with calibrators accurate for low DOAC plasma concentrations are not available to guide antidote administration, a normal TT and the absence of anti-Xa activity measured with LMWH- or UFH-calibrated methods can rapidly avoid unnecessary antidote administration.

Patients who have bled may have an acquired coagulopathy (e.g. polytrauma-induced coagulopathy or dilutional coagulopathy) in addition to anticoagulant therapy. Early administration of hemostatic therapy such as prothrombin complex concentrates (PCCs), fibrinogen concentrates, fresh frozen plasma, platelets and antifibrolytics may be critical for preventing complex coagulopathies and progression to severe, life-threatening hemorrhage [105].

In the absence of an antidote, previously suggested reversal strategies can be considered:

- **reduction of intestinal absorption**: activated charcoal should be considered in the first hours after ingestion [106].
- **increase in DOAC clearance:** ensure adequate diuresis, especially for patients taking dabigatran. Only patients on supratherapeutic level of dabigatran may be candidates for renal replacement therapy (RRT) when an invasive procedure needs to be rapidly planned. However, within 4 h after RRT, a rebound of dabigatran plasma concentration can occur with a potential risk of bleeding [104].
- administration of **coagulation factors**: Prothrombin complex concentrates (PCCs) contain lyophilized human plasma-derived vitamin-K dependent coagulation factors (clotting factors II, VII, IX and X) and are standardised according to their factor IX content. They may also contain anticoagulation proteins such as protein C, protein S, protein Z, antithrombin and heparin. They are categorized as 4-factor PCC if their content of FVII is high and as 3-factor PCC if it is low. Furthermore, aPCCs (FEIBA®) are available which contain non-activated factors II, IX and X, and activated factor VII [104]. Prophylactic administration of PCCs is not recommended. The mechanisms of action of PCCs and aPCCs are similar as both increase thrombin generation and animal studies have not shown any significant differences in the reduction of bleeding. Therefore, it is not useful to switch from one to the other when trying to manage bleeding in a patient on dabigatran [45, 103]. In the pre-clinical setting, PCC or aPCC showed an improvement in coagulation parameters, blood loss and mortality. Dose recommendations are difficult to make with the lack of high-level evidence with PCCs and aPCCs for dabigatran reversal, but it appears necessary to use the minimum effective dose because of the theoretical thromboembolic risk (starting with an initial dose of 25 U/kg). Suggested doses for 4-Factor PCCs and aPCC are 50 U/kg and 80 U/kg respectively.

In a recent prospective cohort study of dabigatran-associated major bleeding, the effectiveness of activated prothrombin complex concentrate (median first dose: 44 units/kg, range: 24–98), was assessed as good in 9/14 patients and moderate in 5/14 patients. No thromboembolic events occurred within 30 days [107].

Concerning recombinant factor VIIa (rVIIa), as it did not provide any advantages over PCC or aPCC, recent guidance has withdrawn rVIIa from potential reversal treatment for DOAC in bleeding patients [22].

Antidotes

The ISTH guidance state that potential indications for antidotes include life-threatening bleeding, bleeding into a critical organ or closed space, prolonged bleeding despite local hemostatic measures, high risk of recurrent bleeding because of overdose or delayed clearance of DOACs, and need for an urgent intervention associated with a high risk of bleeding. Antidotes should not be used when bleeding can be stopped with local hemostatic measures or when interventions can be delayed to enable anticoagulant clearance, especially in patients with normal renal function [108]. Some urgent procedures without bleeding may have antidote administration delayed into the operating room, e.g. for patients with clinically relevant DOAC plasma concentration and unsatisfactory hemostatic conditions.

Antidote for dabigatran etexilate

Idarucizumab is a specific reversal agent for dabigatran [108]. It is a humanized mouse monoclonal antibody fragment (Fab) that specifically binds to dabigatran with high affinity (approximately 350-fold greater than the affinity of dabigatran for thrombin) and neutralizes its anticoagulant effect. Idarucizumab, when attached to dabigatran, prevents the latter binding to thrombin. It has an estimated half-life of 45 min [109].

According to the clinical study REVERSE AD Phase III, idarucizumab should be given at a dose of 5 g once via a 5-min intravenous infusion. At this dosage of idarucizumab, the reversibility period of the anticoagulant effect of dabigatran is complete, immediate and sustained [109, 110].

No specific side effects have been attributed to idarucizumab yet, and no changes in coagulation markers in blood tests in the absence of dabigatran [111].

After publication of the first results of the REVERSE AD phase III trial, idarucizumab received an accelerated marketing approval from the FDA and EMA and is now licensed in the United States and European countries for the reversal of the anticoagulant effect of dabigatran in life-threatening or uncontrolled bleeding and urgent surgery or invasive procedures [112, 113].

Some limitations of the REVERSE AD trial should be considered. First, the primary end point was not patients' clinical outcomes, but normalization of laboratory tests to demonstrate the maximum percentage reversal of the anticoagulant effect of dabigatran (measured with the dilute thrombin time or ecarin clotting time). Two groups of patients on dabigatran were included, 298 patients in group A who had serious bleeding, and 196 patients in group B who required an urgent procedure. The dTT normalized within 4 h in 235/238 patients (98.7%) in group A and 141/143 patients (98.6%) in group B. Clinical outcomes, considered only as secondary endpoints, were assessed by the treating clinician. It is important to note that the median time to the cessation of bleeding in group A was 3.5 h for GI bleeds and 4.5 h for non GI and non ICH bleeds after idarucizumab administration. The authors admitted that this endpoint was difficult to assess in many patients, such as those with intracranial or retroperitoneal bleeding.

Secondly, 51 of the 494 patients who received idarucizumab did not have prolonged dTT in the emergency department, due to dabigatran clearance. Thrombotic events occurred in 31 of 496 patients at 90 days (6.3%). Two thirds received no antithrombotic therapy prior to the event (i.e. VTE, myocardial infarct, ischemic stroke, systemic embolism).

The worrying death rate (18.7% in group A and 18.5% in group B) was, according to the authors, related to the index event or associated with coexisting conditions.

Third, in some patients, there were subsequent increases in dabigatran concentrations 12 h and 24 h after idarucizumab administration. This was probably due to redistribution of extravascular dabigatran into the intravascular compartment, In addition, 7 patients received more than 1 dose of 5 g idarucizumab.

Finally, a major limitation is the lack of a control group with current guidance recommending prothrombin complex concentrates for the management of serious bleeding in dabigatran-treated patients [114].

As this study was not designed to demonstrate a clear benefit in patient outcomes, compared with other reversal strategies, clinicians need to be aware of these limitations and should provide an institutional protocol to guide the administration of idarucizumab and to enable appropriate patient follow-up.

Antidote for oral factor Xa inhibitors

Andexanet alpha is a recombinant modified human factor Xa decoy, which is catalytically inactive but able to bind direct factor Xa inhibitors with high affinity at its active site, as well as LMWH or fondaparinux.

Andexanet alpha causes a rapid and reproducible reversal of anticoagulant effects in healthy volunteers receiving rivaroxaban, apixaban, edoxaban or enoxaparin [115]. It has a half-life of approximately 1 h and the maximum effect is achieved after 2–5 min. The dosing strategies used in the phase II clinical trials were different for rivaroxaban (clinical trial ANNEXA-R) and apixaban (clinical trial ANNEXA-A) due to different pharmacokinetic and pharmacodynamic models. An andexanet alpha bolus injection needs to be followed by a continuous intravenous infusion for 2 h due to a rebound effect of factor Xa inhibitors within 15 min of the bolus.

To reverse the effects of rivaroxaban at a daily dose of 20 mg, the recommended bolus of andexanet alpha is 800 mg IV (30 mg per minute) followed by a continuous infusion of 8 mg/min for 2 h (960 mg in total). For apixaban at a dose of 5 mg twice a day, the recommended bolus of andexanet alpha is 400 mg IV (30 mg per minute) followed by a continuous infusion of 4 mg/min for 2 h (480 mg in total).

No serious adverse events or thrombotic complications were recorded in the ANNEXA-A and ANNEXA-R studies, which included 101 patients receiving andexanet alpha.

Recently, results from the phase III trial, the « Prospective, Open-Label Study of Andexanet Alfa in Patients Receiving a Factor Xa Inhibitor Who Have Acute Major Bleeding » (ClinicalTrials.gov number, NCT02329327) have been published. The authors evaluated 67 patients with acute major bleeding within 18 h of the last FXa inhibitor administration. Most bleeds were from gastrointestinal or intracranial sites. Andexanet alpha was administrated in a mean (+ – SD) time of 4.8 h + – 1.8 h after emergency department admission. After bolus administration and the two hour infusion, the median anti-FXa activity decreased by 86% from baseline among patients on rivaroxaban and by 92% among those receiving apixaban. At 12 h after andexanet alpha administration, the median anti-FXa activity had decreased from baseline by 64% for rivaroxaban, and 31% for apixaban. At this time, the clinical hemostasis was estimated as excellent or good in 37 of 47 patients. Rates of excellent or good efficacy occurred in 84% of cases for gastrointestinal bleeding and 80% for intracranial bleeding.

As for idarucizumab, this study also had limitations due to a lack of control group. Furthermore, the death rate was 15% and the high increase of anti-FXa activity at 4 h raises questions of the real contribution of andexanet alpha to the evaluation of the clinical hemostasis. Finally, 18% of patients had an ischemic event during the 30-day follow-up period after the infusion of andexanet. Only 27% of patients resumed anticoagulant therapy within 30 days after acute major bleeding. Birocchi et al. have asked recently if resuming anticoagulant therapy soon after an effective hemostasis could reduce thrombotic events. In conclusion, additional information needs to be collected about the safety of andexanet alpha.

Universal antidote

The third approach is the small molecule ciraparantag, which antagonizes the effects of all anticoagulants tested, except VKAs and argatroban. Ciraparantag consists of a small, water-soluble, cationic and synthetic molecule that binds LMWH, UFH, FIIa and FXa inhibitors by non-covalent binding. It can be perceived as a universal antidote for many potential anticoagulant molecules [116]. In vitro studies have shown no major interactions with other coagulation factors or albumin. Animal studies showed a reduction in the blood loss induced by DOACs [117]. In an in vivo study of healthy volunteers who were either untreated or pre-treated with 60 mg of edoxaban, ciraparantag did not induce serious adverse events or a procoagulant signal (measured by D-dimer, TFPI, prothrombin fragments 1.2). A single bolus of 100 to 300 mg of IV ciraparantag normalized the whole blood clotting time to less than 10% above baseline within 30 min in volunteers treated with 60 mg of edoxaban with a stable effect lasting for 24 h. Monitoring the reversal effect of ciraparantag will be challenging in clinical practice as blood collected with sodium citrate, oxalate, EDTA or heparin disrupts the ciraparantag anticoagulant complex and frees the anticoagulant in the plasma. Furthermore, kaolin and celite-based assays are insensitive to monitor the reversal effect of ciraparantag as these activators adsorb the antidote and reduce its active concentration in a blood sample [117].

Why should we monitor the anticoagulant effect with antidote administration?

The time since last DOAC intake and laboratory tests (including CrCl) can guide clinicians in administering an antidote. The residual anticoagulant effect can only be accurately estimated with specific laboratory tests. However, even if the antidote is administered before the availability of DOAC plasma estimation, understanding the initial concentration at a later time may help to assess the efficacy of the dosage. Indeed, it is important to assess if a single administration is sufficient to decrease the anticoagulant activity to a safe level and to check for potential rebound effects in patients with initial supra-therapeutic DOAC levels or decreased DOAC clearance.

A recent case report described a patient with a plasma dabigatran concentration of 3337.3 ng/ml (assessed by HemosIL® DTI, Instrumentation Laboratory, United States) which decreased to 513.5 ng/ml a few minutes after the administration of 5 g idarucizumab. Seven hours later, the dabigatran level rebounded to 1126 ng/ml.

DOACs distribute within the intra- and extra-vascular compartments, and rebound anticoagulant levels after antidote administration have been described, especially in patients with impaired renal function taking dabigatran. This rebound effect also applies to dabigatran after hemodialysis [118]. In patients with impaired renal function, the reversal of idarucizumab should be monitored after 24 h to exclude dabigatran reappearance if bleeding reoccurs later or an invasive procedure needs to be planned.

Noting the findings from the phase III trial of andexanet alpha, the increase of FXA inhibitor activity 4 h after the end of the infusion should be carefully monitored, especially if patients are still in the operating room for a high risk bleeding procedure, or if they start to bleed again. Interestingly, in 10% of the patients with the highest anti-Xa activity after antidote reversal (median anti-Xa activity 327 ng/ml at the end of the infusion) clinicians considered their clinical hemostasis to be excellent or good [119].

Specific laboratory tests are the only means to distinguish recurrent bleeding due to anti Xa factors or acquired coagulopathy.

In a recent review Greinacher et al. described the potential issues with the development of immunogenicity due to antidote use with DOACs and argue the need to monitor this [120].

Physicians should keep in mind that despite the ability of antidotes to reverse the anticoagulant effects of DOACs, their impact on survival still needs to be proved. Postmarketing registries are needed to determine their clinical utility, especially before thrombolytic therapy in patients with acute ischemic stroke or when additional dosing is necessary due to incomplete reversal and ongoing bleeding [22, 121].

Conclusions

The correct management of DOACs in the perioperative setting, requires a good understanding of DOAC pharmacokinetics, indications, drug-drug interactions and their effects on laboratory assays. This information should enable clinicians to easily recognize possible problems and solve them.

Decisions in elective situations about when to stop DOACs perioperatively must be based on their half-life, the bleeding risk of the invasive procedures, and on the thromboembolic risk of the patient. Due to the high inter-individual variability of DOAC plasma concentrations, laboratory testing may be useful for specific populations and clinical contexts.

Further perioperative research studies are necessary to confirm previous guidance based on pharmacological and/or laboratory approaches, especially for the management of emergencies or procedures with a high risk of bleeding. The question of whether patients with high TE risks need to be bridged with heparins during prolonged perioperative interruption of DOACs is still not answered. The administration of antidotes needs to be assessed via registries to validate their benefit in outcomes such as survival in patients undergoing emergency procedures with bleeding complications.

Abbreviations

DOACs: Direct oral anticoagulants; VKAs: Vitamin K antagonists; VTE: Venous thromboembolism; NVAF: Non-valvular atrial fibrillation; CrCl: Creatinine clearance; AF: Atrial fibrillation; TE: Thrombo-embolism; ACCP: American College of Chest Physicians; MHV: Mechanical heart valves; GDF-15: Growth differentiation factor-15; cTnT-hs: high-sensitivity cardiac troponin T; GIHP: Groupe d'Intérêt en Hémostase Péri-opératoire – Working Group on Perioperative Haemostasis; EHRA: European Heart Rhythm Association; MDRD: Modified Diet in Renal Disease; P-gp: P-glycoprotein; ASRA: American Society of Regional Anesthesia; CA: Catheter ablation; LMWH: Low Molecular Weight Heparin; UFH: Unfractionated Heparin; ACT: Activated Clotting Time; ESA: European Society of Anaesthesiology; CI: Confidence interval; OR: Odds ratio; aPTT: Activated partial thromboplastin time; PT: Prothrombin time; TT: Thrombin time; POC: Point-of-care; TGA: Thrombin generation assay; PiCT: Prothrombinase induced clotting time; TEG: Thromboelastography; TEM: Thromboelastometry; dTT: diluted Thrombin Time; DRVVT: Dilute Russell viper venom time; ISTH: International Society of Thrombosis and Haemostasis; ECT: Ecarin clotting time; TFPI: Tissue factor pathway inhibitor; RRT: Renal replacement therapy; PCCs: Prothrombin complex concentrates; aPCC: Activated prothrombin complex concentrates

Acknowledgements

The authors thank Dr. Elizabeth Wager for language editing.

Funding

Not applicable.

Authors' contributions

Virginie Dubois, Anne-Sophie Dincq, Jonathan Douxfils, François Mullier and Sarah Lessire each drafted sections of this manuscript. François Mullier and Sarah Lessire coordinated the writing. All the authors reviewed and agreed the final manuscript.

Competing interests

The authors declare that they have no competing interests.

Author details

[1]Université catholique de Louvain, CHU UCL Namur, Department of Anesthesiology, Yvoir, Belgium. [2]Namur Thrombosis and Hemostasis Center (NTHC), NAmur Research Institute of LIfe Sciences (NARILIS), Namur, Belgium. [3]Université de Namur, Department of Pharmacy, Faculty of Medecine, Namur, Belgium. [4]Université Libre de Bruxelles, Erasme University Hospital,Department of Anesthesiology, Brussels, Belgium. [5]Université Paris Descartes, Cochin University Hospital,Department of Anesthesiology and Intensive Care, Paris, France. [6]Université catholique de Louvain, CHU UCL Namur, Hematology Laboratory, Yvoir, Belgium.

References

1. Mega JL, Braunwald E, Wiviott SD, Bassand JP, Bhatt DL, Bode C, Burton P, Cohen M, Cook-Bruns N, Fox KA, et al. Rivaroxaban in patients with a recent acute coronary syndrome. N Engl J Med. 2012;366:9–19.
2. Investigators E, Bauersachs R, Berkowitz SD, Brenner B, Buller HR, Decousus H, Gallus AS, Lensing AW, Misselwitz F, Prins MH, et al. Oral rivaroxaban for symptomatic venous thromboembolism. N Engl J Med. 2010;363:2499–510.
3. Schulman S, Kakkar AK, Goldhaber SZ, Schellong S, Eriksson H, Mismetti P, Christiansen AV, Friedman J, Le Maulf F, Peter N, et al. Treatment of acute venous thromboembolism with dabigatran or warfarin and pooled analysis. Circulation. 2014;129:764–72.
4. Granger CB, Alexander JH, McMurray JJ, Lopes RD, Hylek EM, Hanna M, Al-Khalidi HR, Ansell J, Atar D, Avezum A, et al. Apixaban versus warfarin in patients with atrial fibrillation. N Engl J Med. 2011;365:981–92.
5. Patel MR, Mahaffey KW, Garg J, Pan G, Singer DE, Hacke W, Breithardt G, Halperin JL, Hankey GJ, Piccini JP, et al. Rivaroxaban versus warfarin in nonvalvular atrial fibrillation. N Engl J Med. 2011;365:883–91.
6. Connolly SJ, Ezekowitz MD, Yusuf S, Eikelboom J, Oldgren J, Parekh A, Pogue J, Reilly PA, Themeles E, Varrone J, et al. Dabigatran versus warfarin in patients with atrial fibrillation. N Engl J Med. 2009;361:1139–51.
7. Lassen MR, Gallus A, Raskob GE, Pineo G, Chen D, Ramirez LM. Investigators A-: Apixaban versus enoxaparin for thromboprophylaxis after hip replacement. N Engl J Med. 2010;363:2487–98.
8. Lassen MR, Raskob GE, Gallus A, Pineo G, Chen D, Hornick P, investigators A. Apixaban versus enoxaparin for thromboprophylaxis after knee replacement (ADVANCE-2): a randomised double-blind trial. Lancet. 2010;375:807–15.
9. Eriksson BI, Dahl OE, Rosencher N, Kurth AA, van Dijk CN, Frostick SP, Kalebo P, Christiansen AV, Hantel S, Hettiarachchi R, et al. Oral dabigatran etexilate

vs. subcutaneous enoxaparin for the prevention of venous thromboembolism after total knee replacement: the RE-MODEL randomized trial. J Thromb Haemost. 2007;5:2178–85.

10. Eriksson BI, Dahl OE, Huo MH, Kurth AA, Hantel S, Hermansson K, Schnee JM, Friedman RJ, Group R-NIS. Oral dabigatran versus enoxaparin for thromboprophylaxis after primary total hip arthroplasty (RE-NOVATE II*). A randomized, double-blind, non-inferiority trial. Thromb Haemost. 2011;105:721–9.
11. Eriksson BI, Kakkar AK, Turpie AG, Gent M, Bandel TJ, Homering M, Misselwitz F, Lassen MR. Oral rivaroxaban for the prevention of symptomatic venous thromboembolism after elective hip and knee replacement. J Bone Joint Surg Br. 2009;91:636–44.
12. Sie P, Samama CM, Godier A, Rosencher N, Steib A, Llau JV, Van der Linden P, Pernod G, Lecompte T, Gouin-Thibault I, et al. Surgery and invasive procedures in patients on long-term treatment with direct oral anticoagulants: thrombin or factor-Xa inhibitors. Recommendations of the Working group on Perioperative Haemostasis and the French study group on thrombosis and Haemostasis. Arch Cardiovasc Dis. 2011;104:669–76.
13. Ferrandis R, Castillo J, de Andres J, Gomar C, Gomez-Luque A, Hidalgo F, Llau JV, Sierra P, Torres LM. The perioperative management of new direct oral anticoagulants: a question without answers. Thromb Haemost. 2013;110:515–22.
14. Dincq AS, Lessire S, Douxfils J, Dogne JM, Gourdin M, Mullier F. Management of non-vitamin K antagonist oral anticoagulants in the perioperative setting. Biomed Res Int. 2014;2014:385014.
15. Douketis JD, Wang G, Chan N, Eikelboom JW, Syed S, Barty R, Moffat KA, Spencer FA, Blostein M, Schulman S. Effect of standardized perioperative dabigatran interruption on the residual anticoagulation effect at the time of surgery or procedure. J Thromb Haemost. 2016;14:89–97.
16. Godier A, Martin AC, Leblanc I, Mazoyer E, Horellou MH, Ibrahim F, Flaujac C, Golmard JL, Rosencher N, Gouin-Thibault I. Peri-procedural management of dabigatran and rivaroxaban: duration of anticoagulant discontinuation and drug concentrations. Thromb Res. 2015;136:763–8.
17. Heidbuchel H, Verhamme P, Alings M, Antz M, Diener HC, Hacke W, Oldgren J, Sinnaeve P, Camm AJ, Kirchhof P. Updated European heart Rhythm Association practical guide on the use of non-vitamin K antagonist anticoagulants in patients with non-valvular atrial fibrillation. Europace. 2015;17:1467–507.
18. Faraoni D, Levy JH, Albaladejo P, Samama CM, Groupe d'Interet en Hemostase P. updates in the perioperative and emergency management of non-vitamin K antagonist oral anticoagulants. Crit Care. 2015;19:203.
19. Albaladejo P, Bonhomme F, Blais N, Collet JP, Faraoni D, Fontana P, Godier A, Llau J, Longrois D, Marret E, et al. Management of direct oral anticoagulants in patients undergoing elective surgeries and invasive procedures: updated guidelines from the French Working group on Perioperative Hemostasis (GIHP) - September 2015. Anaesth Crit Care Pain Med. 2017 Feb;36(1):73–6.
20. Healey JS, Eikelboom J, Douketis J, Wallentin L, Oldgren J, Yang S, Themeles E, Heidbuchel H, Avezum A, Reilly P, et al. Periprocedural bleeding and thromboembolic events with dabigatran compared with warfarin: results from the randomized evaluation of long-term anticoagulation therapy (RE-LY) randomized trial. Circulation. 2012;126:343–8.
21. Sherwood MW, Douketis JD, Patel MR, Piccini JP, Hellkamp AS, Lokhnygina Y, Spyropoulos AC, Hankey GJ, Singer DE, Nessel CC, et al. Outcomes of temporary interruption of rivaroxaban compared with warfarin in patients with nonvalvular atrial fibrillation: results from the rivaroxaban once daily, oral, direct factor Xa inhibition compared with vitamin K antagonism for prevention of stroke and embolism trial in atrial fibrillation (ROCKET AF). Circulation. 2014;129:1850–9.
22. Levy JH, Ageno W, Chan NC, Crowther M, Verhamme P, Weitz JI. Subcommittee on control of a: when and how to use antidotes for the reversal of direct oral anticoagulants: guidance from the SSC of the ISTH. J Thromb Haemost. 2016;14:623–7.
23. Weitz JI, Eikelboom JW. Urgent need to measure effects of direct oral anticoagulants. Circulation. 2016;134:186–8.
24. Pradaxa : EPAR - Product Information - 28/01/2016 Pradaxa -EMEA/H/C/000829 -II/0089 [http://www.ema.europa.eu/docs/en_GB/document_library/EPAR_-_Product_Information/human/000829/WC500041059.pdf].
25. Xarelto -EMEA/H/C/000944 -IB/0040/G - Product Information [http://www.ema.europa.eu/docs/en_GB/document_library/EPAR_-_Product_Information/human/000944/WC500057108.pdf].
26. Eliquis -EMEA/H/C/002148 -R/0034 - Product Information [http://www.ema.europa.eu/docs/en_GB/document_library/EPAR_-_Product_Information/human/002148/WC500107728.pdf].
27. Lixiana -EMEA/H/C/002629 -IB/0002 - Product information [http://www.ema.europa.eu/docs/en_GB/document_library/EPAR_-_Product_Information/human/002629/WC500189045.pdf].
28. Lip GY, Nieuwlaat R, Pisters R, Lane DA, Crijns HJ. Refining clinical risk stratification for predicting stroke and thromboembolism in atrial fibrillation using a novel risk factor-based approach: the euro heart survey on atrial fibrillation. Chest. 2010;137:263–72.
29. Lip GY, Andreotti F, Fauchier L, Huber K, Hylek E, Knight E, Lane D, Levi M, Marin F, Palareti G, et al. Bleeding risk assessment and management in atrial fibrillation patients. Executive summary of a position document from the European heart Rhythm Association [EHRA], endorsed by the European Society of Cardiology [ESC] Working group on thrombosis. Thromb Haemost. 2011;106:997–1011.
30. Jacobs V, May HT, Bair TL, Crandall BG, Cutler M, Day JD, Weiss JP, Osborn JS, Muhlestein JB, Anderson JL, et al. The impact of risk score (CHADS2 versus CHA2DS2-VASc) on long-term outcomes after atrial fibrillation ablation. Heart Rhythm. 2015;12:681–6.
31. Kaatz S, Douketis JD, Zhou H, Gage BF, White RH. Risk of stroke after surgery in patients with and without chronic atrial fibrillation. J Thromb Haemost. 2010;8:884–90.
32. Douketis JD, Spyropoulos AC, Spencer FA, Mayr M, Jaffer AK, Eckman MH, Dunn AS, Kunz R. Perioperative management of antithrombotic therapy: antithrombotic therapy and prevention of thrombosis, 9th ed: American College of Chest physicians evidence-based clinical practice guidelines. Chest. 2012;141:e326S–50S.
33. Spyropoulos AC, Al-Badri A, Sherwood MW, Douketis JD. Periprocedural Management of Patients on a vitamin K antagonist or a direct oral anticoagulant requiring an elective procedure or surgery. J Thromb Haemost. 2016 *May*;14(5):875–85.
34. Tafur A, Douketis JD. Perioperative anticoagulant management in patients with atrial fibrillation : practical implications of recent clinical trials. Pol Arch Med Wewn. 2015;125:666–71.
35. Carrier M, Le Gal G, Wells PS, Rodger MA. Systematic review: case-fatality rates of recurrent venous thromboembolism and major bleeding events among patients treated for venous thromboembolism. Ann Intern Med. 2010;152:578–89.
36. Eichinger S, Weltermann A, Minar E, Stain M, Schonauer V, Schneider B, Kyrle PA. Symptomatic pulmonary embolism and the risk of recurrent venous thromboembolism. Arch Intern Med. 2004;164:92–6.
37. Douketis JD, Kearon C, Bates S, Duku EK, Ginsberg JS. Risk of fatal pulmonary embolism in patients with treated venous thromboembolism. JAMA. 1998;279:458–62.
38. Tafur AJ, Wysokinski WE, McBane RD, Wolny E, Sutkowska E, Litin SC, Daniels PR, Slusser JP, Hodge DO, Heit JA. Cancer effect on periprocedural thromboembolism and bleeding in anticoagulated patients. Ann Oncol. 2012;23:1998–2005.
39. Douketis JD. Perioperative management of patients receiving anticoagulant or antiplatelet therapy: a clinician-oriented and practical approach. Hosp Pract. 2011;39:41–54.
40. Cvirn G, Waha JE, Ledinski G, Schlagenhauf A, Leschnik B, Koestenberger M, Tafeit E, Hinghofer-Szalkay H, Goswami N. Bed rest does not induce hypercoagulability. Eur J Clin Investig. 2015;45:63–9.
41. Zhu W, He W, Guo L, Wang X, Hong K. The HAS-BLED score for predicting major bleeding risk in Anticoagulated patients with Atrial fibrillation: a systematic review and meta-analysis. Clin Cardiol. 2015;38:555–61.
42. O'Brien EC, Simon DN, Thomas LE, Hylek EM, Gersh BJ, Ansell JE, Kowey PR, Mahaffey KW, Chang P, Fonarow GC, et al. The ORBIT bleeding score: a simple bedside score to assess bleeding risk in atrial fibrillation. Eur Heart J. 2015;36:3258–64.
43. Hijazi Z, Oldgren J, Lindback J, Alexander JH, Connolly SJ, Eikelboom JW, Ezekowitz MD, Held C, Hylek EM, Lopes RD, et al. The novel biomarker-based ABC (age, biomarkers, clinical history)-bleeding risk score for patients with atrial fibrillation: a derivation and validation study. Lancet. 2016;387:2302–11.
44. Kirchhof P, Benussi S, Kotecha D, Ahlsson A, Atar D, Casadei B, Castella M, Diener HC, Heidbuchel H, Hendriks J, et al: 2016 ESC guidelines for the management of atrial fibrillation developed in collaboration with EACTS: the task force for the management of atrial fibrillation of the European Society

of Cardiology (ESC)developed with the special contribution of the European heart Rhythm Association (EHRA) of the ESCEndorsed by the European stroke organisation (ESO). Eur Heart J *2016 Oct 7;37(38):*2893-2962.

45. Heidbuchel H, Verhamme P, Alings M, Antz M, Diener HC, Hacke W, Oldgren J, Sinnaeve P, Camm AJ, Kirchhof P, Advisors: Updated European heart Rhythm Association practical guide on the use of non-vitamin-K antagonist anticoagulants in patients with non-valvular atrial fibrillation: executive summary. Eur Heart J 2016. *Jun 9. pii:* ehw058.
46. Heidbuchel H, Verhamme P, Alings M, Antz M, Diener HC, Hacke W, Oldgren J, Sinnaeve P, Camm AJ, Kirchhof P, Advisors: Updated European heart Rhythm Association practical guide on the use of non-vitamin K antagonist anticoagulants in patients with non-valvular atrial fibrillation. Europace 2015. *Oct;17(10):*1467-1507.
47. Mauprivez C, Khonsari RH, Razouk O, Goudot P, Lesclous P, Descroix V. Management of dental extraction in patients undergoing anticoagulant oral direct treatment: a pilot study. Oral Surg Oral Med Oral Pathol Oral Radiol. 2016;122:e146–55.
48. Essebag V, Healey JS, Ayala-Paredes F, Kalfon E, Coutu B, Nery P, Verma A, Sapp J, Philippon F, Sandhu RK, et al. Strategy of continued vs interrupted novel oral anticoagulant at time of device surgery in patients with moderate to high risk of arterial thromboembolic events: the BRUISE CONTROL-2 trial. Am Heart J. 2016;173:102–7.
49. Madan S, Muthusamy P, Mowers KL, Elmouchi DA, Finta B, Gauri AJ, Woelfel AK, Fritz TD, Davis AT, Chalfoun NT. Safety of anticoagulation with uninterrupted warfarin vs. interrupted dabigatran in patients requiring an implantable cardiac device. Cardiovasc Diagn Ther. 2016;6:3–9.
50. Douxfils J, Lessire S, Dincq AS, Hjemdahl P, Ronquist-Nii Y, Pohanka A, Gourdin M, Chatelain B, Dogne JM, Mullier F. Estimation of dabigatran plasma concentrations in the perioperative setting. An ex vivo study using dedicated coagulation assays. Thromb Haemost. 2015;113:862–9.
51. Lessire S, Dincq AS, Douxfils J, Devalet B, Nicolas JB, Spinewine A, Larock AS, Dogne JM, Gourdin M, Mullier F. Preventive strategies against bleeding due to nonvitamin K antagonist oral anticoagulants. Biomed Res Int. 2014;2014:616405.
52. Pengo V, Crippa L, Falanga A, Finazzi G, Marongiu F, Palareti G, Poli D, Testa S, Tiraferri E, Tosetto A, et al. Questions and answers on the use of dabigatran and perspectives on the use of other new oral anticoagulants in patients with atrial fibrillation. A consensus document of the Italian Federation of Thrombosis Centers (FCSA). Thromb Haemost. 2011;106:868–76.
53. Jungbauer L, Dobias C, Stollberger C, Weidinger F. The frequency of prescription of P-glycoprotein-affecting drugs in atrial fibrillation. J Thromb Haemost. 2010;8:2069–70.
54. Douketis JD, Wang G, Chan N, Eikelboom JW, Syed S, Barty R, Moffat KA, Spencer FA, Blostein M, Schulman S. Effect of standardized Perioperative Dabigatran interruption on residual anticoagulation effect at the time of surgery or procedure. J Thromb Haemost. 2016 Jan;14(1):89–97.
55. Horlocker TT, Wedel DJ, Rowlingson JC, Enneking FK, Kopp SL, Benzon HT, Brown DL, Heit JA, Mulroy MF, Rosenquist RW, et al. Regional anesthesia in the patient receiving antithrombotic or thrombolytic therapy: American Society of Regional Anesthesia and Pain Medicine evidence-based guidelines (third edition). Reg Anesth Pain Med. 2010;35:64–101.
56. Cappelleri G, Fanelli A. Use of direct oral anticoagulants with regional anesthesia in orthopedic patients. J Clin Anesth. 2016;32:224–35.
57. Bateman BT, Mhyre JM, Ehrenfeld J, Kheterpal S, Abbey KR, Argalious M, Berman MF, Jacques PS, Levy W, Loeb RG, et al. The risk and outcomes of epidural hematomas after perioperative and obstetric epidural catheterization: a report from the multicenter Perioperative outcomes group research consortium. Anesth Analg. 2013;116:1380–5.
58. Moen V, Dahlgren N, Irestedt L. Severe neurological complications after central neuraxial blockades in Sweden 1990-1999. Anesthesiology. 2004;101:950–9.
59. Rosencher N, Bonnet MP, Sessler DI. Selected new antithrombotic agents and neuraxial anaesthesia for major orthopaedic surgery: management strategies. Anaesthesia. 2007;62:1154–60.
60. Gogarten W, Vandermeulen E, Van Aken H, Kozek S, Llau JV, Samama CM. Regional anaesthesia and antithrombotic agents: recommendations of the European Society of Anaesthesiology. Eur J Anaesthesiol. 2010;27:999–1015.
61. Testa S, Tripodi A, Legnani C, Pengo V, Abbate R, Dellanoce C, Carraro P, Salomone L, Paniccia R, Paoletti O, et al. Plasma levels of direct oral anticoagulants in real life patients with atrial fibrillation: results observed in four anticoagulation clinics. Thromb Res. 2016;137:178–83.
62. Narouze S, Benzon HT, Provenzano DA, Buvanendran A, De Andres J, Deer TR, Rauck R, Huntoon MA: Interventional spine and pain procedures in patients on antiplatelet and anticoagulant medications: guidelines from the American Society of Regional Anesthesia and Pain Medicine, the European Society of Regional Anaesthesia and Pain Therapy, the American Academy of pain Medicine, the international Neuromodulation Society, the north American Neuromodulation Society, and the world Institute of Pain. Reg Anesth Pain Med 2015, 40:182-212.
63. Benzon HT, Avram MJ, Green D, Bonow RO. New oral anticoagulants and regional anaesthesia. Br J Anaesth. 2013;111(Suppl 1):i96–113.
64. Di Biase L, Burkhardt JD, Santangeli P, Mohanty P, Sanchez JE, Horton R, Gallinghouse GJ, Themistoclakis S, Rossillo A, Lakkireddy D, et al. Periprocedural stroke and bleeding complications in patients undergoing catheter ablation of atrial fibrillation with different anticoagulation management: results from the role of Coumadin in preventing Thromboembolism in Atrial fibrillation (AF) patients undergoing catheter ablation (COMPARE) randomized trial. Circulation. 2014;129:2638–44.
65. Lakkireddy D, Reddy YM, Di Biase L, Vallakati A, Mansour MC, Santangeli P, Gangireddy S, Swarup V, Chalhoub F, Atkins D, et al. Feasibility and safety of uninterrupted rivaroxaban for periprocedural anticoagulation in patients undergoing radiofrequency ablation for atrial fibrillation: results from a multicenter prospective registry. J Am Coll Cardiol. 2014;63:982–8.
66. Eitel C, Koch J, Sommer P, John S, Kircher S, Bollmann A, Arya A, Piorkowski C, Hindricks G. Novel oral anticoagulants in a real-world cohort of patients undergoing catheter ablation of atrial fibrillation. Europace. 2013;15:1587–93.
67. Nagao T, Inden Y, Shimano M, Fujita M, Yanagisawa S, Kato H, Ishikawa S, Miyoshi A, Okumura S, Ohguchi S, et al. Efficacy and safety of apixaban in the patients undergoing the ablation of atrial fibrillation. Pacing Clin Electrophysiol. 2015;38:155–63.
68. Nagao T, Inden Y, Shimano M, Fujita M, Yanagisawa S, Kato H, Ishikawa S, Miyoshi A, Okumura S, Ohguchi S, et al. Feasibility and safety of uninterrupted dabigatran therapy in patients undergoing ablation for atrial fibrillation. Intern Med. 2015;54:1167–73.
69. Cappato R, Marchlinski FE, Hohnloser SH, Naccarelli GV, Xiang J, Wilber DJ, Ma CS, Hess S, Wells DS, Juang G, et al. Uninterrupted rivaroxaban vs. uninterrupted vitamin K antagonists for catheter ablation in non-valvular atrial fibrillation. Eur Heart J. 2015;36:1805–11.
70. Nagao T, Inden Y, Yanagisawa S, Kato H, Ishikawa S, Okumura S, Mizutani Y, Ito T, Yamamoto T, Yoshida N, et al. Differences in activated clotting time among uninterrupted anticoagulants during the periprocedural period of atrial fibrillation ablation. Heart Rhythm. 2015;12:1972–8.
71. Konduru SV, Cheema AA, Jones P, Li Y, Ramza B, Wimmer AP. Differences in intraprocedural ACTs with standardized heparin dosing during catheter ablation for atrial fibrillation in patients treated with dabigatran vs. patients on uninterrupted warfarin. J Interv Card Electrophysiol. 2012;35:277–84. discussion 284
72. Efremidis M, Vlachos K, Letsas KP, Giannopoulos G, Lioni L, Georgopoulos S, Vadiaka M, Deftereos S, Sideris A. Low dose dabigatran versus uninterrupted acenocoumarol for peri-procedural anticoagulation in atrial fibrillation catheter ablation. J Electrocardiol. 2015;48:840–4.
73. Dincq AS, Lessire S, Chatelain B, Gourdin M, Dogne JM, Mullier F, Douxfils J. Impact of the direct oral anticoagulants on activated clotting time. J Cardiothorac Vasc Anesth. 2017 Feb;31(1):e24–7.
74. Kozek-Langenecker SA, Afshari A, Albaladejo P, Santullano CA, De Robertis E, Filipescu DC, Fries D, Gorlinger K, Haas T, Imberger G, et al. Management of severe perioperative bleeding: guidelines from the European Society of Anaesthesiology. Eur J Anaesthesiol. 2013;30:270–382.
75. Beyer-Westendorf J, Gelbricht V, Forster K, Ebertz F, Kohler C, Werth S, Kuhlisch E, Stange T, Thieme C, Daschkow K, Weiss N: Peri-interventional management of novel oral anticoagulants in daily care: results from the prospective Dresden NOAC registry. Eur Heart J 2014. *Jul 21;35(28):*1888-1896.
76. Steinberg BA, Peterson ED, Kim S, Thomas L, Gersh BJ, Fonarow GC, Kowey PR, Mahaffey KW, Sherwood MW, Chang P, et al. Use and outcomes associated with bridging during anticoagulation interruptions in patients with atrial fibrillation: findings from the outcomes registry for better informed treatment of Atrial fibrillation (ORBIT-AF). Circulation. 2015;131:488–94.
77. Douketis JD, Healey JS, Brueckmann M, Eikelboom JW, Ezekowitz MD, Fraessdorf M, Noack H, Oldgren J, Reilly P, Spyropoulos AC, et al.

Perioperative bridging anticoagulation during dabigatran or warfarin interruption among patients who had an elective surgery or procedure. Substudy of the RE-LY trial. Thromb Haemost. 2015;113:625–32.

78. Garcia D, Alexander JH, Wallentin L, Wojdyla DM, Thomas L, Hanna M, Al-Khatib SM, Dorian P, Ansell J, Commerford P, et al. Management and clinical outcomes in patients treated with apixaban vs warfarin undergoing procedures. Blood. 2014;124:3692–8.
79. Garcia DA, Baglin TP, Weitz JI, Samama MM. American College of Chest P: Parenteral anticoagulants: antithrombotic therapy and prevention of thrombosis, 9th ed: American College of Chest physicians evidence-based clinical practice guidelines. Chest. 2012;141:e24S–43S.
80. Mar PL, Familtsev D, Ezekowitz MD, Lakkireddy D, Gopinathannair R. Periprocedural management of anticoagulation in patients taking novel oral anticoagulants: review of the literature and recommendations for specific populations and procedures. Int J Cardiol. 2016;202:578–85.
81. Flaker GC, Theriot P, Binder LG, Dobesh PP, Cuker A, Doherty JU. Management of Periprocedural Anticoagulation: a survey of contemporary practice. J Am Coll Cardiol. 2016;68:217–26.
82. Tafur AJ, McBane R 2nd, Wysokinski WE, Litin S, Daniels P, Slusser J, Hodge D, Beckman MG, Heit JA. Predictors of major bleeding in peri-procedural anticoagulation management. J Thromb Haemost. 2012;10:261–7.
83. Douxfils J, Mullier F, Dogne JM. Dose tailoring of dabigatran etexilate: obvious or excessive? Expert Opin Drug Saf. 2015;14:1283–9.
84. Martin K, Beyer-Westendorf J, Davidson BL, Huisman MV, Sandset PM, Moll S. Use of the direct oral anticoagulants in obese patients: guidance from the SSC of the ISTH. J Thromb Haemost. 2016;14:1308–13.
85. Testa S, Legnani C, Tripodi A, Paoletti O, Pengo V, Abbate R, Bassi L, Carraro P, Cini M, Paniccia R, et al: Poor comparability of coagulation screening test with specific measurement in patients on direct oral anticoagulants: results from a multicenter/multiplatform study. J Thromb Haemost 2016. *Nov; 14(11)*:2194-2201.
86. Barrett YC, Wang Z, Frost C, Shenker A. Clinical laboratory measurement of direct factor Xa inhibitors: anti-Xa assay is preferable to prothrombin time assay. Thromb Haemost. 2010;104:1263–71.
87. Gouin-Thibault I, Flaujac C, Delavenne X, Quenet S, Horellou MH, Laporte S, Siguret V, Lecompte T. Assessment of apixaban plasma levels by laboratory tests: suitability of three anti-Xa assays. A multicentre French GEHT study. Thromb Haemost. 2014;111:240–8.
88. Douxfils J, Chatelain C, Chatelain B, Dogne JM, Mullier F. Impact of apixaban on routine and specific coagulation assays: a practical laboratory guide. Thromb Haemost. 2013;110:283–94.
89. Cuker A, Siegal DM, Crowther MA, Garcia DA. Laboratory measurement of the anticoagulant activity of the non-vitamin K oral anticoagulants. J Am Coll Cardiol. 2014;64:1128–39.
90. Lessire S, Douxfils J, Baudar J, Bailly N, Dincq AS, Gourdin M, Dogne JM, Chatelain B, Mullier F. Is Thrombin Time useful for the assessment of dabigatran concentrations? An in vitro and ex vivo study. Thromb Res. 2015;136(3):693–6.
91. Douxfils J, Lessire S, Dincq AS, Hjemdahl P, Ronquist-Nii Y, Pohanka A, Gourdin M, Chatelain B, Dogne JM, Mullier F. Estimation of dabigatran plasma concentrations in the perioperative setting. An ex vivo study using dedicated coagulation assays. Thromb Haemost. 2014:113.
92. Mani H, Rohde G, Stratmann G, Hesse C, Herth N, Schwers S, Perzborn E, Lindhoff-Last E. Accurate determination of rivaroxaban levels requires different calibrator sets but not addition of antithrombin. Thromb Haemost. 2012;108:191–8.
93. Konigsbrugge O, Quehenberger P, Belik S, Weigel G, Seger C, Griesmacher A, Pabinger I, Ay C. Anti-coagulation assessment with prothrombin time and anti-Xa assays in real-world patients on treatment with rivaroxaban. Ann Hematol. 2015;94:1463–71.
94. Lessire S, Douxfils J, Pochet L, Dincq AS, Larock AS, Gourdin M, Dogné JM, Chatelain B, Mullier F. Estimation of rivaroxaban plasma concentrations in the perioperative setting in patients with or without heparin bridging. Clin Appl Thromb Hemost. 2016 Jan 1:1076029616675968; doi:10.1177/1076029616675968.
95. Lessire S, Dincq AS, Douxfils J, Mullier F: Periprocedural management of direct oral anticoagulants should be guided by accurate laboratory tests. Reg Anesth Pain Med 2016 *Nov/Dec*;41*(6)*:787-788.
96. Gosselin RC, Francart SJ, Hawes EM, Moll S, Dager WE, Adcock DM. Heparin-calibrated Chromogenic anti-Xa activity measurements in patients receiving rivaroxaban: can this test be used to quantify drug level? Ann Pharmacother. 2015;49:777–83.
97. Douxfils J, Chatelain B, Hjemdahl P, Devalet B, Sennesael AL, Wallemacq P, Ronquist-Nii Y, Pohanka A, Dogne JM, Mullier F. Does the Russell viper venom time test provide a rapid estimation of the intensity of oral anticoagulation? A cohort study. Thromb Res. 2015 *May*;135(5):852–60.
98. Exner T, Ellwood L, Rubie J, Barancewicz A. Testing for new oral anticoagulants with LA-resistant Russells viper venom reagents. An in vitro study. Thromb Haemost. 2013;109:762–5.
99. Altman R, Gonzalez CD. Simple and rapid assay for effect of the new oral anticoagulant (NOAC) rivaroxaban: preliminary results support further tests with all NOACs. Thromb J. 2014;12:7.
100. Altman R, Gonzalez CD. Supporting the use of a coagulometric method for rivaroxaban control: a hypothesis-generating study to define the safety cut-offs. Thromb J. 2015;13:26.
101. Dale BJ, Chan NC, Eikelboom JW. Laboratory measurement of the direct oral anticoagulants. Br J Haematol. 2016;172:315–36.
102. Pernod G, Albaladejo P, Godier A, Samama CM, Susen S, Gruel Y, Blais N, Fontana P, Cohen A, Llau JV, et al. Management of major bleeding complications and emergency surgery in patients on long-term treatment with direct oral anticoagulants, thrombin or factor-Xa inhibitors. Proposals of the Working group on Perioperative Haemostasis (GIHP) - march 2013. Ann Fr Anesth Reanim. 2013;32:691–700.
103. Godier A, Gouin-Thibault I, Rosencher N, Albaladejo P. Groupe d'Interet en Hemostase P: [management of direct oral anticoagulants for invasive procedures]. J Mal Vasc. 2015;40:173–81.
104. Grottke O, Aisenberg J, Bernstein R, Goldstein P, Huisman MV, Jamieson DG, Levy JH, Pollack CV Jr, Spyropoulos AC, Steiner T, et al. Efficacy of prothrombin complex concentrates for the emergency reversal of dabigatran-induced anticoagulation. Crit Care. 2016;20:115.
105. Lohrmann GM, Atwal D, Augoustides JG, Askar W, Patel PA, Ghadimi K, Makar G, Gutsche JT, Shamoun FE, Ramakrishna H. Reversal agents for the new generation of oral anticoagulants: implications for the Perioperative physician. J Cardiothorac Vasc Anesth. 2016;30:823–30.
106. Chai-Adisaksopha C, Hillis C, Lim W, Boonyawat K, Moffat K, Crowther M. Hemodialysis for the treatment of dabigatran-associated bleeding: a case report and systematic review. J Thromb Haemost. 2015;13:1790–8.
107. Schulman S, Ritchie B, Nahirniak S, Gross PL, Carrier M, Majeed A, Hwang HG, Zondag M. Study i: reversal of dabigatran-associated major bleeding with activated prothrombin concentrate: a prospective cohort study. Thromb Res. 2017;152:44–8.
108. Schiele F, van Ryn J, Canada K, Newsome C, Sepulveda E, Park J, Nar H, Litzenburger T. A specific antidote for dabigatran: functional and structural characterization. Blood. 2013;121:3554–62.
109. Glund S, Stangier J, Schmohl M, Gansser D, Norris S, van Ryn J, Lang B, Ramael S, Moschetti V, Gruenenfelder F, et al. Safety, tolerability, and efficacy of idarucizumab for the reversal of the anticoagulant effect of dabigatran in healthy male volunteers: a randomised, placebo-controlled, double-blind phase 1 trial. Lancet. 2015;386:680–90.
110. Glund S, Moschetti V, Norris S, Stangier J, Schmohl M, van Ryn J, Lang B, Ramael S, Reilly P. A randomised study in healthy volunteers to investigate the safety, tolerability and pharmacokinetics of idarucizumab, a specific antidote to dabigatran. Thromb Haemost. 2015;113:943–51.
111. Schmohl M, Glund S, Harada A, Imazu S, De Smet M, Moschetti V, Ramael S, Ikushima I, Grunenfelder F, Reilly P, Stangier J. Idarucizumab does not have procoagulant effects: assessment of thrombosis biomarkers in healthy volunteers. Thromb Haemost. 2017;117:269–76.
112. Pollack CV Jr, Reilly PA, Eikelboom J, Glund S, Verhamme P, Bernstein RA, Dubiel R, Huisman MV, Hylek EM, Kamphuisen PW, et al. Idarucizumab for Dabigatran Reversal. N Engl J Med. 2015;373:511–20.
113. Pollack CV, Reilly PA, van Ryn J, Eikelboom J, Glund S, Bernstein RA, Dubiel R, Huisman MV, Hylek EM, Kamphuisen PW, et al. Idarucizumab for Dabigatran Reversal: Updated Results of the RE-VERSE AD Study. In American Heart Association Scientific Sessions 2016. New Orleans: The American Journal of Managed Care; 2016. http://www.ajmc.com/conferences/aha2016/results-of-the-re-verse-ad-study-confirmidacizumab-efficacy-safety-at-follow-up.
114. Siegal DM, Curnutte JT, Connolly SJ, Lu G, Conley PB, Wiens BL, Mathur VS, Castillo J, Bronson MD, Leeds JM, et al. Andexanet Alfa for the reversal of factor Xa inhibitor activity. N Engl J Med. 2015;373:2413–24.
115. Connors JM. Antidote for Factor Xa Anticoagulants. N Engl J Med. 2015;373:2471–2.

116. Ansell JE, Bakhru SH, Laulicht BE, Steiner SS, Grosso M, Brown K, Dishy V, Noveck RJ, Costin JC. Use of PER977 to reverse the anticoagulant effect of edoxaban. N Engl J Med. 2014;371:2141–2.
117. Ansell JE, Bakhru SH, Laulicht BE, Steiner SS, Grosso MA, Brown K, Dishy V, Lanz HJ, Mercuri MF, Noveck RJ, Costin JC. Single-dose ciraparantag safely and completely reverses anticoagulant effects of edoxaban. Thromb Haemost. 2017;117:238–45.
118. Khadzhynov D, Wagner F, Formella S, Wiegert E, Moschetti V, Slowinski T, Neumayer HH, Liesenfeld KH, Lehr T, Hartter S, et al. Effective elimination of dabigatran by haemodialysis. A phase I single-centre study in patients with end-stage renal disease. Thromb Haemost. 2013;109:596–605.
119. Connolly SJ, Milling TJ Jr, Eikelboom JW, Gibson CM, Curnutte JT, Gold A, Bronson MD, Lu G, Conley PB, Verhamme P, et al. Andexanet Alfa for acute major bleeding associated with factor Xa inhibitors. N Engl J Med. 2016;375:1131–41.
120. Greinacher A, Thiele T, Selleng K. Reversal of anticoagulants: an overview of current developments. Thromb Haemost. 2015;113:931–42.
121. Rottenstreich A, Jahshan N, Avraham L, Kalish Y. Idarucizumab for dabigatran reversal - does one dose fit all? Thromb Res. 2016;146:103–4.

16

Disseminated intravascular coagulation with the fibrinolytic phenotype predicts the outcome of patients with out-of-hospital cardiac arrest

Takeshi Wada, Satoshi Gando*, Yuichi Ono, Kunihiko Maekawa, Kenichi Katabami, Mineji Hayakawa and Atsushi Sawamura

Abstract

Background: We tested the hypothesis that disseminated intravascular coagulation (DIC) during the early phase of post-cardiopulmonary resuscitation (CPR) is associated with systemic inflammatory response syndrome (SIRS), multiple organ dysfunction syndrome (MODS) and affects the outcome of out-of-hospital cardiac arrest (OHCA) patients.

Methods: A review of the computer-based medical records of OHCA patients was retrospectively conducted and included 388 patients who were divided into DIC and non-DIC patients based on the Japanese Association for Acute Medicine DIC diagnostic criteria. DIC patients were subdivided into two groups: those with and without hyperfibrinolysis. Pre-hospital factors, platelet count, coagulation and fibrinolysis markers and lactate levels within 24 h after resuscitation were evaluated. The outcome measure was all-cause hospital mortality.

Results: DIC patients exhibited lower platelet counts, prolonged prothrombin time, decreased levels of fibrinogen and antithrombin associated with increased fibrinolysis than those without DIC. DIC patients more frequently developed SIRS and MODS, followed by worse outcomes than non-DIC patients. The same changes were observed in DIC patients with hyperfibrinolysis who showed a higher prevalence of MODS, leading to worse outcome than those without hyperfibrinolysis. Logistic regression analyses showed that lactate levels predicted hyperfibrinolysis and DIC is an independent predictor of patient death. Survival probabilities of DIC patients during hospital stay were significantly lower than non-DIC patients. The area under the receiver operating characteristic curve of DIC for the prediction of death was 0.704.

Conclusions: The fibrinolytic phenotype of DIC during the early phase of post-CPR more frequently results in SIRS and MODS, especially in patients with hyperfibrinolysis, and affects the outcome of OHCA patients.

Keywords: Cardiac arrest, Disseminated intravascular coagulation (DIC), Fibrinolysis, Outcome, Out-of-hospital

* Correspondence: gando@med.hokudai.ac.jp
Division of Acute and Critical Care Medicine, Department of Anesthesiology and Critical Care Medicine, Hokkaido University Graduate School of Medicine, N15W7, Kita-ku, Sapporo 060-8638, Japan

Background

Whole body ischemia reperfusion due to cardiac arrest constitutes post-resuscitation syndrome resulting from microvascular obstruction-induced tissue hypoxia in many vital organs, which affects the patient's outcome [1]. Microvascular obstruction, referred to as the no reflow phenomenon, in the brain has been attributed to intravascular thrombosis during cardiac arrest [1, 2]. Post-resuscitation syndrome is now referred to as post-cardiac arrest syndrome consisting of four syndromes including systemic ischemia reperfusion responses and post-cardiac arrest brain injury [3]. Main pathophysiologies of the former responses are systemic inflammatory response syndrome (SIRS) and increased coagulation, which clinically manifest as tissue hypoxia/ischemia and multiple organ dysfunctions [3]. Adrie et al. [4] confirmed that successfully resuscitated cardiac arrest was followed by SIRS and activation of coagulation, both of which contributed to organ dysfunction, including the brain. Recent studies have indicated that disseminated intravascular coagulation (DIC) leads to organ dysfunction and affects the prognosis of out-of-hospital cardiac arrest (OHCA) patients [5, 6].

Inflammatory cytokine-initiated activation of tissue-factor-dependent coagulation, insufficient control of the anticoagulation pathways, and plasminogen activator inhibitor-1 (PAI-1)-mediated suppression of fibrinolysis characterize the pathogenesis of DIC [7]. From the first report of DIC following cardiac arrest [8], higher levels of tumor necrosis factor-α (TNF-α), interleukin-6 (IL-6) and IL-8 [4, 9, 10]; increased tissue factor levels [11]; insufficient levels of tissue factor pathway inhibitor (TFPI), antithrombin, protein C and protein S [4, 11]; and increased PAI-1 levels [12, 13] have been repeatedly confirmed during cardiopulmonary resuscitation (CPR) and after return of spontaneous circulation (ROSC). These changes lead to massive thrombin generation and consecutive fibrin formation [4, 6, 12]. Importantly, underlying conditions of DIC occasionally cause a simultaneous increase in fibrinolysis resulting from tissue-type plasminogen activator (t-PA), which is referred to as DIC with the fibrinolytic phenotype, as opposed to the thrombotic phenotype associated with elevated PAI-1 levels [14]. Both types of DIC have been recognized to affect the patient's outcome [7, 14].

Marked increases in t-PA antigen and activity levels were followed by the PAI-1 expression during CPR and immediately after ROSC within 24 h [12]. In this study, therefore, significant imbalances between the levels of t-PA and PAI-1 during the first 24 h after cardiac arrest and resuscitation was noted which was coincided with the definition of DIC with the fibrinolytic phenotype.

According to the results of these previous studies on DIC, we investigated changes in coagulation and fibrinolysis markers during the first 24 h after OHCA and resuscitation. We tested the hypothesis that DIC with the fibrinolytic phenotype during the early phase of post-CPR is associated with SIRS, organ dysfunctions and affects the patient's outcome.

Methods

Patient selection and data collection

From June 2000 to December 2011, all consecutive patients older than 12 years of age with successful ROSC from OHCA who were admitted to the ICU were eligible for this study. Patients who suffered to cardiac arrest due to trauma or burns, those on warfarin therapy, those with end-stage liver diseases, terminal illnesses or profound hypothermia, and those underwent percutaneous cardiopulmonary support (PCPS) were excluded. The Institutional Review Board of our institution approved this study and issued a waiver of informed consent.

A systematic review of the computer-based medical records of these patients was retrospectively conducted to provide baseline characteristics and DIC-related variables. Data regarding the platelet count, prothrombin time, prothrombin time ratio, fibrinogen, antithrombin, fibrin/fibrinogen degradation products (FDP), D-dimer and lactate were obtained at 4 time points within 24 h after successful ROSC: Time Point 01, immediately after ROSC to 4 h after ROSC; Time Point 02, 4 to 8 h after ROSC; Time Point 03, 8 to 16 h after ROSC; and Time Point 04, 16 to 24 h after ROSC. Day 0 data indicates the highest or lowest values of these 4 points measurements. Namely, the maximal worst values during this time period were considered for classfiyng patients with or without DIC and for determining the phenotype. The standard practice in our ICU for all patients is to draw blood several times a day in order to analyze the laboratory data including platelet count, coagulation and fibrinolysis. Blood gas analyses with lactate measurements were also frequently performed.

Study setting and definitions

The levels of care provided by the emergency medical technicians (EMT) in our country are comparable to other advanced countries worldwide. The management of cardiac arrest was based on the 2000, 2005, and 2010 guidelines proposed by the International Liaison Committee on Resuscitation. Detailed pre-hospital care and CPR methods in our department can be found elsewhere [15].

Successful ROSC was defined as measurable blood pressure and pulse for more than 1 h and admission to the ICU, regardless of catecholamine use. Organ dysfunction was assessed by the Sequential Organ Failure Assessment (SOFA) score [16]. Multiple organ dysfunction syndrome (MODS) was defined as a SOFA score ≥ 12 [16]. The SIRS score was calculated according to the

American College of Chest Physicians/Society of Critical Care Medicine consensus conference [17]. The diagnosis of DIC was made based on the Japanese Association for Acute Medicine (JAAM) DIC diagnosis criteria using day 0 data [18]. When the total score was ≥ 4, the DIC was established. The DIC phenotype was defined with reference to the criteria of Asakura, hyperfibrinolysis was defined as an FDP level of ≥ 100 μg/mL, and the FDP/D-dimer ratio was used as a surrogate marker of fibrin (ogen) olysis [14]. Tissue hypoperfusion was defined as a blood lactate level of ≥ 4 mmol/L based on the Surviving Sepsis Campaign Guidelines 2012 [19]. The outcome measure was the hospital all-cause mortality.

Statistical analysis

Data are presented as the median and interquartile range. The IBM SPSS 22.0 for MAC OSX software program (IBM Japan, Tokyo) was used for the statistical analyses and calculations. Comparisons between the two groups were performed with the Mann-Whitney *U* test and either the Chi-square test or Fisher's exact test when required. The relationships between the dependent and the independent variables were analyzed by a logistic regression analysis (the backward stepwise method based on likelihood) and the results were reported as the odds ratio and 95 % confidence intervals. The discriminatory performance for hospital death was evaluated using the area under the receiver operating characteristic (ROC) curve (AUC). Survival curves during hospital stay were derived according to the Kaplan-Meier methods and compared using the log-rank test. Differences with p-values <0.05 were considered to be statistically significant.

Results

Baseline patient characteristics

During the study period, a total of 1243 OHCA patients presented to our Emergency Department. After the exclusion of ineligible patients and patients with incomplete data for calculation of the DIC score, those performed PCPS were further excluded. Finally, 388 eligible patients were identified, who were divided into DIC ($n = 208$) and non-DIC patients ($n = 180$).

Table 1 shows the demographic data of the patients. Cardiac arrest due to a cardiac origin was less frequent in DIC patients. All DIC patients developed SIRS. DIC patients exhibited higher SIRS and SOFA scores associated with MODS, which associated with a significantly higher mortality than non-DIC patients (54.8 % vs. 23.9 %). Although some data were lacking (DIC, $n = 182$; Non DIC, $n = 163$), the Acute Physiology and Chronic

Table 1 Demographic and clinical characteristics of all patients

	Non DIC	DIC	*p* Value
	(180)	(208)	
Age (year)	66 (55–76)	71 (58–80)	0.020
Male sex (*n*,%)	112 (62.2)	124 (59.6)	0.604
Causes of cardiac arrest			
CNS/Cardiac/Respiratory/Asphyxia/Other/Unknown	13/99/24/32/11/1	18/86/30/37/32/5	–
Cardiac (*n*,%)	99 (55.0)	86 (41.3)	0.008
Initial rhythm			
VF/Asystole/PEA/Pulseless VT/Unknown	32/41/33/3/71	24/75/35/6/24	–
Shockable rhythm (*n*,%)	35 (19.4)	30 (14.4)	0.220
Witnessed arrest	75 (41.7)	92 (44.2)	0.681
Bystander CPR (*n*,%)	55 (30.6)	50 (24.0)	0.169
Shock by EMT (*n*,%)	42 (23.3)	44 (21.1)	0.626
Therapeutic hypothermia (*n*,%)	44 (24.4)	40 (19.2)	0.219
DIC score	2 (1–2)	5 (4–6)	0.000
SIRS score	3 (3–4)	4 (3–4)	0.048
SIRS (*n*,%)	178 (98.9)	208 (100)	0.215
SOFA day 0 score	6 (4–8)	9 (6–11)	0.000
MODS day 0 (*n*,%)	7 (3.9)	49 (23.6)	0.000
MODS day 5 (*n*,%)	10 (5.5)	67 (32.2)	0.000
Outcome death (*n*,%)	43 (23.9)	114 (54.8)	0.000

CNS central nervous system, *VF* ventricular fibrillation, *PEA* pulseless electrical activity, *VT* ventricular tachycardia, *CPR* cardiopulmonary resuscitation, *EMT* emergency medical technician, *DIC* disseminated intravascular coagulation, *APACHEII* Acute Physiology and Chronic Health Evaluation II, *SIRS* systemic inflammatory response syndrome, *SOFA* sequential organ failure assessment, *MODS* multiple organ dysfunction syndrome

Health Evaluation II scores of the DIC patients [34 (29–38)] were significantly higher than those of the non-DIC patients [29 (24–33)] ($P < 0.001$), suggesting that conditions of the DIC patients were more severe.

Serial changes in measured variables

DIC patients continuously showed lower platelet counts, more prolonged prothrombin time ratios, and lower levels of fibrinogen and antithrombin than non-DIC patients (Fig. 1). Extremely high levels of FDP and D-dimer associated with marked increases in lactate levels were also observed in DIC patients (Fig. 2). In addition, FDP/D-dimer ratios in DIC patients were significantly higher than in non-DIC patients (Fig. 3). These results suggest consumption coagulopathy, insufficient anticoagulation, fibrin (ogen) olysis, and tissue hypoperfusion in DIC patients and that the DIC belongs to the fibrinolytic phenotype. The numbers of patients at each time point are provided in Additional file 1: Table S1.

Subgroup analyses of DIC patients

DIC patients were subdivided into those with ($n = 73$) and without ($n = 135$) hyperfibrinolysis (Table 2). The markers of fibrinolysis and lactate levels of DIC patients with hyperfibrinolysis are presented in Table 3. Patients with hyperfibrinolysis had higher DIC and SOFA scores. Furthermore, MODS in these patients continued from day 0 to day 5, leading to a higher mortality rate of 68.5 % in comparison to patients without hyperfibrinolysis (41.7 %). The median FDP/D-dimer ratio of 2.0 in patients with hyperfibrinolysis was significantly higher than that in those without hyperfibrinolysis (Table 3). In addition, the lactate levels were significantly higher in those with hyperfibrinolysis than in those without fibrinolysis. These results suggest that DIC with hyperfibrinolysis is considered to be more severe DIC associated with extreme fibrin (ogen) olysis and tissue hypoperfusion, which results in worse outcome.

Outcome analyses

Stepwise logistic regression analyses confirmed that DIC, SOFA scores, and lactate levels are independent predictors of patient death (Table 4). Hyperfibrinolysis also predicted patient death (Table 5). Table 5 shows that tissue hypoperfusion (as indicated by lactate level) is one of the causes of hyperfibrinolysis. ROC curves showed a significant discriminative performance of DIC and SOFA scores and lactate levels for patient death (Fig. 4). These

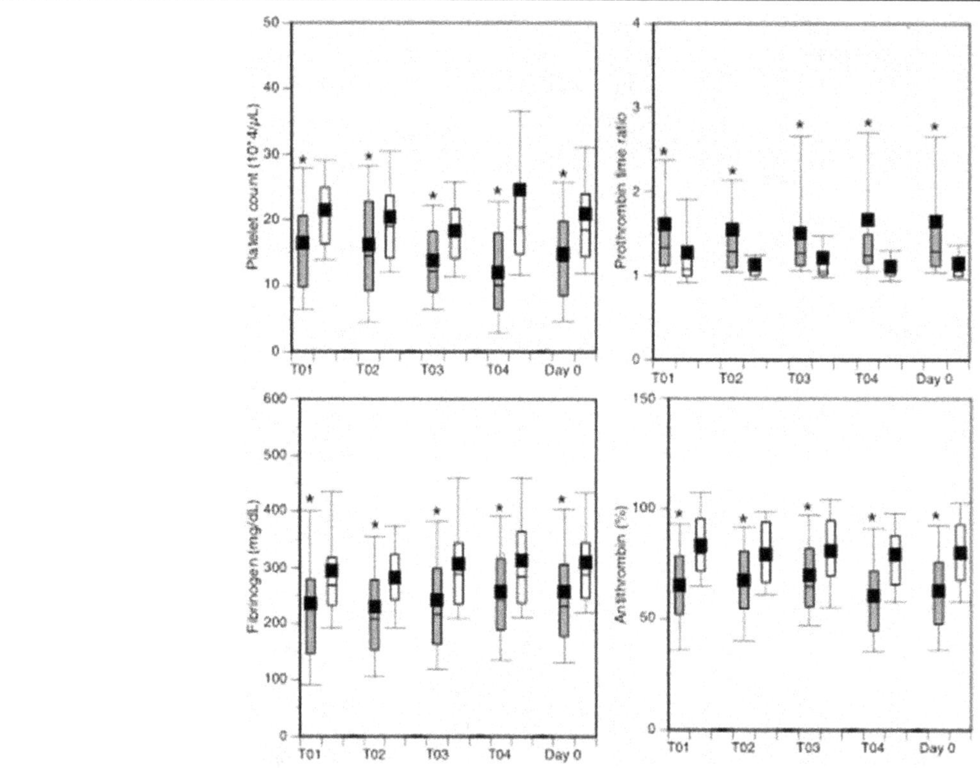

Fig. 1 Box plots showing serial changes in the platelet counts, prothrombin time ratios, fibrinogen and antithrombin levels during the first 24 h in successfully resuscitated patients after OHCA. DIC patients (*grey* boxes) showed significantly lower platelet counts, more prolonged prothrombin time ratios, lower levels of fibrinogen and antithrombin than non-DIC patients (open boxes). Horizontal bars in the box indicate the median (*middle*) and interquartile ranges (*upper* 25 %, *lower* 75 %). Black squares in the box indicate the mean value. Top and bottom bars indicate the maximum and minimum values, respectively. *$p < 0.001$ vs. non-DIC patients

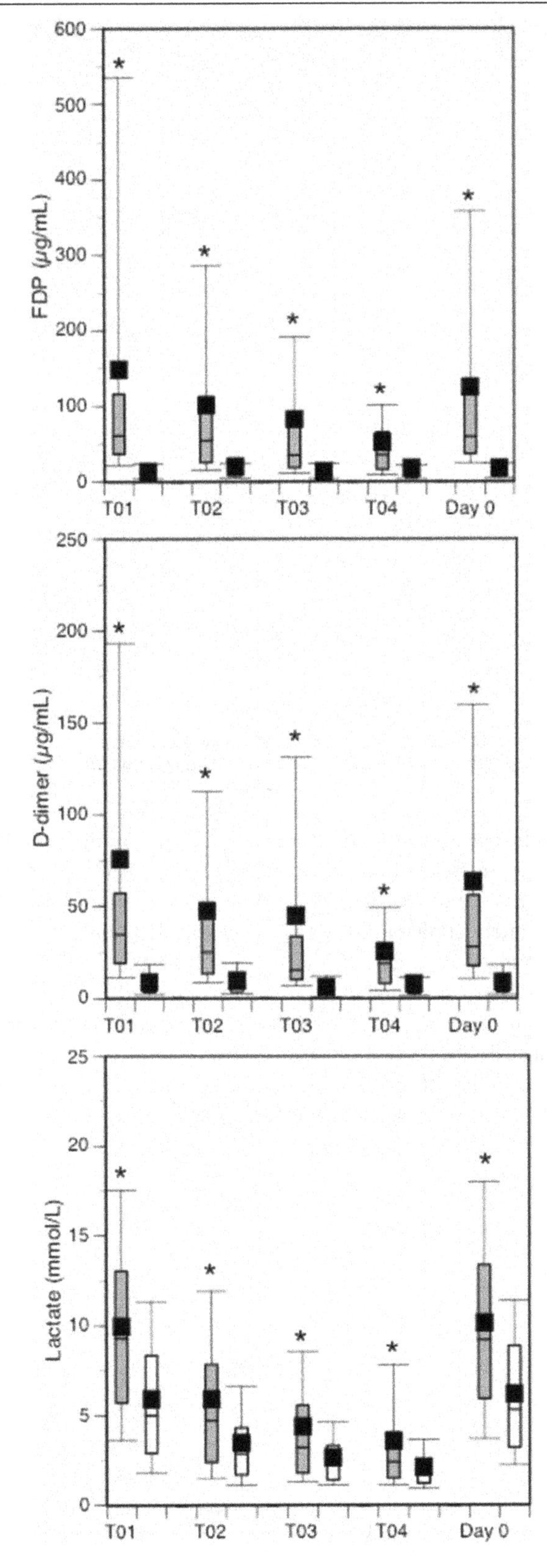

Fig. 2 Box plots showing serial changes in FDP, D-dimer and lactate levels. DIC patients (*grey* boxes) showed significantly higher values of three variables than non-DIC patients (open boxes). Horizontal bars in the box indicate the median (*middle*) and interquartile ranges (*upper* 25 %, *lower* 75 %). Black squares in the box indicate the mean value. Top and bottom bars indicate the maximum and minimum values, respectively. *$p < 0.001$ vs. non-DIC patients

results are important because the DIC score (score of one organ dysfunction [blood]) showed good discriminative power for the outcome compared with the SOFA score (score of multiple organ dysfunction). Kaplan-Meier curves showed that DIC, especially DIC with hyperfibrinolysis, significantly affected patient death (Fig. 5).

Discussion

The results of the present study demonstrate that OHCA patients with DIC during the early phase of post CPR are at risk of SIRS and MODS and that their condition is associated with a poor prognosis. The markedly higher FDP and D-dimer levels, and FDP/D-dimer ratio indicate that this type of DIC belongs to DIC with the fibrinolytic phenotype accompanied by fibrin (ogen) olysis. The outcomes of DIC patients with hyperfibrinolysis were worse than those observed in DIC patients without hyperfibrinolysis. The results of the logistic regression analyses suggest

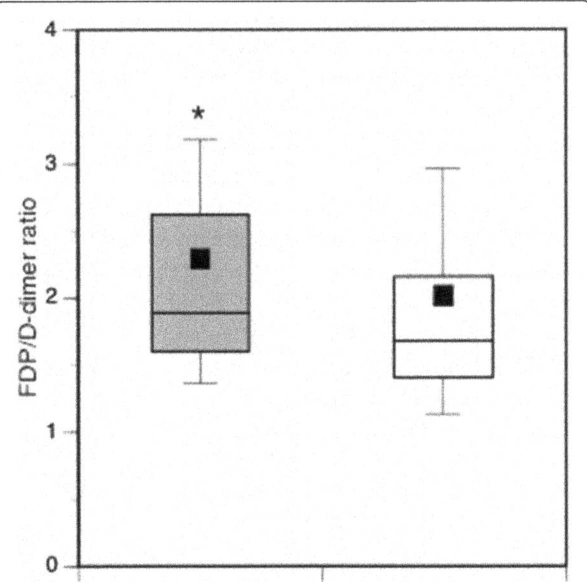

Fig. 3 Box plots showing FDP/D-dimer ratios between DIC (*grey* boxes) and non-DIC patients (open boxes). DIC patients exhibited significantly higher ratios than non-DIC patients. Horizontal bars in the box indicate the median (*middle*) and interquartile ranges (*upper* 25 %, *lower* 75 %). *Black* squares in the box indicate the mean value. Top and bottom bars indicate the maximum and minimum values, respectively. *$p < 0.001$ vs. non-DIC patients

Table 2 Demographic and clinical characteristics of the DIC patients

	DIC		
	Hyperfibrinolysis No (135)	Hyperfibrinolysis Yes (73)	*p* Value
Age (year)	70 (58–79)	73 (59–82)	0.091
Male sex (*n*,%)	78 (57.8)	46 (63.0)	0.554
Causes of cardiac arrest			
Cardiac (*n*,%)	54 (40.0)	32 (43.8)	0.659
Initial rhythm			
Shockable rhythm (*n*,%)	22 (16.3)	8 (11.0)	0.408
Witnessed arrest	59 (43.7)	33 (45.2)	0.884
Bystander CPR (*n*,%)	28 (20.7)	22 (30.1)	0.173
Shock by EMT (*n*,%)	27 (20.0)	17 (23.3)	0.597
Therapeutic hypothermia (*n*,%)	30 (22.2)	10 (13.7)	0.146
DIC score	5 (4–5)	5 (4.5–6)	0.000
SIRS score	3 (3–4)	4 (3–4)	0.359
SIRS (*n*,%)	135 (100)	73 (100)	–
SOFA day 0 score	8 (6–11)	10 (7–13)	0.001
MODS day 0 (*n*,%)	23 (17.0)	26 (35.6)	0.004
MODS day 5 (*n*,%)	36 (26.7)	31 (42.5)	0.029
Outcome death (*n*,%)	64 (47.4)	50 (68.5)	0.004

CNS central nervous system, *VF* ventricular fibrillation, *PEA* pulseless electrical activity, *VT* ventricular tachycardia, *CPR* cardiopulmonary resuscitation, *EMT* emergency medical technician, *DIC* disseminated intravascular coagulation, *SIRS* systemic inflammatory response syndrome, *SOFA* sequential organ failure assessment, *MODS* multiple organ dysfunction syndrome

that tissue hypoperfusion, as evaluated by the lactate level, may be a cause of increased fibrinolysis.

Kim et al. [5] found that an increased initial DIC score in OHCA patients was an independent predictor for poor outcomes and early mortality risk. OHCA patients with a higher D-dimer level on admission had a poor outcome and the D-dimer levels were independent predictor of mortality [20]. Although hyperfibrinolysis was assessed by maximum lysis of rotational thromboelastometry, OHCA patients associated with hyperfibrinolysis showed a higher mortality rate, and hyperfibrinolysis was correlated with markers of tissue hypoperfusion including pH, base excess and lactate levels [21, 22]. Cardiac arrest due to asphyxia by drowning developed DIC with the fibrinolytic phenotype was associated with lower platelet counts and fibrinogen levels, prolonged prothrombin time, and significantly higher D-dimer levels, which led to a worse outcome [23]. The present study has importance in that it validates the previous studies, which separately confirmed the importance of DIC or increased fibrinolysis, and provides a unified concept of DIC with the fibrinolytic phenotype. It also reveals that this DIC phenotype is associated with an increased risk of mortality, especially those with hyperfibrinolysis.

For a long time, anoxia and endothelial injury were believed to be clearly established triggering stimuli for the appearance of circulating fibrinolytic activator and

Table 3 Markers of fibrinolysis and lactate levels between DIC patients with and without hyperfibrinolysis

	Hyperfibrinolysis No (135)	Hyperfibrinolysis Yes (73)	*p* Value
FDP (μg/mL)	42.5 (28.2–57.6)	186.0 (110.3–404.5)	0.000
D-dimer (μg/mL)	20.3 (14.4–28.2)	74.3 (49.9–182.5)	0.000
FDP/D-dimer	1.8 (1.5–2.5)	2.0 (1.7–2.9)	0.007
Lactate (mmol/L)	8.1 (5.3–11.1)	11.3 (8.5–15.6)	0.000

Day 0 data are used for the FDP, D-dimer, and FDP/D-dimer values. The lactate data was obtained using data from time point 01

Table 4 Stepwise logistic regression analyses for prediction of the outcome (death)

	Odds ratio	*p* Value	95 % confidence interval
DIC score	1.171	0.041	1.006–1.364
SOFA score	1.178	0.001	1.073–1.292
Lactate	1.129	0.000	1.065–1.0197
Witnessed arrest	0.637	0.081	0.385–1.057
Cardiac origin	0.449	0.003	0.266–0.756
Shockable rhythm	0.400	0.024	0.180–0.887

The results of the final step of the analyses are shown. The dependent variables on the first steps: age, sex, DIC score (day 0), SOFA score (day 0), SIRS score (day 0), lactate level (time point 01), witnessed arrest, bystander CPR, shock by EMT, cardiac origin, and shockable rhythm
DIC disseminated intravascular coagulation, *SOFA* sequential organ failure assessment, *SIRS* systemic inflammatory response syndrome, *CPR* cardiopulmonary resuscitation, *EMT* emergency medical technician

Table 5 Logistic regression analyses for prediction of the outcome (death) and hyperfibrinolysis in DIC patients

	Odds ratio	*p* Value	95 % confidence interval
Outcome (enter method)			
SOFA score	1.204	0.000	1.094–1.324
Hyperfibrinolysis	1.938	0.038	1.036–3.626
Hyperfibrinolysis (stepwise method)			
Age	1.002	0.030	1.002–1.043
Bystander CPR	0.536	0.083	0.265–1.085
Lactate on time point 01	1.129	0.000	1.062–1.196

The stepwise method shows the results of the final step of the analyses. The dependent variables on the first steps: age, sex, lactate level, witnessed arrest, bystander CPR, shock by EMT, cardiac origin, and shockable rhythm
DIC disseminated intravascular coagulation, *SOFA* sequential organ failure assessment, *CPR* cardiopulmonary resuscitation, *EMT* emergency medical technician

increased fibrinolysis [24–26]. Schneiderman et al. [27, 28] confirmed immediate increases in t-PA activity following arterial occlusion-induced ischemia both in humans and a rat model, which is attributable to the release of preexisting t-PA in Weibel-Palade bodies [29]. PAI-1 mRNA is initially expressed 4 h after hypoxia, followed by the appearance of PAI-1 antigen at 6 h, and reaches its peak levels at 20 to 24 h after hypoxia [30]. These chronological changes in the levels of t-PA and PAI-1 completely coincide with the changes in these variables during CPR and after ROSC in patients with OHCA [12]. These results suggest that hypoxia during pre-cardiac arrest, and ischemia/hypoxia during cardiac arrest and CPR result in whole body tissue hypoperfusion recognized as increased lactate levels, which is followed by increased fibrinolysis in DIC patients, as observed in the present and our previous study and asphyxia-induced OHCA patients [12, 23].

There are pre-cardiac arrest differences in the perfusion pressure and blood flow and the duration and degree of tissue hypoperfusion, which is dependent on the cause of cardiac arrests, such as shock, exsanguination, asphyxia, and ventricular fibrillation [1]. Ventricular fibrillation indicates sudden onset of ischemia without pre-cardiac arrest

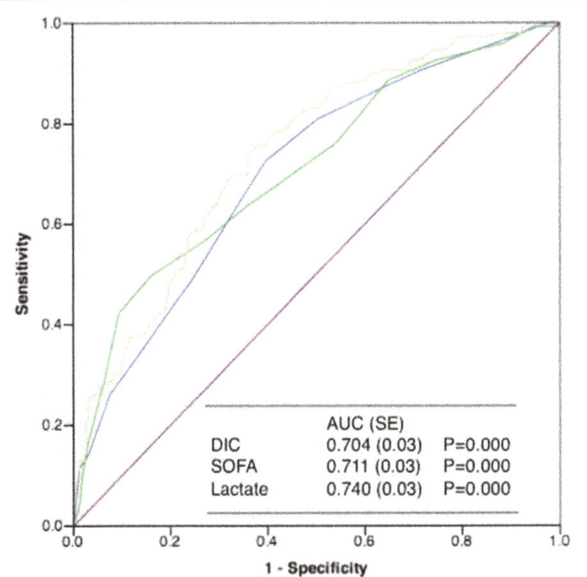

Fig. 4 ROC curves of the DIC scores (*blue* line), SOFA scores (*green* line) and lactate levels (*yellow* line) for the prediction of hospital death of OHCA patients. All of these variables showed a good discriminative power to predict poor outcome of the patients. SE, standard error

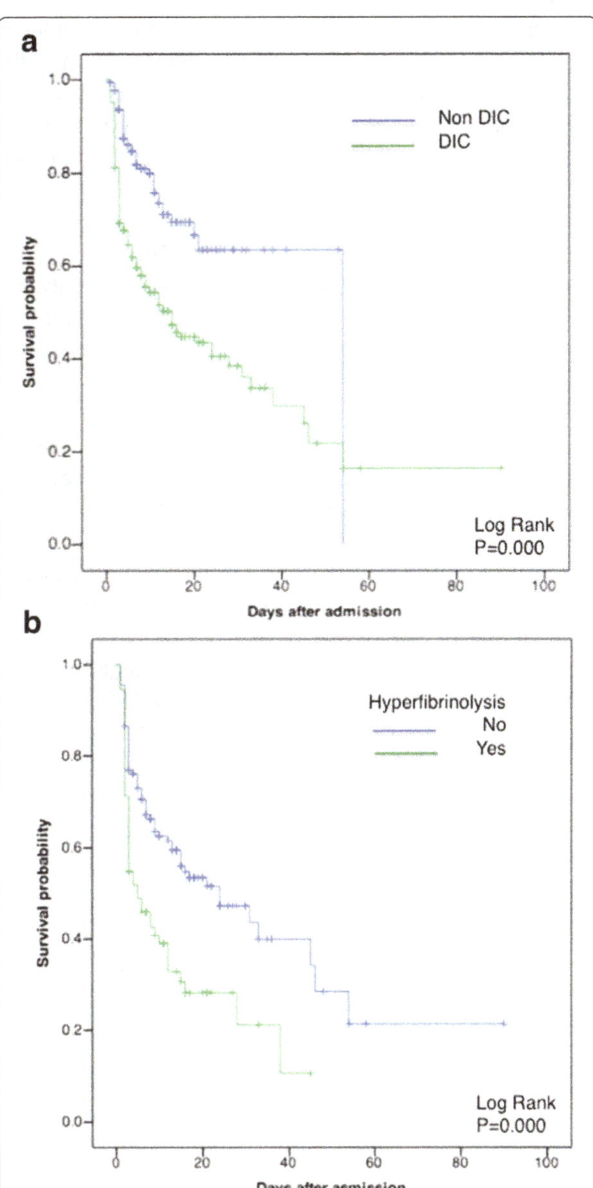

Fig. 5 Kaplan-Meier curves showing the association between DIC (**a**) or hyperfibrinolysis (**b**) with hospital mortality. DIC and DIC with hyperfibrinolysis showed a significantly lower survival probability in the hospital than non-DIC patients and DIC without hyperfibrinolysis

hypoxia. Therefore, in the present study, a low incidence of cardiac arrest due to a presumed cardiac origin in DIC patients might, in part, explain the finding that causes of cardiac arrest influence the degree of fibrinolysis. However, a subgroup analysis of a previous study confirmed that the magnitude of increased risk of a DIC-dependent poor prognosis in cardiac etiology was similar to that of the overall study population [5]. Many studies have reported that the time to first basic life support and duration of CPR were two of the main causes of hyperfibrinolysis [5, 21–23]. Although these parameters were not obtained in the present study, low odds ratio of bystander CPR in Table 5 indirectly suggests that a shortened ischemia period due to bystander CPR may reduce the risk of hyperfibrinolysis. Lastly, evenly distributed therapeutic hypothermia excluded the effects of hypothermia on DIC and increased fibrinolysis in the present study. Taken together, these results suggest that the duration of hypoxia/ ischemia, but not etiologies of cardiac arrest, may be a primary determinant of the development of DIC with the fibrinolytic phenotype in OHCA patients.

Activated protein C did not increase in OHCA patients [22]. Another study confirmed that activated protein C levels are not high enough to inhibit PAI-1 [23]. Neither syndecan-1 nor endothelial heparin sulfate levels were elevated in DIC with the fibrinolytic phenotype observed in asphyxia-induced OHCA [23]. Furthermore, other heparinase-sensitive glycosaminoglycans were not elevated [23]. These results suggest that participations of activated protein C and phenomena referred to as auto-heparinization are highly unlikely during hyperfibrinolysis in patients with OHCA.

Limitations. The results of the present study is based on retrospective analyses of OHCA in a single center and limited by an incomplete data set. Although increased fibrinolysis can be confirmed, the supposed causes of this phenomenon, such as t-PA and PAI-1, were not measured. Bleeding or a bleeding tendency, and the time to ROSC, and outcome scores such as cerebral performance category were not evaluated due to a lack of data. However, the magnitude of the results of this study suggests that a prospective multicenter study is needed to evaluate the effect of DIC on the outcome of OHCA patients.

Conclusions

In OHCA patients, DIC during the early phase of post-CPR exhibited lower platelet counts, consumption coagulopathy, and insufficient antithrombin levels associated with increased fibrin (ogen) olysis assessed by higher FDP/ D-dimer ratios, which can explain DIC of the fibrinolytic phenotype. DIC patients, especially those with hyperfibrinolysis, more gives rise to MODS associated with SIRS, leading to worse outcomes than those without DIC. Tissue hypoperfusion due to hypoxia and ischemia during cardiac arrest and CPR may be considered to be one of the causes of increased fibrinolysis in this type of DIC. The present study has validated previous studies that separately confirmed existence of DIC or increased fibrinolysis during the early post-CPR phase in OHCA patients. This study has further importance in that it unifies DIC and increased fibrinolysis as a single condition in the fibrinolytic phenotype of DIC and it recognized that this phenotype is associated with poor outcome.

Abbreviations

CNS: Central nervous system; CPR: Cardiopulmonary resuscitation; DIC: Disseminated intravascular coagulation; EMT: Emergency medical technician; FDP: Fibrin/fibrinogen degradation products; MODS: Multiple organ dysfunction syndrome; OHCA: Out-of-hospital cardiac arrest; PCPS: Percutaneous cardiopulmonary support; PEA: Pulseless electrical activity; ROSC: Return of spontaneous circulation; SIRS: Systemic inflammatory response syndrome; SOFA: Sequential organ failure assessment; VF: Ventricular fibrillation; VT: Ventricular tachycardia

Acknowledgements

None.

Funding

Departmental funding was used for this study.

Authors' contributions

TW designed the study, interpreted the data, and drafted the manuscript. SG conceived the study, analyzed and interpreted the data, and drafted the manuscript. YO, KM, KK, MH, and AS participated in the study design, helped to draft the manuscript, and proofread the manuscript. All authors read and approved the final manuscript.

Competing interests

Gando S received payment for lectures from Asahi Kasei Pharma. The other authors declare that they have no conflict of interests.

References

1. Safer P, Bircher NG. Prolonged life support. Cardiopulmonary cerebral resuscitation. Basic and advanced cardiac and trauma life support. In: Safer P, Bircher NG, editors. An introduction to resuscitation medicine. 3rd ed. Philadelphia: Saunders Company; 1988. p. 229–78.
2. Fisher M, Hossmann KA. No-reflow after cardiac arrest. Intensive Care Med. 1995;21:132–41.
3. Neumar RW, Nolan JP, Adrie C, Aibiki M, Berg RA, Böttiger BW, et al. Post-cardiac arrest syndrome: epidemiology, pathophysiology, treatment, and prognostication. A consensus statement from the International Liaison Committee on Resuscitation (American Heart Association, Australian and New Zealand Council on Resuscitation, European Resuscitation Council, Heart and Stroke Foundation of Canada, InterAmerican Heart Foundation, Resuscitation Council of Asia, and the Resuscitation Council of Southern Africa); the American Heart Association Emergency Cardiovascular Care Committee; the Council on Cardiovascular Surgery and Anesthesia; the Council on Cardiopulmonary, Perioperative, and Critical Care; the Council on Clinical Cardiology; and the Stroke Council. Circulation. 2008;118:2452–83.

4. Adrie C, Monchi M, Laurrent I, Um S, Yan SB, Thuong M, et al. Coagulopathy after successful cardiopulmonary resuscitation following cardiac arrest. Implication of the protein C anticoagulant pathway. J Am Coll Cardiol. 2005;46:21–8.
5. Kim J, Kim K, Lee JH, Jo YH, Kim T, Rhee JE, et al. Prognostic implication of initial coagulopathy in out-of-hospital cardiac arrest. Resuscitation. 2013;84:48–53.
6. Wada T, Gando S, Mizugaki A, Yanagida Y, Jesmin S, Yokota H, et al. Coagulofibrinolytic changes in patients with disseminated intravascular coagulation associated with post-cardiac arrest syndrome – Fibrinolytic shutdown and insufficient activation of fibrinolysis lead to organ dysfunction. Thromb Res. 2013;132:e64–9.
7. Levi M, ten Cate H. Disseminated intravascular coagulation. N Engl J Med. 1999;341:586–92.
8. Mehta B, Briggs DK, Sommers SC, Karpatkin M. Disseminated intravascular coagulation following cardiac arrest: a study of 15 patients. Am J Med Sci. 1972;264:353–63.
9. Hayakawa H, Sawamura A, Yanagida Y, Sugano M, Kubota M, Hoshino H, et al. Insufficient production of urinary trypsin inhibitor for neutrophil elastase release after cardiac arrest. Shock. 2008;29:549–52.
10. Shyu KG, Chang H, Lin CC, Huang FY, Hung CR. Concentrations of serum interleukin-8 after successful cardiopulmonary resuscitation in patients with cardiopulmonary arrest. Am Heart J. 1997;134:551–6.
11. Gando S, Nanzaki S, Morimoto M, Kobayashi S, Kemmotsu O. Tissue factor and tissue factor pathway inhibitor levels during and after cardiopulmonary resuscitation. Thromb Res. 1999;96:107–13.
12. Gando S, Kameue T, Nanzaki S, Nakanishi Y. Massive fibrin formation with consecutive impairment of fibrinolysis in patients with out-of-cardiac arrest. Thromb Haemost. 1997;77:278–82.
13. Geppert A, Zorn G, Delle-Karth G, Heinz G, Murer G, Siostrzonik P, et al. Plasminogen activator inhibitor type 1 and outcome after successful cardiopulmonary resuscitation. Crit Care Med. 2001;29:1670–7.
14. Asakura H. Classifying types of disseminated intravascular coagulation: clinical and animal models. J Intensive Care. 2014;2:20.
15. Ono Y, Hayakawa M, Wada T, Sawamura A, Gando S. Effects of prehospital epinephrine administration on neurological outcomes in patients with out-of-hospital cardiac arrest. J Intensive Care. 2015;3:29.
16. Ferreira FL, Bota DP, Bross A, Mélot C, Vincent JL. Serial evaluation of the SOFA score to predict outcome in critically ill patients. JAMA. 2001;286:1754–8.
17. Members of the American College of Chest Physicians/Society of Critical Care Medicine Consensus Conference committee. American College of Chest Physicians/Society of Critical Care Medicine Consensus Conference. Definition for sepsis and organ failure and guidelines for the use innovative therapies in sepsis. Crit Care Med. 1992;20:864–74.
18. Gando S, Saitoh D, Ogura H, Mayumi T, Koseki K, Ikeda T, et al. Japanese Association for Acute Medicine disseminated intravascular coagulation (JAAM DIC) study group. Natural history of disseminated intravascular coagulation diagnosed based on the newly established diagnostic criteria for critically ill patients: Results of a multicenter, prospective survey. Crit Care Med. 2008;36:145–50.
19. Dellinger RP, Levy MM, Rhodes A, Annane D, Gerlach H, Opal SM, et al. Surviving sepsis campaign: international guidelines for management of severe sepsis and septic shock: 2012. Crit Care Med. 2013;41:580–637.
20. Szymanski FM, Karpinski G, Filipiak KJ, Platek AE, Hrynkiewicz-Szymanska A, Kotkowski M, et al. Usefulness of the D-dimer concentration as a predictor of mortality in patients with out-of-hospital cardiac arrest. Am J Cardiol. 2013;112:467–71.
21. Viersen VA, Greuters S, Korfage AR, Van der Rijst C, Van Bochove V, Nanayakkara PW, et al. Hyperfibrinolysis in out of cardiac arrest is associated with markers of hypoperfusion. Resuscitation. 2012;83:1451–5.
22. Duvekot A, Viersen VA, Dekkar SE, Geeraedts LMG, Schwarte LA, Spoelstra-Man AME, et al. Low cerebral oxygenation levels during resuscitation in out-of-hospital cardiac arrest are associated with hyperfibrinolysis. Anesthesiology. 2015;123:820–9.
23. Schwameis M, Schober A, Schörgenhofer C, Sperr WR, Schöchl H, Janata-Schwatczek K, et al. Asphyxia by drowning induces massive bleeding due to hyperfibrinolytic disseminated intravascular coagulation. Crit Care Med. 2015;43:2394–402.
24. Clearke RL, Clifton EE. Oxygen saturation and spontaneous fibrinolytic activity. Am J Med Sci. 1962;244:466–71.
25. Todd AS. Endothelium and fibrinolysis. Atherosclerosis. 1972;15:137–40.
26. Bätsch P, Haeberli A, Hauser K, Gubser A, Straub PW. Fibrinogenolysis in the absence of fibrin formation in severe hypobaric hypoxia. Aviat Space Environ Med. 1988;59:428–32.
27. Schneiderman J, Adar R, Savion N. Changes in plasmatic tissue-type plasminogen activator and plasminogen activator inhibitor activity during acute arterial occlusion associated with ischemia. Thromb Res. 1991;62:401–8.
28. Schneiderman J, Eguchi Y, Adar R, Sawdey M. Modulation of fibrinolytic system by major peripheral ischemia. J Vasc Surg. 1994;19:516–24.
29. Lowenstein CJ, Morrell CN, Yamakuchi M. Regulation of Weibel-Palde body exocytosis. Trend Cardiovasc Med. 2005;15:302–8.
30. Pinsky DJ, Liao H, Lawson CA, Yan SF, Chen J, Cameliet P, et al. Coordinated induction of plasminogen activator inhibitor-1 (PAI-1) and inhibition of plasminogen activator gene expression by hypoxia promotes pulmonary vascular fibrin deposition. J Clin Invest. 1998;102:919–28.

17

β_3 phosphorylation of platelet $\alpha_{IIb}\beta_3$ is crucial for stability of arterial thrombus and microparticle formation in vivo

Weiyi Feng[1,3†], Manojkumar Valiyaveettil[1,4†], Tejasvi Dudiki[1†], Ganapati H. Mahabeleshwar[1], Patrick Andre[2], Eugene A. Podrez[1*] and Tatiana V. Byzova[1*]

Abstract

Background: It is well accepted that functional activity of platelet integrin $\alpha_{IIb}\beta_3$ is crucial for hemostasis and thrombosis. The β_3 subunit of the complex undergoes tyrosine phosphorylation shown to be critical for outside-in integrin signaling and platelet clot retraction ex vivo. However, the role of this important signaling event in other aspects of prothrombotic platelet function is unknown.

Method: Here, we assess the role of β_3 tyrosine phosphorylation in platelet function regulation with a knock-in mouse strain, where two β_3 cytoplasmic tyrosines are mutated to phenylalanine (DiYF). We employed platelet transfusion technique and intravital microscopy for observing the cellular events involved in specific steps of thrombus growth to investigate in detail the role of β_3 tyrosine phosphorylation in arterial thrombosis in vivo.

Results: Upon injury, DiYF mice exhibited delayed arterial occlusion and unstable thrombus formation. The mean thrombus volume in DiYF mice formed on collagen was only 50% of that in WT. This effect was attributed to DiYF platelets but not to other blood cells and endothelium, which also carry these mutations. Transfusion of isolated DiYF but not WT platelets into irradiated WT mice resulted in reversal of the thrombotic phenotype and significantly prolonged blood vessel occlusion times. DiYF platelets exhibited reduced adhesion to collagen under in vitro shear conditions compared to WT platelets. Decreased platelet microparticle release after activation, both in vitro and in vivo, were observed in DiYF mice compared to WT mice.

Conclusion: β_3 tyrosine phosphorylation of platelet $\alpha_{IIb}\beta_3$ regulates both platelet pro-thrombotic activity and the formation of a stable platelet thrombus, as well as arterial microparticle release.

Keywords: β_3 integrin phosphorylation, Outside-in integrin signaling, Microparticles, Arterial thrombosis

Background

Platelet activation and aggregation control physiological defense mechanisms such as cessation of bleeding after injury, and also underlie the pathophysiology of ischemic disorders, stroke and myocardial infarction [1, 2]. Several signaling pathways trigger platelet activation in vivo, but the common result is the activation of the major platelet surface glycoprotein, integrin $\alpha_{IIb}\beta_3$ [1, 3–5]. On platelets, integrin $\alpha_{IIb}\beta_3$ is a key receptor whose activity is rapidly induced upon agonist stimulation (ADP, thrombin, etc.), resulting in binding of its major physiological ligand, plasma fibrinogen, and subsequent platelet aggregation [4]. The blockade of $\alpha_{IIb}\beta_3$ with antibodies, peptides, peptidomimetics or small compounds results in reduced thrombotic activity and prolonged occlusion times [6, 7]. Animals deficient for β_3 integrin are characterized by prolonged bleeding times, gastrointestinal hemorrhage, and abnormal platelet aggregation and clot retraction [8, 9].

The $\alpha_{IIb}\beta_3$ cytoplasmic domains serve as docking sites for numerous intracellular adaptors, signaling molecules and cytoskeletal proteins. These interactions are crucial

* Correspondence: podreze@ccf.org; byzovat@ccf.org
†Equal contributors
[1]Department of Molecular Cardiology, The Cleveland Clinic Foundation, Cleveland 44195, OH, USA
Full list of author information is available at the end of the article

for both inside-out and outside-in signaling processes [10, 11]. The β_3 subunit of $\alpha_{IIb}\beta_3$ contains two cytoplasmic tyrosine residues, Tyr747 and Tyr759. Tyrosine phosphorylation of the β_3 was shown to occur during platelet aggregation as a result of fibrinogen binding to the receptor; it is considered to be a process triggered by outside-in integrin signaling [12–14]. Phosphorylation of β_3 was shown to be crucial for recruitment of several adaptor molecules, including Shc, Grb and cytoskeletal myosin, a protein crucial for retraction of the fibrin clot by platelets [4, 15].

The direct role of β_3 tyrosine phosphorylation in the regulation of platelet functions was tested using the knock-in mouse strain DiYF, where both tyrosines were mutated to phenylalanine. The resultant mutant $\alpha_{IIb}\beta_3$ is unable to undergo phosphorylation and interact with adaptor molecules, which severely affects platelet functions. Aggregation of DiYF platelets was reported to be reversible with defective clot retraction responses, resulting in the tendency of DiYF mice to re-bleed in the standard tail bleeding assay [9]. Importantly, the β_3 subunit in complex with α_V is present on several populations of blood cells, including monocytes and T lymphocytes, and also on vascular endothelial cells [16]. Besides platelets, the DiYF mutation affects functions of other cells known to serve as important contributing factors in thrombus formation [17]. Our recent studies showed that the DiYF mutation results in a series of abnormalities in endothelial cell adhesion, spreading, and migration [18]. Thus, endothelial defects in DiYF mice might be critical for thrombus initiation in vivo. Additionally, it is known that heterotypic interactions between platelets and blood mononuclear cells serve as another important mechanism regulating thrombus progression [19].

Accordingly, the aim of this study was to comprehensively analyze the role of β_3 tyrosine phosphorylation within an in vivo model of arterial thrombosis and to dissect the role of the platelet-specific component. For the latter objective, we have developed a new in vivo model involving platelet transfusion which allows analysis of DiYF mutation exclusively on platelets.

Methods

Mice

Eight- to 12-week-old, sex- and age-matched wild type (WT, C57BL/6) or DiYF mice were used in this study. Seven generations of back crossed $GFP^{+/+}$-C57BL/6 mice were purchased from The Jackson Laboratory (Bar Harbor, ME). $GFP^{+/+}$-DiYF mice were bred from DiYF and GFP heterozygous mice. All animal procedures were performed in accordance with an approved institutional protocol according to the guidelines of the Institutional Animal Care and Use Committee of the Cleveland Clinic.

Intravital microscopy

Blood was collected from the abdominal vein of WT or DiYF mice and treated with 1/10 vol of acid-citrate-dextrose anticoagulent containing 1 μg/ml prostaglandin E_1 (Sigma-Aldrich, St. Louis, MO). WT or DiYF platelets were obtained and labeled with calcein green (Invitrogen, Carlsbad, CA), and then infused into the respective WT or DiYF mice (4-5 × 10^6 /g) via tail vein as previously described [20]. Mice were anesthetized and placed on a 37 °C warm platform. The carotid artery was exposed and visualized using a Leica DMLFS fixed stage microscope. Images were recorded with a high speed color cooled digital camera (Q-imaging Retiga Exi Fast 1394) with Streampix[R] high speed acquisition software. Leica water immersion objectives at 10× –63× were used. To initiate thrombosis, a patch (1.5 × 1.5 mm) of filter paper saturated with 10% $FeCl_3$ solution was placed on the carotid artery for 2 min. The blood flow and platelet vessel wall interactions taking place in the carotid artery were monitored continuously for 60 min after vessel wall injury, or until full occlusion occurred and lasted for more than 30 s.

Perfusion chamber experiments

The thrombosis phenotype of WT and DiYF mice was evaluated in the murine ex vivo perfusion chamber protocol exposing fibrillar collagen to non-anticoagulated samples of blood under arterial shear rates as previously described [21]. Briefly, non-anticoagulated blood was collected from the vena cava of anesthetized mice and perfused for 2.5 min through human type III collagen-coated capillary chambers. Capillary chambers with a diameter of 345 μm were used to establish a shear rate of 871/s (flow rate of 212 μl/min). Mean thrombus volume ($\mu m^3/\mu m^2$) was quantified on semi-thin cross section and by mean grey level measurements at 5 mm from the proximal part of the capillary using Simple PCI software.

Irradiation and platelet transfusion model

WT mice were depleted of blood cells by sublethal γ–irradiation (6 Gy) then were subdivided into two groups 14 days later. 5 × 10^8 WT or DiYF platelets (10% of the platelets were labeled fluorescently with calcein green) in 0.3 ml Tyrode's buffer pH 7.4 (composition [mM]: NaCl 134, $NaHCO_3$ 12, KCl 2.9, $MgCl_2$ 1, $CaCl_2$ 2, HEPES 5, supplemented with 5 mM glucose and BSA) were infused into each irradiated mouse through the tail vein in their respective WT and DiYF groups. The in vivo thrombosis procedure was performed and thrombus formation was observed in these mice. Carotid artery occlusion was induced as described above for 3 min using filter paper saturated with 15% $FeCl_3$.

Tail-bleeding measurements

WT mice were infused with 5 × 10^8 WT or DiYF platelets 2 weeks after irradiation as described above. Platelet suspension buffer was injected for the control mice. Two hours after infusion, mice were anaesthetized and placed on a 37 °C warm platform before having 2 mm of the tip of their tails cut with a sharp scalpel. The time required for the flow of blood to cease was recorded.

Clot retraction experiments

Platelet rich plasma (PRP) was obtained from blood of irradiated and WT or DiYF platelet transfused WT mice (WT-WT(platelet) or WT-DiYF(platelet) mice, respectively). Platelet concentration in PRP was adjusted to $2 \times 10^5/\mu l$ with PBS. Clot retraction was measured by mixing the following in an aggregometer tube: 100 µl of PRP, 160 µl of clot retraction buffer (PBS solution containing 1 mM $CaCl_2$ and 1 mM $MgCl_2$), 50 µl of working solution of thrombin (clot retraction buffer with 8 U/ml thrombin). For visualization, 5 µl of WT erythrocytes were added. A glass rod was placed upright in the test tube which was incubated at 37 °C. Clot formation was checked and the volume of remaining solution was measured after 30 min incubation.

Flow cytometry analysis of platelet $\alpha_{IIb}\beta_3$ activation

Gel-filtered platelets (1.0×10^6) from WT-WT(platelet) or WT-DiYF(platelet) mice were resuspended in Tyrode's buffer containing 2 mM Ca^{2+} and 1 mM Mg^{2+}. Platelets were stimulated either with ADP (10 or 2 µM) or thrombin (0.1 or 0.05 U/ml) for 5 min at room temperature. The activated platelets were incubated with PE-conjugated anti-$\alpha_{IIb}\beta_3$ antibody (Emfret Analytics, Germany) for 15 min. Data for 20,000 positive cells were acquired using a FACSCalibur instrument (BD Biosciences, San Jose, CA).

Platelet aggregation

Gel filtered platelets were prepared as described above. Platelet aggregation was monitored using a Lumi-Aggregometer type 500 VS (Chrono-log Corporation, Havertown, PA). Thrombin (0.1, 0.075 and 0.05 U/ml) and collagen (5, 2.5 and 1 µg/ml) were used as agonists.

Platelet adhesion

5×10^7 GFP-transgenic WT or DiYF platelets (in 250 µl Tyrode's/BSA buffer) were added to collagen coated wells of a 6–Well culture plate at 37 °C in an orbital shaker at a maximum speed of either 380 cm/min (36 RPM) or 640 cm/min (60 RPM) and incubated for 1 h. The wells were washed with Tyrode's buffer and the images of bound platelets were acquired by fluorescence microscopy. Image quantification was performed using ImagePro software.

Preparation and flow cytometry analysis of microparticles from platelets

4×10^7 WT or DiYF platelets in suspension were activated by either thrombin (0.5 U/ml) or 200 nM phorbol-12-myristate-13-acetate (PMA, Calbiochem, San Diego, CA) for 15 min at 37 °C. Samples were then centrifuged at 12,000×g for 10 min at 22 °C to remove the platelets. The microparticle-enriched supernatant was harvested and stained with FITC-labeled annexin V (BD Biosciences, San Diego, CA) for 15 min in the dark at room temperature. The positive microparticle population was analyzed using a FACSCalibur instrument.

For in vivo experiments, a modified ferric chloride model of arterial thrombosis was used [22]. Briefly, WT and DiYF mice were anesthetized with ketamine/xylazine, a midline cervical incision was made and the mesentery was exposed by blunt dissection at 37 °C. 0.2 ml of 2% $FeCl_3$ solution in saline was applied to the surface of the vessels in the mesentery. After 5 min, blood was collected from the abdominal vein, labeled with FITC-conjugated annexin V and the positive microparticles in whole blood were measured by flow cytometry.

Statistical analysis

Results are reported as the mean ± SEM. Statistical significance was assessed by unpaired Student's t test. The non-parametric log-rank test was used to analyze occlusion and bleeding times. *P* values <0.05 were considered significant.

Results

Unstable thrombi and prolonged occlusion time in DiYF mice

As Fig. 1a shows, blood vessel injury resulted in the rapid attachment of platelets to the damaged site with the subsequent formation of platelet microaggregates. Adherent platelets and small aggregates of platelets appeared approximately 3-8 min after injury, both in WT and DiYF groups (Fig. 1b). Video analysis revealed that the formation of platelet microaggregates in DiYF mice was slightly but not significantly delayed in the initial stages of thrombus formation. The average times for the first thrombus ≥40 µm size formed in the carotid were 5.8 min in WT mice and 6.5 min in DiYF mice (Fig. 1b). Compared to WT, the subsequent growth rate of the thrombus appeared to be generally normal in DiYF mice. In WT mice the platelet thrombus occluded the blood vessel causing the complete cessation of blood flow around 12 min after injury (Fig. 1a and c). However, in DiYF mice, despite the presence of a thrombus, blood flow still continued for a prolonged period of time. As shown in Fig. 1a and c, the carotid arteries of DiYF mice remained open after 12 min time point with the continuous high shear, whereas the blood flow was

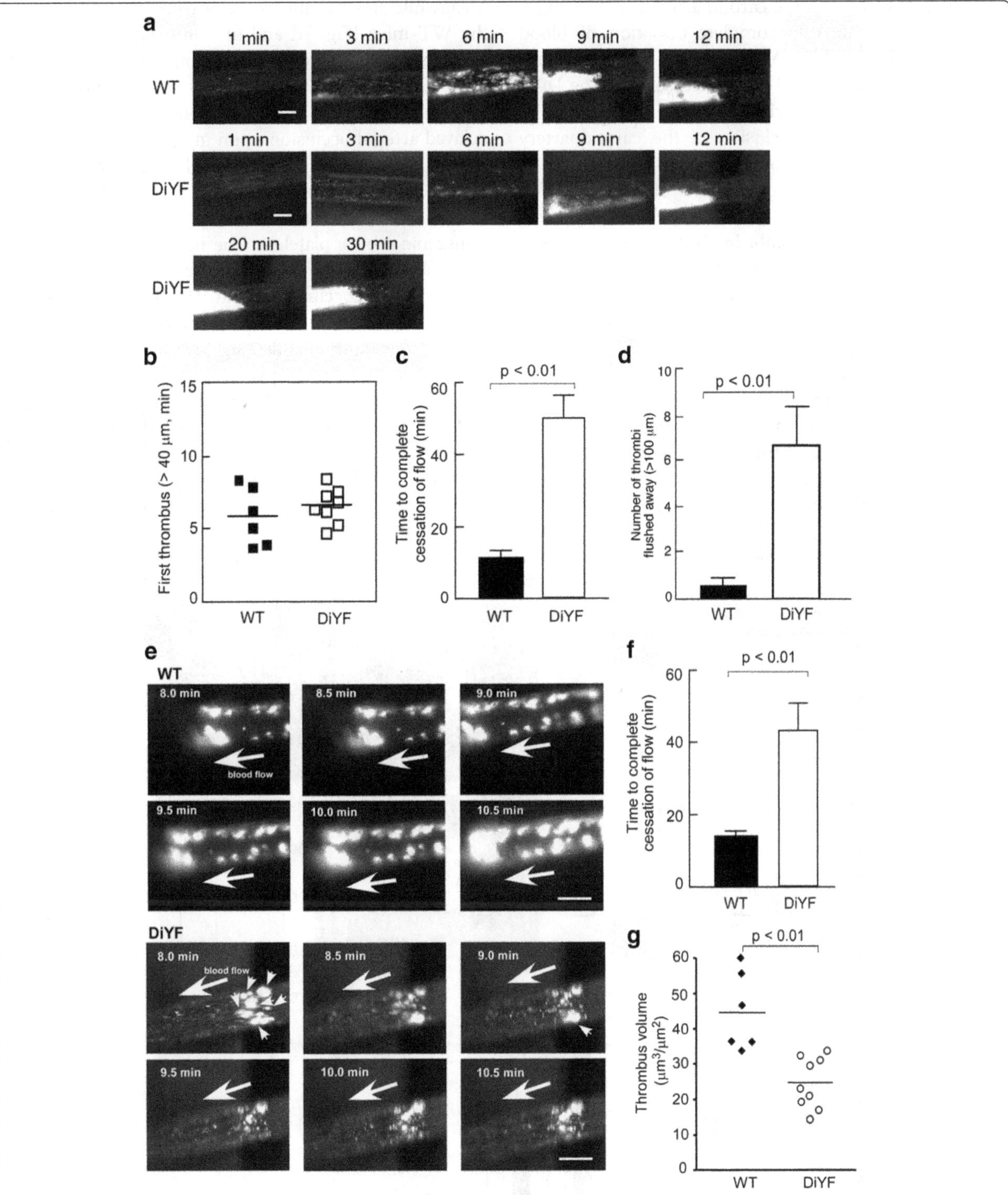

Fig. 1 Delayed thrombosis in DiYF mice. **a** Characteristics of thrombus growth in WT and DiYF mice in the carotid artery after injury. Bars = 500 μm. **b** No significant difference in the time to first thrombus formation (>40 μm) between WT ($n = 6$) and DiYF ($n = 8$) mice. **c** Delayed thrombus formation in DiYF mice ($n = 8$) compared to WT mice ($n = 6$). **d** Numbers of thrombi (>100 μm) removed by blood flow in WT and DiYF mice 10 min after carotid injury. **e** Characteristics of thrombi removed by blood flow in DiYF mice. → show blood flow, → show detached/flushed thrombi. Bars = 500 μm. **f** Delayed thrombus formation in GFP-transgenic DiYF mice ($n = 6$) compared to GFP-transgenic WT mice ($n = 6$). **g** Decreased thrombus volumes from DiYF blood formed on collagen in capillary chambers compared to their WT counterpart. Error bars represent SEM

completely disrupted in the carotid arteries of WT mice. On average, the time to complete cessation of blood flow was prolonged in DiYF mice by ~5 fold as compared to WT mice (Fig. 1c). In most cases with the DiYF mice (6 out of 8), the experiment was stopped at 60 min, even though complete occlusion of the carotid artery was not achieved. Video analysis showed that as thrombus formation progressed, parts of or even entire thrombi formed in DiYF mice were loosely packed. These loosely packed thrombi in DiYF mice were easily detached by flowing blood after they had grown larger, up to 100-200 μm. ImagePro analysis of the video revealed that thrombi formed in DiYF mice were ~50% less stable than that formed in WT mice. This defect resulted in the delayed visual accumulation of aggregated platelets at the site of injury (Fig. 1a) and dramatically prolonged occlusion times in DiYF mice (Fig. 1c). In addition, approximately 7 thrombi (≥100 μm size) were washed away in each DiYF mouse during the 10 min after the first thrombus appeared (Fig. 1d and e). Meanwhile, no thrombi were washed away in most of the WT mice (Fig. 1d and e). Thus, it appears that reversible platelet aggregation previously observed in DiYF mice causes the formation of a fragile and unstable thrombus, which, in turn, is responsible for substantially delayed arterial occlusion upon injury.

To make sure that calcein green labeling was not affecting platelet function, we repeated the same in vivo thrombus experiments by using WT and DiYF GFP-transgenic mouse platelets. The microthrombi formed in DiYF mice were still looser and less stable than in WT. Blood flow was occluded around 15 min in WT mice, but only three out of six DiYF mice reached occlusion before 60 min after injury, confirming the previous observations and the functional activity of platelets (Fig. 1f).

To further investigate the initial stages of thrombosis in DiYF mice, we analyzed thrombus formation on collagen under high shear conditions. The results showed that DiYF thrombi formed on the collagen surface were significantly smaller than their WT counterparts (Fig. 1g),

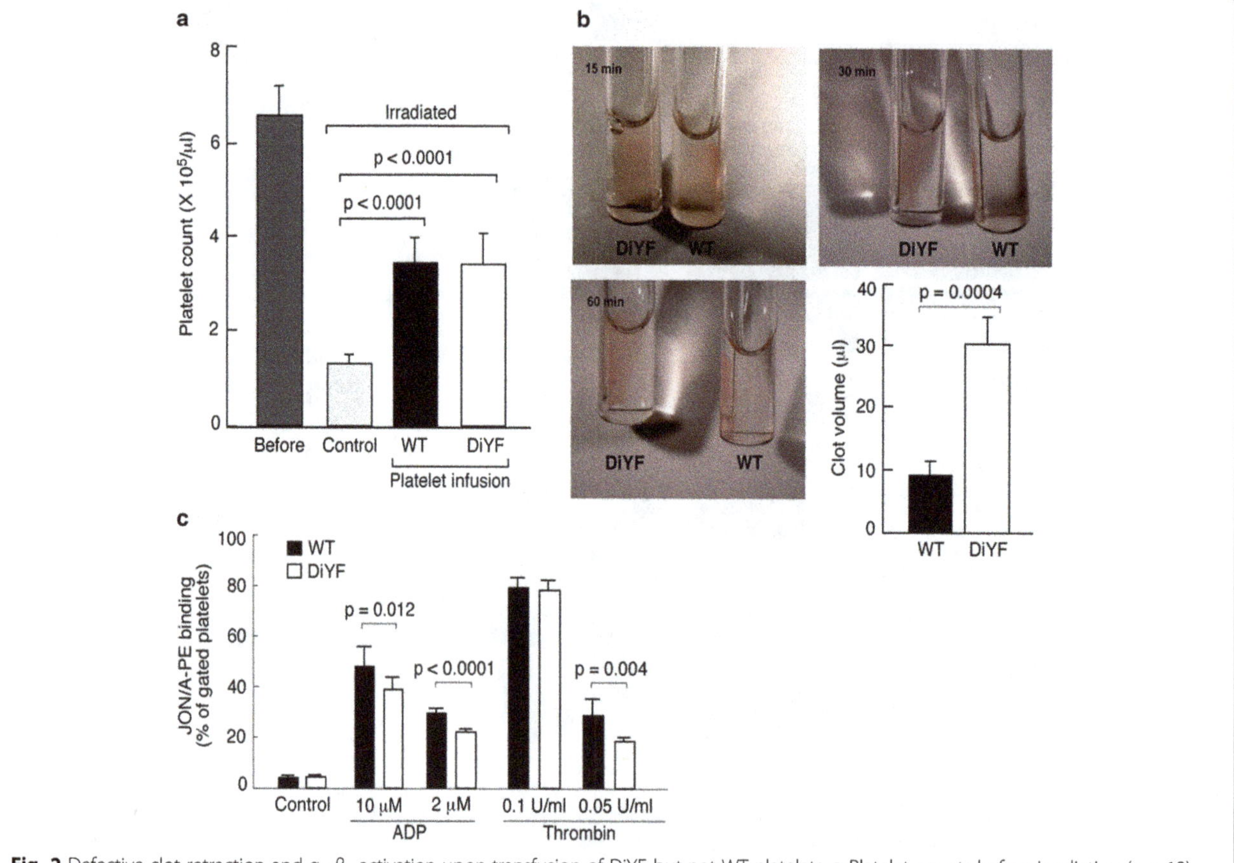

Fig. 2 Defective clot retraction and $\alpha_{IIb}\beta_3$ activation upon transfusion of DiYF but not WT platelets. **a** Platelet counts before irradiation (*n* = 12), after irradiation (control, *n* = 12) and after platelet transfusions (both *n* = 8). **b** Defective platelet retraction function in WT mice with DiYF platelets; Characteristics of clot retraction after 15, 30 and 60 min in transfused WT and DiYF PRP samples. Quantification of significantly increased clot volumes in transfused DiYF platelets compared to WT platelets is shown as a graph in the bottom right panel (mean ± SEM from five independent experiments). **c** Defective platelet $\alpha_{IIb}\beta_3$ activation in WT mice with DiYF platelets (mean ± SEM from three independent experiments)

suggesting that impaired β_3 phosphorylation also affects the process of platelet adhesion to and thrombus formation on collagen substrate.

Delayed thrombus formation in WT mice with DiYF platelets in vivo

As shown in Fig. 2a, irradiation caused at least a 5-fold reduction in platelet counts while transfusion of either WT or DiYF platelets showed a 2.5-fold increase. Clot retraction by the platelets from WT-DiYF(platelet) mice was significantly delayed compared to their WT counterparts (Fig. 2b), indicating defective platelet retraction, consistent with a previous report on WT and DiYF platelets [9]. Moreover, upon stimulation with ADP and thrombin, $\alpha_{IIb}\beta_3$ activation on the surface of platelets from WT-DiYF(platelet) mice was significantly impaired compared to the WT-WT(platelet) group (Fig. 2c; the difference was notable at lower concentrations of agonist). In aggregation assays, platelets from the WT-DiYF(platelet) group failed to aggregate upon stimulation with either 0.05 U/ml of thrombin or 1 μg/ml of collagen, compared to WT-WT(platelet) mice (Fig. 3a and b). At higher concentrations of agonist (0.1 U/ml thrombin or 5 μg/ml collagen), there was no significant difference in the aggregation curves (Fig. 3a and b), similar to previous observations [9]. Thus, transfusion of irradiated WT mice with DiYF platelets produced a platelet-specific DiYF phenotype.

Next, WT-WT(platelet) and WT-DiYF(platelet) mice were tested with the carotid injury model. Around 30% of thrombi formed in WT-DiYF(platelet) mice were unstable and repeatedly detached, in contrast to the WT-WT(platelet) group where thrombi were consistently stable. This phenomenon occurred in most WT-DiYF(platelet) mice but not in WT-WT(platelet) mice. Accordingly, the time to complete cessation of blood flow in WT-DiYF(platelet) mice was significantly longer than in the WT-WT(platelet) group (Fig. 3c).

Measurements of tail bleeding times in mice transfused with WT and DiYF platelets revealed that WT-DiYF(platelet) mice bled 5 times longer than WT-WT(platelet) mice (Fig. 3d). Interestingly, it was previously observed that while DiYF mice exhibited a pronounced tendency to re-bleed after transient hemostasis, the bleeding times were not substantially prolonged [9]. It is possible that in these animals with overall low blood cell counts, the typical tail cut model presents a greater hemostatic challenge and reveals a relatively subtle phenotype caused by the DiYF mutation in platelets.

Thus, it appears that the hemostatic defect observed in DiYF mice is primarily linked to the abnormal

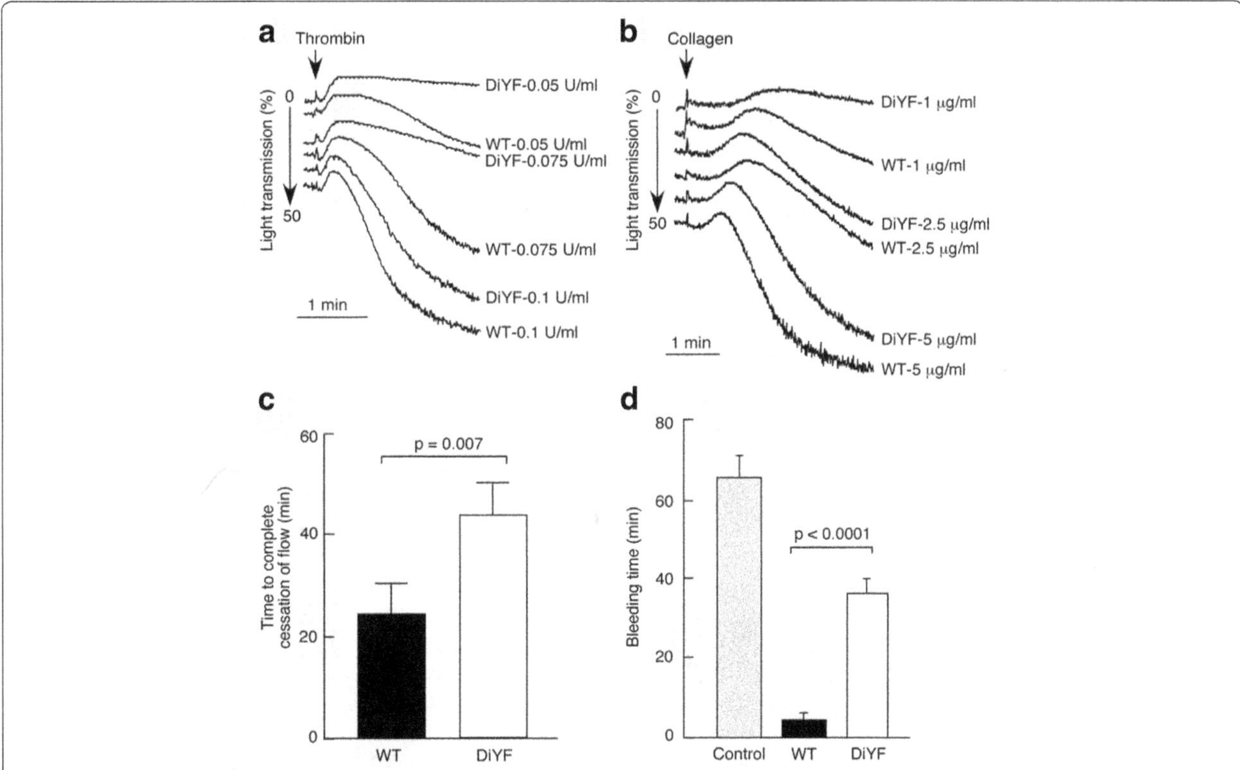

Fig.3 a and **b** Aggregation assays of platelet function in WT mice with WT or DiYF platelets (representative curves from three independent experiments). **c** Delayed thrombus formation in irradiated mice transfused with DiYF but not WT platelets (mean ± SEM from nine independent experiments). **d** Prolonged bleeding time in WT mice with DiYF platelets compared to their WT counterparts (mean ± SEM, *n* = 5)

function of β_3 integrin on platelets rather than on other cell types. Moreover, defective phosphorylation of β_3 in platelets, which impairs outside-in integrin signaling, affects thrombus structure and stability in vivo.

Reduced adhesion of DiYF platelets to type I collagen

Quantitative analysis of platelet adhesion to collagen at a lower velocity (380 cm/min) revealed that the DiYF mutation caused a 40% decrease in the number of adherent platelets compared to WT (Fig. 4a and b). At the same time, the difference in adhesion of WT and DiYF platelets was much more dramatic at higher velocity (640 cm/min; Fig. 4c and d). While WT platelets firmly adhered to collagen coated plates and formed small aggregates, attachment of DiYF platelets was reduced by at least 5-fold. Thus, the defects in firm adhesion of DiYF platelets can only be revealed under conditions of higher velocity, which, in turn, should primarily affect thrombosis at the arterial side of circulation.

Critical role of β_3 tyrosine phosphorylation in platelet microparticle release

In view of increasing evidence that platelet microparticles are particularly important for in vivo thrombosis [23–27], we assessed whether impaired β_3 phosphorylation affected microparticle release by activated platelets in vitro and in vivo. Platelet stimulation with PMA, thrombin or collagen resulted in a substantial release of microparticles and DiYF platelets shed approximately 50% fewer microparticles compared to WT platelets with all the agonists tested (Fig. 5a).

Importantly, reduced circulating microparticle levels were observed in DiYF mice compared to WT when multiple thrombosis processes were triggered by $FeCl_3$in mesenteric blood vessels. The presence of annexin V-positive microparticles in the blood of DiYF mice was decreased by 3-fold compared to WT (Fig. 5b). Thus, it appears that β_3 integrin tyrosine phosphorylation is critical for microparticle release upon platelet activation both in vivo and in vitro.

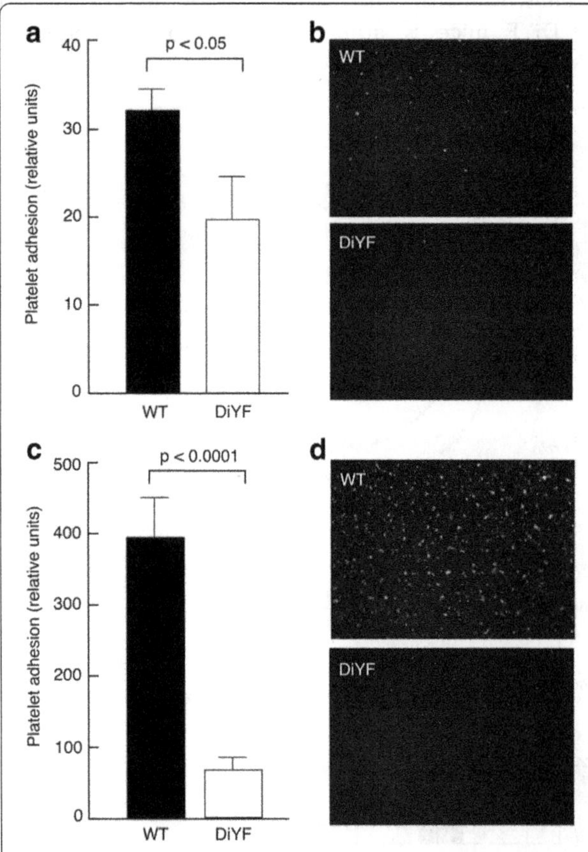

Fig. 4 Reduced DiYF platelet adhesion to collagen type I compared to WT platelets. Platelet adhesion and accumulation on collagen at shaker rates of 380 cm/min (**a**, **b**) and 640 cm/min (**c**, **d**) are shown (mean ± SEM from three independent experiments)

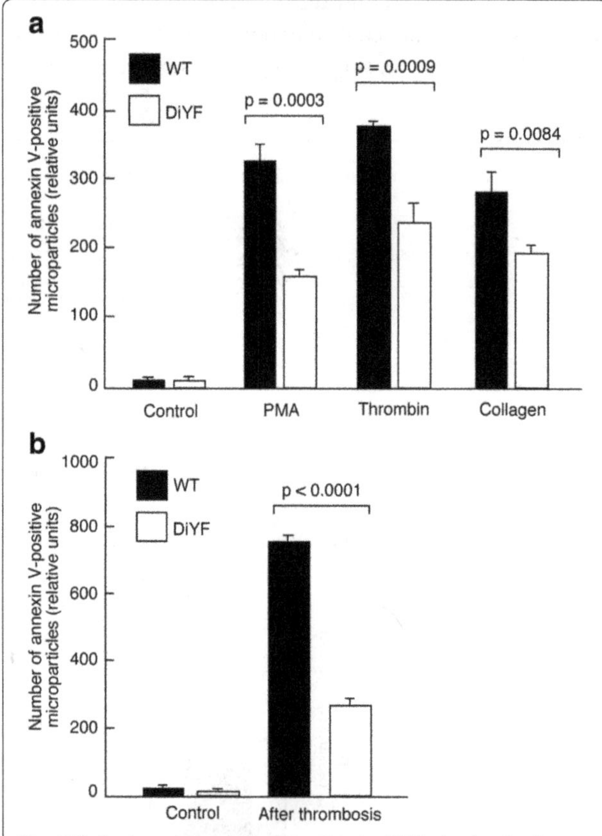

Fig. 5 Defective microparticle formation by DiYF platelets in vitro and in vivo. **a** Decreased annexin V-positive microparticles generated by DiYF platelets compared to WT platelets. **b** Reduced microparticles originating from platelets after thrombus formation in DiYF mice compared to their WT counterparts. Mean ± SEM from three independent experiments

Discussion

Using knock-in DiYF mice we assessed the role of β_3-integrin tyrosine phosphorylation in the regulation of arterial thrombosis in vivo with a particular focus on platelet-specific effects. Our major findings are: 1) the thrombus formed in the DiYF mouse is unstable, thus is easily detached by blood flow resulting in delayed occlusion of injured arteries. 2) Delayed thrombosis is due to impaired β_3 phosphorylation on platelets but not on other cells expressing β_3 integrin. 3) Defective β_3-phosphorylation results in impaired adhesion of DiYF platelets to collagen under shear conditions. 4) β_3-phosphorylation is crucial for microparticle release by activated platelets. Platelet microparticle levels were reduced in DiYF mice compared to WT in vivo and in vitro.

We employed intravital microscopy, a powerful tool for observing the cellular events involved in specific steps of thrombus growth [8], to investigate in detail the role of β_3 tyrosine phosphorylation in arterial thrombosis in vivo. We show that the time required for complete cessation of blood flow was substantially prolonged in DiYF knock-in mice. This phenomenon was not due to delayed or impaired progression of thrombus growth, but due to loose platelet-platelet bonds and an overall reduced stability of platelet aggregates (Fig. 6). Thrombi formed in DiYF but not in WT mice were easily detached and washed away by blood flow in injured arteries. In vivo, only a modest delay in the early stages of thrombus formation was observed in DiYF mice vs WT. However, more detailed ex vivo analysis revealed impaired platelet adhesion and thrombus formation by DiYF platelets on collagen under shear conditions. This defect might be crucial during initiation of thrombotic events when collagen matrix is a strong contributing factor. Although platelet attachment to collagen under flow is mediated by GPVI and $\alpha_2\beta_1$, $\alpha_{IIb}\beta_3$ serves as a crucial mediator of platelet-platelet interactions and the formation of microaggregates [28]. Activation of $\alpha_{IIb}\beta_3$ was reported to serve as a prerequisite for $\alpha_2\beta_1$ activation and interaction with collagen [29]. Interestingly, high shear conditions were able to reveal substantial defects in adhesion of phosphorylation-defective DiYF platelets to collagen, indicating that β_3 phosphorylation is crucial for this process. It is possible that impaired $\alpha_{IIb}\beta_3$ outside-in signaling might affect activation of collagen receptor $\alpha_2\beta_1$.

Integrin β_3 (in combination with αv) is expressed on endothelial cells as well as on circulating blood cells such as monocytes, lymphocytes and neutrophils. These cellular components are known to be critical for thrombus formation in vivo [30–33]. For obvious reasons, DiYF bone marrow transplantation into WT mice was only partially helpful to observe platelet functions in vivo, since it would affect all circulating blood cells. Accordingly, we developed a new platelet transfusion technique which allows the assessment of platelet-specific effects rather than broad platelet-leukocyte-vascular phenotype features of mice with modified function of β_3 integrin. Using this model we demonstrate in DiYF mice that the phenomenon of unstable thrombi is caused by defective platelet function, not endothelial cells or leukocytes. As we reported previously, endothelial cells of DiYF mice display a series of abnormalities including impaired integrin-dependent adhesion and spreading [18, 34]. Although these functions are crucial for angiogenesis, they do not substantially contribute to arterial thrombosis, which appears to be solely dependent on platelet β_3 integrin and its phosphorylation.

Another mechanism responsible for the overall delay of in vivo thrombosis in DiYF mice is the defective shedding of annexin V-positive microparticles by DiYF platelets. Microparticle formation accompanies in vivo platelet activation and greatly promotes the process of thrombin generation, further accelerating platelet activation and aggregation [35–38]. Our finding is further supported by an observation that platelets from Glanzmann thrombasthenia patients also have decreased microparticle release when stimulated with various agonists, as compared with normal human platelets [39], thereby solidifying the role for $\alpha_{IIb}\beta_3$ signaling in microparticle generation. Clinical studies demonstrated that elevated platelet microparticles play an important role in the

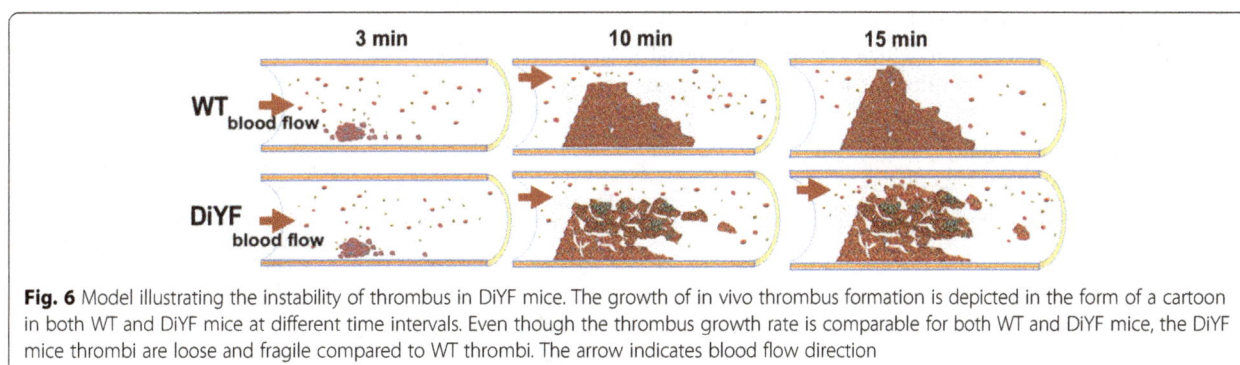

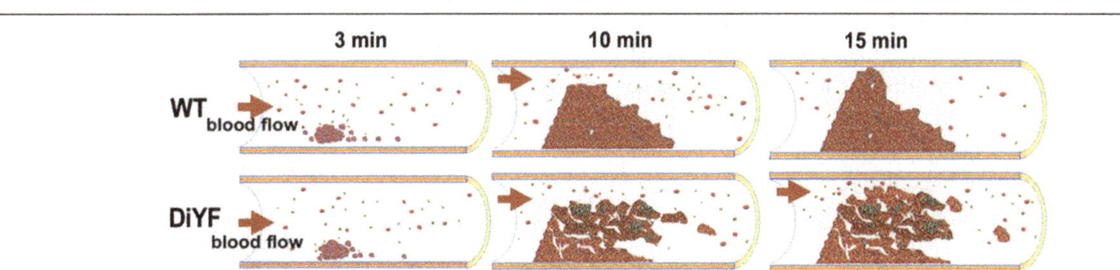

Fig. 6 Model illustrating the instability of thrombus in DiYF mice. The growth of in vivo thrombus formation is depicted in the form of a cartoon in both WT and DiYF mice at different time intervals. Even though the thrombus growth rate is comparable for both WT and DiYF mice, the DiYF mice thrombi are loose and fragile compared to WT thrombi. The arrow indicates blood flow direction

pathogenesis of the prothrombotic state in patients suffering from a number of diseases such as systemic lupus erythematosus. Patients with lupus have a significantly increased risk for thrombosis which affects both venous and arterial vessels [23, 40]. Thus, platelet microparticles, which are highly active in thrombin generation and fibrin clot formation processes as well as in amplification of platelet aggregation, appear to contribute to thrombosis in certain clinical settings [41]. Here we provide evidence that platelet β_3 phosphorylation and outside-in signaling promotes the release of microparticles upon platelet activation, which in turn, might accelerate the later stages of thrombus progression. Thus, not only reversible platelet aggregation in DiYF mice, but also impaired platelet-collagen interactions under shear and reduced shedding of microparticles are factors contributing to the formation of fragile and unstable thrombi in DiYF mice, which in turn, is responsible for substantially delayed arterial occlusion upon injury.

Our study highlights an importance of platelet $\alpha_{IIb}\beta_3$ phosphorylation and outside-in signaling for the formation of a stable platelet thrombus as well as for microparticle release by platelets. These two phosphorylation sites (Y747 and Y759) within the β_3 integrin cytoplasmic domain regulate arterial thrombosis under high sheer, without affecting hemostasis [9]. Therefore, targeting of these sequences within the β_3 integrin might represent an attractive therapeutic strategy with a potential of developing drugs diminishing arterial thrombosis without causing serious bleeding complications, which is one of the main drawbacks of existing anti-platelet strategies. This has major implications for various pathologies associated with platelet hyperreactivity, such as arterial thrombosis leading to myocardial infarction and, especially, stroke, as well as thrombotic complications in cancer patients, where excessive bleeding is associated with a high risk of morbidity. Thus, disruption of integrin function by targeting the β_3 phosphorylation motifs could provide new and potentially safer therapeutic interventions for numerous thrombotic complications.

Conclusion

This study shows that the phosphorylation status of $\alpha_{IIb}\beta_3$ on platelets, but not $\alpha_V\beta_3$ on leukocytes or endothelial cells, is critical for the formation of a stable thrombus. Therefore, β_3 phosphorylation and the resulting outside-in $\alpha_{IIb}\beta_3$ signaling is a primary mechanism regulating not only the consolidation and stabilization of platelet aggregation [13] but also platelet procoagulant activity.

Abbreviations

ADP: Adenosine 5'-diphosphate; DiYF: knock-in mouse strain, where two β_3 cytoplasmic tyrosines are mutated to phenylalanine; PBS: phosphate-buffered saline; PMA: Phorbol-12-myristate-13-acetate; PRP: Platelet rich plasma; WT: Wild type

Acknowledgements

Not applicable.

Funding

This work was supported by NIH grants HL071625 and HL073311 to T. V. Byzova and NIH grants HL077213 to E.A. Podrez.

Authors' contributions

TVB, EAP, WF, MV, PA, and TD, designed the study, analyzed the data, and wrote the manuscript. WF, MV, and GHM designed and performed the experiments; all authors discussed the results and commented on the manuscript. All authors read and approved the final manuscript.

Competing interests

The authors declare that they have no competing interests.

Author details

[1]Department of Molecular Cardiology, The Cleveland Clinic Foundation, Cleveland 44195, OH, USA. [2]Plaint Therapeutics, Redwood City, CA, USA. [3]The First Affiliated Hospital, School of Medicine, Xi'an Jiaotong University, Xi'an, Shaanxi 710061, China. [4]US Army Medical Materiel Development Activity, 1430 Veterans Drive, Fort Detrick, Frederick, MD 21702, USA.

References

1. Jurk K, Kehrel BE. Platelets: physiology and biochemistry. Semin Thromb Hemost. 2005;31:381–92.
2. Ruggeri ZM, Mendolicchio GL. Adhesion mechanisms in platelet function. Circ Res. 2007;100:1673–85.
3. Li Z, Zhang G, Feil R, Han J, Du X. Sequential activation of p38 and ERK pathways by cGMP-dependent protein kinase leading to activation of the platelet integrin alphallb beta3. Blood. 2006;107:965–72.
4. Abrams CS. Intracellular signaling in platelets. Curr Opin Hematol. 2005;12:401–5.
5. Ma YQ, Qin J, Plow EF. Platelet integrin alpha(IIb)beta(3): activation mechanisms. J Thromb Haemost. 2007;5:1345–52.
6. Gruner S, Prostredna M, Schulte V, Krieg T, Eckes B, Brakebusch C, et al. Multiple integrin-ligand interactions synergize in shear-resistant platelet adhesion at sites of arterial injury in vivo. Blood. 2003;102:4021–7.
7. Smyth SS, Reis ED, Vaananen H, Zhang W, Coller BS. Variable protection of beta 3-integrin–deficient mice from thrombosis initiated by different mechanisms. Blood. 2001;98:1055–62.
8. Denis CV, Wagner DD. Platelet adhesion receptors and their ligands in mouse models of thrombosis. Arterioscler Thromb Vasc Biol. 2007;27:728–39.
9. Law DA, DeGuzman FR, Heiser P, Ministri-Madrid K, Killeen N, Phillips DR. Integrin cytoplasmic tyrosine motif is required for outside-in alphallbbeta3 signalling and platelet function. Nature. 1999;401:808–11.
10. Gawaz M, Besta F, Ylanne J, Knorr T, Dierks H, Bohm T, et al. The NITY motif of the beta-chain cytoplasmic domain is involved in stimulated internalization of the beta3 integrin a isoform. J Cell Sci. 2001;114:1101–13.
11. Hynes RO. Integrins: bidirectional, allosteric signaling machines. Cell. 2002;110:673–87.
12. Jenkins AL, Nannizzi-Alaimo L, Silver D, Sellers JR, Ginsberg MH, Law DA, et al. Tyrosine phosphorylation of the beta3 cytoplasmic domain mediates integrin-cytoskeletal interactions. J Biol Chem. 1998;273:13878–85.
13. Phillips DR, Prasad KS, Manganello J, Bao M, Nannizzi-Alaimo L. Integrin tyrosine phosphorylation in platelet signaling. Curr Opin Cell Biol. 2001;13:546–54.
14. Xi X, Flevaris P, Stojanovic A, Chishti A, Phillips DR, Lam SC, et al. Tyrosine phosphorylation of the integrin beta 3 subunit regulates beta 3 cleavage by calpain. J Biol Chem. 2006;281:29426–30.
15. Law DA, Nannizzi-Alaimo L, Phillips DR. Outside-in integrin signal transduction. Alpha IIb beta 3-(GP IIb IIIa) tyrosine phosphorylation induced by platelet aggregation. J Biol Chem. 1996;271:10811–5.
16. Zhao R, Pathak AS, Stouffer GA. Beta(3)-Integrin cytoplasmic binding proteins. Arch Immunol Ther Exp. 2004;52:348–55.
17. Siegel-Axel DI, Gawaz M. Platelets and endothelial cells. Semin Thromb Hemost. 2007;33:128–35.

18. Mahabeleshwar GH, Feng W, Phillips DR, Byzova TV. Integrin signaling is critical for pathological angiogenesis. J Exp Med. 2006;203:2495–507.
19. Murohara T, Ikeda H, Otsuka Y, Aoki M, Haramaki N, Katoh A, et al. Inhibition of platelet adherence to mononuclear cells by alpha-tocopherol: role of P-selectin. Circulation. 2004;110:141–8.
20. Podrez EA, Byzova TV, Febbraio M, Salomon RG, Ma Y, Valiyaveettil M, et al. Platelet CD36 links hyperlipidemia, oxidant stress and a prothrombotic phenotype. Nat Med. 2007;13:1086–95.
21. Andre P, Delaney SM, LaRocca T, Vincent D, DeGuzman F, Jurek M, et al. P2Y12 regulates platelet adhesion/activation, thrombus growth, and thrombus stability in injured arteries. J Clin Invest. 2003;112:398–406.
22. Westrick RJ, Winn ME, Eitzman DT. Murine models of vascular thrombosis (Eitzman series). Arterioscler Thromb Vasc Biol. 2007;27:2079–93.
23. Flaumenhaft R. Formation and fate of platelet microparticles. Blood Cells Mol Dis. 2006;36:182–7.
24. Mause SF, von Hundelshausen P, Zernecke A, Koenen RR, Weber C. Platelet microparticles: a transcellular delivery system for RANTES promoting monocyte recruitment on endothelium. Arterioscler Thromb Vasc Biol. 2005;25:1512–8.
25. Morel O, Toti F, Hugel B, Bakouboula B, Camoin-Jau L, Dignat-George F, et al. Procoagulant microparticles: disrupting the vascular homeostasis equation? Arterioscler Thromb Vasc Biol. 2006;26:2594–604.
26. Piccin A, Murphy WG, Smith OP. Circulating microparticles: pathophysiology and clinical implications. Blood Rev. 2007;21:157–71.
27. Ardoin SP, Shanahan JC, Pisetsky DS. The role of microparticles in inflammation and thrombosis. Scand J Immunol. 2007;66:159–65.
28. Goto SY, Tamura N, Handa S, Arai M, Kodama K, Takayama H. Involvement of glycoprotein VI in platelet thrombus formation on both collagen and von Willebrand factor surfaces under flow conditions. Circulation. 2002;106:266–72.
29. Van de Walle GR, Schoolmeester A, Iserbyt BF, Cosemans JMEM, Heemskerk JWM, Hoylaerts MF, et al. Activation of alpha(IIb)beta(3) is a sufficient but also an imperative prerequisite for activation of alpha(2)beta(1) on platelets. Blood. 2007;109:595–602.
30. Gross PL, Furie BC, Merrill-Skoloff G, Chou J, Furie B. Leukocyte-versus microparticle-mediated tissue factor transfer during arteriolar thrombus development. J Leukoc Biol. 2005;78:1318–26.
31. Badlou BA, Wu YP, Smid MW, Akkerman JWN. Metabolic arrest suppresses platelet binding to and phagocytosis by macrophages. Blood. 2004;104:988a-a.
32. Weyrich A, Cipollone F, Mezzetti A, Zimmerman G. Platelets in atherothrombosis: new and evolving roles. Curr Pharm Design. 2007;13:1685–91.
33. Verhamme P, Hoylaerts MF. The pivotal role of the endothelium in haemostasis and thrombosis. Acta Clin Belg. 2006;61:213–9.
34. Mahabeleshwar GH, Feng WY, Reddy K, Plow EF, Byzova TV. Mechanisms of integrin-vascular endothelial growth factor receptor cross-activation in angiogenesis. Circ Res. 2007;101:570–80.
35. Berckmans RJ, Nieuwland R, Boing AN, Romijn FPHTM, Hack CE, Sturk A. Cell-derived microparticles circulate in healthy humans and support low grade thrombin generation. Thromb Haemost. 2001;85:639–46.
36. Nieuwland R, Berckmans RJ, RotteveelEijkman RC, Maquelin KN, Roozendaal KJ, Jansen PGM, et al. Cell-derived microparticles generated in patients during cardiopulmonary bypass are highly procoagulant. Circulation. 1997;96:3534–41.
37. Owens MR. The role of platelet microparticles in Hemostasis. Transfus Med Rev. 1994;8:37–44.
38. Perez-Pujol S, Marker PH, Key NS. Platelet microparticles are heterogeneous and highly dependent on the activation mechanism: studies using a new digital flow cytometer. Cytom Part A. 2007;71A:38–45.
39. Gemmell CH, Sefton MV, Yeo EL. Platelet-derived microparticle formation involves glycoprotein IIb-IIIa. Inhibition by RGDS and a Glanzmann's thrombasthenia defect. J Biol Chem. 1993;268:14586–9.
40. Pereira J, Alfaro G, Goycoolea M, Quiroga T, Ocqueteau M, Massardo L, et al. Circulating platelet-derived microparticles in systemic lupus erythematosus - association with increased thrombin generation and procoagulant state. Thromb Haemost. 2006;95:94–9.
41. Jy W, Horstman LL, Arce M, Ahn YS. Clinical-significance of platelet microparticles in autoimmune Thrombocytopenias. J Lab Clin Med. 1992;119:334–45.

18

Poor outcomes associated with antithrombotic undertreatment in patients with atrial fibrillation attending Gondar University Hospital: a retrospective cohort study

Eyob Alemayehu Gebreyohannes[*], Akshaya Srikanth Bhagavathula and Henok Getachew Tegegn

Abstract

Background: Atrial fibrillation (AF) is a major risk factor for stroke as it increases the incidence of stroke nearly fivefold. Antithrombotic treatment is recommended for the prevention of stroke in AF patients. However, majorly due to fear of risk of bleeding, adherence to recommendations is not observed. The aim of this study was to investigate the impact of antithrombotic undertreatment, on ischemic stroke and/or all-cause mortality in patients with AF.

Methods: A retrospective cohort study was conducted from January 7, 2017 to April 30 2017 using medical records of patients with AF attending Gondar University Hospital (GUH) between November 2012 and September 2016. Patients receiving appropriate antithrombotic management and those on undertreatment, were followed for development of ischemic stroke and/or all-cause mortality. Kaplan-Meier and a log-rank test was used to plot the survival analysis curve. Cox regression was used to determine the predictors of guideline-adherent antithrombotic therapy.

Results: The final analysis included 159 AF patients with a median age of 60 years. Of these, nearly two third (64.78%) of patients were receiving undertreatment for antithrombotic medications. Upon multivariate analysis, history of ischemic stroke/transient ischemic attack (TIA) was associated with lower incidence of antithrombotic undertreatment. A significant increase (HR: 8.194, 95% CI: 2.911–23.066)] in the incidence of ischemic stroke and/or all-cause mortality was observed in patients with undertreatment. Up-on multivariate analysis, only increased age was associated with a statistically significant increase incidence of ischemic stroke and/or all-cause mortality, while only history of ischemic stroke/TIA was associated with a decrease in the risk of ischemic stroke and/or all-cause mortality.

Conclusion: Adherence to antithrombotic guideline recommendations was found to be crucial in reducing the incidence of ischemic stroke and/or all-cause mortality in patients with AF without increasing the risk of bleeding. However, undertreatment to antithrombotic medications was found to be high (64.78%) and was associated with poorer outcomes in terms of ischemic stroke and/or all-cause mortality. Impact on practice: This research highlighted the magnitude of antithrombotic undertreatment and its impact on ischemic stroke and/or all-cause mortality in patients with AF. This article has to alert prescribers to routinely evaluate AF patients' risk for ischemic stroke and provide appropriate interventions based on guideline recommendations.

Keywords: Atrial fibrillation, Antithrombotic, Anticoagulant, Ischemic stroke, Ethiopia

* Correspondence: justeyob@gmail.com
Department of Clinical Pharmacy, University of Gondar, Gondar, Ethiopia

Background

Atrial fibrillation (AF) is one of the most common cardiovascular problems worldwide the prevalence of which has been increasing over the years with an estimated 33.5 million people affected globally [1, 2]. It is a major risk factor for stroke as it increases the incidence of stroke nearly fivefold. It nearly doubles the risk of mortality when compared to non-AF stroke and is associated with increased frequency and functional deficits secondary to ischemic stroke [3]. Its prevalence increases with older age; however, unlike other risk factors of stroke such as hypertension and coronary heart disease, the effect of AF on the risk of stroke doesn't weaken with advancing age [2, 4].

Earlier studies identified mitral stenosis (MS) as a high risk factor for arterial embolization in patients with AF [5–8] and such patients along with those having mechanical or bioprosthetic heart valves and mitral valve repair have been commonly referred to as having valvular AF [9]. In these patients, a significant reduction in the incidence of systemic embolization has been achieved with oral anticoagulants and withdrawal of anticoagulants has been associated with recurrence of thromboembolic events [6, 10, 11]. Thus, anticoagulation with vitamin K antagonists has been recommended for such patients. As a result these patients have since been generally excluded from studies that evaluated the outcomes of anticoagulation [12–21].

AF patients other than those having "valvular AF" are known to have non-valvular AF (NVAF). As stroke risk among NVAF patients vary, different stroke risk stratification tools including the $CHADS_2$ score have been used over the years and currently the CHA_2DS_2-VASc score is recommended [9, 22, 23]. NVAF patients can be stratified into low, intermediate, and high risk to stroke depending on whether their CHA_2DS_2-VASc scores are 0, 1, or ≥ 2, respectively. A similar categorization may be done using the $CHADS_2$ score, however, patients with a $CHADS_2$ score of 0 may not all be low risk when stratified using CHA_2DS_2-VASc score. Therefore, the CHA_2DS_2-VASc has an important advantage of identifying patients who are truly low risk [24].

Oral anticoagulation therapy is the standard management recommended for the prevention of stroke in AF patients with valvular-AF [9, 12] and high risk NVAF patients [9, 22, 23]. However, majorly due to fear of risk of bleeding, adherence to recommendations is not observed and underprescription is now a major barrier to effective anticoagulation. Hence, variability in practice and underutilization of antithrombotic agents as a result of non-adherence to guidelines recommendations can increase the risk of stroke, thromboembolic events, and death [2, 25–29].

The prevalence of cardiovascular diseases including AF in Ethiopia is on the rise. In 2014, cardiovascular diseases were estimated to account to 9% of total deaths in the country [30]. To the best of the authors' knowledge studies that assessed the impact of undertreatment with antithrombotic agents with AF patients on clinical outcomes are lacking. Therefore, we aimed to measure the adequacy of antithrombotic medication use and to investigate the impact of antithrombotic undertreatment, on ischemic stroke and/or all-cause mortality in patients with AF.

Methods

Study setting and period

The study was conducted from January 7, 2017 to April 30 2017 at Gondar University Hospital (GUH). GUH is a teaching and referral hospital located in the northwest Ethiopia 727 k meter from the capital Addis Ababa. The hospital gives service to estimated 7 million people. The medical inpatient ward comprises of 62 beds, 34 beds for males and 28 beds for females.

Study design

A census using retrospective cohort study was conducted using medical records of patients, 18 years and older, with AF attending the medical inpatient ward and chronic ambulatory clinic of GUH between November 2012 and September 2016. Patients' medical records were selected based on diagnosis of AF regardless of the presence or absence of other comorbid diseases. The CHA_2DS_2-VASc score [9, 31] was calculated to estimate the risk of stroke in patients with NVAF and classify patients into high, moderate, and low risk categories. This score was used to determine the appropriateness of antithrombotic agents. However, as anticoagulation is recommended for all patients with valvular AF, no score was calculated for these patients. Based on this, patients were classified into two groups: guideline adherent treatment vs undertreatment according to the "2016 European Society of Cardiology (ESC) Guidelines for the management of atrial Fibrillation" [9] and the "2014 2014 American Heart Association/American College of Cardiology (AHA/ACC) Guideline for the Management of Patients With Valvular Heart Disease" [12]. The two groups were then followed for occurrence ischemic stroke and/or all-cause mortality. Predictors of ischemic stroke and/or all-cause mortality will then be assessed.

Statistical analysis

Descriptive statistics were used to summarize sociodemographic and other baseline information. Categorical variables were expressed as frequencies (percentage) and quantitative variables as mean ± standard deviation or median + interquartile range (IQR)/range. Baseline intergroup comparisons were made using a X^2 test (or a Fisher's exact test if any expected cell count was < 5) and

Pearson's correlation. Patients in the two groups, i.e. those receiving appropriate antithrombotic management and those on undertreatment, were followed for development of clinical events (ischemic stroke and/or all-cause mortality). Kaplan-Meier and a log-rank test was used to plot the survival analysis curve. A stepwise cox hazard regression was used to determine the predictors of guideline-adherent antithrombotic therapy use including into the model all the candidate variables (variables with $p \leq 0.10$ in univariate, except those with a high number of missing data). A two-sided statistical tests at 5% level of significance was used. All of the analyses were performed using statistical package for social sciences (SPSS) version 20 (IBM Corp., Armonk, NY).

Definition of terms and operational definitions

NVAF: AF in the absence of rheumatic mitral stenosis, a mechanical or bioprosthetic heart valve, or mitral valve repair; *Paroxysmal AF: AF that terminates spontaneously or with intervention within 7 days of onset; Persistent AF:* Continuous AF that is sustained > 7 days; *Longstanding persistent AF:* Continuous AF > 12 months in duration; *Permanent AF:* The term *"permanent AF"* is used when the patient and clinician make a joint decision to stop further attempts to restore and/or maintain sinus rhythm; *Guideline adherent treatment*: prescribing OAC for patients with valvular AF; or prescribing OAC in NVAF patients with CHA2DS2-VASc score ≥ 2; or prescribing an antithrombotic medication (OAC or ASA) in NVAF patients with CHA2DS2-VASc score of 1; or not prescribing any antithrombotic medication in NVAF patients with a CHA2DS2-VASc score of 0; *undertreatment*: prescribing ASA only or not prescribing any antithrombotic medication at all in NVAF patients with CHA2DS2-VASc score ≥ 2;; or not prescribing any antithrombotic agent at all in NVAF patients with CHA2DS2-VASc score of 1; or prescribing ASA only or not prescribing any antithrombotic medication at all in patients with valvular AF.

Results

Patients' characteristics

The study identified a total of 231 patients with AF during the study period. Of these, 72 patients were excluded because either the diagnoses of AF were made once they had developed ischemic stroke with no further follow-up, were with incomplete records, or the medical records were lost from the medical record room. The final analysis included 159 patients with AF. The median (range) age of the patients was 60 (18–90) years with female majority (67.9%). All patients with valvular AF (*N* = 38) have rheumatic MS but none of them had mechanical or bioprosthetic heart valves, or mitral valve repair. On the other hand, patients with NVAF (*N* = 121) had a median CHA_2DS_2-VASc score of 3 (range = 0–9) [Fig. 1]. Of these patients, 2 (1.7%), 12 (9.9%), and 108

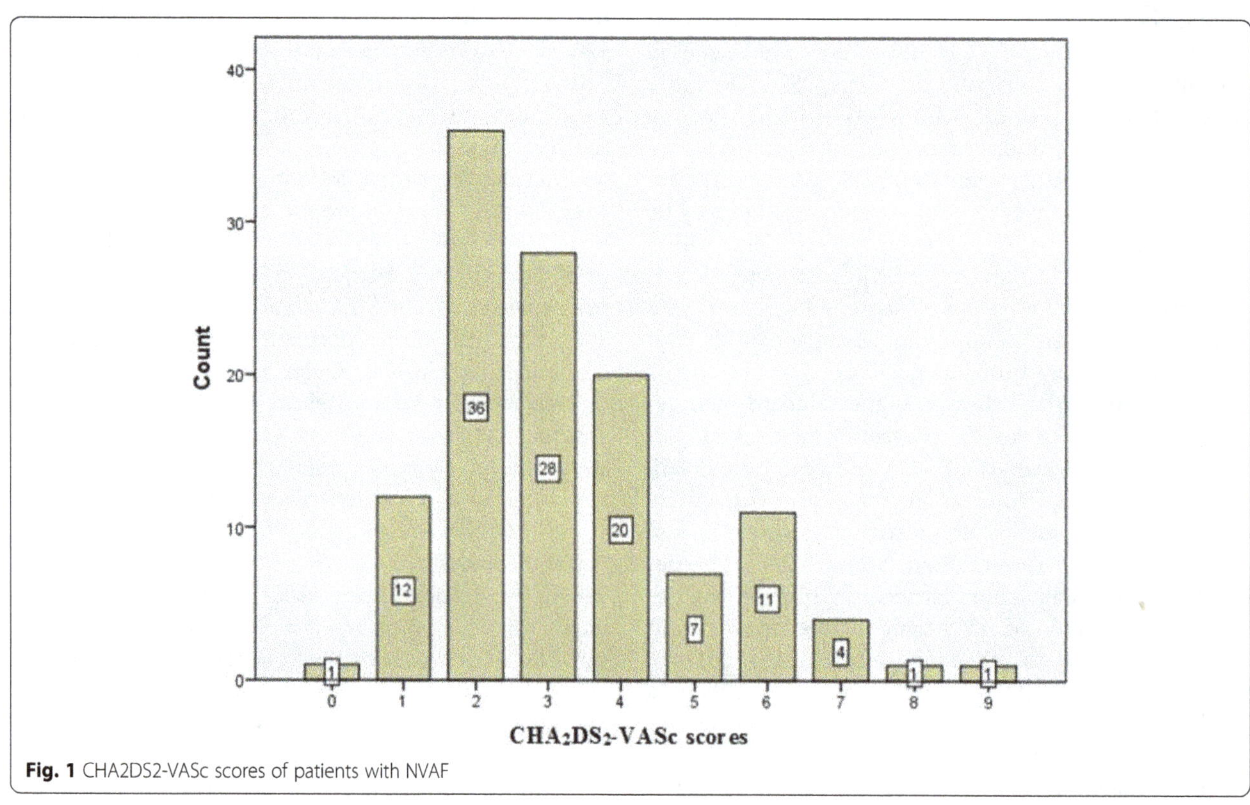

Fig. 1 CHA2DS2-VASc scores of patients with NVAF

(89.26%) patients were at low, intermediate, and high risk for the development of ischemic stroke, respectively. Ten (6.3%), 98 (61.6%), 51 (32.1%) patients were having paroxysmal, persistent, and longstanding persistent AF, respectively [Table 1]. For 117 (73.6%) patients, ECG documentation of AF was found.

Antithrombotic undertreatment/guideline-adherent treatment

One hundred forty five patients, 38 with valvular AF and 107 NVAF patients with CHA_2DS_2-VASc score of 2 or more, needed anticoagulation. Twelve of the patients with NVAF also needed at least antiplatelet agents (CHA_2DS_2-VASc score of 1). Of these, nearly two third (64.78%) of patients were receiving undertreatment for antithrombotic medications, while the rest were treated according to guideline recommendations. Proportion of antithrombotic undertreatment was higher in patients with NVAF (70.5%) when compared to patients with valvular AF (44.74%).

Compared with those treated according to guideline, patients with undertreatment were but less likely to have a history of ischemic stroke. The two groups have otherwise comparable baseline characteristics. HF and Hypertension were the two most common co-morbidities (Tables 1 and 2) while furosemide and digoxin were the two most commonly prescribed medications in these patients. Of the antithrombotic medications, aspirin ($N=66$) and warfarin ($N=53$) were most commonly utilized (Table 3).

Predictors of antithrombotic undertreatment in patients with AF

Valvular AF, older age, hypertension, history of stroke/TIA, higher serum creatinine, VHD, and medications such as atenolol and monthly benzathine penicillin were identified in a univariate analysis as factors that decrease in the incidence antithrombotic undertreatment. However, upon multivariate analysis, only history of ischemic stroke/TIA and prescription of atenolol and enalapril were associated with lower incidence of antithrombotic undertreatment (Table 4).

Survival analysis

The median duration of follow-up was 15.00 months for undertreatment group and 74.00 months for according to guideline treatment, respectively. During the follow-up period, a total of 52 (32.7%) patients developed ischemic stroke, 47 patients from the undertreatment group and 5 from the guideline-adherent group. Five cases of bleeding were reported but there was no statistically significant difference between the two groups

Table 1 Baseline characteristics of AF patients attending GUH, 2017 ($N=159$)

Variable	All patients $N=159$	Undertreatment $N=103$	According to guideline treatment $N=56$	*P*-value
Age in years				0.09
Mean ± SD	58.50 ± 19.082	62.175 ± 16.215	51.732 ± 22.057	
Median (range)	60 (18–90)	65 (18–89)	51 (18–90)	
IQR	30	18.75	41.75	
Sex				0.989
Males	51 (32.1%)	33 (32.04%)	18 (32.14%)	
Hemoglobin				
Mean ± SD	13.328 ± 2.019	13.226 ± 2.246	13.518 ± 1.574	0.384
Serum creatinine				
Median (IQR)	0.850 (0.32)	0.890 (0.42)	0.765 (0.34)	0.026
SGOT				
Median (IQR)	26.0 (26.95)	27.100 (24.50)	24.55 (38.75)	0.668
SGPT				
Median (IQR)	19.0 (24.3)	18.00 (22.55)	20.00 (33.53)	0.214
AF clinical type				0.003
Valvular AF	38 (23.9%)	17 (16.5%)	21 (37.5%)	
NVAF	121 (76.1%)	86 (83.5%)	35 (62.5%)	
AF pattern				
Paroxysmal	10 (6.3%)	10 (9.7%)	0 (0%)	
Persistent	98 (61.6%)	71 (68.9%)	27 (48.2%)	
Longstanding Persistent	51 (32.1%)	22 (21.4%)	29 (51.8%)	

Table 2 Co-morbidities in patients with AF attending GUH, 2017 ($N = 159$)

	All patients $N = 159$	Potential Undertreatment $N = 103$	According to guideline treatment $N = 56$	*P*-value
CHF	101 (63.5)	63 (61.2%)	38 (67.9%)	0.402
Hypertension	54 (34)	41 (39.8%)	13 (23.2%)	0.080
History of stroke/TIA	30 (18.9)	10 (9.7%)	20 (35.7%)	0.000
Vascular disease	36 (22.6)	21 (20.4%)	15 (26.8%)	0.357
DM	8 (5.0)	6 (5.8%)	2 (3.6%)	0.714
Anemia (Hemoglobin< 12/13)	33 (20.8)	22 (21.4%)	11 (19.64%)	0.799
IHD/ACS	14 (8.8)	10 (9.7%)	4 (7.1%)	0.772
Hyperthyroidism	22 (13.8)	16 (15.5%)	6 (10.7%)	0.400
Cardiomyopathy	5 (3.1)	3 (2.9%)	2 (3.6%)	1.000
Cardiomegaly	43 (27.0)	23 (22.3%)	20 (35.7%)	0.070
Increased LV wall thickness	5 (3.1)	1 (1.0%)	4 (7.1%)	0.052
LVH	18 (11.3)	12 (11.7%)	6 (10.7%)	0.859
LA enlargement	10 (6.3)	6 (5.8%)	4 (7.1%)	0.742
Liver disease (LFT > 3XULN)	11 (6.9%)	6 (5.8%)	5 (8.9%)	0.461
History of bleeding	5 (3.1%)	2 (1.9%)	3 (5.4%)	0.236

($p = 0.980$). Eight patients died during the follow-up period 7 of which were receiving undertreatment. Kaplan-Meier (log Rank test, $p = 0.000$) and Cox regression analyses (AHR: 8.194, 95% CI: 2.911–23.066) showed a significant increase in the incidence of ischemic stroke and/or all-cause mortality in patients with undertreatment [Fig. 2]. A sub-group analysis of patients with NVAF also revealed a similar result (AHR: 7.511, 95% CI: 2.295–24.580, $p = 0.001$).

Predictors of ischemic stroke and/or all-cause mortality in patients with AF

Up-on univariate analysis, cox proportional hazard regression revealed that NVAF, older age, hypertension were associated with higher risk of ischemic stroke and/or all-cause mortality. On the other hand, the presence of CHF, history of ischemic stroke/TIA, cardiomegaly, presence of any type of valvular disease, and use of medications such as ASA, warfarin,

Table 3 Commonly prescribed medications in patients with AF attending GUH, 2017 ($N = 159$)

	All patients $N = 159$	Potential Undertreatment $N = 103$	According to guideline treatment $N = 56$
ASA	66 (41.5%)	39 (37.9%)	27 (48.2%)
Warfarin	53 (33.3%)	1 (1.0%)	52 (92.9%)
Clopidogrel	5 (3.1%)	3 (2.9%)	2 (3.6%)
Digoxin	74 (46.5%)	43 (41.7%)	30 (53.6%)
Atenolol	58 (36.5%)	29 (28.2%)	29 (51.8%)
Metoprolol	17 (10.7%)	8 (7.8%)	9 (16.1%)
Carvedilol	2 (1.3%)	2 (1.9%)	0 (0%)
Propranolol	10 (6.3%)	8 (7.8%)	2 (3.6%)
Simvastatin	21 (13.2%)	12 (11.7%)	9 (16.1%)
Atorvastatin	20 (12.6%)	10 (9.7%)	10 (17.9%)
Captopril	1 (0.6%)	0 (0%)	1 (1.8%)
Enalapril	33 (20.8%)	17 (16.5%)	16 (28.6%)
Furosemide	89 (56.0%)	53 (51.5%)	36 (64.3%)
Spironolactone	72 (45.3%)	43 (41.7%)	29 (51.8%)
Hydrochlorothiazide	14 (8.8%)	9 (8.7%)	5 (8.9%)
Nifedipine/amlodipine	3 (1.9%)	2 (1.9%)	1 (1.8%)
Monthly benzathine penicillin	17 (10.7%)	3 (2.9%)	14 (25.0%)
PTU	19 (11.9%)	12 (11.7%)	7 (12.5%)

Table 4 Predictors of antithrombotic undertreatment among AF patients attending GUH, 2017 ($N = 159$)

Variables		COR (95% CI)	p-value	AOR (95% CI)	*p*-value
Clinical type	Valvular AF	0.329 (0.156–0.698)	0.004	1.116 (0.285–4.367)	0.875
Age	in years	1.030 (1.011–1.048)	0.001	1.009 (0.979–1.040)	0.575
Hypertension	Yes	2.187 (1.049–4.562)	0.037	2.849 (0.926–8.770)	0.068
History of stroke/TIA	Yes	0.194 (0.083–0.453)	0.000	0.054 (0.017–0.175)	0.000
Serum creatinine	mg/dL	3.328 (1.135–9.753)	0.028	1.901 (0.582–6.208)	0.287
Cardiomegaly	Yes	0.518 (0.253–1.060)	0.072	0.657 (0.239–1.807)	0.416
Increased LV wall thickness	Yes	0.127 (0.014–1.170)	0.069	0.135 (0.003–5.344)	0.286
ECG documentation	Yes	0.507 (0.230–1.121)	0.093	0.351 (0.120–1.029)	0.056
VHD	Yes	0.377 (0.188–0.757)	0.006	0.392 (0.149–1.036)	0.059
Atenolol	Yes	0.365 (0.185–0.718)	0.004	0.362 (0.144–0.910)	0.031
Enalapril	Yes	0.494 (0.227–1.077)	0.076	0.317 (0.107–0.942)	0.039
Monthly benzathine penicillin	Yes	0.090 (0.025–0.330)	0.000	0.186 (0.030–1.167)	0.073

digoxin, atenolol, enalapril, furosemide and spironolactone were associated with a decrease in the risk of ischemic stroke and/or all-cause mortality. However, up-on multivariate analysis, only increased age was associated with a modest but statistically significant increase risk for ischemic stroke and/or all-cause mortality (AHR: 1.035, 95% CI = 1.004–1.067), while only history of ischemic stroke/TIA was associated with a decrease in the risk of ischemic stroke and/or all-cause mortality (AHR: 0.038, 95% CI: 0.002–0.596) (Table 5).

Discussion

This retrospective analysis of medical records of AF patients assessed adequacy of antithrombotic treatment using 2016 ESC [7] and 2014 AHA/ACC [8] guidelines to evaluate outcomes of undertreatment. The findings of this study showed that adherence to guideline recommendations was associated with significantly better outcomes. Incidence of the primary endpoint (ischemic stroke and/or all-cause mortality) was increased by more than eight-folds (AHR: 8.194, 95% CI: 2.911–23.066) in patients with antithrombotic undertreatment.

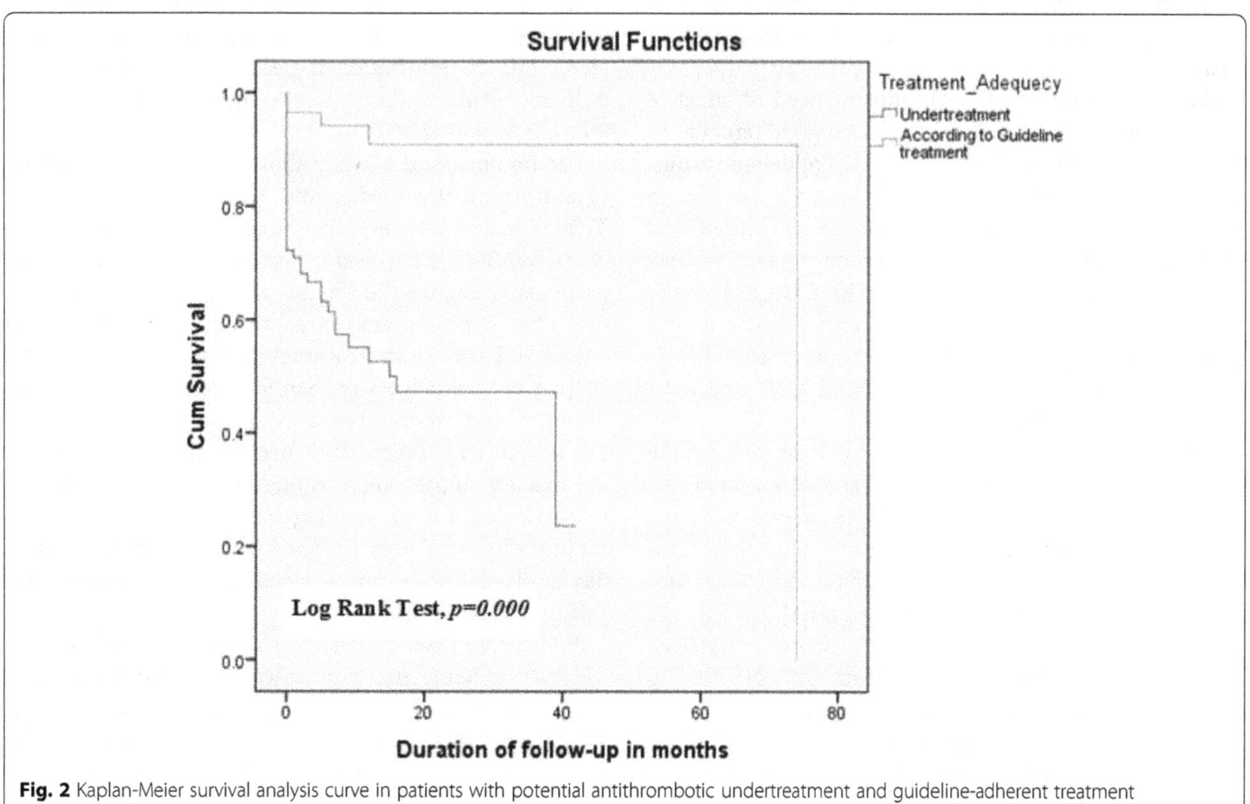

Fig. 2 Kaplan-Meier survival analysis curve in patients with potential antithrombotic undertreatment and guideline-adherent treatment

Table 5 Predictors of ischemic stroke and/or all-cause mortality in patients with AF attending GUH, 2017 ($N = 159$)

Variables		CHR (95% CI)	*p*-value	AHR (95% CI)	*p*-value
Clinical type	NVAF	3.374 (1.321–8.614)	0.011	0.784 (0.194–3.167)	0.733
Age	in years	1.039 (1.019–1.060)	0.000	1.035 (1.004–1.067)	0.029
CHF	Yes	0.223 (0.119–0.416)	0.000	0.347 (0.105–1.141)	0.081
Hypertension	Yes	1.970 (1.097–3.536)	0.023	1.117 (0.410–3.042)	0.828
History of stroke/TIA	Yes	0.371 (0.133–1.036)	0.058	0.038 (0.002–0.596)	0.020
Cardiomegaly	Yes	0.484 (0.225–1.040)	0.063	0.843 (0.316–2.244)	0.732
LVEF	in %	1.033 (1.006–1.061)	0.017	1.051 (0.998–1.106)	0.059
Any type of Valvular disease	Yes	0.429 (0.234–0.788)	0.006	1.757 (0.660–4.679)	0.259
AF pattern					
Paroxysmal		–	–	–	–
Persistent		0.361 (0.158–0.826)	0.016	1.293 (0.287–5.830)	0.738
Longstanding persistent		0.016 (0.003–0.074)	0.000	0.002 (0.000–1.875)	0.075
ASA	Yes	0.443 (0.231–0.850)	0.014	1.179 (0.256–5.426)	0.832
Warfarin	Yes	0.099 (0.030–0.320)	0.000	0.294 (0.033–2.642)	0.275
Digoxin	Yes	0.300 (0.151–0.597)	0.001	1.259 (0.678–2.337)	0.465
Atenolol	Yes	0.146 (0.057–0.373)	0.000	0.139 (0.017–1.125)	0.064
Enalapril	Yes	0.364 (0.143–0.926)	0.034	1.395 (0.087–22.248)	0.814
Furosemide	Yes	0.201 (0.101–0.397)	0.000	0.416 (0.057–3.008)	0.385
Spironolactone	Yes	0.149 (0.063–0.354)	0.000	0.121 (0.013–1.134)	0.064

A statistically significant ($p = 0.000$) difference in the duration of follow-up between patients with guideline-adherent treatment (median: 74 months) and undertreatment (median: 15 months) was also observed up-on Kaplan-Meier analysis.

These observations stress the urgent need of effective antithrombotic treatment by practicing adherence to 2016 ESC [7] and 2014 AHA/ACC [8] guideline recommendations. Prevention of ischemic stroke should be an integral part in the management of patients with AF and clinicians should routinely evaluate their patients for risk of ischemic stroke. NVAF patients with CHA_2DS_2-VASc score of 2 or more and all patients with valvular AF are particularly at high risk for the development of ischemic stroke and as such should be provided with oral anticoagulant medications.

Earlier studies identified a substantial increase in the incidence of ischemic stroke in patients with valvular AF that was shown to be significantly decreased with the use of oral anticoagulants, particularly vitamin k antagonists, and recurrence of thromboembolic events was observed upon withdrawal of anticoagulants [5, 8, 10, 11]. On the other hand, CHA_2DS_2-VASc score has proven useful in the management of patients with NVAF. Lip et al. reported that guideline non-adherence was associated with an increase in the incidence of ischemic stroke and thromboembolic events (AHR: 1.679, 95% CI: 1.202–2.347) [32] in patients with NVAF. Similarly, the CHA_2DS_2-VASc score was also found very important in the current study stratifying patients with NVAF into different risk categories. Accordingly, non-adherence to antithrombotic guideline recommendations was associated with an enormous increase in the incidence of ischemic stroke and/or all-cause mortality (AHR: 7.511, 95% CI: 2.295–24.580).

The findings of this study showed that undertreatment of antithrombotic medications was very high (64.78%). This was much higher than that was reported by Lip et al. (17.3%) [32]. Proportion of undertreatment was particularly higher (70.5%) in patients with NVAF. On the other hand, Basaran et al. reported a 30.5% rate of antithrombotic undertreatment in patients with NVAF [33] which is much lower than the present study. Fear of bleeding and underestimation of the benefit of antithrombotic treatment have been mentioned as major reasons for antithrombotic undertreatment [9, 30, 34]. In particular, fear of bleeding might be the main reason for the observed high proportion of undertreatment in our study; however, our study didn't assess reasons for this undertreatment.

Predictors of ischemic stroke and/or all-cause mortality and guideline non-adherence were also assessed in this study. On a multivariate analysis, only older age was associated with a statistically significant increase in the incidence of ischemic stroke and/or all-cause mortality upon cox regression [AHR (95% CI): 1.035 (1.004–

1.067), $p = 0.029$]. In other studies, history of ischemic stroke, older age, vascular disease, diabetes, female gender, and hypertension were identified as predictors of ischemic stroke and/or thromboembolic events on multivariate analyses [28, 35]. Similar to the Firberg et al. study [35], heart failure and thyroid disease were not identified as predictors of ischemic stroke and/or all-cause mortality in the present study. Older age, female sex, first detected and paroxysmal AF have been identified as predictors of poor adherence to guidelines in other studies [28, 32, 36]. However, none of these factors were identified as predictors of adherence to guideline recommendations in the present study. On the other hand, history of ischemic stroke/TIA was associated with at lower incidence of ischemic stroke in the present study. This might be explained by the fact that, physicians' tendency to prescribe antithrombotic medications once patients develop ischemic stroke/TIA with thinking the risk of developing ischemic stroke outweighs any potential adverse event especially the risk of bleeding. This justification was supported by the fact that history of stroke/TIA was associated with lower incidence of undertreatment in our study. Mochalina et al. also identified history of ischemic stroke as a factor that increase the odds of oral anticoagulant prescription in patients with NVAF [28]. He also reported that oral anticoagulant use didn't strictly follow stroke risk assessment as only three (history of ischemic stroke, hypertension, and older age) of the seven risk factors in the CHA_2DS_2-VASc score were associated with increased odds of oral anticoagulant medication use. In the present study, in addition to history of ischemic stroke, use of medications such as atenolol [AHR (95% CI): 0.362 (0.144–0.910), $p = 0.031$] and enalapril [AHR (95% CI): 0.317 (0.107–0.942), $p = 0.039$] was also associated with better guideline adherence.

Five patients (3.14%) experienced bleeding. Of these, one patient experienced GIB while on ASA. Four patients experienced epistaxis and/or blood in sputum of which 3 patients were receiving both ASA and warfarin while the remaining patient was receiving ASA. 5.03% ($N = 8$) of the study participants died. Of these, 1 patient was with valvular AF while the remaining 7 patients were with NVAF. This gave us an all-cause mortality rate of 5.79% in patients with NVAF.

In our study, warfarin was the only oral anticoagulant used by any of the patients. A number of novel oral anticoagulants are now currently in use world-wide. Several studies that compared these medications indicated that this medications have at least comparable efficacy with more or less similar, if not better, safety profile in terms of bleeding and mortality particularly in patients with NVAF [37–39]. In addition, they showed better persistence than warfarin [40]. These advantages makes the novel oral anticoagulants alternatives to these patients especially those with NVAF as they haven't extensively studied in patients with valvular AF. These medications were also suggested to be cost-effective in terms of life-years gained and quality-adjusted life years in developed countries [41, 42], however, this might not be the case in developing countries like Ethiopia as the cost-effectiveness studies were based on willingness to pay which definitely will not be the same depending on the income status of the countries.

Study limitations

Though the study clearly assessed adequacy of antithrombotic treatment and outcomes of undertreatment, it is not without limitations. The sample size was small which may obscure the impact of some predictors that would have been evident with a larger sample size. It was a retrospective study design and suffered from incompleteness and even loss of patients' medical records. The study also didn't assess the bleeding risk of patients. Therefore, interpretation of the results of these study should be in light of these limitations.

Conclusion

Adherence to 2016 ESC and 2014 AHA/ACC antithrombotic guideline recommendations was found to be crucial in reducing the incidence of ischemic stroke and/or all-cause mortality in patients with AF without increasing the risk of bleeding. However, undertreatment to antithrombotic medications was found to be high and was associated with poorer outcomes in terms of composite end points of thromboembolic events and/or. Even if increased age was associated with a statistically significant increase risk for ischemic stroke and/or all-cause mortality, it was very modest. On the other hand, a tendency to prescribe antithrombotic medications in AF patients with a history of ischemic stroke/TIA was observed and was associated with a decrease in the risk of composite end points of stroke and/or mortality as well as undertreatment.

Abbreviations

ACC: American College of Cardiology; ACS: Acute Coronary Syndrome; AF: Atrial Fibrillation; AHA: American Heart Association; ASA: Aspirin; DM: Diabetes Mellitus; ESC: European Society of Cardiology; GUH: Gondar University Hospital; HF: Heart Failure; HR: Hazard Ratio; IHD: Ischemic Heart Disease; IQR: Interquartile Range; LA: Left Atrium; LVEF: Left Ventricular Ejection Fraction; LVH: Left Ventricular Hypertrophy; MS: Mitral Stenosis; NVAF: Non-valvular Atrial Fibrillation; OAC: Oral Anticoagulant; OR: Odds Ratio; SD: Standard Deviation; SPSS: Statistical Package for Social Sciences; TIA: Transient Ischemic Attack; ULN: Upper Limit of the Normal; VHD: Valvular Heart Disease

Acknowledgements

We would like to acknowledge staffs from medical records departments for their support in organizing and searching patients' medical charts. We also would like to thank the University of Gondar and the Gondar University Hospital for their permission and support in conducting this study.

Ethics approval and consent for participation

A proposal was submitted to the department of clinical pharmacy. After getting acceptance from the department of clinical pharmacy, ethical clearance was obtained from the ethical clearance committee of school of pharmacy, college of medicine and health sciences (CMHS), University of Gondar (UOG). Permission to access the medical records of patients was then obtained from GUH clinical directorate. Confidentiality of the information regarding patients was ensured in such a way that the data will only be used for the study purpose only. Moreover, the information obtained from the patients' medical records is presented only in collective manner. As the study participants were not directly involved in the study, informed consent was not sought from them.

Funding

No funding source.

Authors' contributions

EAG conceived the study, designed the study protocol, collected, entered, analyzed, and interpreted the data, conducted literature review, and drafted the final manuscript. HGT reviewed the study protocol, supervised the study, and conducted literature review. ASB reviewed the study protocol and conducted literature review. All authors read and approved the final manuscript.

Competing interests

The authors declare that they have no competing interests.

References

1. Chugh SS, Havmoeller R, Narayanan K, Singh D, Rienstra M, Benjamin EJ, et al. Worldwide epidemiology of atrial fibrillation: a Global Burden of Disease 2010 Study. Circulation. 2013;CirculationAHA:113.005119.
2. Lin AH, Oakley LS, Phan HL, Shutt BJ, Birgersdotter-Green U, Francisco GM. Prevalence of stroke and the need for thromboprophylaxis in young patients with atrial fibrillation: a cohort study. J Cardiovasc Med. 2014;15(3):189–93.
3. Lin HJ, Wolf PA, Kelly-Hayes M, Beiser AS, Kase CS, Benjamin EJ, D'agostino RB. Stroke severity in atrial fibrillation. Stroke. 1996;27(10):1760–4.
4. Wolf PA, Abbott RD, Kannel WB. Atrial fibrillation as an independent risk factor for stroke: the Framingham study. Stroke. 1991;22(8):983–8.
5. Olesen KH. The natural history of 271 patients with mitral stenosis under medical treatment. Br Heart J. 1962;24(3):349.
6. Szekely P. Systemic embolism and anticoagulant prophylaxis in rheumatic heart disease. Br Med J. 1964;1(5392):1209.
7. Coulshed N, Epstein EJ, McKendrick CS, Galloway RW, Walker E. Systemic embolism in mitral valve disease. Br Heart J. 1970;32(1):26.
8. Casella L, Abelmann WH, Ellis LB. Patients with mitral stenosis and systemic emboli: hemodynamic and clinical observations. Arch Intern Med. 1964;114(6):773–81.
9. Kirchhof P, Benussi S, Kotecha D, Ahlsson A, Atar D, Casadei B, Castella M, Diener HC, Heidbuchel H, Hendriks J, Hindricks G. 2016 ESC Guidelines for the management of atrial fibrillation developed in collaboration with EACTS. Eur Heart J. 2016;37(38):2893–962.
10. Pérez-Gómez F, Salvador A, Zumalde J, Iriarte JA, Berjón J, Alegría E, Almería C, Bover R, Herrera D, Fernández C. Effect of antithrombotic therapy in patients with mitral stenosis and atrial fibrillation: a sub-analysis of NASPEAF randomized trial. Eur Heart J. 2006;27(8):960–7.
11. Wood JC, Conn HL. Prevention of systemic arterial embolism in chronic rheumatic heart disease by means of protracted anticoagulant therapy. Circulation. 1954;10(4):517–23.
12. Nishimura RA, Otto CM, Bonow RO, Carabello BA, Erwin JP, Guyton RA, O'Gara PT, Ruiz CE, Skubas NJ, Sorajja P, Sundt TM. 2014 AHA/ACC guideline for the management of patients with valvular heart disease: a report of the American College of Cardiology/American Heart Association Task Force on Practice Guidelines. J Am College Cardiol. 2014;63(22):e57–185.
13. Leef G, Qin D, Althouse A, Alam MB, Rattan R, Munir MB, Patel D, Khattak F, Vaghasia N, Adelstein E, Jain SK. Risk of stroke and death in atrial fibrillation by type of anticoagulation: a propensity-matched analysis. Pacing Clin Electrophysiol. 2015;38(11):1310–6.
14. Ezekowitz MD, Nagarakanti R, Noack H, Brueckmann M, Litherland C, Jacobs M, Clemens A, Reilly PA, Connolly SJ, Yusuf S, Wallentin L. Comparison of Dabigatran and warfarin in patients with atrial fibrillation and Valvular heart DiseaseClinical perspective. Circulation. 2016;134(8):589–98.
15. Halperin JL, Hankey GJ, Wojdyla DM, et al. Efficacy and safety of rivaroxaban compared with warfarin among elderly patients with nonvalvular atrial fibrillation in the Rivaroxaban Once Daily, Oral, Direct Factor Xa Inhibition Compared With Vitamin K Antagonism for Prevention of Stroke and Embolism Trial in Atrial Fibrillation (ROCKET AF). Circulation 2014;130:138–46.
16. Executive Steering Committee, ROCKET AF study investigators. Rivaroxaban—once daily, oral, direct factor Xa inhibition compared with vitamin K antagonism for prevention of stroke and embolism trial in atrial fibrillation: rationale and design of the ROCKET AF study. Am Heart J. 2010;159(3):340–7.
17. Hori M, Matsumoto M, Tanahashi N, Momomura SI, Uchiyama S, Goto S, Izumi T, Koretsune Y, Kajikawa M, Kato M, Ueda H. Rivaroxaban versus warfarin in Japanese patients with Nonvalvular atrial fibrillation in relation to the CHADS 2 score: a subgroup analysis of the J-ROCKET AF trial. J Stroke Cerebrovasc Dis. 2014;23(2):379–83.
18. Sherwood MW, Douketis JD, Patel MR, Piccini JP, Hellkamp AS, Lokhnygina Y, Spyropoulos AC, Hankey GJ, Singer DE, Nessel CC, Mahaffey KW, Fox KA, Califf RM, Becker RC, on behalf of the RAFI. Outcomes of Temporary Interruption of Rivaroxaban Compared with Warfarin in Patients with Nonvalvular Atrial Fibrillation: Results from ROCKET AF. Circulation. 2014;129:1850–9.
19. Lip GY, Halperin JL, Petersen P, Rodgers GM, Pall D, Renfurm RW. A phase II, double-blind, randomized, parallel group, dose-finding study of the safety and tolerability of darexaban compared with warfarin in patients with non-valvular atrial fibrillation: the oral factor Xa inhibitor for prophylaxis of stroke in atrial fibrillation study 2 (OPAL-2). J Thromb Haemost. 2015;13(8):1405–13.
20. Mao L, Li C, Li T, Yuan K. Prevention of stroke and systemic embolism with rivaroxaban compared with warfarin in Chinese patients with atrial fibrillation. Vascular. 2014;22(4):252–8.
21. Avezum A, Lopes RD, Schulte PJ, Lanas F, Gersh BJ, Hanna M, Pais P, Erol C, Diaz R, Bahit MC, Bartunek J. Apixaban compared with warfarin in patients with atrial fibrillation and valvular heart disease: findings from the ARISTOTLE trial. Circulation. 2015:CirculationAHA-114.
22. January CT, Wann LS, Alpert JS, Calkins H, Cigarroa JE, Conti JB, et al. 2014 AHA/ACC/HRS guideline for the management of patients with atrial fibrillation: executive summary: a report of the American College of Cardiology/American Heart Association task force on practice guidelines and the Heart Rhythm Society. J Am Coll Cardiol. 2014;64(21):2246–80.
23. Xiong Q, Chen S, Senoo K, Proietti M, Hong K, Lip GY. The CHADS 2 and CHA 2 DS 2-VASc scores for predicting ischemic stroke among east Asian patients with atrial fibrillation: a systemic review and meta-analysis. Int J Cardiol. 2015;195:237–42.
24. Chen J-Y, Zhang A-D, Lu H-Y, Guo J, Wang F-F, Li Z-C. CHADS2 versus CHA2DS2-VASc score in assessing the stroke and thromboembolism risk stratification in patients with atrial fibrillation: a systematic review and meta-analysis. J Geriatr Cardiol. 2013;10(3):258–66.
25. Gross CP, Vogel EW, Dhond AJ, Marple CB, Edwards RA, Hauch O, et al. Factors influencing physicians' reported use of anticoagulation therapy in nonvalvular atrial fibrillation: a cross-sectional survey. Clin Ther. 2003;25(6):1750–64.
26. Vallakati A, Lewis WR. Underuse of anticoagulation in patients with atrial fibrillation. Postgrad Med. 2016;128(2):191–200.
27. Kakkar AK, Mueller I, Bassand J-P, Fitzmaurice DA, Goldhaber SZ, Goto S, et al. Risk profiles and antithrombotic treatment of patients newly diagnosed with atrial fibrillation at risk of stroke: perspectives from the international, observational, prospective GARFIELD registry. PLoS One. 2013;8(5):e63479.
28. Mochalina N, Jöud A, Carlsson M, Sandberg ME, Själander A, Juhlin T, Svensson PJ. Antithrombotic therapy in patients with non-valvular atrial fibrillation in southern Sweden: a population-based cohort study. Thromb Res. 2016;140:94–9.
29. Potter BJ, Andò G, Cimmino G, Ladeiras-Lopes R, Frikah Z, et al. Time trends in antithrombotic management of patients with atrial fibrillation treated with coronary stents: results from TALENT-AF (the internAtionaL stENT – atrial fibrillation study) multicenter registry. Clin Cardiol. 2018;41(4):470–5.
30. Riley L, Cowan M. Noncommunicable diseases country profiles 2014. Geneva: World Health Organization; 2014.

31. Lip GY, Nieuwlaat R, Pisters R, Lane DA, Crijns HJ. Refining clinical risk stratification for predicting stroke and thromboembolism in atrial fibrillation using a novel risk factor-based approach: the euro heart survey on atrial fibrillation. Chest Journal. 2010;137(2):263–72.
32. Lip GY, Laroche C, Popescu MI, Rasmussen LH, Vitali-Serdoz L, Dan GA, Kalarus Z, Crijns HJ, Oliveira MM, Tavazzi L, Maggioni AP. Improved outcomes with European Society of Cardiology guideline-adherent antithrombotic treatment in high-risk patients with atrial fibrillation: a report from the EORP-AF general pilot registry. Europace. 2015 Dec 1; 17(12):1777–86.
33. Başaran Ö, Dogan V, Biteker M, Karadeniz FÖ, Tekkesin Aİ, Çakıllı Y, Türkkan C, Hamidi M, Demir V, Gürsoy MO, Öztürk MT. Guideline-adherent therapy for stroke prevention in atrial fibrillation in different health care settings: results from RAMSES study. Eur J Intern Med. 2017;40:50–5.
34. Merli G, Weitz HH. The decision to anticoagulate: assessing whether benefits outweigh the risks for patients with atrial fibrillation. Clin Cardiol. 2004 Jun 1;27(6):313–20.
35. Friberg L, Rosenqvist M, Lip GY. Evaluation of risk stratification schemes for ischaemic stroke and bleeding in 182 678 patients with atrial fibrillation: the Swedish atrial fibrillation cohort study. Eur Heart J. 2012 Jun 1;33(12):1500–10.
36. Tulner LR, Van Campen JP, Kuper IM, Gijsen GJ, Koks CH, Mac Gillavry MR, van Tinteren H, Beijnen JH, Brandjes DP. Reasons for undertreatment with oral anticoagulants in frail geriatric outpatients with atrial fibrillation. Drugs Aging. 2010 Jan 1;27(1):39–50.
37. Romanelli RJ, Nolting L, Dolginsky M, Kym E, Orrico KB. Dabigatran versus warfarin for atrial fibrillation in real-world clinical practice. Circulation. 2016; 9(2):126–34.
38. Aslan O, Yaylali YT, Yildirim S, Yurtdas M, Senol H, Ugur-Yildiz M, Ozdemir M. Dabigatran versus warfarin in atrial fibrillation: multicenter experience in Turkey. Clin Appl Thromb Hemost. 2016;22(2):147–52.
39. Uchiyama S, Hori M, Matsumoto M, Tanahashi N, Momomura SI, Goto S, Izumi T, Koretsune Y, Kajikawa M, Kato M, Ueda H. Net clinical benefit of rivaroxaban versus warfarin in Japanese patients with nonvalvular atrial fibrillation: a subgroup analysis of J-ROCKET AF. J Stroke Cerebrovasc Dis. 2014;23(5):1142–7.
40. Zalesak M, Siu K, Francis K, Yu C, Alvrtsyan H, Rao Y, Walker D, Sander S, Miyasato G, Matchar D, Sanchez H. Higher persistence in newly diagnosed nonvalvular atrial fibrillation patients treated with dabigatran versus warfarin. Circ Cardiovasc Qual Outcomes. 2013;6(5):567–74.
41. Ademi Z, Pasupathi K, Liew D. Cost-effectiveness of apixaban compared to warfarin in the management of atrial fibrillation in Australia. Eur J Prev Cardiol. 2015;22(3):344–53.
42. Lanitis T, Kongnakorn T, Jacobson L, De Geer A. Cost-effectiveness of apixaban versus warfarin and aspirin in Sweden for stroke prevention in patients with atrial fibrillation. Thromb Res. 2014;134(2):278–87.

19

NOACs replace VKA as preferred oral anticoagulant among new patients: a drug utilization study in 560 pharmacies in The Netherlands

J. M. van den Heuvel[1,2], A. M. Hövels[1], H. R. Büller[3], A. K. Mantel-Teeuwisse[1], A. de Boer[1] and A. H. Maitland-van der Zee[1,2*]

Abstract

Background: In 2012, around 400.000 patients in the Netherlands were treated with Vitamin K Antagonists (VKA) for thromboembolic diseases. Since 2011, non-VKA oral anticoagulants (NOACs) are available. NOACs do not require frequent INR monitoring which benefits patients, but also imposes a risk of reduced therapy adherence. The objective of this study is to describe uptake and patient adherence of NOACs in The Netherlands until October 2016.

Methods: Prescription data for 247.927 patients across 560 pharmacies were used to describe patient profiles, uptake of NOACs among new naive patients and switch between VKA and NOACs, and calculate therapy adherence as the Proportion of Days Covered (PDC).

Results: During the studied period the share of NOACs in oral anticoagulants has grown to 57% of prescriptions to new patients. More than 70% of new NOAC users were new naive patients and around 26% switched from VKA. The overall share of NOACs among starters is largest in the group of patients of 50-80 years. Calculated compliance rate for NOAC patients shows that 88% of all users are adherent with a PDC higher than 80%.

Conclusions: NOAC have overtaken VKA as the major treatment prescribed to new oral anticoagulant patients, and the number of starters on VKA is decreasing. Patients are generally adherent to NOACs during the implementation phase, the period that the medication is used. Fear for inadherence by itself does not need to be a reason for not prescribing NOACs instead of VKA.

Background

Oral anticoagulants (OAC) are used to prevent and treat a range of thromboembolic diseases. The main indications for oral anticoagulants are atrial fibrillation (AF), venous thromboembolism (VTE) (comprising of deep vein thrombosis (DVT), pulmonary embolism (PE)) and mechanical heart valves [1–3] and for the prevention of thromboembolism after hip or knee replacement surgery [4]. The oral anticoagulants that are currently available in The Netherlands include the vitamin K antagonists (VKA) acenocoumarol and phenprocoumon and the newer oral anticoagulants (dabigatran, rivaroxaban, apixaban, and edoxaban), also called direct oral anticoagulants (DOACs) or non-VKA oral anticoagulants (NOACs) [5]. One NOAC (rivaroxaban) is also registered to be prescribed in triple therapy after acute coronary syndrome (ACS) [5].

In 2012, nearly 400,000 people in the Netherlands were treated with Vitamin K antagonists (VKAs) [4]. VKAs have a small therapeutic window. Treating patients with VKAs requires titration of the dose, and the required dosage can differ largely among patients [6, 7]. If the dose is too low, clots may form in the bloodstream and if the dose is too high, hemorrhages can occur [4].

* Correspondence: a.h.maitland@amc.uva.nl
[1]Utrecht Institute for Pharmaceutical Sciences (UIPS), Division of Pharmacoepidemiology and Clinical Pharmacology, Utrecht University, Utrecht, The Netherlands
[2]Department of Respiratory Medicine, Academic Medical Center, University of Amsterdam, Amsterdam, The Netherlands
Full list of author information is available at the end of the article

For this reason International Normalized Ratio (INR) must be frequently monitored to adjust the dose if necessary. For this intensive supervision, a system of Thrombosis Services exists in the Netherlands [4].

Recently, NOACs have proven to be an effective and safe alternative to VKA for prevention of stroke and systemic embolism in patients with AF and patients with VTE [6, 7]. Compared to VKAs, NOACs offer simplification of long-term anticoagulation therapy because they do not require frequent INR monitoring and less frequent dose adjustments. However, also NOACs may require dose adjustments according to age, body weight, renal function and concomitant use of glycoprotein inhibitors [8]. Absence of frequent monitoring may lead to an increased risk of undetected reduced therapy adherence, with potentially severe consequences [6].

Up until now, it is not known what the uptake of NOACs in the Netherlands is. The aim of the present study is therefore to describe uptake and patient adherence of the NOACs dabigatran, rivaroxaban, apixaban and edoxaban in The Netherlands between July 2011 and October 2016, based on pharmacy prescription data.

The following research questions are addressed: how many patients are treated with oral anticoagulants, and what is the percentage that receives NOACs? How many patients are newly initiated on NOACs? What is the impact of the introduction of NOACs on the usage of VKA? Are there patients already treated with VKA that switch to using NOACs? Are there differences in characteristics between patients that use VKA and patients that use NOACs? Finally, are patients therapy adherent during the period in which they are treated with a NOAC?

Methods

Data collection and study population

For this study, data from the NControl database were obtained. Our dataset contains data of 544 pharmacies, spread across The Netherlands with data for the complete study period. The total number of public pharmacies in The Netherlands is approximately 1900. Since 2011, the NControl database contains data related to over 557 million prescriptions and 7.2 million patients.

The database contains (not exhaustive) the following information about the prescriptions, the dispensed medication and quantity, dispensing date, prescribed daily dosage, prescriber type and the patient's age and gender. Patients in the database cannot be identified, but can be tracked over time across pharmacies in the database. Prescribers are anonymized and cannot be identified nor tracked over time. NControl is allowed to use these prescription data for research purposes. NControl adheres to data protection and privacy regulations, as established in amongst others the Personal Data Protection Act in The Netherlands as well as the Netherlands Norm (NEN) 7510 standard, related to information protection in healthcare, which is derived from International Organisation for Standardization (ISO) norm 27,001 and 27,002. Because most patients in The Netherlands are registered with a single community pharmacy, dispension records in the Ncontrol database contain a (virtually) complete view of patient history of prescription drugs [9].

All patients who received at least one prescription for VKAs or NOACs between 1 July 2011 and 30 September 2016 were included in the study.

Data analysis

We analysed the uptake of NOACs versus VKAs by measuring the number of prescriptions per month. The proportions of NOACs and VKAs in the total amount of prescribed anticoagulants and the proportion prescribed to new naive patients were calculated separately. A naive starter was defined as a patient who received a first prescription for an OAC, and had a history of other medications in the NControl database for at least 1 year before this OAC initiation. Any other first OAC prescription has been excluded from the analyses of new naive patients.

A patient who did not receive an OAC for 365 days or more, is labelled a stopper. We took 365 days to limit misclassification of inadherent patients or patients that missed a prescription at the public pharmacy e.g. because of hospitalization as a stopper.

For any patient a switch was defined as a first prescription for an OAC in a particular anatomical, therapeutical and chemical (ATC) medication cluster that was preceded by an anticoagulant drug from another ATC cluster. There are four switching categories: switch from VKA to NOAC, from NOAC to VKA, between VKAs and between NOACs.

We analyzed if prescribers of NOACs targeted specific patient groups in terms of age, gender and number of co-medications used. This number was used as a proxy for a patient's general health status.

Therapy adherence consists of three phases: initiation, implementation and discontinuation [10]. We specifically looked that therapy adherence during treatment with NOACs, i.e. the implementation phase. For this reason we calculated adherence as the Proportion of Days Covered (PDC) [11, 12]. In literature, more than one definition for PDC can be found [11–15]. Our definition of PDC can also be referred to as Compliance Ratio (CR) [13, 14]. This metric is calculated through the following formula:

$$PDC = \frac{100\% * \text{Number of days of supply (excl. last dispension)}}{\text{Number of days between first and last dispension}}$$

The number of days of supply equals the quantity dispensed divided by the daily dosage indicated on the prescription. To calculate PDC, we only included patients with dispensions on two or more different dates. Patients that did not get a refill after their first NOAC dispension were excluded from the adherence analyses. We also excluded patients that received weekly dispensions, because PDC for these patients will always be close to 100%. Patients with a PDC of 80% or higher are considered adherent. This cut-off is supported by the International Society for Pharmaceutical and Outcomes Research [15].

Differences between groups were tested by analysis of variance (ANOVA) and t-tests.

For analysis and reporting SQL server 2014 and Excel 2013 were used.

Unless mentioned otherwise, year totals refer to the period of the 12 months ending 1 October of that year, e.g. 2016 means 1 October 2015 to 30 September 2016.

Results

The total number of OAC users included in this study was 256,641 across 544 pharmacies and they received a total of 3,029,294 VKA or NOAC prescriptions between 1 July 2011 and 30 September 2016.

Uptake

In our panel, the total number of patients on OACs grew from 126,638 in 2012 to 159,291 in 2016, with an average yearly growth rate of 5.9%. The number of naive starters per month oscillated around an average of 2553.

During the past 5 years, the number of NOAC starters has increased steadily, from 4000 in 2012 to 40,000 in 2016. Rivaroxaban is most used in terms of absolute patients, followed by dabigatran and apixaban. However, apixaban has the fastest growth rate (119% in 2016) and an equal number of naive starters as dabigatran in 2016 (Figs. 1, 2 and 3). In recent months, the share of dabigatran and apixaban in naive starters on NOAC each oscillate around 25%. From June 2013, when apixaban received a reimbursement status for the AF indication, the total number of naive starters on NOACs also started to grow and apixaban quickly gained market share from rivaroxaban and mainly dabigatran. The share of dabigatran in naive starters stabilized from June 2015, when the indications for dabigatran were extended from AF and the prevention of VTE after knee or hip replacement surgery to include also DVT and PE. Since the introduction of apixaban, the share of rivaroxaban in naive starters has also declined somewhat, but less than that of dabigatran, and remained relatively stable until January 2016, when the share of dabigatran in naive starters slightly increased again (Fig. 4). Overall, the share of NOACs in naive starters is growing at an increasing speed and was 57% in September 2016 (Fig. 5).

For VKA, during this same studied period, we have seen the number of patients grow at a declining pace up until 2015. In 2016 the number of VKA patients declined for the first time. These last 12 months, the

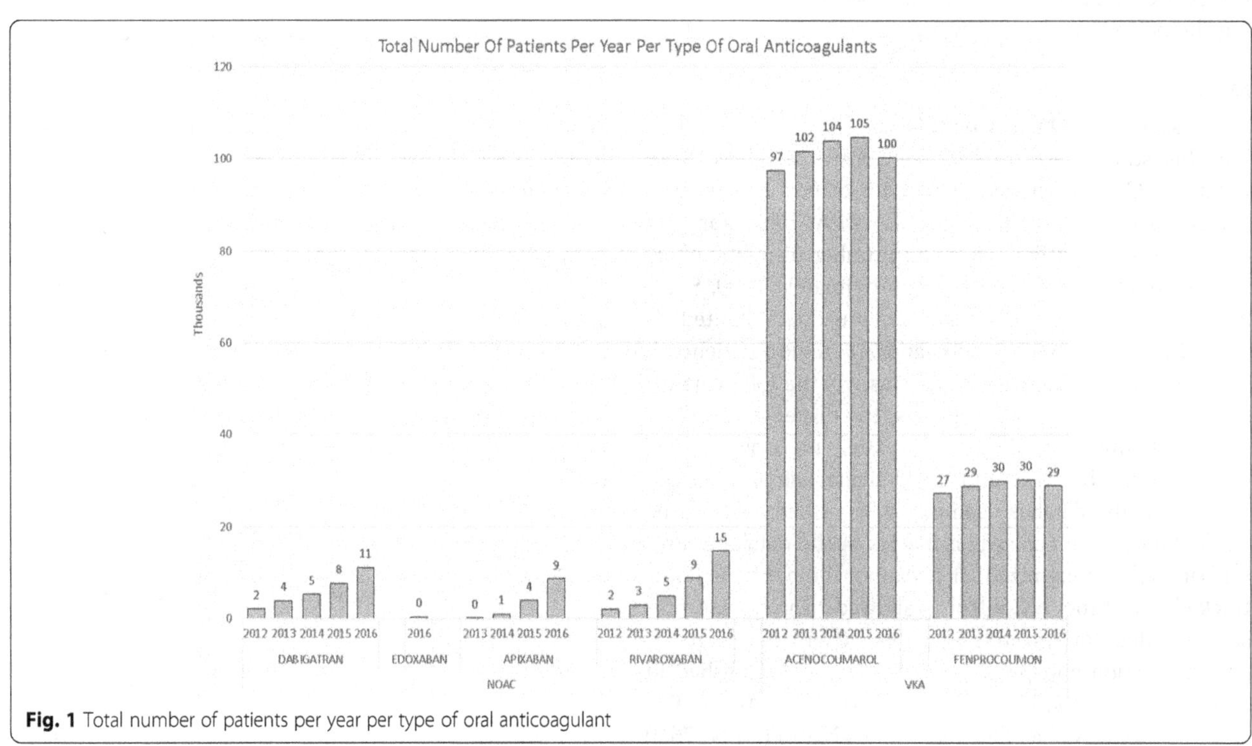

Fig. 1 Total number of patients per year per type of oral anticoagulant

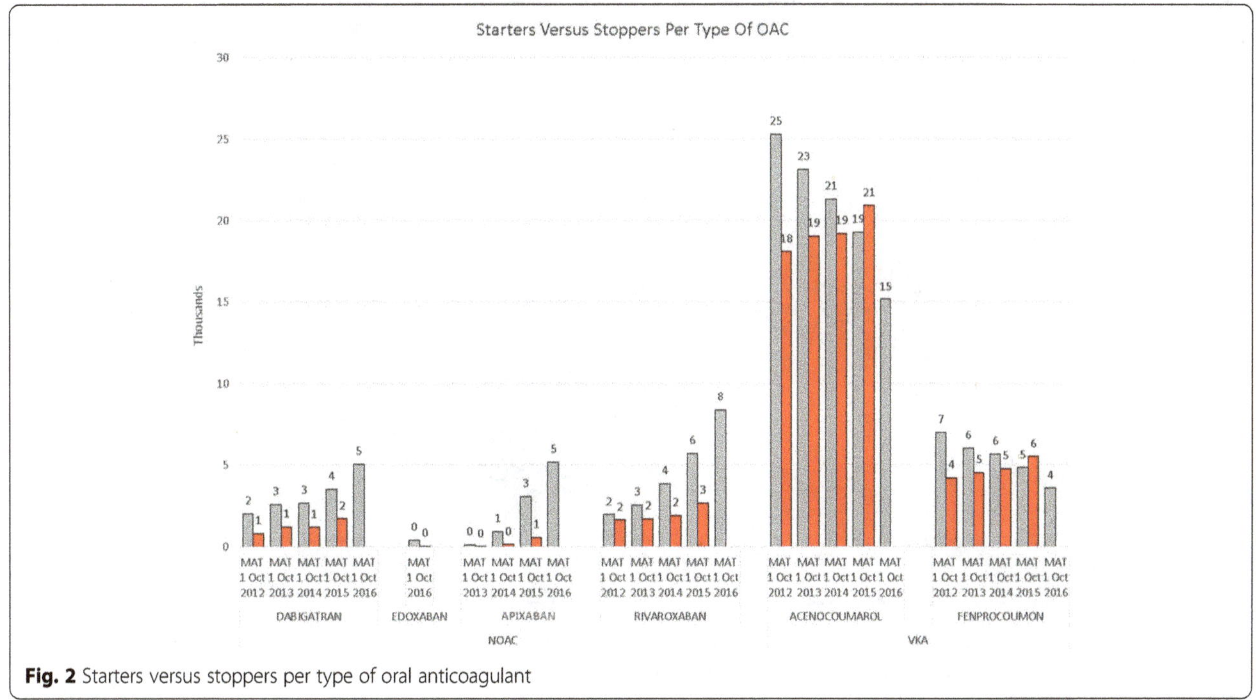

Fig. 2 Starters versus stoppers per type of oral anticoagulant

population of VKA patients decreases with 6000 patients (-4.4%) (Fig. 1). In 2015, the number of patients stopping VKA treatment is increasing, while the number of starters in 2016 decreases, resulting in a net decline of patients (Fig. 3). (We have no information on stoppers for 2016 yet: we need 365 days after a last dispensing to label a patient as stopper.)

Source of NOAC patients

During the studied period, 48,291 patients started with a NOAC. 70% of this group where new naive patients and 30% were switchers from either VKA or another NOAC. A total of 12,769 (26% of NOAC starters) were patients switching from VKA. In comparison, during that same period, 3437 patients switched from a NOAC to VKA. 2480 patients switched between NOACs.

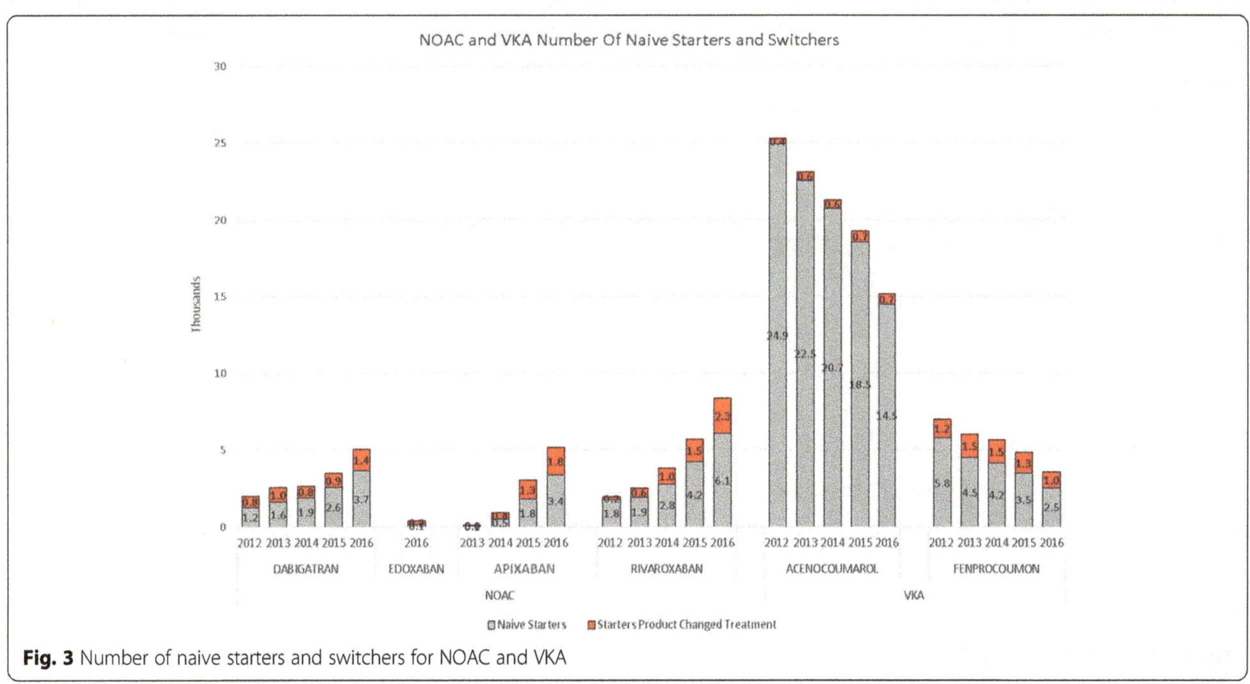

Fig. 3 Number of naive starters and switchers for NOAC and VKA

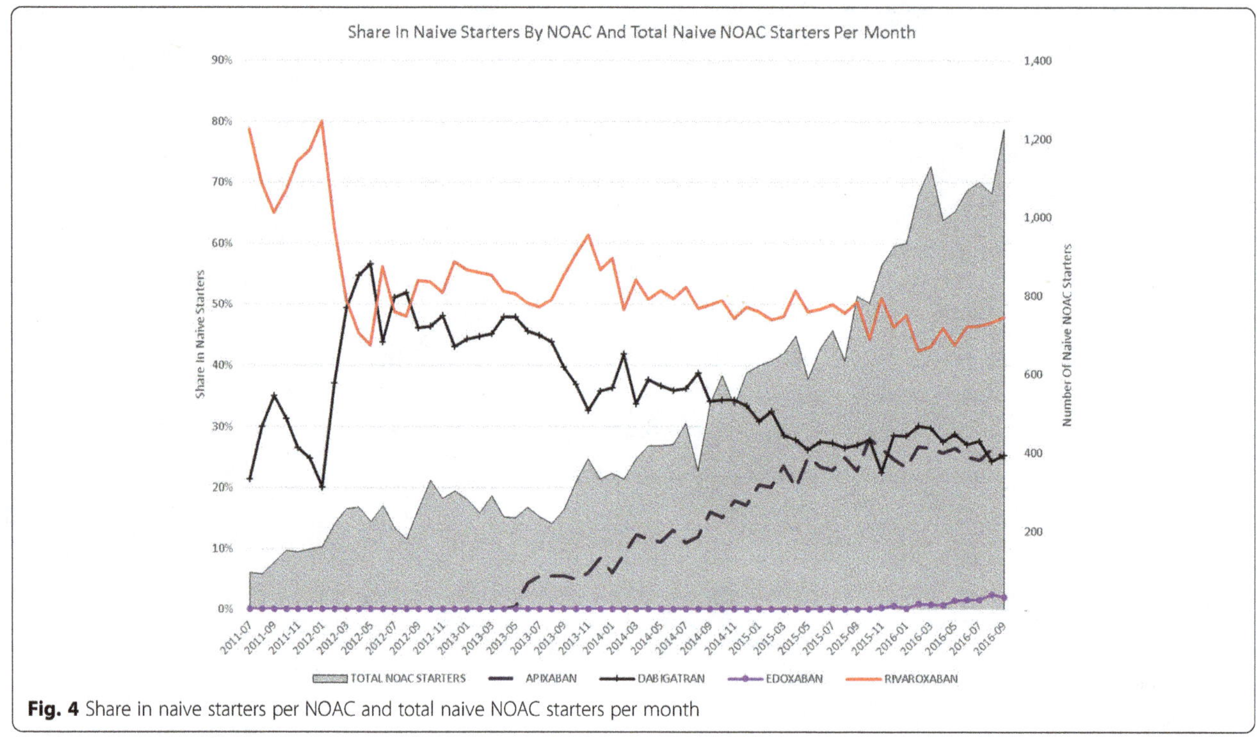

Fig. 4 Share in naive starters per NOAC and total naive NOAC starters per month

Patient targeting

To analyze if prescribers of NOACs targeted specific patient groups, age, gender and the number of co-medications used were extracted. OACs were mainly prescribed to adults. During the study period, there were only 181 initiations of OACs to patients under the age of 18, and only 6 of those (3.3%) received a NOAC.

The proportion of NOAC prescriptions was highest (29%) in the group of new users aged between 60 and 69, whereas the average proportion of NOACs in naive starters on OACs was 22% (Fig. 6). Share of NOACs in naive starters was also above average in the age groups 50-59 (24%) and 70-79 (25%).

The share of female starters in NOACs was 48% on average. However this proportion differed somewhat across age categories: the largest group of females (34% of all females) starting on NOACs was between 70 and 79 years old. This was also the age group with most starters on OACs in general. In the group of patients aged 80 and older, share of women was over 60%, and in

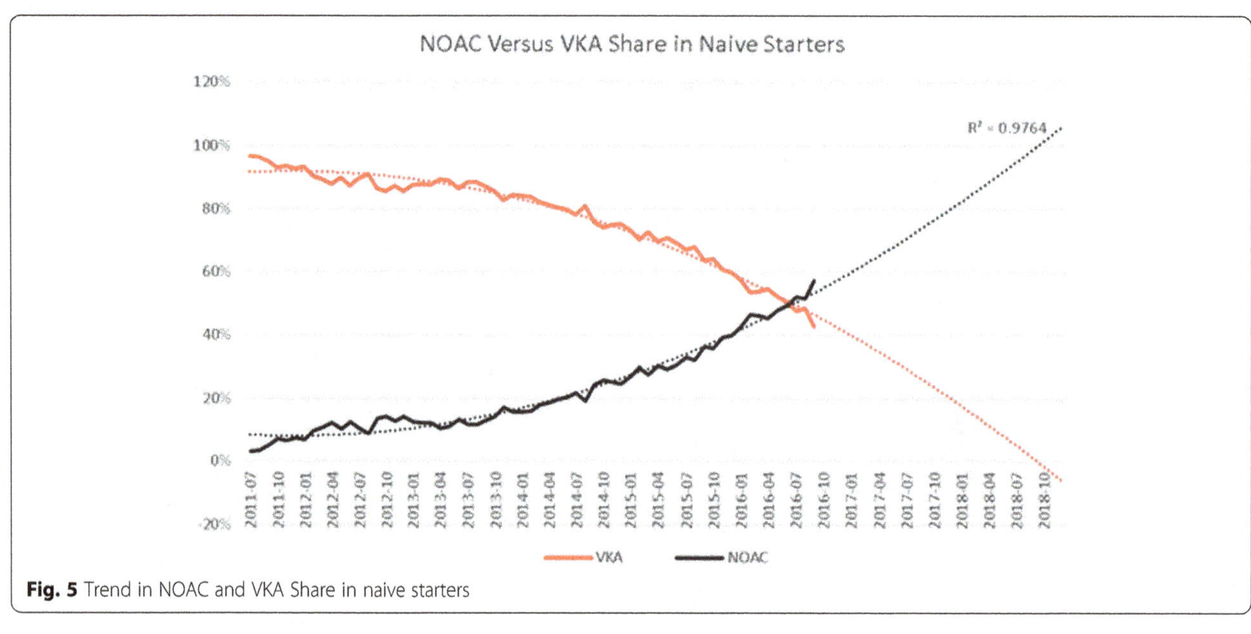

Fig. 5 Trend in NOAC and VKA Share in naive starters

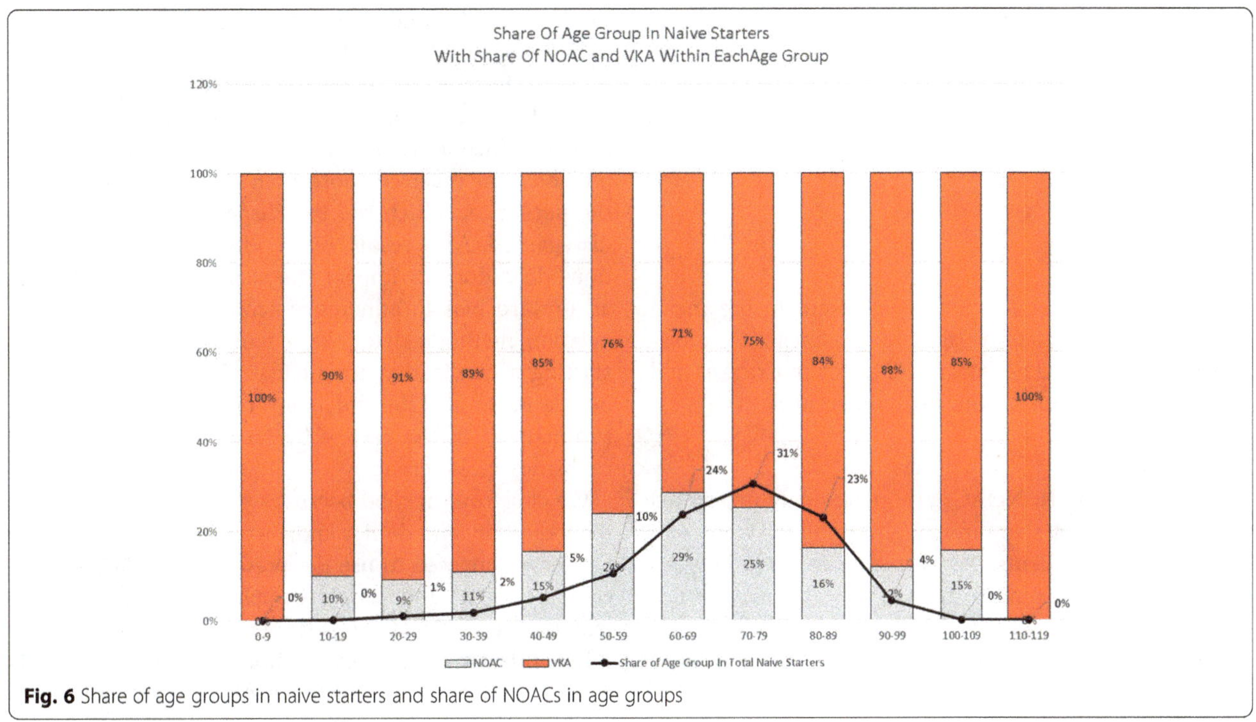

Fig. 6 Share of age groups in naive starters and share of NOACs in age groups

the group below 70, they represented 44%. The largest group of male starters was aged between 60 and 69 (34%) (Table 1) (Fig. 6).

On average, VKA patients used 9.4, and NOAC users used 8.2 different medications during the 6 months before their first oral anticoagulant prescription ($p < 0.0001$)). There was a difference across age categories: 8.6 different medications for NOAC patients versus 10.0 for VKA patients aged above 65 ($p < 0.0001$), and 7.0 ATCs for NOAC starters versus 7.6 for VKA starters aged below 65 ($p < 0.0001$).

Adherence

88% of NOAC users had a PDC above 80% (Table 2). Mean PDC was 108% for dabigatran, 107% for apixaban and 112% for rivaroxaban (Table 3). Only the PDC

Table 1 Patients by age and gender

Age group	NOAC					VKA				
	Male		Female		Total	Male		Female		Total
	Nr of patients	pct in age group	Nr of patients	pct in age group	Nr of patients	Nr of patients	pct in age group	Nr of patients	pct in age group	Total
0-9						34	59%	24	41%	58
10-19	14	41%	20	59%	34	117	36%	206	64%	323
20-29	66	46%	76	54%	142	386	29%	925	71%	1311
30-39	170	53%	148	47%	318	950	40%	1451	60%	2401
40-49	762	59%	539	41%	1301	3276	49%	3343	51%	6619
50-59	2343	58%	1671	42%	4014	7691	64%	4297	36%	11,988
60-69	5656	54%	4791	46%	10,447	15,638	62%	9759	38%	25,397
70-79	5228	49%	5428	51%	10,656	17,509	54%	15,211	46%	32,720
80-89	1906	40%	2831	60%	4737	10,212	40%	15,063	60%	25,275
90-99	193	33%	389	67%	582	1100	27%	3039	73%	4139
100-109	1	17%	5	83%	6	7	19%	29	81%	36
110-119						1	50%	1	50%	2
Total	16,339	51%	15,898	49%	32,237	56,921	52%	53,348	48%	110,269

Table 2 Percentage of adherent patients per NOAC

	Pct of patients	
	PDC* > =80	Nr of patients
Apixaban	92%	7094
Dabigatran	88%	11,782
Rivaroxaban	88%	13,975
Total	89%	32,851

for rivaroxaban was significantly different to the mean of dabigatran ($p = 0.0026$) and to the mean of apixaban ($p = 0.0331$). The mean PDC for apixaban and dabigatran were not significantly different.

Discussion

In The Netherlands, NOACs are increasingly prescribed and gained market share from VKA among existing and especially new patients. Patients treated with NOACs are in general adherent to their therapy, during the implementation phase of their treatment. NOACs represented 57% of all new prescriptions in the month of September 2016, even though the introduction of NOACs in the Netherlands has met some resistance, [4, 16, 17]). The introduction has been gradual, as was advised by the Health Council of the Netherlands, but now the share of NOACs in starters increases every month, and the number of VKA patients is decreasing since 2016. If the current trend continues, within 24 months we expect virtually all naive starters to receive a NOAC, and that only a limited number of patients with a contra-indication for NOAC will still start on VKA. We did not find evidence that NOACs were targeted to specific patient groups, except for some specific age groups. The fact that patients treated with NOACs are generally adherent to their therapy during the implementation phase is specifically important because unlike VKA patients, they are not under continuous supervision of the Thrombosis Service in The Netherlands. The therapy adherence that we measured is high compared to adherence to other medications measured in other studies [12] and in line with high adherence to NOACs in other comparable studies [14, 18, 19]. Borne et al. [18] use a comparable method for calculating PDC, only exclude patients with less than 1 year follow-up and find that 74.2 patients have a PDC > = 80%. Schulman et al. use the same method for calculating PDC and arrive at 89% of all patients with a PDC > = 80% [19]. Mueller et al. find that 90.6% of all patients have a compliance ratio of >80% [14], also using this method of calculation. Our method, as is the case for the above mentioned studies, only includes patients that received more than one dispension. Also, the period for which the last dispension was valid was disregarded. As a result, (early) discontinuation (cessation) does dot not impact the score. This may lead to an upward bias in adherence scores, compared to calculation methods that take a fixed time interval after starting a medication to calculate PDC, like the study by Maura et al. [20] and many of the studies that are summarized in the review by Obamiro et al. [21] and report lower adherence.

Table 3 Average PDC per NOAC

PDC[a]	Apixaban	Dabigatran	Rivaroxaban
Mean	109	108	113
Std.dev.	81	141	120
Median	102	101	103

[a] All patients with more than 1 dispensing
Excluding patients with weekly dispensings

We chose our method because we have no knowledge of the indication, and do not know with certainty how long a patient is supposed to use the prescribed NOAC, and because we wanted to assess compliance explicitly during treatment, excluding the impact of discontinuation.

Like other studies of medication adherence, our study is also limited by the accuracy of assessing adherence from pharmacy prescription data, which may misclassify the adherence of patients who fill prescriptions but do not actually take them.

Multiple studies have shown that the use of NOACs appears to be as efficacious as and safer than the use of VKAs [6, 7] and the number of NOAC prescriptions is increasing also in other countries. From other national level database studies, we know that the number of NOAC prescriptions in Canada increased annually between 2008 and 2014, from 1% to 33% of all OAC prescriptions [22]. In the US, NOACs have had a modest but growing uptake (from 0.04 in the beginning of 2011 to 12% in second quarter of 2012) among atrial fibrillation patients hospitalized with stroke or transient ischemic attack [23]. Other, smaller studies have shown an increasing uptake of NOACs among patients using oral anticoagulants in specific hospitals [24, 25].

Some arguments mentioned against introducing NOACs in The Netherlands state that with the Thrombosis Services, The Netherlands has an excellent infrastructure to monitor patients using VKA, and the use of NOACs in clinical practice has both positive and negative aspects. Initially, in the media and in politics, there has been criticism around the benefits of NOACs over VKA. Until recently no antidote for NOACs was available - idarucizumab, an antidote for dabigatran was introduced only in January 2016 - and the benefit that NOACs are to be used without constant supervision of the Thrombosis Service could be countered by the argument that this reduced supervision could lead to a lower therapy adherence, accompanied with health risks.

Also, in the period following the introduction of dabigatran and rivaroxaban, NOACs met opposition for reasons associated with healthcare budgets [16] and increased risk of gastrointestinal bleeding [17], contrary to the results of more recent studies [6, 7]. This may have hampered the uptake of NOACs. Our study showed that NOAC users are generally very therapy adherent, which could be an argument in favor of prescribing NOACs in the future. We found that the largest percentage of adherent patients was found under rivaroxaban users. Even though our t-tests showed statistically significant differences with dabigatran and apixaban, we believe that these are not clinically relevant.

Dabigatran was the first NOAC on the market and had the largest market share during the first period after its introduction, but it lost market share first to rivaroxaban, and then to apixaban. We observed an immediate start in uptake of apixaban from June 2013, when it received reimbursement status for AF, and since then apixaban gained share almost every month until June 2015. We suspect that the steady growth of apixaban, introduced years after dabigatran and rivaroxaban, was caused at least partly because it was welcomed as a perceived safe alternative to the existing NOACs on the market. Apixaban, like dabigratran needs to be taken twice per day, but has no contraindication for patients with kidney deficiency, and may therefore also be considered a safer alternative to dabigatran [5]. In this context of the perceived safety of specific NOACs, it is also interesting to note that the share of dabigatran in naive starters increased in January 2016, after the introduction of idarucizumab, its antidote, albeit only for a few months.

Approximately three quarters of patients starting on NOACs were new naive patients. 27% of NOAC starters have switched from VKA and the number of switchers from VKA to NOAC was 3.5 times higher than the number of patients switching from NOAC to VKA, resulting in a net flow of patients from VKA to NOAC. The number of patients switching between NOACs was smaller than the number of patients switching from NOAC to VKA. This suggests that patients experiencing problems caused by their treatment with a NOAC were more likely to switch (back) to VKA than to try another NOAC. The reason for switching back to VKA cannot be explained by our data, but may partly be the result of unfamiliarity of general practitioners with NOACs. Until October 2016, NOACs could only be prescribed by medical specialists. Starting November 2016, also GPs can prescribe NOACs. This might result in an additional acceleration of the speed of uptake of NOACs.

It does not appear that physicians were targeting a specific group of patients in terms of age and gender. Based on the number of co-medications used, it cannot be concluded that NOAC starters were in a significantly better or worse state of health than starters on VKA. The reason why the percentage of patients starting NOACs above the age of 74 was lower may be associated with co-morbidities (among others renal insufficiency and higher bleeding risk, higher risk of falling) [26], even though a meta-analysis clearly showed that those above 75 years of age mostly benefit from using NOACs, both in terms of efficacy and safety [6].

We acknowledge that there are some limitations that may have influenced the results. Pharmacies included in this study are only public pharmacies, no hospital pharmacies. Outpatient pharmacies (4% of all public pharmacies in The Netherlands) were underrepresented. Patients that start NOACs in the hospital may appear only in our panel after discharge. Adherence results can be negatively affected by patients that spend time in a hospital between receiving dispensions from their public pharmacy. Also related to adherence, we analysed adherence only during the period that NOAC was used: the implementation phase. The impact of early cessation is not included in our metric which may lead to a higher calculated adherence. Another limitation is our inability to analyse the reasons for prescribing medication and therefore we have not been able to describe the uptake of NOACs for different indications. We used the number of ATCs prescribed to a patient to infer the general health status of that patient, and we acknowledge that this number by itself is no firm measure of health status, however, it is the only information available to us. Lastly, we analyzed the medication that was dispensed to the patient only. We do not know with certainty whether the patient took all received medication. An important strength of our study is that the population, with almost one third of all public pharmacies in The Netherlands is very large. We consider it representative for public pharmacies in The Netherlands as a whole.

NOACs have gained a solid position in the market in The Netherlands. At present, the majority of new patients are prescribed NOACs, and some VKA users switch to NOACs. NOACs are being used across all adult patient groups in terms of age, gender and health status. We expect that almost all oral anticoagulants prescribed to new patients will be NOAC, even though a number of (new) patients on VKA will likely remain.

The high therapy adherence measured among patients that use NOACs should be considered one of the most relevant outcomes of this study. At the introduction of NOACs in The Netherlands, fear of patients not being adherent to their treatment and the related health risks as a result of absent supervision of NOAC patients by the thrombosis service has been the most important caveat of the Health Council of the Netherlands, related to the prescription of NOACs. Based on our results, fear for inadherence by itself does not need to be a reason for not prescribing NOACs instead of VKA. However, monitoring adherence and identifying (early) discontinuation should remain important.

Conclusions

NOAC have overtaken VKA as the major treatment prescribed to new oral anticoagulant patients, and the number of starters on VKA is decreasing. Patients are generally adherent to NOACs during the implementation phase, the period that the medication is used. Fear for inadherence by itself does not need to be a reason for not prescribing NOACs instead of VKA.

Abbreviations

ACS: Acute coronary syndrome; AF: Atrial fibrillation; ANOVA: Analysis of variance; ATC: Anatomical, therapeutical and chemical medication cluster; CR: Compliance ratio; DOAC: Direct oral anticoagulants; DVT: Deep vein thrombosis; INR: International normalized ratio; ISO: International organisation for standardization; NEN: Netherlands Norm; NOAC: Non-VKA oral anticoagulants; OAC: Oral anticoagulants; PDC: Proportion of days covered; PE: Pulmonary embolism; VKA: Vitamin K Antagonists; VTE: Venous thromboembolism

Acknowledgements

Not applicable

Funding

Not applicable

Authors' contributions

JMvdH analyzed and interpreted the patient data regarding the uptake of NOACs in The Netherlands. All authors read and approved the final manuscript.

Ethics approval and consent to participate

For this study, data from the NControl database were obtained. Our dataset contains data of 544 pharmacies, spread across The Netherlands. Since 2011, the NControl database contains data related to over 557 million prescriptions and 7.2 million patients.

Patients in the database cannot be identified, but can be tracked over time across pharmacies in the NControl database. Prescribers are anonymized and cannot be identified nor tracked over time. NControl is allowed to use these prescription data for research purposes. NControl adheres to data protection and privacy regulations, as established in amongst others the Personal Data Protection Act in The Netherlands as well as the NEN 7510 standard, related to information protection in healthcare, which is derived from ISO 27001 and 27,002.

Competing interests

The authors declare that they have no competing interests.

Author details

[1]Utrecht Institute for Pharmaceutical Sciences (UIPS), Division of Pharmacoepidemiology and Clinical Pharmacology, Utrecht University, Utrecht, The Netherlands. [2]Department of Respiratory Medicine, Academic Medical Center, University of Amsterdam, Amsterdam, The Netherlands. [3]Department of Vascular Medicine, Academic Medical Center, University of Amsterdam, Amsterdam, The Netherlands.

References

1. Riley R, Tiddwell A. An introduction to Thromboembolic disease. 1st ed. Richmond, VA: Virginia Commonwealth University; 2016. [cited 1 Mar 2016]. Available from: https://pdfs.semanticscholar.org/5a93/304bbcf7e995ef14d006b8a44bc55d64744b.pdf.
2. Ansell J, Hirsh J, Hylek E, et al. Pharmacology and Management of the Vitamin K Antagonists: American College of Chest Physicians Evidence-Based Clinical Practice Guidelines (8th edition). https://doi.org/10.1378/chest.08-0670.
3. Bruni-Fitzgerald K. Venous thromboembolism: an overview. J Vasc Nurs. 2015;33:95–9. https://doi.org/10.1016/j.jvn.2015.02.001.
4. Health Council of the Netherlands. New Anticoagulants: A well-dosed introduction. The Hague: Health Council of the Netherlands; 2012. publication no. 2012/07E. ISBN 978-90-5549-940-3.
5. Farmacotherapeutisch Kompas. bladeren-volgens-boek/inleidingen/inl-overige-anticoagulantia. 2016 [cited 1 Mar 2016]. Available from: https://www.farmacotherapeutischkompas.nl/bladeren/indicatieteksten/trombo_embolie__behandeling.
6. van Es N, Coppens M, Schulman S, et al. Direct oral anticoagulants compared with vitamin K antagonists for acute venous thromboembolism: evidence from phase 3 trials. Blood. 2014;124:1968–75. https://doi.org/10.1182/blood-2014-04-571232.
7. Nairooz R, Ayoub K, Sardar P, et al. Uninterrupted new oral anticoagulants compared with uninterrupted vitamin K antagonists in ablation of Atrial fibrillation: a meta-analysis. Can J Cardiol. 2016;32:814–23. https://doi.org/10.1016/j.cjca.2015.09.012.
8. Dillinger JG, Aleil B, Cheggour S et al. Dosing issues with non-vitamin K antagonist oral anticoagulants for the treatment of non-valvular atrial fibrillation: Why we should not underdose our patients. Archives of Cardiovascular Diseases 2017, available on-line. https://doi.org/10.1016/j.acvd.2017.04.008
9. Buurma H, Bouvy ML, De Smet PA, et al. Prevalence and determinants of pharmacy shopping behaviour. J Clin Pharm Ther. 2008;33:17–23. https://doi.org/10.1111/j.1365-2710.2008.00878.x.
10. Vrijens B, De Geest S, Hughes DA, et al. A new taxonomy for describing and defining adherence to medications. Br J Clin Pharmacol. 2012 May;73(5):691–705. https://doi.org/10.1111/j.1365-2125.2012.04167.x.
11. Nau DP. Proportion of Days Covered (PDC) as a Preferred Method of Measuring Medication Adherence, Research & Performance Measurement Pharmacy Quality Alliance, http://www.pqaalliance.org/images/uploads/files/PQA%20PDC%20vs%20%20MPR.pdf.
12. Choudry NK, Shrank WH, Levin RL, et al. Measuring concurrent adherence to multiple related medication. Am J Manag Care. 2009;15:457–64.
13. Hess L, Raebel M, Conner D. Measurement of adherence in pharmacy administrative databases: a proposal for standard definitions and preferred measures measurement of adherence in pharmacy administrative databases: a proposal for standard definitions and preferred measures. Ann Pharmacother. 2006;40:1280–8. 2006
14. Mueller T, Alvarez-Madrazo S, Robertson C, Bennie M. Use of direct oral anticoagulants in patients with atrial fibrillation in Scotland: applying a coherent framework to drug utilisation studies. Pharmacoepidemiol Drug Saf. 2017;26:1378–86. https://doi.org/10.1002/pds.4272
15. Karve S, Cleves MA, Helm M, et al. Good and poor adherence: optimal cut-point for adherence measures using administrative claims data. Curr Med Res Opin. 2009;25:2303–10. https://doi.org/10.1185/03007990903126833.
16. Government of The Netherlands.https://www.rijksoverheid.nl/documenten/kamerstukken/2015/03/24/beantwoording-kamervragen-over-uitblijven-onderzoek-naar-veiligheid-nieuwe-antistollingsmiddelen.
17. Government of The Netherlands. https://www.rijksoverheid.nl/documenten/kamerstukken/2013/08/28/beantwoording-kamervragen-over-het-bericht-dat-nieuwe-bloedverdunners-dodelijke-maag-darmbloedingen-kunnen-veroorzaken.

18. Borne R, O'Donnel C, Turakhia M, et al. Adherence and outcomes to direct oral anticoagulants among patients with atrial fibrillation: findings from the veterans health administration. BMC Cardiovasc Disord. 2017;17:236. https://doi.org/10.1186/s12872-017-0671-6.
19. Schulman S, Shortt B, Robinson M et al.. Adherence to anticoagulant treatment with dabigatran in a real-world setting, Journal of thrombosis and haemostasis 2013 https://doi.org/10.1111/jth.122411.
20. Maura G, Pariente A, Alla F, et al. Adherence with direct oral anticoagulants in nonvalvular atrial fibrillation new users and associated factors: a French nationwide cohort study. Pharmacoepidemiol Drug Saf. 2017;26:1367–77. https://doi.org/10.1002/pds.4268.
21. Obamiro KO, Chlmers L, LRE B. A summary of the literature evaluating adherence and persistence with oral anticoagulants in Atrial fibrillation. Am J Cardiovasc Drugs. 2016;16:349. https://doi.org/10.1007/s40256-016-0171-6.
22. Weitz J, Semchuk W, Turpie A, et al. Trends in prescribing oral anticoagulants in Canada, 2008–2014. Clin Ther. 2015;37:2506–2514.e4. https://doi.org/10.1016/j.clinthera.2015.09.008.
23. Patel P, Zhao X, Fonarow G, et al. Novel oral anticoagulant use among patients with Atrial fibrillation hospitalized with ischemic stroke or transient ischemic attack. Circ Cardiovasc Qual Outcomes. 2015;8:383–92. https://doi.org/10.1161/CIRCOUTCOMES.114.000907.
24. Baker D, Wilsmore B, Narasimhan S. The adoption of direct oral anticoagulants for stroke prevention in atrial fibrillation. Intern Med J 2016 https://doi.org/10.1016/j.hlc.2015.06.657.
25. Al-Khalili F, Lindström C, Benson L. The safety and persistence of non-vitamin-K-antagonist oral anticoagulants in atrial fibrillation patients treated in a well structured atrial fibrillation clinic. Curr Med Res Opin. 2016;32:779–85. https://doi.org/10.1185/03007995.2016.1142432.
26. Factor Xa remmers en directe trombine remmers (nieuwe orale anticoagulantia, NOAC) bij kwetsbare ouderen? Standpunt van de Werkgroep Klinische Gerontofarmacologie (WKGF) van de Nederlandse Vereniging van Klinische Geriatrie en et Expertise Centrum Pharmacotherapie bij Ouderen (Ephor). Aug 2013.

20

Association between plasminogen activator inhibitor-1 and cardiovascular events

Richard G. Jung[1,2,3†], Pouya Motazedian[1†], F. Daniel Ramirez[1,4,5], Trevor Simard[1,2,3,4], Pietro Di Santo[1,4], Sarah Visintini[6], Mohammad Ali Faraz[1], Alisha Labinaz[1], Young Jung[7] and Benjamin Hibbert[1,2,3,4*]

Abstract

Background: Small studies have implicated plasminogen activator inhibitor-1 (PAI-1) as a predictor of cardiovascular events; however, these findings have been inconsistent.
We sought out to examine the potential role of PAI-1 as a marker for major adverse cardiovascular events (MACE).

Methods: We systematically reviewed all indexed studies examining the association between PAI-1 and MACE (defined as death, myocardial infarction, or cerebrovascular accident) or restenosis. EMBASE, Web of Science, Medline, and the Cochrane Library were searched through October 2016 to identify relevant studies, supplemented by letters to authors and review of citations. Studies reporting the results of PAI-1 antigen and/or activity levels in association with MACE in human subjects were included.

Results: Of 5961 articles screened, we identified 38 articles published between 1991 to 2016 that reported PAI-1 levels in 11,557 patients. In studies that examined PAI-1 antigen and activity levels, 15.1% and 29.6% of patients experienced MACE, respectively. Patients with MACE had higher PAI-1 antigen levels with a mean difference of 6. 11 ng/mL (95% CI, 3.27-8.96). This finding was similar among patients with and without known coronary artery disease. Comparatively, studies that stratified by PAI-1 activity levels were not associated with MACE. In contrast, studies of coronary restenosis suggest PAI-1 antigen and activity levels are negatively associated with MACE.

Conclusions: Elevated plasma PAI-1 antigen levels are associated with MACE. Definitive studies are needed to ascertain if PAI-1 acts simply as a marker of risk or if it is indeed a bona fide therapeutic target.

Keywords: Plasminogen activator inhibitor-1, Biomarkers, Mortality, Myocardial infarction, Meta-analysis

Background

Obstructive coronary artery disease (CAD) is the leading cause of mortality in the western world. The cornerstone of therapy for CAD remains revascularization and secondary medical therapy to modify risk factors. The fibrinolytic system has implications for both approaches to disease management. First, percutaneous coronary intervention (PCI) with implantation of a coronary stent remains the predominant method of coronary revascularization [1]. However, complications such as in-stent restenosis and stent thrombosis following PCI limit its efficacy. Thus, in the peri-revascularization period, preventing thrombotic events is paramount until the vessel's endothelial lining and function are restored. Second, long term therapy with antiplatelet and/or oral anticoagulation is an integral part of secondary preventive medical therapy. Thus, dysregulation of the fibrinolytic pathways may increase the risk of complications from revascularization therapy *and* diminish the efficacy of long term medical therapy to reduce the risk of recurrent events.

The fibrinolytic system is activated by the conversion of plasminogen to plasmin by serine proteases such as tissue or urokinase-type plasminogen activator (t-PA and

* Correspondence: bhibbert@ottawaheart.ca
†Equal contributors
[1]CAPITAL Research Group, University of Ottawa Heart Institute, 40 Ruskin Street, H-4238, Ottawa, ON K1Y 4W7, Canada
[2]Department of Cellular and Molecular Medicine, University of Ottawa, Ottawa, ON, Canada
Full list of author information is available at the end of the article

u-PA, respectively). In contrast, fibrinolysis is inhibited by plasminogen activator inhibitor-1 (PAI-1), which is a member of the serine protease inhibitor (serpin) family. Ultimately, thrombosis risk is influenced by the balance between PAI-1 and t-PA. Thus, an increase in the PAI-1 levels in plasma can induce a hypercoagulable state [2]. PAI-1 is released by vascular endothelial cells, hepatocytes, adipocytes, cardiomyocytes, fibroblasts, and platelets [3, 4]. In healthy humans, plasma levels of PAI-1 exceed t-PA by a ratio of over 4:1 with most of PAI-1 being cleared by the liver [5]. In pathologic conditions, PAI-1 production can be upregulated by pro-inflammatory factors such as TNFα, TGFβ, and insulin [6]. Elevated plasma PAI-1 levels have been associated with impaired fibrinolytic activity in stroke and coronary artery disease [7]. Moreover, PAI-1 antigen and activity levels are elevated in patients with type 2 diabetes [8], hyperinsulinemia [9], and those with insulin resistance [10, 11]. Yet, a definitive assessment of the impact of elevated PAI-1 as a biomarker or therapeutic target has yet to be evaluated. Accordingly, we performed a systematic review and meta-analysis of PAI-1 antigen and activity levels and their relationship with major adverse cardiovascular events (MACE) in humans.

Methods

Literature search strategy

Literature searches were guided by a medical librarian with expertise in systematic reviews (S.V.) using a combination of key terms and index headings related to PAI-1, coronary disease (informed by the Cochrane review search strategy for coronary heart disease in exercise-based cardiac rehabilitation [12]), and the Cochrane Highly Sensitive search strategy to eliminate articles on animal studies in Medline. The search was additionally peer-reviewed by a second medical librarian (R.S.). Once finalized, the search strategy was then translated to other bibliographic databases (see Additional file 1 for the full Medline search). The final search was conducted on October 2016 in Medline (Ovid) (In-Process & Other Non-Indexed Citations and Ovid MEDLINE(R) 1946-), Embase (Ovid) (Embase Classic + Embase 1947-), Cochrane Library (Ovid) (from inception), and Web of Science (Thomson Reuters) (all indexes, from inception). Search results were exported to EndNote X7 (Thomson Reuters, New York, USA) and duplicates eliminated using the program's duplicate identification feature and manual inspection. A review protocol was produced but not registered in a database.

Titles and abstracts were screened by two independent reviewers (R.J. and P.M.) using Covidence (Melbourne, Australia). Full articles were retrieved in cases of missing abstracts. Corresponding authors were contacted for additional information when necessary.

Inclusion and exclusion criteria and quality assessment

Studies were included if they met the following criteria: (1) PAI-1 antigen or activity levels were reported; (2) the population studied comprised individuals aged 18 years or older; (3) components of MACE (death, myocardial infarction, and cerebrovascular events including stroke and transient ischemic attacks) or restenosis were reported; (4) articles were published in English. Exclusion criteria included: (1) PAI-1 polymorphism studies examining the association between 4G/5G and adverse events; (2) animal or in vitro studies; and (3) studies reporting hazard ratios only. Full text data extraction was conducted by two independent evaluators (R.J. and P.M.). Each reviewer independently extracted patient population characteristics, group sizes, PAI-1 antigen and activity levels, follow-up duration, and MACE and restenosis. All discrepancies were resolved by consensus prior to locking the database for analysis (Tables 1 and 2). Included observational studies were evaluated for quality and risk of bias using the Newcastle-Ottawa Quality Assessment Scale [13] by two independent evaluators (R.J. and P.M.) with disagreements resolved by consensus. Visual funnel plot inspection was used to screen for publication bias.

Statistical analysis

The primary clinical endpoint for this study was MACE – a composite of death, myocardial infarction, or cerebrovascular events. The secondary endpoint included components of the primary as well as coronary restenosis in patients undergoing coronary revascularization. Mean circulating PAI-1 antigen (ng/mL) and activity (IU/mL) levels and their associated standard deviations were used for analyses. Fourteen studies reported median and interquartile ranges, which were converted to approximated means and standard deviations using the method described by Wan et al. [14].

All analyses were performed using Review Manager (RevMan) 5.3 (Cochrane Collection, Copenhagen, Denmark). PAI-1 antigen and activity levels were compared between patients with or without the outcomes of interest either as absolute values or dichotomized as high vs. low. Random effects models stratified by study design and study quality were used to generate pooled mean differences with 95% confidence intervals. *Post-hoc* meta regression was performed to account for timing of blood draw and acute phase reactions in studies of patients presenting with acute myocardial infarction or stroke.

Results

Included studies

Study selection

After excluding duplicate articles, 5961 titles and abstracts were screened, of which 340 underwent full

Table 1 Studies reporting PAI-1 antigen levels (ng/mL) and major adverse cardiovascular events and restenosis

					Event								No Event	
Reference	Year	Study Design	Follow-up (months)	Population of interest	N	PAI-1 (IU/mL)	Range	Death	MI	Restenosis	CVA	N	PAI-1 (IU/mL)	Range
Sane et al. [50]	1991	Cohort	24	Fibrinolytics	24	57	58	24	n/a	n/a	n/a	315	54	53
Cortellaro et al. [51]	1993	Case-Control	24	Subgroups Combined	58	11.3	0.7	13	17	n/a	20	87	7.3	0 5
Brannstrom et al. [52]	1995	Cohort	46	Anticoagulant	38	21.9	15.1	38	n/a	n/a	n/a	167	16.7	11.8
Juhan-Vague et al. [53]	1996	Cohort	24	MI	106	18.2	8 2	40	66	n/a	n/a	2700	14.8	8.9
Nordt et al. [54]	1998	Cohort	12	Fibrinolytics	5	28.8	14.3	n/a	n/a	5	n/a	26	27.1	15.4
Alaigh et al. [55]	1998	Cohort	6	Elective PCI	28	20.75	11.06	n/a	n/a	28	n/a	45	24.5	13.85
Moss et al. [56]	1999	Cohort	26	MI	81	25	18	25	56	n/a	n/a	964	29	28
Redondo et al. [57]	2001	Cohort	24	MI	37	40.725	22.28	2	5	30	n/a	157	42.65	21.02
Fornitz et al. [58]	2001	Cohort	6	Elective PCI	7	82.6	26.6	n/a	n/a	7	n/a	12	72.2	27
Bogaty et al. [59]	2001	Case-Control	48	MI	23	23.83	19.04	n/a	8	n/a	n/a	77	18.9	16.24
Ganti et al. [60]	2002	Cohort	n/a	MI	4	80.68	16.38	4	n/a	n/a	n/a	38	61	21.95
Lip et al. [61]	2002	Cohort	12	Stroke	27	56.5	30.7	27	n/a	n/a	n/a	59	45.9	23.3
Inoue et al. [62]	2003	Cohort	6	MI	24	28	4	n/a	n/a	24	n/a	42	29	4
Christ et al. [20]	2005	Cohort	6	Elective PCI	25	14.8	0.7	n/a	n/a	25	n/a	55	16.8	2.1
Robinson et al. [63]	2007	Cohort	5 to 51	Coronary Heart Disease	19	36.3	17.9	2	2	n/a	2	79	45.4	25.6
Katsaros et al. [24]	2008	Cohort	6 to 8	Elective PCI	12	11.69	8.05	n/a	n/a	12	n/a	61	22.78	18.76
Thogersen et al. [64]	2009	Case-Control	n/a	Healthy	50	38.27	16.79	n/a	50	n/a	n/a	56	29	15.75
Akkus et al. [65]	2009	Cohort	12	Cardiogenic Shock	33	116.5	97.26	33	n/a	n/a	n/a	27	71.33	54.79
Pineda et al. [66]	2010	Cohort	36	MI	25	65.13	53.3	4	21	n/a	n/a	117	70.1	48.34
Wennberg et al. [67]	2012	Case-Control	168	Healthy	469	57.28	25.83	n/a	469	n/a	n/a	895	51.23	25.11
Yano et al. [68]	2013	Cohort	20	Smokers	66	65.73	64.57	n/a	11	n/a	55	744	42.97	36.54
Yano et al. [69]	2014	Cohort	30	Hypertension	42	31.67	16.12	4	13	n/a	16	548	28.33	14.87
Knudsen et al. [70]	2014	Case-Control	12	HIV	54	111	8.5	3	51	n/a	n/a	54	92	7
Golukhova et al. [71]	2015	Cohort	28	Elective PCI	23	72.75	29.86	2	9	11	n/a	71	49.75	23.16

CVA cerebrovascular accident

Table 2 Studies reporting PAI-1 activity levels (IU/mL) and major adverse cardiovascular events and restenosis

					Event						No Event		
Reference	Year	Study Design	Follow-up (months)	Population of interest	N	PAI-1 Activity (U/mL)	Range	Death	MI	Restenosis	N	PAI-1 Activity (U/mL)	Range
Sane et al. [50]	1991	Cohort	24	Fibrinolytics	28	17	16	n/a	n/a	28	328	19	21
Shah et al. [72]	1992	Cohort	9	Elective PCI	28	8	7.1	n/a	n/a	28	40	12	8
Gray et al. [73]	1993	Cohort	0.1	MI	13	20.6	11	n/a	13	n/a	85	20.1	7.9
Malmberg et al. [74]	1994	Case-Control	90	MI	53	23.75	13.34	20	33	n/a	55	18	10.97
Brack et al. [75]	1994	Cohort	4	Elective PCI	16	4.63	4.71	n/a	n/a	16	30	5.77	5.06
Nordt et al. [54]	1998	Cohort	12	Fibrinolytics	5	8.7	8.3	n/a	5	n/a	26	9.9	8.2
Jansson et al. [76]	1998	Cohort	120	MI	54	9.1	5.1	54	n/a	n/a	69	10.6	7.1
Wiman et al. [77]	2000	Case-Control	3	MI	61	22.1	17.5	n/a	61	n/a	95	18.2	16.5
Wiman et al. [77]	2000	Case-Control	3	MI	25	15.4	13.6	n/a	25	n/a	38	17.8	12.4
Prisco et al. [78]	2001	Cohort	18	MI	18	11.27	7.64	n/a	n/a	18	36	15.8	27.49
Prisco et al. [78]	2001	Cohort	18	Elective PCI	6	8.33	8.1	n/a	n/a	6	42	7.57	9.52
Sargento et al. [79]	2003	Cohort	12	MI	7	6.34	1.56	5	2	n/a	80	4.47	1.84
Marcucci et al. [19]	2006	Case-Control	22 2	MI	109	22	9.09	54	55	n/a	411	24.25	10.63
Schoebel et al. [80]	2008	Cohort	2	MI	18	3.7	1.8	n/a	n/a	18	42	5.3	3.2

Wiman et al. [77] is presented twice as data for men and women were reported separately

review and 38 were ultimately included (Fig. 1, Tables 1 and 2). Study populations were heterogeneous, including patients presenting with stable angina, acute coronary syndrome, and non-cardiac diseases. Study sample sizes ranged from 19 to 2806. Most studies were of moderate quality (see Additional file 1: Tables S1 and S2 for details of study quality assessments). Funnel plots are shown in Additional file 1: Figures S1 and S2. In pooled analyses of all studies reporting PAI-1 antigen levels ($n = 8999$), 1362 events were reported, including 234 deaths, 795 myocardial infarctions, 101 cerebrovascular events, and 142 restenoses (Table 1). In all studies that examined PAI-1 activity levels ($n = 1490$), 441 events were reported, including 133 deaths, 194 myocardial infarctions, and 114 cases of restenosis (Table 2).

PAI-1 and clinical outcomes

Major adverse cardiovascular events

PAI-1 antigen levels were higher in those with MACE with a mean difference of 6.11 ng/mL (95% CI, 3.27-8.96, $P < 0.001$) – a difference that was present irrespective of study design (Fig. 2). When restricted to high-quality studies, PAI-1 antigen levels in patients with MACE were 5.22 ng/mL (95% CI, 2.97-7.54, P < 0.001; Additional file 1: Figure S3). Among seven studies reporting morning blood draws between 7:00 and 10:00 am, PAI-1 antigen levels were higher in those with MACE with a mean difference of 4.61 ng/mL (95% CI, 1.49-7.74, $P = 0.004$; Additional file 1: Figure S4). Meta-regression analysis of timing of the blood draw and acute phase studies was not predictive of the heterogeneity in our selected studies nor did it contribute to a greater understanding of the impact of PAI-1 in its association with MACE (Additional file 1: Table S3).

In contrast to PAI-1 plasma antigen levels, there was no significant difference in PAI-1 activity levels between those with vs. without MACE (mean difference 0.59 IU/mL (95% CI, – 1.63-2.80, $P = 0.60$; Fig. 3). No association between PAI-1 activity levels and MACE was observed when the analysis was restricted to three high-quality studies with a mean difference of 1.14 IU/mL (95% CI, – 3.37-5.65, $P = 0.62$; Additional file 1: Figure S5).

Major adverse cardiovascular events: Pre-existing versus no known coronary artery disease

Overall, among patients without prior coronary artery disease, 12.2% had an event. PAI-1 antigen levels in those without previously known coronary artery disease were on average 6.44 ng/mL higher in those with MACE relative to those without (95% CI, 2.64-10.25, $P < 0.001$; Fig. 4a). In studies that included patients with known CAD, 19.3% had MACE. PAI-1 antigen levels in those with known CAD were on average 5.49 ng/mL higher in those with MACE than those without (95% CI, 0.36-10.63, $P = 0.04$; Fig. 4b). No difference in PAI-1 activity levels between event and control groups was observed in the five studies reporting PAI-1 activity levels and MACE (Additional file 1: Figure S6).

Death

In the five studies that reported mortality data, 126 deaths were observed (17.2% of patients). PAI-1 antigen levels were higher among patients who died (mean difference: 10.34 ng/mL (95% CI, 1.90-18.79, $P = 0.02$; Additional file 1: Figure S7).

Restenosis

In the six studies that examined restenosis following percutaneous coronary intervention (with and without coronary stent implantation), 101 events were observed (29.5% of patients). PAI-1 antigen levels were lower in those with restenosis with a mean difference of – 2.43 ng/mL (95% CI, – 4.48-(– 0.37), $P = 0.02$; Fig. 5a). An additional six studies provided restenosis rates and PAI-1 activity levels. These studies reported restenosis in 119 patients (17.9%). PAI-1 activity was lower in those with restenosis with a mean difference of – 1.73 IU/mL (95% CI: -2.80-(– 0.67), $P = 0.001$; Fig. 5b).

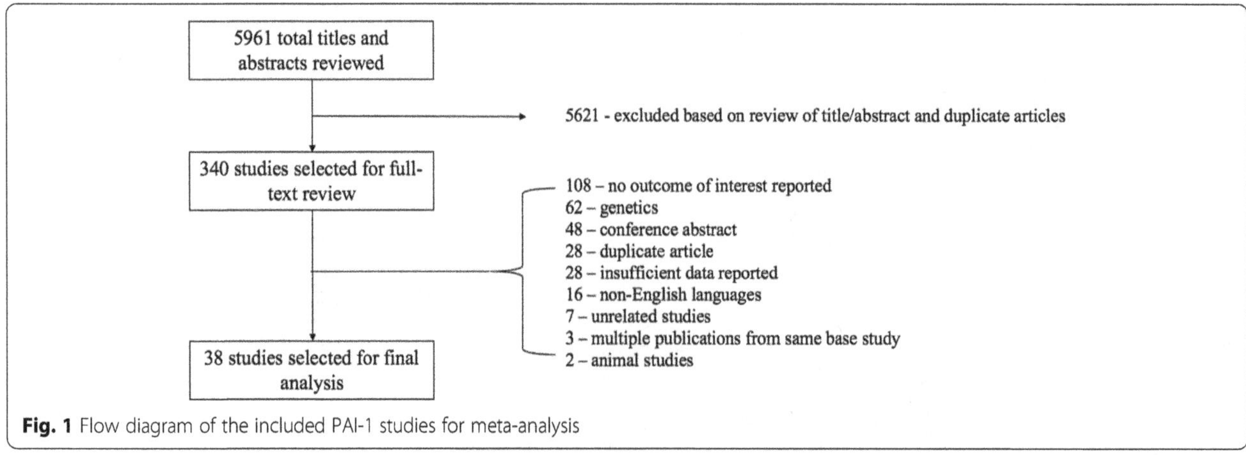

Fig. 1 Flow diagram of the included PAI-1 studies for meta-analysis

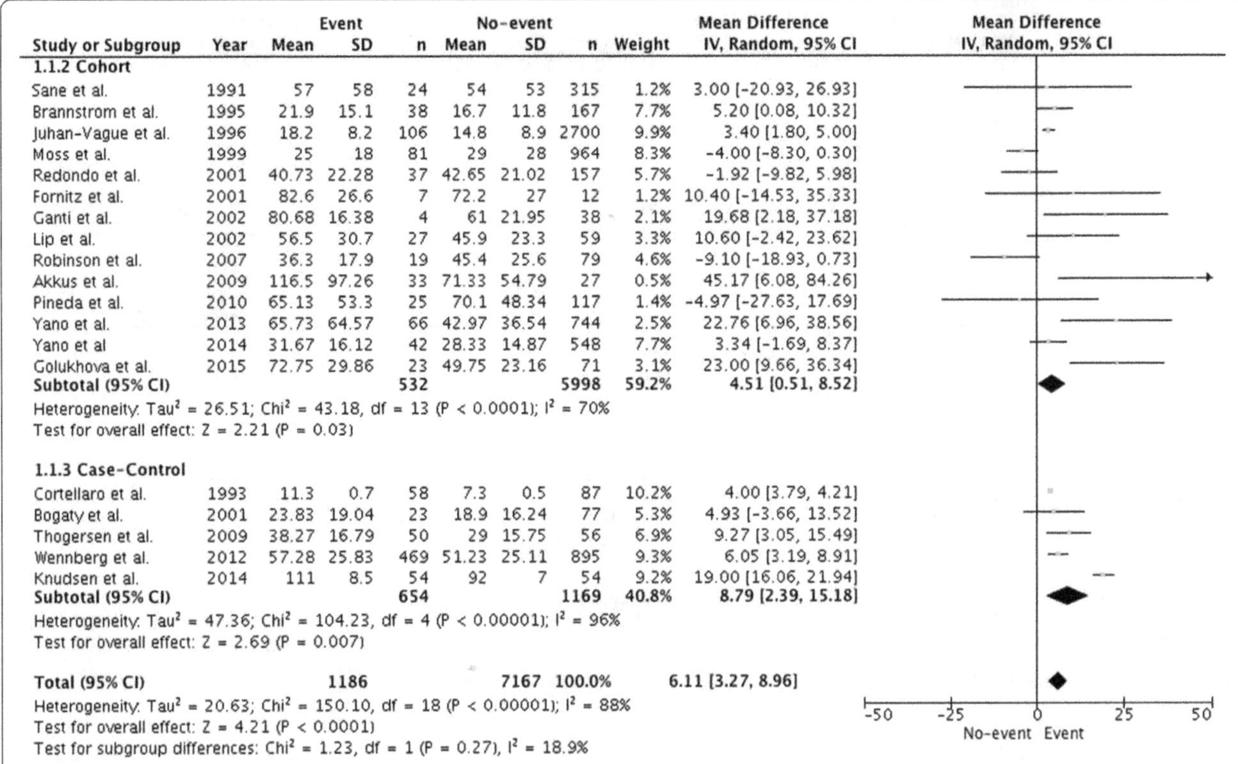

Study or Subgroup Year Event Mean SD n No-event Mean SD n Weight Mean Difference IV, Random, 95% CI
1.1.2 Cohort
Sane et al. 1991 57 58 24 54 53 315 1.2% 3.00 [-20.93, 26.93]
Brannstrom et al. 1995 21.9 15.1 38 16.7 11.8 167 7.7% 5.20 [0.08, 10.32]
Juhan-Vague et al. 1996 18.2 8.2 106 14.8 8.9 2700 9.9% 3.40 [1.80, 5.00]
Moss et al. 1999 25 18 81 29 28 964 8.3% -4.00 [-8.30, 0.30]
Redondo et al. 2001 40.73 22.28 37 42.65 21.02 157 5.7% -1.92 [-9.82, 5.98]
Fornitz et al. 2001 82.6 26.6 7 72.2 27 12 1.2% 10.40 [-14.53, 35.33]
Ganti et al. 2002 80.68 16.38 4 61 21.95 38 2.1% 19.68 [2.18, 37.18]
Lip et al. 2002 56.5 30.7 27 45.9 23.3 59 3.3% 10.60 [-2.42, 23.62]
Robinson et al. 2007 36.3 17.9 19 45.4 25.6 79 4.6% -9.10 [-18.93, 0.73]
Akkus et al. 2009 116.5 97.26 33 71.33 54.79 27 0.5% 45.17 [6.08, 84.26]
Pineda et al. 2010 65.13 53.3 25 70.1 48.34 117 1.4% -4.97 [-27.63, 17.69]
Yano et al. 2013 65.73 64.57 66 42.97 36.54 744 2.5% 22.76 [6.96, 38.56]
Yano et al 2014 31.67 16.12 42 28.33 14.87 548 7.7% 3.34 [-1.69, 8.37]
Golukhova et al. 2015 72.75 29.86 23 49.75 23.16 71 3.1% 23.00 [9.66, 36.34]
Subtotal (95% CI) 532 5998 59.2% 4.51 [0.51, 8.52]
Heterogeneity. Tau² = 26.51; Chi² = 43.18, df = 13 (P < 0.0001); I² = 70%
Test for overall effect: Z = 2.21 (P = 0.03)
1.1.3 Case-Control
Cortellaro et al. 1993 11.3 0.7 58 7.3 0.5 87 10.2% 4.00 [3.79, 4.21]
Bogaty et al. 2001 23.83 19.04 23 18.9 16.24 77 5.3% 4.93 [-3.66, 13.52]
Thogersen et al. 2009 38.27 16.79 50 29 15.75 56 6.9% 9.27 [3.05, 15.49]
Wennberg et al. 2012 57.28 25.83 469 51.23 25.11 895 9.3% 6.05 [3.19, 8.91]
Knudsen et al. 2014 111 8.5 54 92 7 54 9.2% 19.00 [16.06, 21.94]
Subtotal (95% CI) 654 1169 40.8% 8.79 [2.39, 15.18]
Heterogeneity. Tau² = 47.36; Chi² = 104.23, df = 4 (P < 0.00001); I² = 96%
Test for overall effect: Z = 2.69 (P = 0.007)
Total (95% CI) 1186 7167 100.0% 6.11 [3.27, 8.96]
Heterogeneity. Tau² = 20.63; Chi² = 150.10, df = 18 (P < 0.00001); I² = 88%
Test for overall effect: Z = 4.21 (P < 0.0001)
Test for subgroup differences: Chi² = 1.23, df = 1 (P = 0.27), I² = 18.9%
-50 -25 0 25 50
No-event Event

Fig. 2 Comparison of mean PAI-1 antigen levels (ng/mL) in patients with major adverse cardiac events and control patients. Data is expressed as a mean difference and analyzed using a random effects model

High versus low PAI-1 levels

Three studies stratified their data by high versus low PAI-1 antigen levels. These studies reported a MACE rate of 54.4% [15–17]. High PAI-1 antigen levels were associated with a 58% greater risk of MACE compared to low PAI-1 antigen levels (RR 1.58, 95% CI: 1.42-1.76, $P < 0.0001$; Fig. 6).

Discussion

Incident and recurrent cardiovascular events remain important adverse outcomes despite major advances in revascularization and medical therapy. PAI-1 has been associated with MACE, but whether it is solely a marker for these events or a mediator with the potential of representing a unique therapeutic target is uncertain.

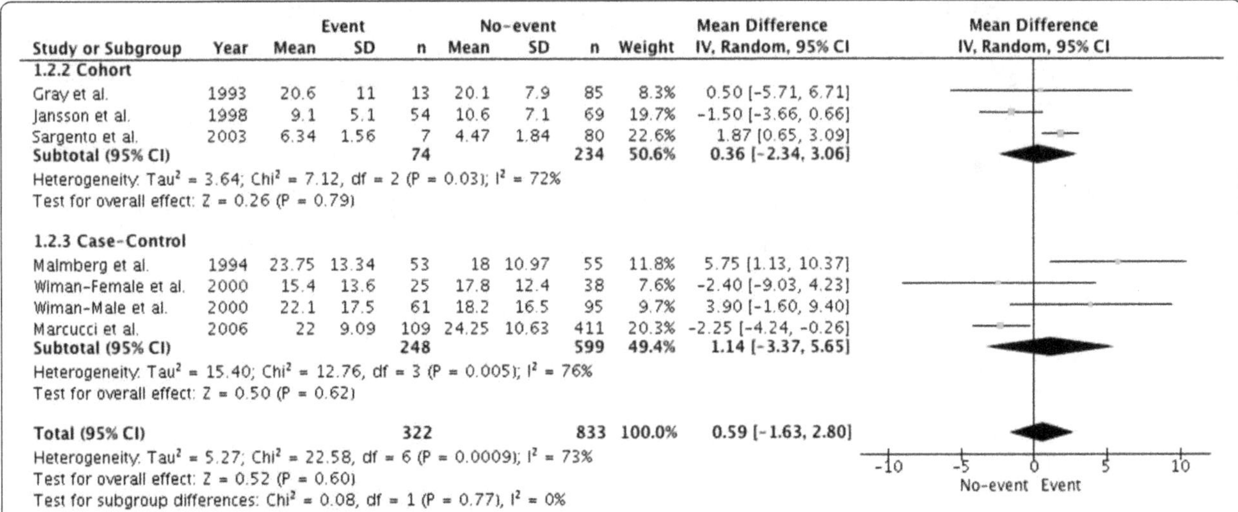

Study or Subgroup Year Event Mean SD n No-event Mean SD n Weight Mean Difference IV, Random, 95% CI
1.2.2 Cohort
Gray et al. 1993 20.6 11 13 20.1 7.9 85 8.3% 0.50 [-5.71, 6.71]
Jansson et al. 1998 9.1 5.1 54 10.6 7.1 69 19.7% -1.50 [-3.66, 0.66]
Sargento et al. 2003 6.34 1.56 7 4.47 1.84 80 22.6% 1.87 [0.65, 3.09]
Subtotal (95% CI) 74 234 50.6% 0.36 [-2.34, 3.06]
Heterogeneity. Tau² = 3.64; Chi² = 7.12, df = 2 (P = 0.03); I² = 72%
Test for overall effect: Z = 0.26 (P = 0.79)
1.2.3 Case-Control
Malmberg et al. 1994 23.75 13.34 53 18 10.97 55 11.8% 5.75 [1.13, 10.37]
Wiman-Female et al. 2000 15.4 13.6 25 17.8 12.4 38 7.6% -2.40 [-9.03, 4.23]
Wiman-Male et al. 2000 22.1 17.5 61 18.2 16.5 95 9.7% 3.90 [-1.60, 9.40]
Marcucci et al. 2006 22 9.09 109 24.25 10.63 411 20.3% -2.25 [-4.24, -0.26]
Subtotal (95% CI) 248 599 49.4% 1.14 [-3.37, 5.65]
Heterogeneity. Tau² = 15.40; Chi² = 12.76, df = 3 (P = 0.005); I² = 76%
Test for overall effect: Z = 0.50 (P = 0.62)
Total (95% CI) 322 833 100.0% 0.59 [-1.63, 2.80]
Heterogeneity. Tau² = 5.27; Chi² = 22.58, df = 6 (P = 0.0009); I² = 73%
Test for overall effect: Z = 0.52 (P = 0.60)
Test for subgroup differences: Chi² = 0.08, df = 1 (P = 0.77), I² = 0%
-10 -5 0 5 10
No-event Event

Fig. 3 Comparison of mean PAI-1 activity levels (IU/mL) in patients with major adverse cardiac events and control patients. Data is expressed as a mean difference and analyzed using a random effects model

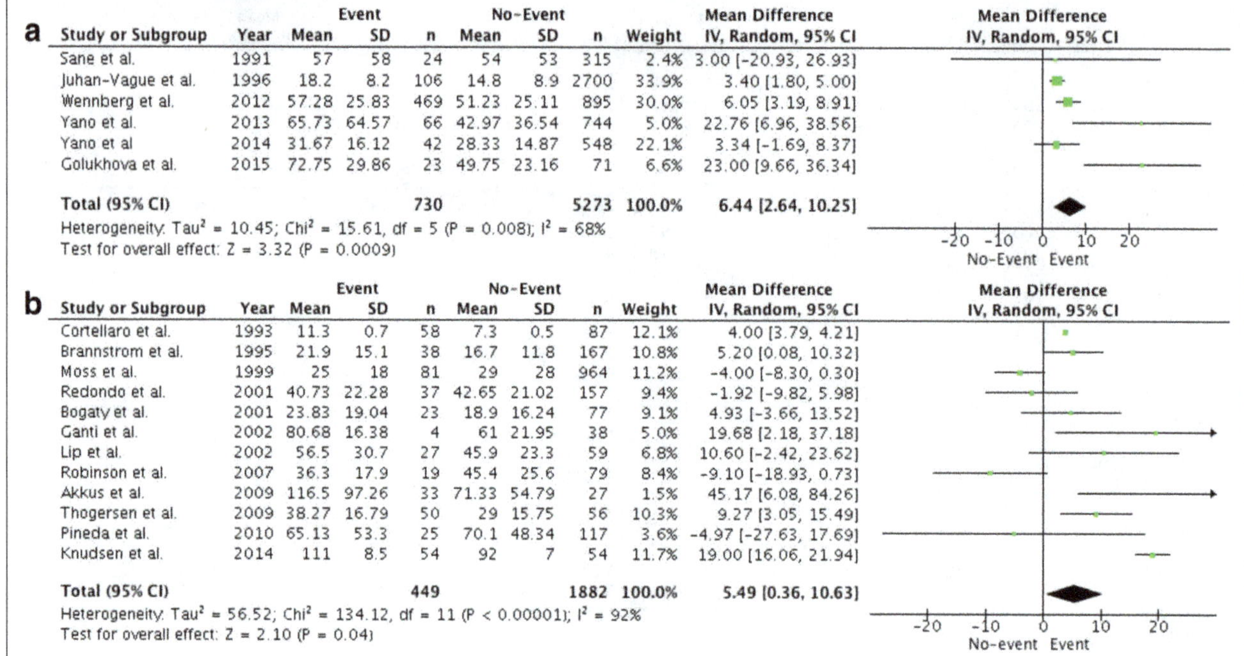

a

Study or Subgroup	Year	Event Mean	Event SD	Event n	No-Event Mean	No-Event SD	No-Event n	Weight	Mean Difference IV, Random, 95% CI
Sane et al.	1991	57	58	24	54	53	315	2.4%	3.00 [-20.93, 26.93]
Juhan-Vague et al.	1996	18.2	8.2	106	14.8	8.9	2700	33.9%	3.40 [1.80, 5.00]
Wennberg et al.	2012	57.28	25.83	469	51.23	25.11	895	30.0%	6.05 [3.19, 8.91]
Yano et al.	2013	65.73	64.57	66	42.97	36.54	744	5.0%	22.76 [6.96, 38.56]
Yano et al	2014	31.67	16.12	42	28.33	14.87	548	22.1%	3.34 [-1.69, 8.37]
Golukhova et al.	2015	72.75	29.86	23	49.75	23.16	71	6.6%	23.00 [9.66, 36.34]
Total (95% CI)				**730**			**5273**	**100.0%**	**6.44 [2.64, 10.25]**

Heterogeneity: Tau² = 10.45; Chi² = 15.61, df = 5 (P = 0.008); I² = 68%
Test for overall effect: Z = 3.32 (P = 0.0009)

b

Study or Subgroup	Year	Event Mean	Event SD	Event n	No-Event Mean	No-Event SD	No-Event n	Weight	Mean Difference IV, Random, 95% CI
Cortellaro et al.	1993	11.3	0.7	58	7.3	0.5	87	12.1%	4.00 [3.79, 4.21]
Brannstrom et al.	1995	21.9	15.1	38	16.7	11.8	167	10.8%	5.20 [0.08, 10.32]
Moss et al.	1999	25	18	81	29	28	964	11.2%	-4.00 [-8.30, 0.30]
Redondo et al.	2001	40.73	22.28	37	42.65	21.02	157	9.4%	-1.92 [-9.82, 5.98]
Bogaty et al.	2001	23.83	19.04	23	18.9	16.24	77	9.1%	4.93 [-3.66, 13.52]
Ganti et al.	2002	80.68	16.38	4	61	21.95	38	5.0%	19.68 [2.18, 37.18]
Lip et al.	2002	56.5	30.7	27	45.9	23.3	59	6.8%	10.60 [-2.42, 23.62]
Robinson et al.	2007	36.3	17.9	19	45.4	25.6	79	8.4%	-9.10 [-18.93, 0.73]
Akkus et al.	2009	116.5	97.26	33	71.33	54.79	27	1.5%	45.17 [6.08, 84.26]
Thogersen et al.	2009	38.27	16.79	50	29	15.75	56	10.3%	9.27 [3.05, 15.49]
Pineda et al.	2010	65.13	53.3	25	70.1	48.34	117	3.6%	-4.97 [-27.63, 17.69]
Knudsen et al.	2014	111	8.5	54	92	7	54	11.7%	19.00 [16.06, 21.94]
Total (95% CI)				**449**			**1882**	**100.0%**	**5.49 [0.36, 10.63]**

Heterogeneity: Tau² = 56.52; Chi² = 134.12, df = 11 (P < 0.00001); I² = 92%
Test for overall effect: Z = 2.10 (P = 0.04)

Fig. 4 Comparison of mean PAI-1 antigen levels (ng/mL) in patients with primary and secondary major adverse cardiac events and control patients. Data is expressed as a mean difference and analyzed using a random effects model. **a** PAI-1 levels (ng/mL) in patients with primary major adverse cardiac events. **b** PAI-1 levels (ng/mL) in patients with secondary major adverse cardiac events

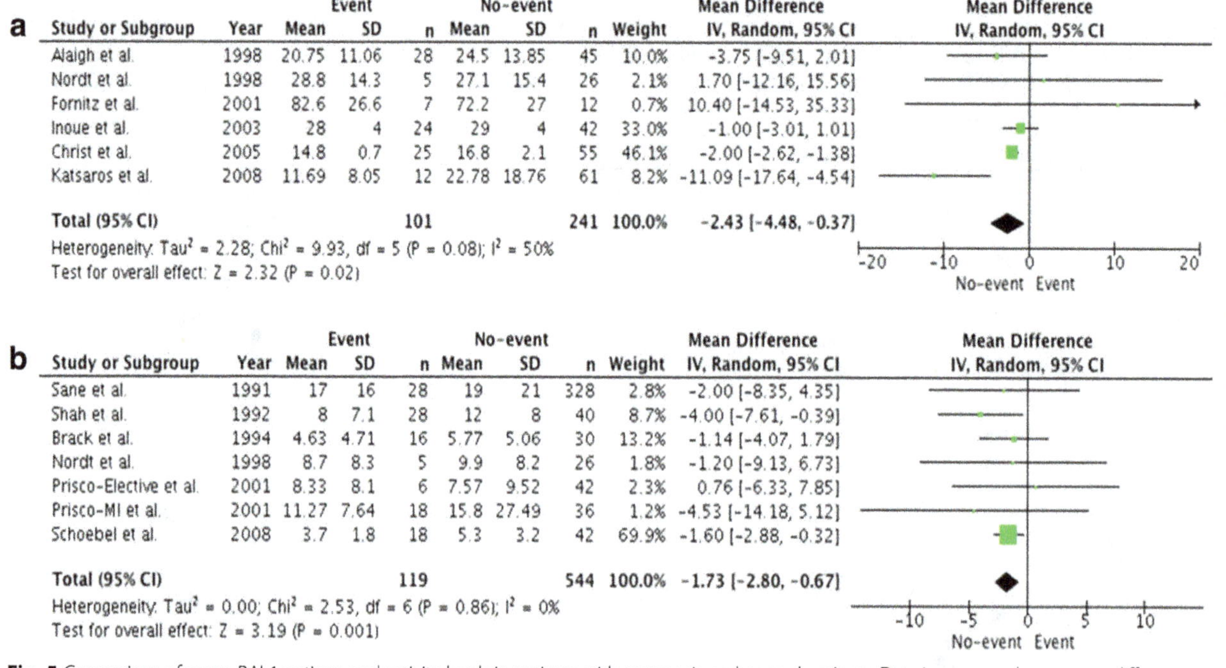

a

Study or Subgroup	Year	Event Mean	Event SD	Event n	No-event Mean	No-event SD	No-event n	Weight	Mean Difference IV, Random, 95% CI
Alaigh et al.	1998	20.75	11.06	28	24.5	13.85	45	10.0%	-3.75 [-9.51, 2.01]
Nordt et al.	1998	28.8	14.3	5	27.1	15.4	26	2.1%	1.70 [-12.16, 15.56]
Fornitz et al.	2001	82.6	26.6	7	72.2	27	12	0.7%	10.40 [-14.53, 35.33]
Inoue et al.	2003	28	4	24	29	4	42	33.0%	-1.00 [-3.01, 1.01]
Christ et al.	2005	14.8	0.7	25	16.8	2.1	55	46.1%	-2.00 [-2.62, -1.38]
Katsaros et al.	2008	11.69	8.05	12	22.78	18.76	61	8.2%	-11.09 [-17.64, -4.54]
Total (95% CI)				**101**			**241**	**100.0%**	**-2.43 [-4.48, -0.37]**

Heterogeneity: Tau² = 2.28; Chi² = 9.93, df = 5 (P = 0.08); I² = 50%
Test for overall effect: Z = 2.32 (P = 0.02)

b

Study or Subgroup	Year	Event Mean	Event SD	Event n	No-event Mean	No-event SD	No-event n	Weight	Mean Difference IV, Random, 95% CI
Sane et al.	1991	17	16	28	19	21	328	2.8%	-2.00 [-8.35, 4.35]
Shah et al.	1992	8	7.1	28	12	8	40	8.7%	-4.00 [-7.61, -0.39]
Brack et al.	1994	4.63	4.71	16	5.77	5.06	30	13.2%	-1.14 [-4.07, 1.79]
Nordt et al.	1998	8.7	8.3	5	9.9	8.2	26	1.8%	-1.20 [-9.13, 6.73]
Prisco-Elective et al.	2001	8.33	8.1	6	7.57	9.52	42	2.3%	0.76 [-6.33, 7.85]
Prisco-MI et al.	2001	11.27	7.64	18	15.8	27.49	36	1.2%	-4.53 [-14.18, 5.12]
Schoebel et al.	2008	3.7	1.8	18	5.3	3.2	42	69.9%	-1.60 [-2.88, -0.32]
Total (95% CI)				**119**			**544**	**100.0%**	**-1.73 [-2.80, -0.67]**

Heterogeneity: Tau² = 0.00; Chi² = 2.53, df = 6 (P = 0.86); I² = 0%
Test for overall effect: Z = 3.19 (P = 0.001)

Fig. 5 Comparison of mean PAI-1 antigen and activity levels in patients with restenosis and control patients. Data is expressed as a mean difference and analyzed using a random effects model. **a** Comparison of mean PAI-1 antigen levels (ng/mL) in patients with restenosis. **b** Comparison of mean PAI-1 activity levels (IU/mL) in patients with restenosis

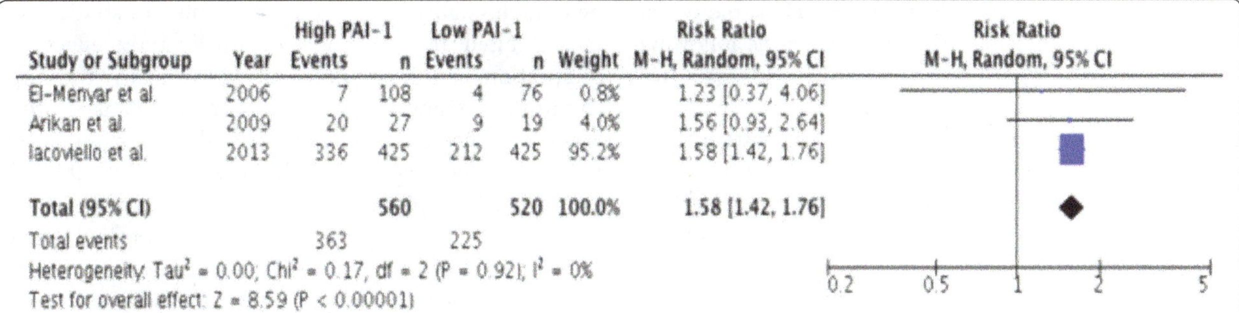

Fig. 6 Comparison of risk of major adverse cardiac events in patients stratified by PAI-1 antigen levels (ng/mL). Data is expressed as a risk ratio and analyzed using a random effects model

Our analysis set out to evaluate the current state of evidence linking PAI-1 antigen and activity levels with these outcomes. Our study suggests that elevated PAI-1 antigen levels are associated with major adverse cardiac events in both primary and secondary event populations. In addition, elevated PAI-1 antigen levels were associated with all-cause mortality. While the populations studied were heterogeneous, the robustness of the association suggests that PAI-1 warrants further study as a marker and potential mediator of adverse cardiovascular events.

Our findings build upon the growing evidence that PAI-1 is a biomarker for MACE in patients with CAD. Tofler et al. identified elevated PAI-1 antigen levels to be predictive of cardiovascular disease [18]. In addition, previous studies of elevated PAI-1 antigen and activity levels predicted acute coronary syndrome after coronary stenting [15, 19–22]. Furthermore, Song et al. recently identified a causal relationship between elevated PAI-1 levels and incident CAD [23]. Our study expands on these findings by identifying elevated PAI-1 antigen levels as being associated with MACE in both primary (incident) and secondary event populations thereby suggesting a broader relevance of PAI-1 antigen levels. In addition, we demonstrate the potential applicability of PAI-1 antigen levels in predicting restenosis, consistent with a previous report by Katsaros et al. [24], which identified that patients with the lowest PAI-1 antigen tertile had a 9.5-fold increased risk of in-stent restenosis in patients managed with modern drug-eluting stents. However, our study, as with those mentioned above, are unable to ascertain if PAI-1 is a mediator or simply a marker of these events. Further study is needed to establish this important distinction.

The association of PAI-1 activity with MACE did not meet our pre-specified thresholds for significance. Although this finding suggests that PAI-1 antigen levels may be more robust as a biomarker, PAI-1 activity is a functional measure of the entire PAI-1 content in the plasma. The measurement of PAI-1 antigen captures the entire PAI-1 content in the sample in the form of free and active PAI-1 (which we refer to as PAI-1 activity), PAI-1 complexed to t-PA or u-PA, and latent PAI-1. Although PAI-1 antigen and activity levels are correlated, antigen levels will not necessarily reflect PAI-1 activity levels [25]. Indeed, at time of acute trauma such as plaque rupture, t-PA will complex with PAI-1 at a 1:1 ratio reducing detectable PAI-1 activity but not PAI-1 antigen levels. In addition, PAI-1 activity is influenced by experimental techniques during sample isolation such as freeze-thaw or sonication [26], low temperature, low pH, and high salt concentrations [27]. Factors which influence PAI-1 activity levels which impacted the significance of our findings include the method of PAI-1 extraction and isolation [26–30], time of blood draw [31], intra- and inter-assay variability in PAI-1 activity and antigen levels [32], and baseline risk factors which influences PAI-1 levels such as smoking [33, 34], high-fat diet [35], and maximal exercise [36]. Finally, in addition to important biological differences, manifest differences in the quality and power of studies examining antigen and activity levels existed which may explain the divergent results.

In-stent restenosis (ISR) is a result of neointimal formation or intimal thickening that narrows the vascular lumen following PCI [37]. The detailed molecular mechanism behind the pathophysiology of ISR has been reviewed elsewhere [38]. Briefly, studies have revealed that the initial recruitment of inflammatory cells is subsequently followed by smooth muscle cells (SMC) and myofibroblasts recruitment, which creates the extracellular matrix that narrows the vascular lumen [38]. SMCs achieve their peak proliferation at 48-96 h post-injury in the media and intima and return to their baseline following re-endothelialization of that artery within 8 weeks [39]. Conflicting evidence exists in the literature in the role of PAI-1 in cell migration. PAI-1 binding to low-density lipoprotein receptor-related protein 1 (LRP1) in SMCs promotes cell migration [40]. However, PAI-1 complexed to vitronectin has been demonstrated to inhibit cell migration and adhesion [41]. Thus, biological plausibility exists to link PAI-1 and restenosis following coronary intervention.

Clinically, low PAI-1 antigen and activity levels have been found to be associated with increased restenosis in our study; however, several limitations exist in these studies. First, these selected studies range from 1991 to 2008, during which time the intervention of choice evolved from balloon angioplasty to bare-metal stents to drug-eluting stents, which reduced the rate of ISR observed today [1]. Second, anti-proliferative agents that coat drug-eluting stents such as paclitaxel promote PAI-1 transcription and translation, impacting PAI-1 levels at the site of injury [42]. Third, PAI-1 activity cannot detect PAI-1 complexed to LRP1 found on smooth muscle cells and endothelial cells as they are no longer in circulation. Finally, since ISR occurs months following intervention, it remains unclear if baseline levels alone would be as predictive as repeated measurements. Repeat measurements of PAI-1 levels in these patients which would provide a comprehensive assessment of temporal PAI-1 levels from baseline to follow-up angiography or re-intervention. Nonetheless, despite these limitations we were able to link basal PAI-1 levels and restenosis. Future studies looking at modern revascularization techniques and temporal patterns of PAI-1 are warranted.

The value of PAI-1 as a biomarker has been questioned. First, PAI-1 expression is influenced by multiple pro-inflammatory conditions and is associated with various cardiovascular risk factors [6, 43]. For example, metabolic syndrome, obesity [44] and hyperinsulinemia [9]/insulin resistance [10] have all been linked with increased PAI-1 levels. In adjusted analysis, the predictive ability of elevated PAI-1 levels has not been independent of other cardiovascular risk factors and its additive benefit in risk prediction models has been lacking [45]. For example, Yarmolinsky et al. [3] reported that patients with diabetes had a significantly higher level of plasma PAI-1, which was associated with MACE. However, diabetics are at increased risk of both index and recurrent events. Accordingly, further studies are needed in more homogenous populations to ascertain the performance of PAI-1 in each individual cohort.

Our study is not without limitations. Relevant data could not be obtained from certain studies and patient level data were not available. In addition, the broad inclusion criteria resulted in a heterogeneous study population with differing PAI-1 measurement techniques. Variations in assays and standardizations as well as natural variations in PAI-1 levels may have influenced our results. For instance, considerable PAI-1 diurnal changes have been observed in previous studies [46, 47]. Most selected studies were of modest sample size and of low or moderate quality with only seven studies deemed to be of high quality [48]. The small number of studies may have limited the detection of small study effects or publication bias in funnel plots [49]. Finally, the large variation in study dates (1991 to 2016) spans a broad range of pharmacologic and revascularization practices, particularly coronary stent development, the introduction of dual antiplatelet therapy, and broadening indications for oral anticoagulation therapy. Accordingly, these findings may not be applicable in patients with specific risk profiles or those on contemporary medical therapy. Finally, while our study is provocative in the association demonstrated interventional studies are needed to link PAI-1 levels mechanistically to MACE.

Conclusion

PAI-1 plasma levels are promising markers for MACE; however, high quality studies in well-defined populations are still needed to robustly evaluate the performance of PAI-1 as a clinical biomarker. Whether PAI-1 is a bona fide therapeutic target remains to be established.

Abbreviations

CAD: Coronary artery disease; MACE: Major adverse cardiovascular events; PAI-1: Plasminogen activator inhibitor-1; PCI: Percutaneous coronary intervention; t-PA: Tissue-type plasminogen activator; u-PA: Urokinase-type plasminogen activator

Acknowledgements

We thank Risa Shorr (R.S.), MLIS (The Ottawa Hospital, General Campus, Ottawa, Ontario, Canada) for peer-review of the MEDLINE literature search strategy.

Funding

R.J. was funded by the Vanier CIHR Canada Graduate Scholarship for his graduate studies.

Authors' contributions

R.J. and B.H. participated in the design, data extraction and analysis, and drafted the manuscript. P.M. participated in data extraction and analysis, and drafted the manuscript. F.D.R. helped design and drafted the manuscript. T.S., P.S., and Y.J. participated in data extraction. S.V. helped design the search strategy utilized for the systematic review. M.A.F. and A.L. was involved in critical revision of the manuscript. Finally, all authors read and approved the final draft of the manuscript.

Competing interests

The authors declare that they have no competing interests.

Author details

[1]CAPITAL Research Group, University of Ottawa Heart Institute, 40 Ruskin Street, H-4238, Ottawa, ON K1Y 4W7, Canada. [2]Department of Cellular and Molecular Medicine, University of Ottawa, Ottawa, ON, Canada. [3]Vascular Biology and Experimental Medicine Laboratory, University of Ottawa Heart Institute, Ottawa, ON, Canada. [4]Division of Cardiology, University of Ottawa Heart Institute, Ottawa, ON, Canada. [5]School of Epidemiology, Public Health and Preventive Medicine, University of Ottawa, Ottawa, ON, Canada. [6]Berkman Library, University of Ottawa Heart Institute, Ottawa, ON, Canada. [7]Department of Health Research Methods, Evidence, and Impact, McMaster University, Hamilton, ON, Canada.

References

1. Simard T, Hibbert B, Ramirez FD, Froeschl M, Chen YX, O'Brien ER. The evolution of coronary stents: a brief review. Can J Cardiol. 2014;30:35–45.
2. Lucore CL, Sobel BE. Interactions of tissue-type plasminogen activator with plasma inhibitors and their pharmacologic implications. Circulation. 1988;77: 660–9.
3. Yarmolinsky J, Bordin Barbieri N, Weinmann T, Ziegelmann PK, Duncan BB, Ines Schmidt M. Plasminogen activator inhibitor-1 and type 2 diabetes: a systematic review and meta-analysis of observational studies. Sci Rep. 2016; 6:17714.
4. Ghosh AK, Vaughan DE. PAI-1 in tissue fibrosis. J Cell Physiol. 2012; 227:493–507.
5. De Taeye B, Smith LH, Vaughan DE. Plasminogen activator inhibitor-1: a common denominator in obesity, diabetes and cardiovascular disease. Curr Opin Pharmacol. 2005;5:149–54.
6. Srikanthan K, Feyh A, Visweshwar H, Shapiro JI, Sodhi K. Systematic review of metabolic syndrome biomarkers: a panel for early detection, management, and risk stratification in the west Virginian population. Int J Med Sci. 2016;13:25–38.
7. Thogersen AM, Jansson JH, Boman K, Nilsson TK, Weinehall L, Huhtasaari F, Hallmans G. High plasminogen activator inhibitor and tissue plasminogen activator levels in plasma precede a first acute myocardial infarction in both men and women - evidence for the fibrinolytic system as an independent primary risk factor. Circulation. 1998;98:2241–7.
8. Meigs JB, O'Donnell CJ, Tofler GH, Benjamin EJ, Fox CS, Lipinska I, Nathan DM, Sullivan LM, D'Agostino RB, Wilson PW. Hemostatic markers of endothelial dysfunction and risk of incident type 2 diabetes: the Framingham offspring study. Diabetes. 2006;55:530–7.
9. Trost S, Pratley R, Sobel B. Impaired fibrinolysis and risk for cardiovascular disease in the metabolic syndrome and type 2 diabetes. Curr Diab Rep. 2006;6:47–54.
10. Sobel BE, Taatjes DJ, Schneider DJ. Intramural plasminogen activator inhibitor type-1 and coronary atherosclerosis. Arterioscler Thromb Vasc Biol. 2003;23:1979–89.
11. Brazionis L, Rowley K, Jenkins A, Itsiopoulos C, O'Dea K. Plasminogen activator inhibitor-1 activity in type 2 diabetes - a different relationship with coronary heart disease and diabetic retinopathy. Arterioscler Thromb Vasc Biol. 2008;28:786–91.
12. Anderson L, Oldridge N, Thompson DR, Zwisler AD, Rees K, Martin N, Taylor RS. Exercise-based cardiac rehabilitation for coronary heart disease: Cochrane systematic review and Meta-analysis. J Am Coll Cardiol. 2016;67:1–12.
13. G Wells, B Shea, D O'Connell, J Peterson, V Welch, M Losos, P Tugwell. The Newcastle-Ottawa Scale (NOS) for assessing the quality of nonrandomised studies in meta-analyses, 2010. http://www.ohri.ca/programs/clinical_epidemiology/oxford.asp. Accessed 4 Jan 2017.
14. Wan X, Wang W, Liu J, Tong T. Estimating the sample mean and standard deviation from the sample size, median, range and/or interquartile range. BMC Med Res Methodol. 2014;14:135.
15. Iacoviello L, Agnoli C, De Curtis A, di Castelnuovo A, Giurdanella MC, Krogh V, Mattiello A, Matullo G, Sacerdote C, Tumino R, et al. Type 1 plasminogen activator inhibitor as a common risk factor for cancer and ischaemic vascular disease: the EPICOR study. BMJ Open. 2013;3:e003725.
16. El-Menyar AA, Altamimi OM, Gomaa MM, Dabdoob W, Abbas AA, Abdel Rahman MO, Bener A, Albinali HA. Clinical and biochemical predictors affect the choice and the short-term outcomes of different thrombolytic agents in acute myocardial infarction. Coronary artery disease. 2006;17:431–7.
17. Arikan H, Koc M, Tuglular S, Ozener C, Akoglu E. Elevated Plasma Levels of PAI-1 Predict Cardiovascular Events and Cardiovascular Mortality in Prevalent Peritoneal Dialysis Patients. Ren Fail. 2009;31:438–45.
18. Tofler GH, Massaro J, O'Donnell CJ, Wilson PW, Vasan RS, Sutherland PA, Meigs JB, Levy D, D'Agostino RB Sr. Plasminogen activator inhibitor and the risk of cardiovascular disease: the Framingham heart study. Thromb Res. 2016;140:30–5.
19. Marcucci R, Brogi D, Sofi F, Giglioli C, Valente S, Liotta AA, Lenti M, Gori AM, Prisco D, Abbate R, Gensini GF. PAI-1 and homocysteine, but not lipoprotein (a) and thrombophilic polymorphisms, are independently associated with the occurrence of major adverse cardiac events after successful coronary stenting. Heart. 2006;92:377–81.
20. Christ G, Nikfardjam M, Huber-Beckmann R, Gottsauner-Wolf M, Glogar D, Binder BR, Wojta J, Huber K. Predictive value of plasma plasminogen activator inhibitor-1 for coronary restenosis: dependence on stent implantation and antithrombotic medication. J Thromb Haemost. 2005;3:233–9.
21. Garg N, Goyal N, Strawn TL, Wu J, Mann KM, Lawrence DA, Fay WP. Plasminogen activator Inhibitor-1 and Vitronectin expression level and stoichiometry regulate vascular smooth muscle cell migration through physiological collagen matrices. J Thromb Haemost. 2010;8:1847–54.
22. Sinkovic A. Prognostic role of plasminogen-activator-inhibitor-1 levels in treatment with streptokinase of patients with acute myocardial infarction. Clin Cardiol. 2000;23:486–9.
23. Song C, Burgess S, Eicher JD, O'Donnell CJ, Johnson AD. Causal effect of plasminogen activator inhibitor type 1 on coronary heart disease. J Am Heart Assoc. 2017;6. https://doi.org/10.1161/JAHA.116.004918.
24. Katsaros KM, Speidl WS, Kastl SP, Zorn G, Huber K, Maurer G, Glogar D, Wojta J, Christ G. Plasminogen activator inhibitor-1 predicts coronary in-stent restenosis of drug-eluting stents. J Thromb Haemost. 2008;6:508–13.
25. Sakata Y, Murakami T, Noro A, Mori K, Matsuda M. The specific activity of plasminogen activator inhibitor-1 in disseminated intravascular coagulation with acute promyelocytic leukemia. Blood. 1991;77:1949–57.
26. Brogren H, Wallmark K, Deinum J, Karlsson L, Jern S. Platelets retain high levels of active plasminogen activator inhibitor 1. PLoS One. 2011;6:e26762.
27. Sancho E, Tonge DW, Hockney RC, Booth NA. Purification and characterization of active and stable recombinant plasminogen-activator inhibitor accumulated at high levels in Escherichia coli. Eur J Biochem. 1994;224:125–34.
28. Hekman CM, Loskutoff DJ. Endothelial cells produce a latent inhibitor of plasminogen activators that can be activated by denaturants. J Biol Chem. 1985;260:11581–7.
29. Gils A, Declerck PJ. Modulation of plasminogen activator inhibitor 1 by triton X-100–identification of two consecutive conformational transitions. Thromb Haemost. 1998;80:286–91.
30. Andreasen PA, Egelund R, Jensen S, Rodenburg KW. Solvent effects on activity and conformation of plasminogen activator inhibitor-1. Thromb Haemost. 1999;81:407–14.
31. Scheer FA, Shea SA. Human circadian system causes a morning peak in prothrombotic plasminogen activator inhibitor-1 (PAI-1) independent of the sleep/wake cycle. Blood. 2014;123:590–3.
32. Declerck PJ, Alessi MC, Verstreken M, Kruithof EK, Juhan-Vague I, Collen D. Measurement of plasminogen activator inhibitor 1 in biologic fluids with a murine monoclonal antibody-based enzyme-linked immunosorbent assay. Blood. 1988;71:220–5.
33. Scarabin PY, Aillaud MF, Amouyel P, Evans A, Luc G, Ferrieres J, Arveiler D, Juhan-Vague I. Associations of fibrinogen, factor VII and PAI-1 with baseline findings among 10,500 male participants in a prospective study of myocardial infarction–the PRIME study. Prospective epidemiological study of myocardial infarction. Thromb Haemost. 1998;80:749–56.
34. Simpson AJ, Gray RS, Moore NR, Booth NA. The effects of chronic smoking on the fibrinolytic potential of plasma and platelets. Br J Haematol. 1997;97:208–13.
35. Byrne CD, Wareham NJ, Martensz ND, Humphries SE, Metcalfe JC, Grainger DJ. Increased PAI activity and PAI-1 antigen occurring with an oral fat load: associations with PAI-1 genotype and plasma active TGF-beta levels. Atherosclerosis. 1998;140:45–53.
36. Cooper JA, Nagelkirk PR, Coughlin AM, Pivarnik JM, Womack CJ. Temporal changes in tPA and PAI-1 after maximal exercise. Med Sci Sports Exerc. 2004;36:1884–7.
37. Jung RG, Simard T, Labinaz A, Ramirez FD, Di Santo P, Motazedian P, Rochman R, Gaudet C, Faraz MA, Beanlands RSB, Hibbert B. Role of plasminogen activator inhibitor-1 in coronary pathophysiology. Thrombosis Res. 2018;164:54-62.
38. Pourdjabbar A, Hibbert B, Simard T, Ma X, O'Brien ER. Pathogenesis of Neointima formation following vascular injury. Cardiovasc Hematol Disord Drug Targets. 2011;11:30–9.
39. Clowes AW, Reidy MA, Clowes MM. Kinetics of cellular proliferation after arterial injury. I. Smooth muscle growth in the absence of endothelium. Lab Investig. 1983;49:327–33.
40. Luo M, Ji Y, Luo Y, Li R, Fay WP, Wu J. Plasminogen activator Inhibitor-1 regulates the vascular expression of Vitronectin. J Thromb Haemost. 2017; 15:2451-60.
41. Czekay RP, Wilkins-Port CE, Higgins SP, Freytag J, Overstreet JM, Klein RM, Higgins CE, Samarakoon R, Higgins PJ. PAI-1: an integrator of cell signaling and migration. Int J Cell Biol. 2011;2011:562481.

42. Muldowney JA 3rd, Stringham JR, Levy SE, Gleaves LA, Eren M, Piana RN, Vaughan DE. Antiproliferative agents alter vascular plasminogen activator inhibitor-1 expression: a potential prothrombotic mechanism of drug-eluting stents. Arterioscler Thromb Vasc Biol. 2007;27:400–6.
43. Iacoviello L, Agnoli C, De Curtis A, Cutrone A, Giurdanella MC, Guarrera S, Krogh V, Matullo G, Panico S, Sacerdote C, et al. Type 1 plasminogen activator inhibitor (PAI-1) and risk of acute coronary syndrome in the european prospective investigation into cancer (EPIC)-Italy cohort. Blood Transfus. 2012;10:s37.
44. Alessi MC, Juhan-Vague I. PAI-1 and the metabolic syndrome: links, causes, and consequences. Arterioscler Thromb Vasc Biol. 2006;26:2200–7.
45. Johansson L, Jansson JH, Boman K, Nilsson TK, Stegmayr B, Hallmans G. Tissue plasminogen activator, plasminogen activator inhibitor-1, and tissue plasminogen activator/plasminogen activator inhibitor-1 complex as risk factors for the development of a first stroke. Stroke. 2000;31:26–32.
46. Angleton P, Chandler WL, Schmer G. Diurnal variation of tissue-type plasminogen activator and its rapid inhibitor (PAI-1). Circulation. 1989;79:101–6.
47. Chong NW, Codd V, Chan D, Samani NJ. Circadian clock genes cause activation of the human PAI-1 gene promoter with 4G/5G allelic preference. FEBS Lett. 2006;580:4469–72.
48. Bae JM. A suggestion for quality assessment in systematic reviews of observational studies in nutritional epidemiology. Epidemiol Health. 2016;38:e2016014.
49. Lau J, Ioannidis JP, Terrin N, Schmid CH, Olkin I. The case of the misleading funnel plot. BMJ. 2006;333:597–600.
50. Sane DC, Stump DC, Topol EJ, Sigmon KN, Kereiakes DJ, George BS, Mantell SJ, Macy E, Collen D, Califf RM. Correlation between baseline plasminogen activator inhibitor levels and clinical outcome during therapy with tissue plasminogen activator for acute myocardial infarction. Thrombosis and haemostasis. 1991;65:275–9.
51. Cortellaro M, Cofrancesco E, Boschetti C, Mussoni L, Donati MB, Cardillo M, Catalano M, Gabrielli L, Lombardi B, Specchia G, et al. Increased Fibrin Turnover and High Pai-1 Activity as Predictors of Ischemic Events in Atherosclerotic Patients - a Case-Control Study. Arterioscler Thromb. 1993;13:1412–7.
52. Brannstrom M, Jansson JH, Boman K, Nilsson TK. Endothelial Hemostatic Factors May Be Associated with Mortality in Patients on Long-Term Anticoagulant Treatment. Thromb Haemost. 1995;74:612–5.
53. JuhanVague I, Pyke SDM, Alessi MC, Jespersen J, Haverkate F, Thompson SG. Fibrinolytic factors and the risk of myocardial infarction or sudden death in patients with angina pectoris. Circulation. 1996;94:2057–63.
54. Nordt TK, Moser M, Kohler B, Ruef J, Peter K, Kubler W, Bode C. Augmented platelet aggregation as predictor of reocclusion after thrombolysis in acute myocardial infarction. Thromb Haemost. 1998;80:881–6.
55. Alaigh P, Hoffman CJ, Korlipara G, Neuroth A, Dervan JP, Lawson WE, Hultin MB. Lipoprotein(a) level does not predict restenosis after percutaneous transluminal coronary angioplasty. Arterioscler Thromb Vasc Biol. 1998;18:1281–6.
56. Moss AJ, Goldstein RE, Marder VJ, Sparks CE, Oakes D, Greenberg H, Weiss HJ, Zareba W, Brown MW, Liang CS, et al. Thrombogenic factors and recurrent coronary events. Circulation. 1999;99:2517–22.
57. Redondo M, Carroll VA, Mauron T, Demarmels Biasiutti F, Binder BR, Lammle B, Wuillemin WA. Hemostatic and fibrinolytic parameters in survivors of myocardial infarction: A low plasma level of plasminalpha2-antiplasmin complex is an independent predictor of coronary re-events. Blood Coagulation and Fibrinolysis. 2001;12:17–24.
58. Fornitz GG, Nielsen P, Amtorp O, Kassis E, Abildgard U, Sloth C, Winther K, Orskov H, Dalsgard J, Husted S. Impaired fibrinolysis determines the outcome of percutaneus transluminal coronary angioplasty (PTCA). Eur J Clin Invest. 2001;31:586–92.
59. Bogaty P, Poirier P, Simard S, Boyer L, Solymoss S, Dagenais GR. Biological profiles in subjects with recurrent acute coronary events compared with subjects with long-standing stable angina. Circulation. 2001;103:3062–8.
60. Ganti AK, Potti A, Yegnanarayan R. Plasma tissue plasminogen activator and plasminogen activator inhibitor-1 levels in acute myocardial infarction. Pathophysiol Haemost Thromb. 2002;32:80–4.
61. Lip GYH, Blann AD, Farooqi IS, Zarifis J, Sagar G, Beevers DG. Sequential alterations in haemorheology, endothelial dysfunction, platelet activation and thrombogenesis in relation to prognosis following acute stroke: The West Birmingham Stroke Project. Blood Coagul Fibrinolysis. 2002;13:339–47.
62. Inoue T, Yaguchi I, Mizoguchi K, Uchida T, Takayanagi K, Hayashi T, Morooka S, Eguchi Y. Accelerated plasminogen activator inhibitor may prevent late restenosis after coronary stenting in acute myocardial infarction. Clin Cardiol. 2003;26:153–7.
63. Robinson SD, Ludlam CA, Boon NA, Newby DE. Endothelial fibrinolytic capacity predicts future adverse cardiovascular events in patients with coronary heart disease. Arterioscler Thromb Vasc Biol. 2007;27:1651–6.
64. Thogersen AM, Nilsson TK, Weinehall L, Boman K, Eliasson M, Hallmans G, Jansson J-H. Changes in plasma C-reactive protein and hemostatic factors prior to and after a first myocardial infarction with a median follow-up time of 8 years. Blood coagulation & fibrinolysis : an international journal in haemostasis and thrombosis. 2009;20:340–6.
65. Akkus MN, Polat G, Yurtdas M, Akcay B, Ercetin N, Cicek D, Doven O, Sucu N. Admission Levels of CReactive Protein and Plasminogen Activator Inhibitor-1 in Patients With Acute Myocardial Infarction With and Without Cardiogenic Shock or Heart Failure on Admission. Int Heart J. 2009;50:33–45.
66. Pineda J, Marin F, Marco P, Roldan V, Valencia J, Ruiz-Nodar JM, Sogorb F, Lip GYH. Premature coronary artery disease in young (age < 45) subjects: Interactions of lipid profile, thrombophilic and haemostatic markers. Int J Cardiol. 2009;136:222–5.
67. Wennberg P, Wensley F, Di Angelantonio E, Johansson L, Boman K, Rumley A, Lowe G, Hallmans G, Danesh J, Jansson JH. Haemostatic and inflammatory markers are independently associated with myocardial infarction in men and women. Thromb Res. 2012;129:68–73.
68. Yano Y, Hoshide S, Shimada K, Kario K. The Impact of Cigarette Smoking on 24-Hour Blood Pressure, Inflammatory and Hemostatic Activity, and Cardiovascular Risk in Japanese Hypertensive Patients. J Clin Hypertens. 2013;15:234–40.
69. Yano Y, Nakazato M, Toshinai K, Inokuchi T, Matsuda S, Hidaka T, Hayakawa M, Kangawa K, Shimada K, Kario K. Circulating Des-acyl Ghrelin Improves Cardiovascular Risk Prediction in Older Hypertensive Patients. Am J Hypertens. 2014;27:727–33.
70. Knudsen A, Katzenstein TL, Benfield T, Jorgensen NR, Kronborg G, Gerstoft J, Obel N, Kjaer A, Lebech A-M. Plasma plasminogen activator inhibitor-1 predicts myocardial infarction in HIV-1-infected individuals. AIDS (London, England). 2014;28:1171–9.
71. Golukhova EZ, Grigorian MV, Ryabinina MN, Bulaeva NI, Fortmann S, Serebruany VL. Independent Predictors of Major Adverse Events following Coronary Stenting over 28 Months of Follow-Up. Cardiology. 2015;132:176–81.
72. Shah PK, Amin J. Low high density lipoprotein level is associated with increased restenosis rate after coronary angioplasty. Circulation. 1992;85: 1279–85.
73. Gray RP, Yudkin JS, Patterson DL. Enzymatic evidence of impaired reperfusion in diabetic patients after thrombolytic therapy for acute myocardial infarction: a role for plasminogen activator inhibitor? British heart journal. 1993;70:530–6.
74. Malmberg K, Bavenholm P, Hamsten A. Clinical and biochemical factors associated with prognosis after myocardial infarction at a young age. Journal of the American College of Cardiology. 1994;24:592–9.
75. Brack MJ, More RS, Pringle S, Gershlick AH. Absence of a Prothrombotic State in Restenotic Patients. Coronary Artery Dis. 1994;5:501–6.
76. Jansson JH, Nilsson TK, Johnson O, et al. Heart (British Cardiac Society). 1998; 80:334–7.
77. Wiman B, Andersson T, Hallqvist J, Reuterwall C, Ahlbom A, deFaire U. Plasma levels of tissue plasminogen activator/plasminogen activator inhibitor-1 complex and von willebrand factor are significant risk markers for recurrent myocardial infarction in the Stockholm Heart Epidemiology Program (SHEEP) study. Arterioscler Thromb Vasc Biol. 2000;20:2019–23.
78. Prisco D, Antonucci E, Fedi S, Margheri M, Giglioli C, Comeglio M, Lombardi A, Chioccioli M, Abbate R, Gensini GF. D-Dimer increase after percutaneous transluminal angioplasty and clinical recurrence after primary revascularization in acute myocardial infarction? A pilot study. Clin Exper Med. 2001;1:219–24.
79. Sargento L, Saldanha C, Monteiro J, Perdigao C, Martins e Silva J. Evidence of prolonged disturbances in the haemostatic, hemorheologic and inflammatory profiles in transmural myocardial infarction survivors. Thrombosis and haemostasis. 2003;89:892–903.
80. Schoebel FC, Peters AJ, Kreis I, Gradaus F, Heins M, Jax TW. Relevance of hemostasis on restenosis in clinically stable patients undergoing elective PTCA. Thromb Res. 2008;122:229–36.

21

Decreased antithrombin activity in the early phase of trauma is strongly associated with extravascular leakage, but not with antithrombin consumption

Hironori Matsumoto*, Jun Takeba, Kensuke Umakoshi, Satoshi Kikuchi, Muneaki Ohshita, Suguru Annen, Naoki Moriyama, Yuki Nakabayashi, Norio Sato and Mayuki Aibiki

Abstract

Background: We conducted a prospective observational study for investigating coagulofibrinolytic changes and mechanisms of antithrombin (AT) alternations in trauma.

Methods: Trauma patients hospitalized for more than seven days were analyzed for coagulofibrinolytic biomarkers. The patients were stratified into two groups according to AT activity level on admission (day 0), comprising normal AT and low AT patients.

Results: Thirty-nine patients (median Injury Severity Score 20) exhibited initial coagulatory activation and triphasic fibrinolytic changes. AT activity did not show a negative linear correlation with levels of thrombin-antithrombin complex (TAT), a marker of coagulation activity and AT consumption, but was strongly correlated with levels of albumin (Alb), an index of vascular permeability, on day 0 ($r = 0.702$, $p < 0.001$). Furthermore, Alb was one of the independent predictors for AT on day 0. IL-6 on day 0 and thrombomodulin (TM) levels during the study period, reflecting systemic inflammation and endothelial cell injury, respectively, were significantly higher in the lower AT group ($n = 10$) than in the normal group ($n = 29$) (IL-6, $p = 0.004$; TM, $p = 0.017$). On days 2 and 4, TAT levels in the lower AT group were significantly higher than in the normal group.

Conclusions: Trauma caused clear triphasic coagulofibrinolytic changes. Decreased AT in the later phase might lead to a prolonged hypercoagulation. AT reduction in the initial phase of trauma is strongly associated with extravascular leakage as suggested by the association of Alb depletion with IL-6 and TM elevation, but not with AT consumption.

Keywords: Albumin, Antithrombin, Coagulofibrinolysis, Consumption coagulopathy, Extravascular leakage, Thrombin activation, Trauma induced coagulopathy

* Correspondence: matsumotohiro0611@yahoo.co.jp
Department of Emergency and Critical Care Medicine, Ehime University, Graduate School of Medicine, Shitsukawa 454, Toon City, Ehime 791-0295, Japan

Background

Trauma is well known to induce dynamic coagulofibrinolytic changes, which increase bleeding tendency in the initial phase of trauma when the hemostasis becomes uncontrollable [1, 2]. Coagulofibrinolytic disorder has been termed trauma-induced coagulopathy (TIC). The mechanisms of this disorder are still controversial, though they may include disseminated intravascular coagulation (DIC) with a fibrinolytic phenotype or acute traumatic coagulopathy (ATC) [3–5].

The pathophysiology of DIC in the early phase of trauma consists of coagulation activation, hyperfibrinolysis and consumption coagulopathy. Tissue injury due to trauma leads to systemic coagulation activation and thrombin generation via procoagulants such as damage-associated molecular patterns (DAMPs), microparticles or tissue factors. Trauma also induces impairment in anticoagulant activities, which causes dysregulation of coagulation activation and promotes systemic hypercoagulation. Simultaneously, hyperfibrinolysis occurs through the expression of tissue plasminogen activator (t-PA). In the first hours after trauma, plasminogen activator inhibitor-1 (PAI-1) activity has not increased sufficiently to counteract this, and hyperfibrinolysis consumes α_2-plasmin inhibitor (α_2PI), which accelerates further fibrinolysis. This pattern of hypercoagulation and hyperfibrinolysis causes consumption of platelets and coagulation factors, resulting in DIC with a fibrinolytic phenotype characterized by bleeding tendency when hemostasis becomes dysregulated [3]. On the other hand, ATC is a state of activation of the anticoagulant protein C (PC) pathway caused by shock and tissue hypoperfusion, leading to hypocoagulation and subsequent fibrinolysis. Activated PC pathway also abrogates PAI-1 and increases t-PA, resulting in further hyperfibrinolysis [4, 5].

Antithrombin (AT) plays an important role in anticoagulation against intravascular thrombin formation through its ability to bind and inactivate thrombin by forming a thrombin-antithrombin complex (TAT). A decrease in AT level is well known to occur in the early phase of trauma as one of the factors impairing anticoagulation. It is especially notable that AT depletion occurs immediately after trauma [6–9]. Some reports have suggested that decreased AT levels are associated with persistent thrombin generation which could be a potential risk of subsequent thromboembolic complications in trauma patients [7, 10, 11]. Thus in the initial phase of trauma we need to manage not only bleeding tendency, but also hypercoagulation due to the impairment of the anticoagulation system in the subsequent phase. Several studies addressing sepsis or septic DIC have suggested that decreased AT levels occur due to extravascular leakage, increased AT consumption, decreased protein synthesis or degradation by enzymes released from neutrophils [12–15]. Nevertheless, the mechanism of AT depletion in trauma is still unclear. Furthermore, coagulofibrinolytic responses in patients who survive bleeding or organ damage in the early phase of trauma have not been well evaluated. Accordingly, in this study we focused on the impairment in anticoagulation that develops subsequent to the initial coagulopathy in patients who were admitted for longer than seven days as an inclusion criterion. We hypothesized that impaired anticoagulation in trauma would lead to problems even after the initial coagulopathy and organ damage had been overcome. Thus, we carried out a prospective observational study to survey dynamic changes in coagulofibrinolytic responses and to investigate the mechanisms as well as the influence of AT reduction.

Methods

Study design

We performed a prospective observational study collecting the data of trauma patients admitted to the tertiary Ehime University Hospital in Japan commencing in January 2015 and ending in April 2016. This study was approved by the Institutional Local Ethics Committee for Clinical Studies. Informed consent was obtained from all patients or next of kin in accordance with the Declaration of Helsinki.

Patient selection and criteria

All adult trauma patients (≥18 years) who were admitted to our hospital either immediately following trauma or after transfer from another hospital with basically no therapeutic intervention and who were subsequently hospitalized for more than seven days were enrolled. We excluded patients who had received therapeutic interventions, including transfusion, more than 500 mL of fluid administration or medication, before admission to our hospital; those who died during initial treatment at the emergency department; those who had at least one episode of cardiac arrest; those who received anticoagulant therapy; and those who had clotting disorders such as liver cirrhosis or advanced malignancies.

Demographic data, examination findings, treatment history and mortality were recorded. Systemic inflammatory response syndrome (SIRS) was defined according to the consensus conference of the American College of Chest Physicians/Society of Critical Care Medicine [16]. Diagnoses of DIC were made based on the Japanese Association for Acute Medicine (JAAM) DIC criteria [17], by which patients were diagnosed with DIC if they had a score of 4 or higher.

The normal range of plasma AT activity is reported as 80–130% [18, 19], so we stratified the patients into two groups according to their AT levels on arrival (Day 0): normal AT group; ≥80% and lower AT group; < 80%.

Blood sampling and measurement

Blood sampling was performed immediately upon arrival (day 0) and on days 1, 2, 4 and 6. We routinely measured blood counts and biochemistries including albumin (Alb) with TBA-c16000 (Toshiba Medical Systems, Tochigi, Japan) and XE-5000 (Sysmex, Hyogo, Japan) devices. We also used CP-2000 (Sekisui Medical, Tokyo, Japan) and STACIA (LSI Medience, Tokyo, Japan) devices to measure the biomarkers of coagulofibrinolysis, namely, prothrombin time (PT), activated partial thromboplastin time (APTT), hepaplastin test (HPT), fibrinogen (Fbg), fibrin/fibrinogen degradation product (FDP), D-dimer, thrombin-antithrombin complex (TAT), plasmin-α_2-plasmin inhibitor complex (PIC), antithrombin (AT), protein C (PC), α_2-plasmin inhibitor (α_2PI) and plasminogen (PLG). After sampling, the blood samples were centrifuged at 3300 rpm for 15 min at 4 °C, and serum and plasma samples were stored at − 80 °C for subsequent analyses. We also measured total plasminogen activator inhibitor-1 (tPAI-1) on days 0, 1, 2 and 6, thrombomodulin (TM) on days 0, 2 and 6, and IL-6 on day 0 (LSI Medience). We also evaluated the development of deep vein thrombosis (DVT), which was diagnosed by ultrasonography on day 6.

Statistical analysis

Statistical analysis was performed using the IBM SPSS 22 statistics package (IBM, Tokyo, Japan). All data are expressed as median (interquartile range: IQR) or mean ± standard deviation, as appropriate. The statistical significances of differences in patients' clinical features, laboratory values and outcomes were assessed with Student's t test, Mann-Whitney U test or Fisher exact test as appropriate. Time course changes of values of coagulofibrinolytic markers during the study period were tested by one-way repeated measures analysis of variance (ANOVA). The longitudinal differences in various factors between the subgroups stratified according to AT values on day 0 were analyzed by two-way repeated measures ANOVA, and pairwise comparisons were made by Student's t test or Mann-Whitney U test as appropriate. Relationships between AT values and the other values of coagulofibrinolytic markers on day 0 were analyzed by means of linear regression analysis. A multiple regression analysis with stepwise method was applied to predict independent factors for AT levels on day 0. Covariates were selected based on coagulofibrinolytic parameters including hemoglobin, platelet, PT, APTT, HPT, Fbg, FDP, D-dimer, TAT, PIC, tPAI-1, PC, α_2PI, PLG, TM, IL-6, Lactate acid and Alb. Variance Inflation Factor (VIF) was used to check for multicollinearity. A p value less than 0.05 was considered to indicate as significance.

Results

Patients' clinical features and outcomes (Table 1)

Fifty-nine trauma patients were admitted to our hospital during the study period. Twenty patients were excluded according to the exclusion criteria. Thus this present study included thirty-nine trauma patients with median ISS (Injury Severity Score) of 20 (10–27) , and the baseline characteristics and coagulofibrinolytic parameters on day 0 are presented in Table 1. The traumatic mechanism in all the patients was blunt injury, so most of them received several organ injuries. All of the patients had no significant medical histories such as liver cirrhosis or malnutrition which could affect coagulofibrinolytic parameters and serum albumin levels. The parameters reflecting systemic immune response and coagulofibrinolytic activation were notably elevated on day 0 (IL-6, 108.5 [40.8–250.3] pg/mL; TAT, 88.0 [30.1–200.0] μg/L; PIC, 9.1 [2.8–17.8] μg/mL). The median AT activity was 96.2 (79.8–108.3)%, which was within the normal range (80–130%) in spite of TAT elevation.

During the study period, seventeen patients of all patients (43.5%) underwent transfusion, sixteen of whom (94.1%) received transfusion on day 0. Therapeutic interventions such as interventional radiology (IVR), craniotomy, laparotomy or open reduction and internal fixation (ORIF) were performed on twenty-one patients (53.8%), ten of whom (47.6%) received these interventions on day 0. The development of DVT without associated symptoms was observed in six patients (15.3%). Two patients (5.1%) died after the study period of seven days from brain swelling due to severe head injury.

Time course changes in coagulofibrinolytic markers (Fig. 1)

The time courses of the mean values of coagulofibrinolitic biomarkers are presented in Fig. 1. *a) Coagulatory parameters:* Levels of TAT increased to their maximum levels just after trauma on day 0, then remarkably decreased over time ($p < 0.05$). *Anticoagulants:* AT and PC decreased from day 0 to 1 (AT, $p = 0.042$; PC, $p = 0.038$). *b) Fibrinolytic parameters:* PIC reached its maximum level on day 0, drastically dropped to its minimum level on day 2 ($p < 0.0001$), then significantly increased ($p < 0.001$). The time course changes of FDP were similar to those of PIC. PLG was at its minimum level on day 1 ($p < 0.0001$). *Inhibitors of fibrinolysis:* α_2PI showed a trend of decreasing from day 0 to day 1 ($p = 0.18$). tPAI-1 increased from day 0 to 1; this change was preceded by the increases in TAT and PIC on day 0. After that, tPAI-1 dropped on day 2 ($p < 0.0001$), then gradually increased in a pattern of similar to that of PIC ($p < 0.01$).

Table 1 Patient clinical features and outcomes

		All ($n = 39$)	AT activity on day 0		
			lower AT group AT < 80% ($n = 10$)	normal AT group AT ≥80% ($n = 29$)	*P* value
Patient characteristics					
Age	years	61 (38–73)	69 (57–80)	56 (34–72)	0.079
Sex: male / female	n (%)	26 (66.7) / 13 (33.3)	8 (80.0) / 2 (20.0)	18 (62.1) / 11 (37.9)	0.299
Injury Severity Score		20 (10–27)	26 (13–37)	17 (10–26)	0.091
JAAM DIC (+)	n (%)	11 (28.4)	6 (60.0)	5 (17.2)	0.016
Duration of injury to blood sampling					
	min	68 (31–180)	71 (42–205)	68 (30–187)	0.469
Laboratory data					
Hemoglobin	g/L	128 (118–136)	116 (91–129)	132 (120–140)	0.035
Platelet	$\times 10^9$/L	216 (168–253)	130 (86–246)	220 (182–261)	0.033
Prothrombin time (INR)		1.07 (1.00–1.12)	1.16 (1.10–1.33)	1.03 (0.99–1.08)	< 0.001
Activated partial thromboplastin time	sec	24.7 (23.2–27.1)	27.2 (26.1–34.0)	24.3 (22.7–26.3)	0.001
Hepaplastin test	%	112.7 (91.6–126.8)	93.2 (82.1–112.4)	117.0 (96.3–127.8)	0.088
Fibrinogen	g/L	2.4 (1.9–2.8)	1.8 (1.2–2.4)	2.5 (2.3–2.8)	0.024
FDP	µg/mL	63.0 (31.4–168.1)	161.3 (100.4–292.8)	47.7 (22.6–111.7)	0.005
D-dimer	µg/mL	36.4 (16.0–96.6)	92.0 (53.5–136.5)	21.6 (10.7–59.1)	0.010
TAT	µg/L	88.0 (30.1–200.0)	99.4 (74.7–200.5)	64.0 (21.1–200.0)	0.403
PIC	µg/mL	9.1 (2.8–17.8)	15.1 (7.7–23.6)	5.8 (2.2–14.3)	0.022
tPAI-1	ng/mL	30 (3–602)	27 (19.7–113.3)	29 (16–47.5)	0.551
AT activity	%	96.2 (79.8–108.3)	69.9 (66.2–76.9)	102.5 (91.1–109.7)	< 0.001
Protein C	%	90.6 (75.8–101.5)	69.5 (54.6–83.0)	95.3 (82.1–108.8)	0.001
α_2-plasmin inhibitor	%	90.5 (79.6–101.6)	73.8 (62.6–81.8)	95.8 (85.1–105.6)	< 0.001
Plasminogen	%	93.8 (81.5–102.6)	81.4 (64.0–88.2)	99.7 (86.9–106.7)	0.003
Thrombomodulin	ng/mL	2.9 (2.3–3.7)	3.9 (2.5–5.0)	2.9 (2.3–3.7)	0.076
Interleukin-6[a]	pg/mL	108.5 (40.8–250.3)	241.0 (145.5–411.0)	69.5 (33.0–175.5)	0.004
Lactate acid	mmol/L	1.7 (1.2–2.4)	2.2 (1.1–2.9)	1.7 (1.2–2.1)	0.281
Albumin	g/L	39 (34–43)	31 (29–36)	42 (38–43)	< 0.001
Transfusion Day 0 / Day 0-6					
Packed red blood cells	mL	0 (0–0) / 0 (0–560)	140 (0–560) / 280 (280–770)	0 (0–0) / 0 (0–0)	0.094 / 0.011
Fresh frozen plasma	mL	0 (0–480) / 0 (0–480)	480 (0–840) / 480 (0–1680)	0 (0–0) / 0 (0–0)	0.015 / 0.018
Platelets	mL	0 (0–0) / 0 (0–0)	0 (0–0) / 0 (0–100)	0 (0–0) / 0 (0–0)	0.640 / 0.014
Intervention Day 0 / Day 0–6					
Interventional radiology	n (%)	6 (15.3) / 6 (15.3)	3 (30.0) / 3 (30.0)	3 (10.3) / 3 (10.3)	0.162 / 0.162
Craniotomy	n (%)	3 (7.6) / 3 (7.6)	1 (10.0) / 1 (10.0)	2 (6.8) / 2 (6.8)	0.600 / 0.600
Laparotomy	n (%)	1 (2.5) / 1 (2.5)	1 (10.0) / 1 (10.0)	0 (0.0) / 0 (0.0)	0.256 / 0.256
Open reduction and Internal fixation	n (%)	0 (0.0) / 14 (35.9)	0 (0.0) / 4 (40.0)	0 (0.0) / 10 (34.4)	none / 0.519
Outcome					
DVT (+)	n (%)	6 (15.4)	2 (20.0)	4 (13.7)	0.490
In-hospital Mortality	n (%)	2 (5.1)	0 (0.0)	2 (6.8)	0.547

Values are presented as median (interquartile range: IQR) or number (%), if appropriate

AT antithrombin, *JAAM* Japanese Association for Acute Medicine, *DIC* disseminated intravascular coagulation, *FDP* fibrin/fibrinogen degradation product, *TAT* thrombin-antithrombin complex, *PIC* plasmin-α_2-plasmin inhibitor complex, *tPAI-1* total plasminogen activator inhibitor-1, *DVT* deep vein thrombosis; n, numbers of patients

[a]measurements of 38 patients. We started to measure IL-6 from the second patient of this study

Correlations between AT and the other parameters including coagulofibrinolytic biomarkers on day 0 (Fig. 2 and Table 2)

We performed linear regression analyses to evaluate the relationships between AT activities and the other parameters on day 0. As Fig. 2 shows, various parameters such as PLT or D-dimer showed correlations with AT activities (PLT, standard regression coefficient [r] = 0. 534, $p <$ 0.001; D-dimer, $r = 0.349$, $p = 0.029$), but TAT and PIC did not show negative linear correlations with AT (TAT, regression coefficient [B] = 0.008, standard error [SE] = 0.004, $r = 0.349$, $p = 0.029$; PIC, $p = 0.097$). There was a strong linear correlation between AT and Alb values on day 0 ($r = 0.702$, $p < 0.001$). PC and α_2PI were also strongly correlated with AT (PC, $r = 0.681$, $p < 0.001$; α_2PI, $r = 0.704$, $p < 0.001$). IL-6 and TM, reflecting systemic inflammatory responses and endothelial injury, respectively, also showed significant negative linear correlations with AT (IL-6, $r = 0.394$, $p = 0.014$; TM, $r = 0.500$, $p = 0.001$). A multiple linear regression analysis was performed for which the covariates were selected based on the laboratory parameters presented in Table 1. The analysis showed that Alb, α_2PI and PC were independent predictors of AT changes on day 0 (Table 2). None of the VIF values reached as high as 10, indicating that there was no collinearity in the model.

Comparisons of coagulofibrinolytic biomarkers depending on AT activities on day 0 (Table 1 and Fig. 3)

As shown in Table 1, ten patients showed decreased AT activity levels below the lower limit of the normal range on day 0. The median AT activity in this lower AT group ($n = 10$) was 69.9 (66.2–76.9)%, whereas that in the normal group ($n = 29$) was 102.5 (91.1–109.7)%. The lower AT group showed significantly lower AT levels as well as lower levels of PC, another anticoagulant, compared to the normal group throughout the study period.

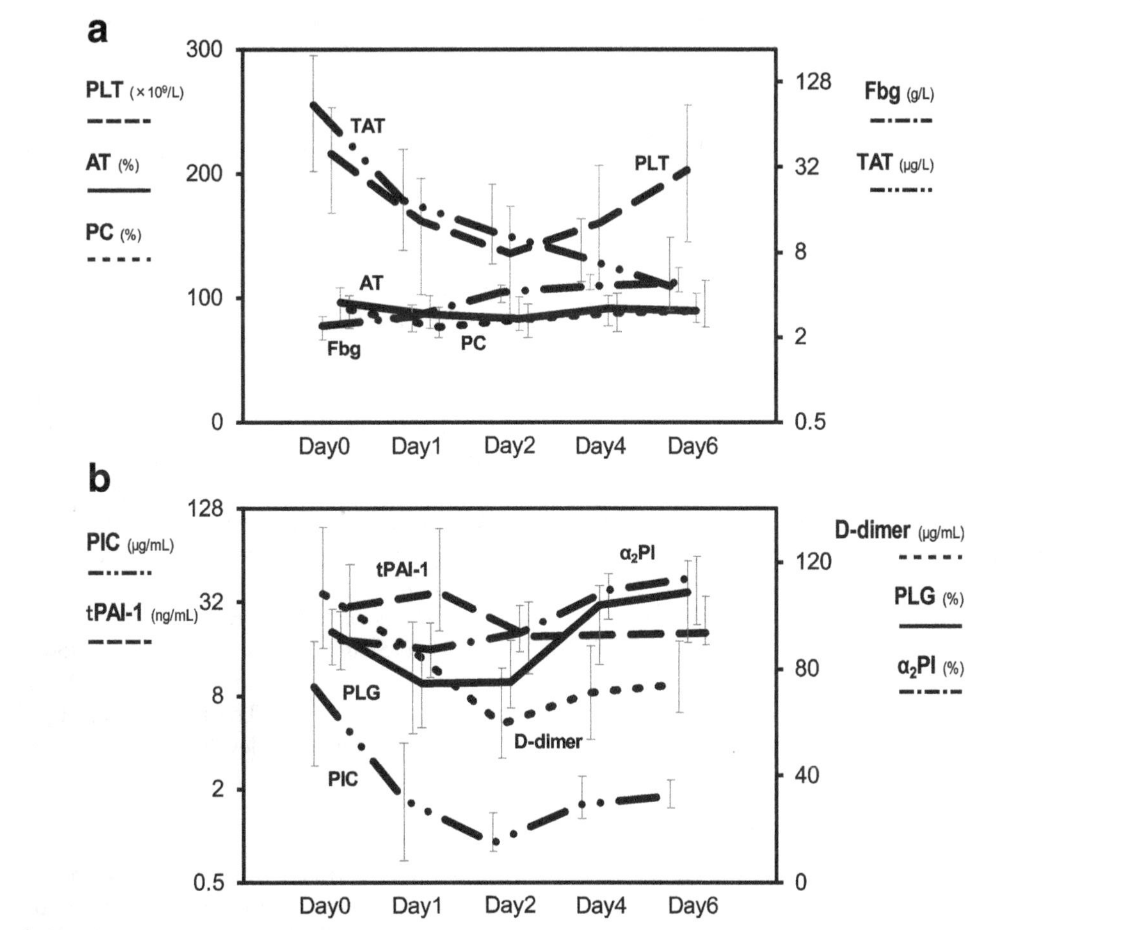

Fig. 1 Time course of coagulofibrinolytic markers. **a**) coagulatory parameters and anticoagulants: TAT increased to the maximum level just after trauma on day 0, then remarkably decreased over time ($p < 0.05$). AT and PC slightly decreased from day 0 to 1 ($p < 0.05$). **b**) fibrinolytic parameters and inhibitors of fibrinolysis: PIC reached its maximum level on day 0, which was followed by a drastic drop to the minimum level on day 2 ($p < 0.0001$), then another increase ($p < 0.001$). α_2PI showed a trend of decreasing from day 0 to day 1 ($p = 0.18$). tPAI-1 increased from day 0 to 1, then dropped on day 2 ($p < 0.0001$), and gradually increased along with PIC ($p < 0.01$)

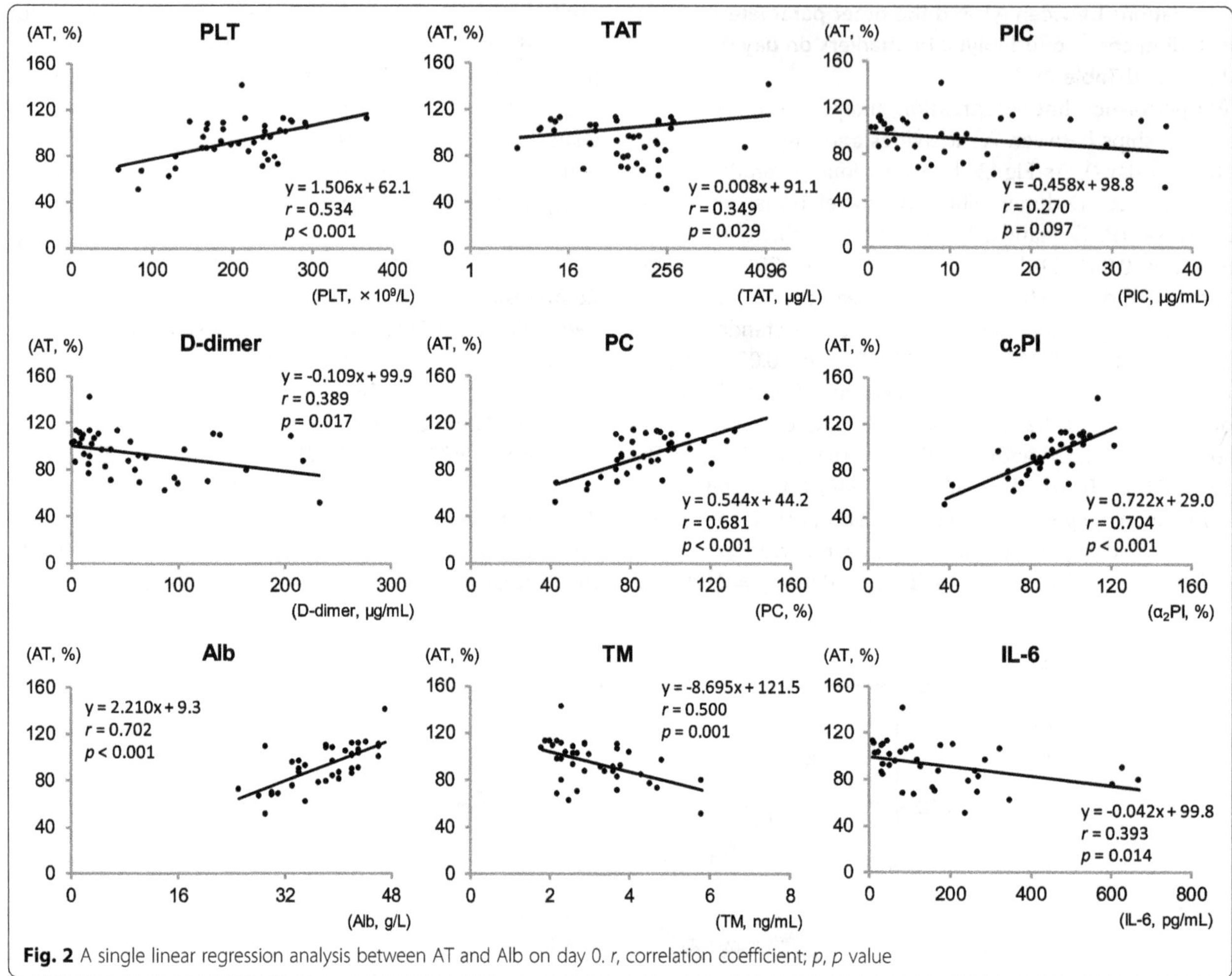

Fig. 2 A single linear regression analysis between AT and Alb on day 0. *r*, correlation coefficient; *p*, *p* value

TAT on day 0 was not significantly different between the two groups ($p = 0.403$ in Table 1). Although the rates of DVT development were not different between the two groups (Table 1), by days 2 and 4, TAT levels were significantly higher than in the normal group ($p < 0.05$, in Fig. 3), suggesting sustained intravascular coagulation.

PLT (Fig. 3) and coagulation factors (PT, Fbg, not shown in the Figure) were significantly lower in the lower AT group than in the normal group ($p < 0.05$). Regarding fibrinolytic parameters, the lower AT group exhibited a significantly greater decrease in α_2PI and greater increases in PIC, D-dimer (Fig. 3) and FDP (not shown in the Figure) as compared to the normal group ($p < 0.05$). The frequency of transfusion during the study period was greater in the lower AT group than in the normal group (packed red blood cells, $p = 0.011$; fresh frozen plasma, $p = 0.018$; platelets, $p = 0.014$, as seen in Table 1), though there were no differences between the two groups regarding the frequencies of other treatments.

IL-6 levels on day 0 and TM levels during the study period were significantly higher in the lower AT group than in the normal group (IL-6, $p = 0.004$; TM, $p < 0.05$ in Table 1 and Fig. 3). The lower AT group showed significantly lower Alb levels than the normal group throughout the study period ($p < 0.05$ in Fig. 3).

Table 2 A multiple linear regression analysis for predicting AT activity on day 0 ($N = 39$)

	B (*SE*)	95% CI	β	*p*	R^2
Alb	1.097 (0.409)	0.266–1.928	0.349	0.011	
PC	0.286 (0.094)	0.094–0.477	0.358	0.030	0.679
α_2PI	0.277 (0.141)	−0.010–0.564	0.270	0.058	

B regression coefficient, *SE* standard error, *CI* confidence interval, β standard regression coefficient, *p* *p* value, R^2 coefficient of determination

Discussion

It is known that the evaluation of physiological hemostatic responses to trauma through the measurement of coagulofibrinolytic biomarkers can be compromised if the measurement is taken during one of three events: fibrinolytic activation, fibrinolytic shutdown and fibrinolytic reactivation [20]. Just after a trauma insult, fibrinolytic activation occurs simultaneously with

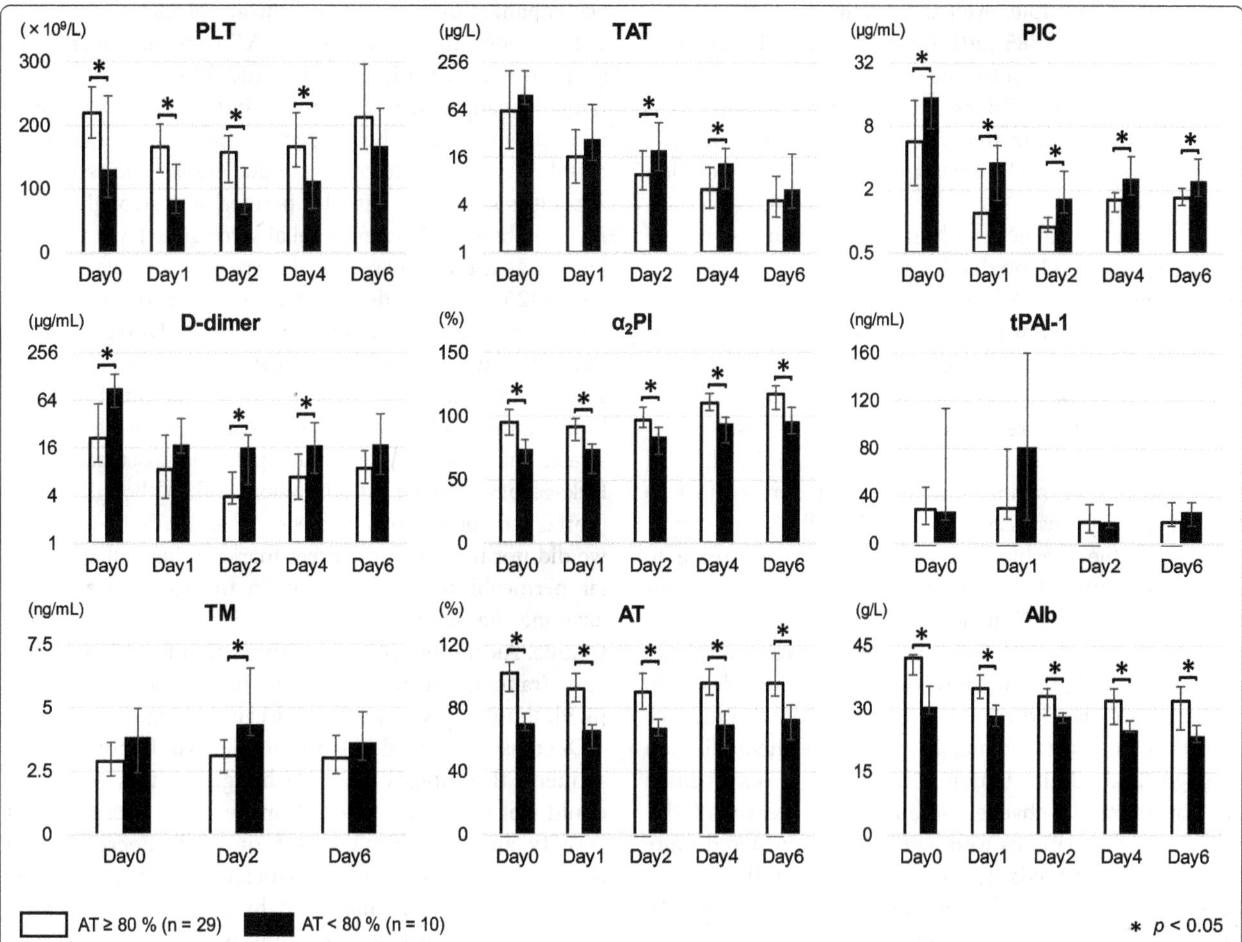

Fig. 3 Comparisons of coagulofibrinolytic biomarkers stratified with AT activity on day 0. TAT did not show any differences on days 0 and 1, but TAT on days 2 and 4 was significantly higher in the lower AT group than in the normal group ($p < 0.05$). TM levels throughout the study period were significantly higher in the lower AT group than in the normal group ($p < 0.05$). *$p < 0.05$

coagulatory activation. This is followed by fibrinolytic inhibition (also known as fibrinolytic shutdown) due to increasing tPAI-1, a controller for excessive fibrinolysis; fibrinolytic shutdown lasts from several to 24 h after a trauma insult or even for several days. After the repair of injured vessels and tissues, tPAI-1 decreases, reactivating fibrinolysis to allow the removal of the fibrin attached to the vessels for hemostasis. In this study, each of these three phases of physiological hemostatic response to trauma was actually observed. This shows that trauma- induced hypercoagulation and the triphasic changes of fibrinolytic activation will occur even in mild trauma patients such as those included in this study. Thus we should be aware of these time course changes to ensure the appropriate timing of treatments such as transfusions, antifibrinolytics or anticoagulants.

This study also focused on impairment in anticoagulation and decreased AT activity in the early phase of trauma. On day 0, which is thought to lie within the fibrinolytic activation phase, AT levels altered along with complex changes in coagulation factors and anticoagulants as well as fibrinolytic factors and their inhibitors. In particular, coagulofibrinolytic markers such as TAT and PIC changed simultaneously and in parallel with one another, even shortly after trauma. Nevertheless, AT did not linearly correlate with TAT and PIC on day 0, which means that, even if coagulation and fibrinolysis are activated, as evidenced by elevated TAT and PIC levels, AT levels do not decrease in response to their activation. AT inactivates thrombin's effects by forming a covalent stable stoichiometric 1:1 complex, TAT. Thus, TAT levels directly reflect the consumption of AT against intravascular thrombin formation. Indeed, TAT value is used as a marker of coagulation activity in the diagnosis of DIC. The normal concentration of AT in human plasma is approximately 125 to 160 μg/mL, which corresponds to 80 to 130% AT activity [18, 19]. Actually, Aibiki et al. have demonstrated a very strong linear correlation between AT activity level and its concentration [15]. Regarding the association between AT and TAT, for example, even the maximum level of TAT in this study was 4385 μg/L (approximately 4.4 μg/mL), an amount much smaller than the AT levels in plasma as mentioned above. Taking these findings together, it is reasonable to assume that decreased AT levels do not result merely from AT consumption even if coagulation is activated.

In this study, changes in plasma Alb, which was one of the predictors of AT on day 0, showed a very strong linear correlation with AT. Alb, a 66-kDa protein synthesized in the liver, is well known as a parameter reflecting an impairment in liver function or extravascular leakage when vascular permeability increases resulting from acute systemic inflammatory responses [21, 22]. Our results suggest that the decrease in AT activity in the initial phase of trauma could be mainly due to systemic responses to trauma strongly associated with Alb values on day 0. Previously, the mechanisms underlying the decrease in AT during trauma have been thought to be related to increased AT consumption, decreased synthesis, extravascular leakage or degradation by enzymes released from neutrophils [3, 8, 9, 23]. However, as presented clearly in this study, AT level does not decrease merely through AT consumption. Furthermore, in this study, hemodilution through fluid administration is not likely to have caused AT concentration changes because one criterion of this study excluded patients who had been administered more than 500 mL of fluids before admission (day 0), and because the blood samples on admission were generally drawn before the initial infusion was started.

Previous studies analyzing septic or obstetrical DIC have demonstrated strong correlations between AT and Alb and revealed that one of the main causes of decreasing AT is leakage from the capillary vessels [14, 15, 24]. Although there is a possibility of impaired synthesis of AT and Alb in the liver, it is highly unlikely if not impossible that liver dysfunction would occur immediately after trauma such that it could simultaneously cause decreased AT and Alb levels just after the insult. Although we were unable to obtain measurements of Alb values in our study subjects before their trauma insults, there were no medical histories of malnutrition or comorbidities that might affect Alb levels as far as we know. On the other hand, it is well known that vascular permeability to plasma contents is restricted to around 70 kDa, so Alb (66 kDa) is mostly retained in the intravascular space under normal conditions. In inflammatory situations, however, vascular permeability increases such that even high molecular weight proteins including Alb become permeable [25]. The molecular weight of AT is 64 kDa, similar to that of Alb, so it is reasonable to presume that AT exhibits similar dynamics in extravascular leakage depending on vascular permeability. Our results clearly show that AT levels decreased immediately after trauma and that this decrease was accompanied by a very strong linear correlation with Alb. Furthermore, these decreases in AT were significantly associated with elevations of IL-6 and TM, markers of systemic inflammatory responses and endothelial injury, respectively. Thus, the present results indicate that AT could decrease due to trauma-induced systemic responses. Also, it is likely that vascular permeability strongly affects AT metabolism. The endothelial glycocalyx layer (EGL) is known as a major player in determining vascular permeability [26, 27]. EGL decreases in response to elevatied IL-6 levels during sepsis and trauma [28, 29]. Di Battista et al. have reported that endotheliopathy, which is associated with glycocalyx breakdown, occurs in the initial phase of brain injury [30]. Furthermore, Rodriguez et al. demonstrated that traumatic endotheliopathy was associated with leakage of Alb even on admission [31]. Although we explored the correlations between AT and Alb, IL-6 or TM, we did not measure any direct markers that reflect vascular permeability in this study. In the future we aim to examine the relationship between EGL and AT activity in trauma. As another plausible explanation for AT depletion after trauma, neutrophil elastase involvement is possible [3, 9], though this awaits further clarification.

Decreased AT could be a potential risk factor for subsequent thrombosis [32]. Although in this study we could not detect an association between decreased AT activity and the development of DVT, decreased AT levels were found to be associated with subsequent thrombin activation indicated by increases in TAT on days 2 and 4. A previous study in patients with AT deficiency showed a persistent elevated thrombin activation [33]. In hereditary AT deficiency, AT levels are typically 40–60% of normal levels and patients have a lifetime risk of venous thromboembolism (VTE) [18]. Furthermore, an increased risk of recurrence of VTE has been reported even in mild AT deficiency (70–80%) [34]. These reports suggest that a reduction in AT levels should be recognized as a cause of thromboembolic complications even when AT levels are not severely decreased. In trauma patients, previous studies have demonstrated systemic increases in thrombin generation in connection with depleted AT levels [7, 10], which supports the present results. Furthermore, low AT levels in trauma patients have been reported to be associated with thromboembolic complications [11]. We need to explore the necessity and the timing of anticoagulant therapy including AT supplementation with regard to vascular permeability for patients with decreased AT activity due to trauma.

Limitations of the study

Several limitations of the present study should be addressed. Firstly, the sample size of this study was small. This means that, although we obtained the present results using the appropriate statistics, in the future we will need larger scale studies to test the hypothesis that has arisen from the present study. Secondarily, we included cases with mild trauma severity who were hospitalized for more than seven days. As one of the aims of this study was to examine time course changes in coagulofibrinolytic markers during the study period, we needed to include patients with mild severity. Yet even in patients with mild severity, we detected clear coagulofibrinolytic responses. However, further studies, including more severe cases, might be required to disclose the hemostatic conditions in different situations. Thirdly, we did not sufficiently address issues related to the trauma site, since many patients included in this study suffered from multiple organ damage due to blunt trauma. Thus there is a possibility that coagulofibrinolytic responses differ depending on the injured organs, especially if the brain is involved. Therefore, future studies must consider specific trauma sites.

Conclusions

Coagulofibrinolytic responses occurred even in mild trauma patients who survived initial coagulopathy and organ injuries. In such situations our results showed an impairment in anticoagulation due to decreased AT activity, which could result in prolonged hypercoagulation. This is the first report examining the mechanisms of decreased AT levels in the early phase of trauma. The observed decrease in AT levels in the initial phase of trauma is unlikely to occur through AT consumption accompanied by coagulofibrinolytic activation. One important cause of decreased AT levels could be trauma-induced systemic responses such as vascular leakage as suggested by Alb depletion along with elevated IL-6 and TM.

Abbreviations

Alb: Albumin; APTT: Activated partial thromboplastin time; AT: Antithrombin; ATC: Acute traumatic coagulopathy; DIC: Disseminated intravascular coagulation; DVT: Deep vein thrombosis; EGL: Endothelial glycocalyx layer; Fbg: Fibrinogen; FDP: Fibrin/fibrinogen degradation product; HPT: Hepaplastin test; ISS: Injury Severity Score; IVR: Interventional radiology; JAAM: the Japanese Association for Acute Medicine; ORIF: Open reduction and internal fixation; PAI-1: Plasminogen activator inhibitor-1; PC: Protein C; PIC: Plasmin-α_2-plasmin inhibitor complex; PLG: Plasminogen; PT: Prothrombin time; SIRS: Systemic inflammatory response syndrome; TAT: Thrombin-antithrombin complex; TIC: Trauma-induced coagulopathy; TM: Thrombomodulin; t-PA: Tissue plasminogen activator; VTE: Venous thromboembolism; α_2PI: α_2-plasmin inhibitor

Acknowledgements

The authors thank the nursing staff of the Intensive Care Unit 2 in Ehime University Hospital for their assistance.

Authors' contributions

HM conceived and designed the study. HM, JT, KU, SK, MO, SA, NM and YN prepared the data for analysis. HM conducted the data analysis. JT, UK, NS and MA assisted with the interpretation of the results and supervised the study. HM and MA drafted the article. All authors read and approved the manuscript. HM and MA take responsibility for the paper as a whole.

Competing interests

The authors declare that they have no competing interests.

References

1. Brohi K, Singh J, Heron M, Coats T. Acute traumatic coagulopathy. J Trauma. 2003;54:1127–30.
2. Macleod JB, Lynn M, McKenney MG, Cohn SM, Murtha M. Early coagulopathy predicts mortality in trauma. J Trauma. 2003;55:39–44.
3. Gando S, Otomo Y. Local hemostasis, immunothrombosis, and systemic disseminated intravascular coagulation in trauma and traumatic shock. Crit Care. 2015;19:72.
4. Hess JR, Brohi K, Dutton RP, Hauser CJ, Holcomb JB, Kluger Y, et al. The coagulopathy of trauma: a review of mechanisms. J Trauma. 2008;65:748–54.
5. Brohi K, Cohen MJ, Ganter MT, Matthay MA, Mackersie RC, Pittet JF. Acute traumatic coagulopathy: initiated by hypoperfusion: modulated through the protein C pathway? Ann Surg. 2007;245:812–8.
6. Oshiro A, Yanagida Y, Gando S, Henzan N, Takahashi I, Makise H. Hemostasis during the early stages of trauma: comparison with disseminated intravascular coagulation. Crit Care. 2014;18:R61.
7. Yanagida Y, Gando S, Sawamura A, Hayakawa M, Uegaki S, Kubota N, et al. Normal prothrombinase activity, increased systemic thrombin activity, and lower antithrombin levels in patients with disseminated intravascular coagulation at an early phase of trauma: comparison with acute coagulopathy of trauma-shock. Surgery. 2013;154:48–57.
8. Liener UC, Brückner UB, Strecker W, Steinbach G, Kinzl L, Gebhard F. Trauma severity-dependent changes in AT III activity. Shock. 2001;15:344–7.
9. Hayakawa M, Sawamura A, Gando S, Kubota N, Uegaki S, Shimojima H, et al. Disseminated intravascular coagulation at an early phase of trauma is associated with consumption coagulopathy and excessive fibrinolysis both by plasmin and neutrophil elastase. Surgery. 2011;149:221–30.
10. Dunbar NM, Chandler WL. Thrombin generation in trauma patients. Transfusion. 2009;49:2652–60.
11. Owings JT, Bagley M, Gosselin R, Romac D, Disbrow E. Effect of critical injury on plasma antithrombin activity: low antithrombin levels are associated with thromboembolic complications. J Trauma. 1996;41:396–406.
12. Levi M, Ten Cate H. Disseminated intravascular coagulation. N Engl J Med. 1999;341:586–92.
13. Ilias W, List W, Decruyenaere J, Lignian H, Knaub S, Schindel F, et al. Antithrombin III in patients with severe sepsis: a pharmacokinetic study. Intensive Care Med. 2000;26:704–15.
14. Asakura H, Ontachi Y, Mizutani T, Kato M, Ito T, Saito M, et al. Decreased plasma activity of antithrombin or protein C is not due to consumption coagulopathy in septic patients with disseminated intravascular coagulation. Eur J Haematol. 2001;67:170–5.
15. Aibiki M, Fukuoka N, Umakoshi K, Ohtsubo S, Kikuchi S. Serum albumin levels anticipate antithrombin III activities before and after antithrombin III agent in critical patients with disseminated intravascular coagulation. Shock. 2007;27:139–44.
16. Bone RC, Balk RA, Cerra FB, Dellinger RP, Fein AM, Knaus WA, et al. Definitions for sepsis and organ failure and guidelines for the use of innovative therapies in sepsis. The ACCP/SCCM consensus conference committee. American College of Chest Physicians/Society of Critical Care Medicine. Chest. 1992;101:1644–55.
17. Gando S, Saitoh D, Ogura H, Mayumi T, Koseki K, Ikeda T, et al. Japanese Association for Acute Medicine Disseminated Intravascular Coagulation (JAAM DIC) Study Group: natural history of disseminated intravascular coagulation diagnosed based on the newly established diagnostic criteria for critically ill patients: results of a multicenter, prospective survey. Crit Care Med. 2008;36:145–50.
18. Rodgers GM. Role of antithrombin concentrate in treatment of hereditary antithrombin deficiency. An update Thromb Haemost. 2009;101:806–12.
19. Levy JH, Sniecinski RM, Welsby IJ, Levi M. Antithrombin: anti-inflammatory properties and clinical applications. Thromb Haemost. 2016;115:712–28.

20. Gando S. Disseminated intravascular coagulation in trauma patients. Semin Thromb Hemost. 2001;27:585–92.
21. Margarson MP, Soni N. Serum albumin: touchstone or totem? Anaesthesia. 1998;53:789–803.
22. Boldt J. Use of albumin: an update. Br J Anaesth. 2010;104:276–84.
23. Miller RS, Weatherford DA, Stein D, Crane MM, Stein M. Antithrombin III and trauma patients: factors that determine low levels. J Trauma. 1994;37:442–5.
24. Kobayashi A, Matsuda Y, Mitani M, Makino Y, Ohta H. Assessment of the usefulness of antithrombin-III in the management of disseminated intravascular coagulation in obstetrically ill patients. Clin Appl Thromb Hemost. 2010;160:688–93.
25. Egawa G, Nakamizo S, Natsuaki Y, Doi H, Miyachi Y, Kabashima K. Intravital analysis of vascular permeability in mice using two-photon microscopy. Sci Rep. 2013;3:1932.
26. Weinbaum S, Tarbell JM, Damiano ER. The structure and function of the endothelial glycocalyx layer. Annu Rev Biomed Eng. 2007;9:121–67.
27. Myburgh JA, Mythen MG. Resuscitation fluids. N Engl J Med. 2013;369:1243–51.
28. Levick JR, Michel CC. Microvascular fluid exchange and the revised Starling principle. Cardiovasc Res. 2010;87:198–210.
29. Chignalia AZ, Yetimakman F, Christiaans SC, Unal S, Bayrakci B, Wagener BM, et al. The glycocalyx and trauma: a review. Shock. 2016;45:338–48.
30. Di Battista AP, Rizoli SB, Lejnieks B, Min A, Shiu MY, Peng HT, et al. Sympathoadrenal activation is associated with acute traumatic coagulopathy and Endotheliopathy in isolated brain injury. Shock. 2016;46: 96–103.
31. Rodriguez EG, Cardenas JC, Lopez E, Cotton BA, Tomasek JS, Ostrowski SR, et al. Early Identification of the Patient with Endotheliopathy of Trauma by Arrival Serum Albumin [Epub ahead of print: Oct. 18, 2017]. Shock. 2017; https://doi.org/10.1097/SHK.0000000000001036.
32. Ornaghi S, Barnhart KT, Frieling J, Streisand J, Paidas MJ. Clinical syndromes associated with acquired antithrombin deficiency via microvascular leakage and the related risk of thrombosis. Thromb Res. 2014;133:972–84.
33. Bauer KA, Rosenberg RD. The pathophysiology of the prethrombotic state in humans: insights gained from studies using markers of hemostatic system activation. Blood. 1987;70:343–50.
34. Di Minno MN, Dentali F, Lupoli R, Ageno W. Mild antithrombin deficiency and risk of recurrent venous thromboembolism: a prospective cohort study. Circulation. 2014;129:497–503.

22

vWF/ADAMTS13 is associated with on-aspirin residual platelet reactivity and clinical outcome in patients with stable coronary artery disease

Ellen M. K. Warlo[1,2,3*], Alf-Åge R. Pettersen[1,3,4], Harald Arnesen[1,2,3] and Ingebjørg Seljeflot[1,2,3]

Abstract

Background: The mechanisms behind residual platelet reactivity (RPR) despite aspirin treatment are not established. It has been shown that coronary artery disease (CAD) patients with high on-aspirin RPR have elevated levels of von Willebrand factor (vWF). ADAMTS13 is a metalloprotease cleaving ultra large vWF multimers into less active fragments. Our aim was to investigate whether ADAMTS13 and vWF/ADAMTS13 ratio were associated with high RPR, and further with clinical endpoints after 2 years.

Methods: Stable aspirin-treated CAD patients ($n = 999$) from the ASCET trial. RPR was assessed by PFA-100. ADAMTS13 antigen and activity were analysed using chromogenic assays. Endpoints were a composite of acute myocardial infarction, stroke and death.

Results: The number of patients with high RPR was 258 (25.8%). Their serum thromboxane B_2 (TxB_2) levels were low, indicating inhibition of COX-1. They had significantly lower levels of ADAMTS13 antigen compared to patients with low RPR (517 vs 544 ng/mL, $p = 0.001$) and significantly lower ADAMTS13 activity (0.99 vs 1.04 IU/mL, $p = 0.020$). The differences were more pronounced when relating RPR to ratios of vWF/ADAMTS13 antigen and vWF/ADAMTS13 activity ($p < 0.001$, both). We found an inverse correlation between vWF and ADAMTS13 antigen ($r = -0.14$, $p < 0.001$) and ADAMTS13 activity ($r = -0.11$, $p < 0.001$). No correlations between TxB_2 and ADAMTS13 antigen or activity, were observed, implying that ADAMTS13 is not involved in TxB2 production. Patients who experienced endpoints ($n = 73$) had higher vWF level (113 vs 105%, $p = 0.032$) and vWF/ADAMTS13 antigen ratio (0.23 vs 0.20, $p = 0.012$) compared to patients without. When dichotomizing vWF/ADAMTS13 antigen at median level we observed that patients above median had higher risk for suffering endpoints, with an adjusted OR of 1.86 (95% CI 1.45, 2.82).

Conclusion: These results indicate that ADAMTS13 is of importance for RPR, and that it in combination with vWF also is associated with clinical endpoints in stable CAD patients on aspirin.

Keywords: ADAMTS13, Von Willebrand factor, Aspirin, Residual platelet reactivity, Cardiovascular disease

* Correspondence: e.m.k.warlo@studmed.uio.no
[1]Center for Clinical Heart Research, Department of Cardiology, Oslo University Hospital, Ullevaal, Pb 4956 Nydalen, 0424 Oslo, Norway
[2]Faculty of Medicine, University of Oslo, Oslo, Norway
Full list of author information is available at the end of the article

Background

Von Willebrand factor (vWF) is an established marker of endothelial activation, and patients with elevated plasma levels of the ultra large vWF molecules are at high risk for future cardiovascular events [1–4].

vWF is a glycoprotein involved in both platelet activation and aggregation through its binding sites for GpIb and GpIIb/IIIa, respectively [5]. It is released to the circulation as ultra-large multimers from Weibel-Palade bodies in the endothelial cells, as well as from α-granules in platelets. vWF occurs in different lengths in the circulation and its thrombotic properties differ depending on its size [6]. It is involved in haemostasis when released as ultra-large multimers, and the activity decreases as the size abates [5]. vWF's activity is also enhanced by shear stress, promoting conformational changes of the molecule to expose important binding sites [6]. vWF is cleaved into smaller fragments with reduced thrombotic activity by a metalloproteinase, ADAMTS13, "A Disintegrin And Metalloprotease with TromboSpondin type 1 motif, member 13" [7]. Reduced amount and activity of ADAMTS13 lead to less fragmentation of vWF with subsequent higher amount of the ultra-large vWF molecules, thus potentially a more prothrombotic state.

The role of ADAMTS13 in coronary artery disease (CAD) has not been established, and inconclusive results have been reported [3]. A recent meta-analysis showed low ADAMTS13 levels, both amount and activity, with concomitant ultra-large vWF, to be a risk factor for myocardial infarction [8]. The importance of ADAMTS13 for platelet reactivity, indirectly by acting on vWF or directly, is limited described.

Aspirin is a cornerstone in treatment of cardiovascular disease (CVD), but patients on aspirin may still experience new cardiovascular events. The phenomenon of residual platelet reactivity (RPR) despite use of aspirin has been extensively studied with diverging results [9]. The prevalence of high RPR and any predictive value vary considerably depending on the laboratory methods used [10, 11]. Thus, there is no recommendation to introduce platelet function testing in clinical practice. Regardless of this, the mechanisms behind high RPR assessed by platelet function testing are still not known in details. In the Aspirin Nonresponsiveness and Clopidogrel Endpoint Trial (ASCET) [12], it was shown that patients with high on-aspirin RPR had significantly elevated levels of vWF compared to patients with low RPR [13].

The aim of the present study was to investigate whether ADAMTS13 alone and as a vWF/ADAMTS13 ratio were associated with the presence of high RPR in aspirin treated CAD patients. We hypothesised that low ADAMTS13 would contribute to high RPR. We further explored whether ADAMTS13 and the vWF/ADAMTS13 ratio were associated with disease entities and risk factors and further with clinical outcome after 2 years follow-up.

Methods

Study population

This is a substudy of the ASCET trial which was performed at Center for Clinical Heart Research, Oslo University Hospital, Ullevaal, Oslo, Norway, from March 2003 until July 2010 [12]. The design of the trial has previously been published [14], and it is registered at https://www.clinicaltrials.gov/ (identification No. NCT00222261).

Patients ($n = 1001$) with stable CAD, previously verified by angiography, were included. All patients were on single antiplatelet therapy with aspirin 160 mg/d for at least 1 week prior to inclusion. Patients were randomized to either continue on aspirin 160 mg/d or change to clopidogrel 75 mg/d and were followed for 2 years for clinical endpoints. Patients in need of dual antiplatelet therapy or warfarin were excluded. The ASCET study was approved by the regional ethics committee and all patients gave their written consent.

Current smokers were defined as patients still smoking or former smokers who had quit less than 3 months ago. Hypertensives included patients with treated hypertension. The criteria for diabetes were patients with treated T1DM and T2DM or fasting blood glucose > 7 mmol/L.

Clinical endpoints in the main ASCET study included unstable angina pectoris, myocardial infarction (MI), non-haemorrhagic stroke and death. For the purpose of the present investigation we excluded the group of unstable angina pectoris as this is a less defined diagnosis. Thus, the recorded endpoints were MI, non-haemorrhagic stroke and death. Endpoints were recorded at study visits and on request for patients unable to attend the final visit. An endpoint committee performed the evaluation of endpoints and internationally accepted diagnostic criteria were used.

Blood sampling

Blood samples were drawn at inclusion in fasting condition between 08.00 and 10.30 AM, 24 h after last intake of aspirin. Citrated plasma (0.129 M in dilution 1:10) was stored on ice and separated within 30 min by centrifugation at 4 °C and 3000 g for 20 min, and stored at -80 °C until analysed for ADAMTS13 antigen and activity, performed by commercial methods (IMUBIND® (Seksui Diagnostics GmbH, Pfungstadt, Germany and TECHNOZYM® ADAMTS-13 activity assay, Technoclone, Vienna, Austria, respectively). We have previously reported on vWF, determined in citrated plasma by use of Asserachrom vWF Ag (Stago Diagnostica, Asnieres, France), and Thromboxane B_2, analysed in serum prepared from whole blood without anticoagulants and kept at 37° for 1 h before centrifugation at 2500×g for 10 min (Amersham Thromboxane B_2 Biotrak Assay, GE Healthcare, Buckinghamshire, UK) [12, 13].

Residual platelet reactivity (RPR)

The method has been described in details previously [12]. Briefly, citrated whole blood (0.129 M in dilution 1:10) was analysed within 2 h by the PFA100 system (Siemens Healthcare Diagnostics, Germany). This system stimulates platelet-based haemostasis in vitro by use of cartridges with collagen and epinephrine. Closure time (CT) was recorded to determine platelet function. The cut-off value, determined by testing 200 CAD patients not on antiplatelet therapy, was set at 196 s based on the 95 percentile in this cohort [15]. Patients with CT below this level were classified with high RPR and patients above this level with low RPR.

Statistical analysis

Continuous variables are presented as mean ± SD or median (25th, 75th percentiles) when appropriate. Categorical data are presented as numbers or percentages. Students unpaired t-test or Mann-Whitney U test were used to compare continuous variables between groups, and group comparisons for categorical variables were performed by Pearson's chi-squared test. Correlation analyses were performed by Spearman's rho. Logistic regression analysis was used to adjust for relevant covariates, estimated from Additional file 1 Table S1. A p-value < 5% was considered statistically significant. SPSS version 22 (SPSS Inc., IL, USA) was used.

Results

Baseline characteristics of the total population and according to the presence of low or high RPR are shown in Table 1. Blood samples from two patients were not available for ADAMTS13 analyses, thus all results are given for 999 patients. The number of patients with high RPR was 258 (25.8%). TxB_2 levels were low in all patients, compared to levels in individuals not on aspirin [15]. There was a significantly lower percentage of hypertensives, and a higher

Table 1 Baseline characteristics of the total populating and according to the presence of low or high RPR

	Total population	Low RPR ($n = 741$)	High RPR ($n = 258$)	p-value[§]
Age (years)[a]	62.4 (36–81)	62.6 (36–81)	61.7 (41–80)	0.154
Sex, female, n (%)	218 (21.8)	159 (21.5)	58 (22.5)	0.731
Caucasian, n (%)	968 (96.8)	724 (97.7)	243 (94.2)	**0.006**
Cardiovascular risk factors, n (%)				
Current smoking	203 (20.3)	136 (18.4)	67 (26.0)	**0.009**
Hypertension	556 (55.7)	433 (58.4)	123 (47.9)	**0.003**
Diabetes mellitus	200 (20.0)	148 (20.0)	52 (20.2)	0.950
Previous CVD[d]	635 (63.6)	462 (62.3)	172 (66.9)	0.189
- Previous myocardial infarction	436 (43.7)	314 (42.4)	121 (47.1)	0.195
Systolic blood pressure (mmHg)[b]	140 ± 19	141 ± 19	136 ± 19	**< 0.001**
Diastolic blood pressure (mmHg)[b]	82 ± 10	82 ± 10	81 ± 9	**0.040**
Body mass index (kg/m^2)[b]	27.4 ± 3.7	27.5 ± 3.8	27.2 ± 3.5	0.237
Blood tests				
Total cholesterol (mmol/L)[b]	4.55 ± 0.98	4.55 ± 0.99	4.53 ± 0.96	0.793
LDL cholesterol (mmol/L)[b]	2.53 ± 0.83	2.53 ± 0.83	2.53 ± 0.83	0.998
HDL cholesterol (mmol/L)[b]	1.33 ± 0.41	1.34 ± 0.42	1.31 ± 0.37	0.277
Triglycerides (mmol/L)[c]	1.31 (0.93, 1.84)	1.29 (0.91, 1.84)	1.35 (0.97, 1.85)	0.144
Residual platelet reactivity, n (%)	258 (25.8)			
TxB_2 (ng/mL)[a]	2.7 (0–21)	2.6 (0–21)	3.0 (0–15)	0.102
Medication, n (%)				
Statins	982 (98.3)	727 (98.2)	254 (98.4)	0.825
B-blockers	755 (75.8)	561 (76.1)	193 (74.8)	0.672
Calcium channel blockers	255 (25.6)	196 (26.5)	59 (23.0)	0.272
ACE-inhibitors	263 (26.5)	200 (27.1)	63 (24.7)	0.455
ARB	239 (24.0)	187 (25.3)	52 (20.4)	0.111

CVD cardiovascular disease, *MI* myocardial infarction, *PCI* percutaneous coronary intervention, *CABG* coronary artery bypass graft, *TxB_2* thromboxane B_2, *ACE* angiotensin-converting enzyme, *ARB* angiotensin II receptor blockers

[§] p-values refer to differences between the groups with high or low RPR

[a] mean (range) [b] mean ± SD [c] median (25th, 75th percentiles) [d] Previous MI, PCI, CABG, non-haemorrhagic stroke

Significant p-values are highlighted with boldface

Table 2 Baseline levels of the measured markers in the total population and according to the presence of low or high RPR

	Total population	Low RPR ($n = 741$)	High RPR ($n = 258$)	p-value[§]
vWF (%)	105 (82, 133)	100 (79, 126)	124 (94, 145)	**< 0.001**
ADAMTS13 antigen (ng/mL)	532 (461, 606)	537 (469, 613)	511 (448, 580)	**0.001**
ADAMTS13 activity (IU/mL)	1.03 (0.83, 1.19)	1.04 (0.84, 1.19)	0.99 (0.76, 1.16)	**0.020**
Ratio vWF/ADAMTS13 antigen	0.20 (0.15, 0.26)	0.19 (0.14, 0.25)	0.23 (0.18, 0.31)	**< 0.001**
Ratio vWF/ADAMTS13 activity	107 (77, 152)	101 (73, 137)	127 (93, 192)	**< 0.001**
Platelet count (× 10^9/L)	227 (195, 264)	224 (192, 261)	236 (200, 273)	**0.010**

Values are given as median (25th, 75th percentiles)
[§]p-values refer to differences between the groups with high or low RPR
Significant p-values are highlighted with boldface

proportion of smokers in the high RPR group compared to the group with low RPR. There was no significant difference in clinical endpoints with regard to high and low RPR. These data on patients with high and low RPR have previously been published [12, 13].

ADAMTS13 as related to RPR

Levels of ADAMTS13 antigen and activity are shown in Table 2, in the total cohort and according to the RPR status. Patients with high RPR had significantly higher levels of vWF ($p < 0.001$) and platelet count ($p = 0.010$) compared to those with low RPR, as previously published [13]. In the present investigation we observed that patients with high RPR had significantly lower levels of both ADAMTS13 antigen and activity compared to individuals with low RPR ($p = 0.001$, $p = 0.020$, respectively). When calculating ratios of vWF/ADAMTS13 antigen and vWF/ADAMTS13 activity the differences were even more pronounced, showing both ratios to be significantly higher in patients with high RPR ($p < 0.001$ for both).

Statistically significant, but weak inverse correlations were found between the levels of vWF and ADAMTS13 antigen ($r = -0.14$, $p < 0.001$) and ADAMTS13 activity ($r = -0.11$, $p < 0.001$). ADAMTS13 antigen and activity were significantly inter-correlated ($r = 0.47$, $p < 0.001$).

ADAMTS13 as related to disease entities

Table 3 shows ADAMTS13 antigen and activity as related to different cardiovascular risk factors. When dichotomizing age at median level, we found that patients

Table 3 Baseline levels of the measured markers according to different clinical conditions

		n	vWF (%)	ADAMTS13 antigen (ng/mL)	ADAMTS13 activity (IU/mL)	Ratio antigen	Ratio activity
Age > median (62 years)	+	500	110 (88, 137)	519 (455, 581)	1.00 (0.79, 1.15)	0.21 (0.17, 0.29)	117 (86, 170)
	−	500	100 (79, 127)	547 (467, 627)	1.05 (0.90, 1.21)	0.19 (0.14, 0.25)	97 (70, 136)
	p		**< 0.001**	**< 0.001**	**< 0.001**	**< 0.001**	**< 0.001**
Sex (female)	+	218	106 (82, 136)	549 (463, 622)	1.04 (0.84, 1.19)	0.20 (0.14, 0.26)	111 (76, 157)
	−	782	106 (83, 133)	525 (460, 596)	1.02 (0.82, 1.19)	0.20 (0.15, 0.27)	106 (77, 150)
	p		0.840	0.052	0.877	0.611	0.726
Diabetes	+	200	111 (83, 141)	557 (465, 639)	1.05 (0.81, 1.18)	0.20 (0.15, 0.27)	117 (84, 170)
	−	800	105 (83, 131)	524 (459, 596)	1.02 (0.83, 1.19)	0.20 (0.15, 0.26)	106 (76, 147)
	p		**0.023**	**0.003**	0.931	0.602	0.059
Hypertension	+	556	104 (80, 132)	530 (463, 606)	1.01 (0.79, 1.16)	0.20 (0.15, 0.26)	107 (76, 150)
	−	443	108 (86, 134)	533 (458, 607)	1.05 (0.86, 1.21)	0.20 (0.16, 0.28)	106 (77, 153)
	p		**0.033**	0.959	**0.034**	0.081	0.962
Previous CVD	+	635	110 (86, 137)	534 (463, 608)	1.02 (0.82, 1.19)	0.20 (0.16, 0.27)	110 (82, 160)
	−	364	98 (78, 126)	525 (456, 602)	1.04 (0.85, 1.18)	0.19 (0.14, 0.25)	103 (72, 136)
	p		**< 0.001**	0.453	0.663	**0.001**	**0.002**
Smokers	+	203	107 (88, 134)	520 (441, 590)	1.03 (0.86, 1.19)	0.20 (0.16, 0.28)	108 (78, 151)
	−	796	105 (83, 133)	532 (466, 607)	1.02 (0.82, 1.18)	0.20 (0.15, 0.26)	107 (77, 152)
	p		0.621	0.100	0.306	0.515	0.796

Values are given as median (25th, 75th percentiles)
p-values refer to differences in the measured marker between patients having the specified clinical condition or not
Significant p-values are highlighted with boldface

above median (62 years) had higher levels of vWF, lower ADAMTS13 antigen and activity, and higher ratios ($p < 0.001$, for all). No sex differences were observed in the measured markers. Diabetic patients had significantly higher levels of both vWF ($p = 0.023$) and ADAMTS13 antigen ($p = 0.003$), whereas hypertensive patients had significantly lower levels of vWF ($p = 0.033$) and lower ADAMTS13 activity ($p = 0.034$) compared to normotensives. Patients with previous CVD had significantly higher levels of vWF ($p < 0.001$) and also higher vWF/ADAMTS13, both antigen ratio ($p = 0.001$) and activity ratio ($p = 0.002$). We observed no differences between smokers and non-smokers.

ADAMTS13 as related to clinical endpoints

After 2 years follow-up 73 clinical endpoints (MI, stroke or death) were recorded. These patients had higher levels of vWF and vWF/ADAMTS13 antigen ratio at inclusion compared to patients without endpoints (Table 4). We found no significant differences in the levels of ADAMTS13, neither antigen nor activity.

When dividing vWF and vWF/ADAMTS13 antigen ratio levels into quartiles, there were no significant trends for frequency of endpoints ($p = 0.135$, $p = 0.071$, respectively) (Fig. 1). Nevertheless, we observed a potential cut-off level at the lowest quartile for vWF (Fig 1a). When dichotomizing vWF at this level, a higher event rate was demonstrated in patients with levels in the three upper quartiles compared to those in the lowest quartile with an OR of 2.18 (95% CI 1.10, 4.31). The significance was, however, lost after adjusting for the covariates age, sex, diabetes, and previous CVD ($p = 0.077$).

When dichotomizing vWF/ADAMTS13 antigen at the median value (Fig 1b), an OR of 1.89 (95% CI 1.15, 3.11) for suffering an event when having levels above the median was observed ($p = 0.011$). After adjustments for covariates the OR was 1.68 (95% CI 1.01, 2.80) and the significance was retained ($p = 0.045$). Additional adjustment for the randomized treatment principle did not influence the results.

Discussion

This study was performed in a stable CAD population where 258 (25.8%) patients had high RPR, determined by the PFA-100 method. TxB_2 levels were low, indicating adequate aspirin compliance. High RPR patients had higher levels of vWF compared to patients with low RPR as previously published [13].

Our main findings were that patients with high RPR had significantly lower levels of ADAMTS13, both antigen and activity, and higher vWF/ADAMTS13 ratios, and further significantly higher vWF levels and vWF/ADAMTS13 antigen ratio in patients who experienced a clinical endpoint after 2 years compared to patients who did not.

To our knowledge, this is the first study reporting on the importance of ADAMTS13 on RPR in stable aspirin-treated CAD patients. Our results are mostly in line with a similar study by Marcucci et al. using other methods for RPR in a smaller CAD population, however, performed in the acute phase [16]. They observed significantly higher vWF and lower ADAMTS13 activity, but no difference in ADAMTS13 antigen in patients with high RPR. The different results on ADAMTS13 antigen might be due to different population sizes, but also the acute phase with a high degree of inflammation, which is known to affect both vWF and ADAMTS13 levels [17].

In our study RPR was related to both the amount and the activity of ADAMTS13. A possible mechanism is that low ADAMTS13 levels cause less fragmentation of vWF, resulting in more long vWF molecules that can activate platelets, thereby a higher RPR. We do not know whether high vWF levels per se cause high RPR or only act as a covariate. In the present situation the association between vWF and ADAMTS13 may be due to the reciprocal course of these molecules, i.e. high vWF may lead to low ADAMTS13 as a result of the increased availability of vWF which may lead to an "exhaustion" or elimination of ADAMTS13 by unknown mechanisms [17].

We observed only a weak correlation between vWF and ADAMTS13 which is in accordance with other reports, showing either weak or no correlation [18–20]. Even though it is well established that ADAMTS13

Table 4 Baseline levels of the measured markers according to clinical endpoint or no endpoint

	Endpoint ($n = 73$)	No endpoint ($n = 927$)	P-value[§]
vWF, %	113 (93, 141)	105 (81, 133)	**0.032**
ADAMTS-13 antigen, ng/mL	506 (452, 576)	533 (462, 607)	0.147
ADAMTS-13 activity, IU/mL	1.00 (0.73, 1.13)	1.03 (0.83, 1.19)	0.212
Ratio antigen	0.23 (0.17, 0.29)	0.20 (0.15, 0.26)	**0.012**
Ratio activity	119 (88, 175)	107 (77, 150)	0.051
Platelet count (× 10^9/L)	221 (181, 272)	228 (196, 263)	0.446

Values are given as median (25th, 75th percentiles)

[§]p-values refer to differences between the groups with high or low RPR

Significant p-values are highlighted with boldface

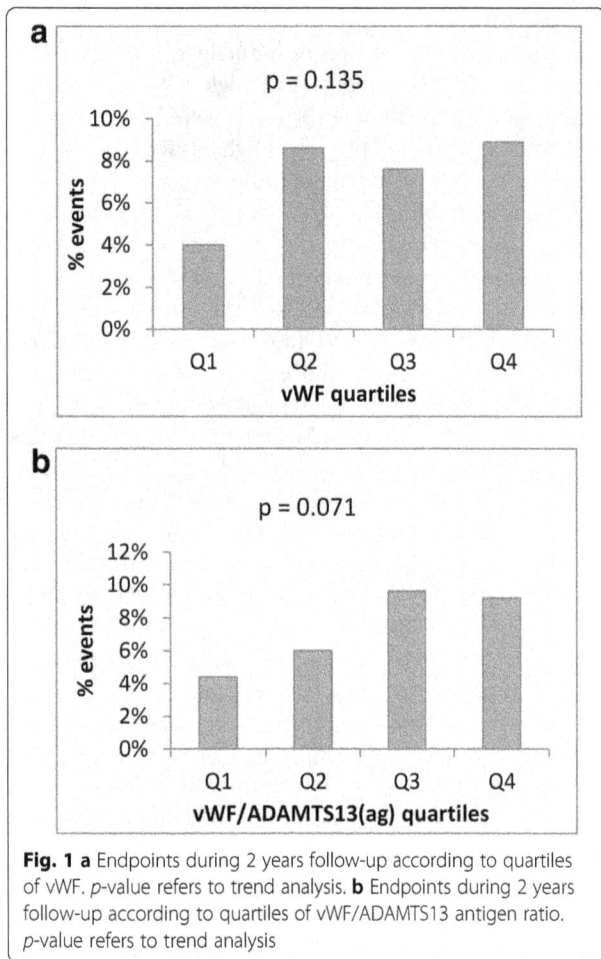

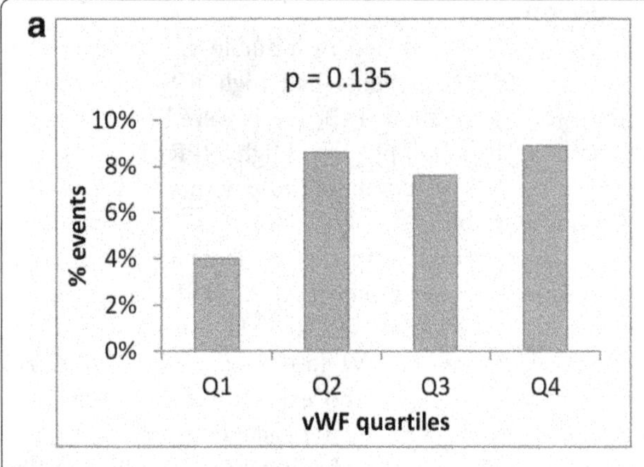

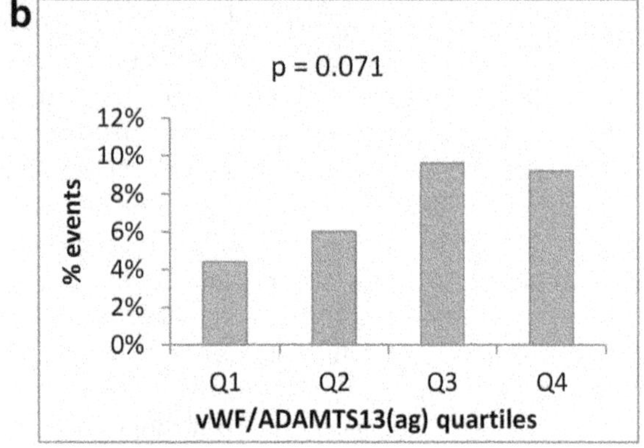

Fig. 1 a Endpoints during 2 years follow-up according to quartiles of vWF. *p*-value refers to trend analysis. **b** Endpoints during 2 years follow-up according to quartiles of vWF/ADAMTS13 antigen ratio. *p*-value refers to trend analysis

cleaves vWF, both are affected by other factors that might weaken this correlation [21–23]. It has also been suggested that the two molecules, independent of each other, are associated with clinical endpoints, and that ADAMTS13 have cardioprotective properties beyond vWF cleavage [20, 24, 25].

Both vWF and ADAMTS13, as well as the ratios were significantly associated with age, in line with other reports [26–30]. No significant sex differences were observed. Lower ADAMTS13, both antigen and activity have previously been shown in men [27–30]. Higher levels of both vWF and ADAMTS13 antigen were observed in diabetic patients. High vWF have generally been associated with diabetes, but the results for ADAMTS13 are more diverging [20, 29–31]. In the Rotterdam study higher ADAMTS13 activity in patients with diabetes compared to those without was reported [29], and they also showed ADAMTS13 activity to be an independent risk factor for both prediabetes and diabetes type 2 [32]. In hypertensive patients higher vWF and lower ADAMTS13 activity were found, which to some degree is in accordance with other reports, although varying results exist [26, 31]. Also, patients with previous CVD had higher vWF levels in our study. There are some case-control studies supporting this result, whereas the observations on ADAMTS13 are diverging [19, 20]. We found no differences between smokers and non-smokers which is in accordance with previous reports [20, 31].

Our observations of vWF and ADAMTS13 to be associated with clinical endpoints are partly in accordance with previous reports. vWF have repeatedly been associated with increased risk of coronary heart disease [3]. We observed higher levels of vWF in patients experiencing clinical endpoints, however, the significance was lost when adjusting for covariates. This might strengthen the recent suggestion that vWF is more modestly associated with coronary heart disease than previously estimated [32].

Previous reports on ADAMTS13, both antigen and activity as related to clinical outcome are inconclusive, and we could not demonstrate any association between ADAMTS13 and clinical endpoints. The meta-analysis by Maino et al. concluded that ADAMTS13 levels below the 5th percentile was associated with increased risk of MI [8], whereas Sonneveld et al. concluded an uncertainty on whether ADAMTS13 increases the risk of arterial thrombosis due to diverging results and lack of prospective studies [3].

We could, however, demonstrate that patients who suffered a clinical endpoint had significantly higher levels of vWF/ADAMTS13 antigen ratio. Patients with ratio above median level had an OR of 1.68 for suffering an event, significant also after adjustments for relevant covariates, indicating that the combination of vWF and ADAMTS13 antigen might be a better prognostic marker than vWF alone. To the best of our knowledge this is the first report on vWF/ADAMTS13 antigen ratio in relation to future cardiovascular events.

Study limitations

The platelet function test used in this study, PFA-100 with collagen and epinephrine cartridges, has been questioned with regard to response to aspirin. It is a COX-1-non-specific test, and therefore not quite suitable to detect real aspirin-resistance. High RPR by this method is not necessarily due to insufficient inhibition of COX-1, but might be caused by platelet activation through other pathways. Although high RPR by the PFA-100 method have, in some studies shown to be associated with increased risk of clinical endpoints [11], in our population, as well as in other studies, PFA-100 was not able to identify these high-risk patients [12, 33, 34]. RPR was determined only at baseline without re-testing during the follow-up period. It should also be emphasized that the method is dependent of vWF levels [13, 35]. However, in our population very few had levels below or above the reference values. vWF varies with blood type and the coagulation factors VIII and fibrinogen concentrations [21, 36, 37]. It is also uncertain whether the vWF antigen levels measured reflect vWF length.

Conclusion

In our population of stable CAD patients on aspirin treatment, low ADAMTS13 levels were associated with high RPR and in combination with vWF associated with clinical outcome after 2 years. Beyond the properties of ADAMTS13 to cleave vWF, other mechanisms behind these associations are not clear and further investigations are needed.

Abbreviations

ACE: Angiotensin-converting enzyme; ADAMTS13: A Disintegrin And Metalloprotease with TromboSpondin type 1 motif, member 13; ARB: Angiotensin II receptor blockers; ASCET: Aspirin Nonresponsiveness and Clopidogrel Endpoint Trial; CABG: Coronary artery bypass graft; CAD: Coronary artery disease; CT: Closure time; CVD: Cardiovascular disease; MI: Myocardial infarction; PCI: Percutaneous coronary intervention; RPR: Residual platelet reactivity; TxB_2: Thromboxane B_2; vWF: Von Willebrand Factor

Acknowledgements

The authors would like to thank medical laboratory technologist Sissel Åkra for excellent technical assistance.

Funding

The study was financially supported by The Research Council of Norway through the Medical Student Research Program at the University of Oslo, specified to the first author, and Stein Erik Hagens Foundation for Clinical Heart Research, Oslo Norway by unrestricted grants to the research milieu (recipients HA and IS).

Authors' contributions

EW performed laboratory and statistically analyses, contributed to interpretation of results and drafting the manuscript. AP was the principal investigator in the ASCET study, involved in planning of the study, the recruitment and follow-up of the study participants and acquisition of clinical data. IS and HA contributed to the overall design of the study, the interpretation of the results and the intellectual content of the manuscript. All authors read and approved the final manuscript.

Competing interests

The authors declare that they have no competing interest.

Author details

[1]Center for Clinical Heart Research, Department of Cardiology, Oslo University Hospital, Ullevaal, Pb 4956 Nydalen, 0424 Oslo, Norway. [2]Faculty of Medicine, University of Oslo, Oslo, Norway. [3]Center for Heart Failure Research, University of Oslo, Oslo, Norway. [4]Department of Medicine, Vestre Viken HF, Ringerike Hospital, Hønefoss, Norway.

References

1. Morange PE, Simon C, Alessi MC, Luc G, Arveiler D, Ferrieres J, et al. Endothelial cell markers and the risk of coronary heart disease: the prospective epidemiological study of myocardial infarction (PRIME) study. Circulation. 2004;109:1343–8. https://doi.org/10.1161/01.cir.0000120705.55512.ec.
2. Thompson SG, Kienast J, Pyke SD, Haverkate F, van de Loo JC. Hemostatic factors and the risk of myocardial infarction or sudden death in patients with angina pectoris. European concerted action on thrombosis and disabilities angina pectoris study group. N Engl J Med. 1995;332:635–41. https://doi.org/10.1056/nejm199503093321003.
3. Sonneveld MA, de Maat MP, Leebeek FW. Von Willebrand factor and ADAMTS13 in arterial thrombosis: a systematic review and meta-analysis. Blood Rev. 2014;28:167–78. https://doi.org/10.1016/j.blre.2014.04.003.
4. Folsom AR, KK W, Shahar E, Davis CE. Association of hemostatic variables with prevalent cardiovascular disease and asymptomatic carotid artery atherosclerosis. The atherosclerosis risk in communities (ARIC) study investigators. Arterioscler Thromb. 1993;13:1829–36. http://atvb.ahajournals.org/content/atvbaha/13/12/1829.full.pdf
5. Stockschlaeder M, Schneppenheim R, Budde U. Update on von Willebrand factor multimers: focus on high-molecular-weight multimers and their role in hemostasis. Blood Coagul Fibrinolysis. 2014;25:206–16. https://doi.org/10.1097/mbc.0000000000000065.
6. Reininger AJ. The function of ultra-large von Willebrand factor multimers in high shear flow controlled by ADAMTS13. Hamostaseologie. 2015;35:225–33. https://doi.org/10.5482/hamo-14-12-0077.
7. Eerenberg ES, Levi M. The potential therapeutic benefit of targeting ADAMTS13 activity. Semin Thromb Hemost. 2014;40:28–33. https://doi.org/10.1055/s-0033-1363156.
8. Maino A, Siegerink B, Lotta LA, Crawley JT, le Cessie S, Leebeek FW, et al. Plasma ADAMTS-13 levels and the risk of myocardial infarction: an individual patient data meta-analysis. J Thromb Haemost. 2015;13:1396–404. https://doi.org/10.1111/jth.13032.
9. Pettersen AA, Arnesen H, Seljeflot I. A brief review on high on-aspirin residual platelet reactivity. Vasc Pharmacol. 2015;67-69:6–9. https://doi.org/10.1016/j.vph.2015.03.018.
10. Hovens MM, Snoep JD, Eikenboom JC, van der Bom JG, Mertens BJ, Huisman MV. Prevalence of persistent platelet reactivity despite use of aspirin: a systematic review. Am Heart J. 2007;153:175–81. https://doi.org/10.1016/j.ahj.2006.10.040.
11. Wisman PP, Roest M, Asselbergs FW, de Groot PG, Moll FL, van der Graaf Y, et al. Platelet-reactivity tests identify patients at risk of secondary cardiovascular events: a systematic review and meta-analysis. J Thromb Haemost. 2014;12:736–47. https://doi.org/10.1111/jth.12538.
12. Pettersen AA, Seljeflot I, Abdelnoor M, Arnesen H. High on-aspirin platelet reactivity and clinical outcome in patients with stable coronary artery disease: results from ASCET (aspirin nonresponsiveness and Clopidogrel endpoint trial). J Am Heart Assoc. 2012;1:e000703. https://doi.org/10.1161/jaha.112.000703.
13. Pettersen AA, Arnesen H, Opstad TB, Bratseth V, Seljeflot I. Markers of endothelial and platelet activation are associated with high on-aspirin platelet reactivity in patients with stable coronary artery disease. Thromb Res. 2012;130:424–8. https://doi.org/10.1016/j.thromres.2012.06.016.
14. Pettersen AA, Seljeflot I, Abdelnoor M, Arnesen H. Unstable angina, stroke, myocardial infarction and death in aspirin non-responders. A prospective, randomized trial. The ASCET (ASpirin non-responsiveness and Clopidogrel endpoint trial) design. Scand Cardiovasc J. 2004;38(6):353. https://doi.org/10.1080/14017430410024324.
15. Andersen K, Hurlen M, Arnesen H, Seljeflot I. Aspirin non-responsiveness as measured by PFA-100 in patients with coronary artery disease. Thromb Res. 2002;108:37–42.
16. Marcucci R, Cesari F, Cinotti S, Paniccia R, Gensini GF, Abbate R, et al. ADAMTS-13 activity in the presence of elevated von Willebrand factor levels as a novel mechanism of residual platelet reactivity in high risk coronary patients on antiplatelet treatment. Thromb Res. 2008;123:130–6. https://doi.org/10.1016/j.thromres.2008.05.017.
17. Reiter RA, Varadi K, Turecek PL, Jilma B, Knobl P. Changes in ADAMTS13 (von-Willebrand-factor-cleaving protease) activity after induced release of von Willebrand factor during acute systemic inflammation. Thromb Haemost. 2005;93:554–8. https://doi.org/10.1160/th04-08-0467.
18. Andersson HM, Siegerink B, Luken BM, Crawley JT, Algra A, Lane DA, et al. High VWF, low ADAMTS13, and oral contraceptives increase the risk of ischemic stroke and myocardial infarction in young women. Blood. 2012;119:1555–60. https://doi.org/10.1182/blood-2011-09-380618.
19. Bongers TN, de Bruijne EL, Dippel DW, de Jong AJ, Deckers JW, Poldermans D, et al. Lower levels of ADAMTS13 are associated with cardiovascular disease in young patients. Atherosclerosis. 2009;207:250–4. https://doi.org/10.1016/j.atherosclerosis.2009.04.013.

20. Crawley JT, Lane DA, Woodward M, Rumley A, Lowe GD. Evidence that high von Willebrand factor and low ADAMTS-13 levels independently increase the risk of a non-fatal heart attack. J Thromb Haemost. 2008;6:583–8. https://doi.org/10.1111/j.1538-7836.2008.02902.x.
21. Gallinaro L, Cattini MG, Sztukowska M, Padrini R, Sartorello F, Pontara E, et al. A shorter von Willebrand factor survival in O blood group subjects explains how ABO determinants influence plasma von Willebrand factor. Blood. 2008;111:3540–5. https://doi.org/10.1182/blood-2007-11-122945.
22. Zheng XL. Structure-function and regulation of ADAMTS-13 protease. J Thromb Haemost. 2013:11 Suppl 1:11–23. https://doi.org/10.1111/jth.12221.
23. Tersteeg C, Fijnheer R, Pasterkamp G, de Groot PG, Vanhoorelbeke K, de Maat S, et al. Keeping von Willebrand factor under control: alternatives for ADAMTS13. Semin Thromb Hemost. 2016;42:9–17. https://doi.org/10.1055/s-0035-1564838.
24. Feng Y, Li X, Xiao J, Li W, Liu J, Zeng X, et al. ADAMTS13: more than a regulator of thrombosis. Int J Hematol. 2016;104:534–9. https://doi.org/10.1007/s12185-016-2091-2.
25. Chion CK, Doggen CJ, Crawley JT, Lane DA, Rosendaal FR. ADAMTS13 and von Willebrand factor and the risk of myocardial infarction in men. Blood. 2007;109:1998–2000. https://doi.org/10.1182/blood-2006-07-038166.
26. Enooku K, Kato R, Ikeda H, Kurano M, Kume Y, Yoshida H, et al. Inverse correlations between serum ADAMTS13 levels and systolic blood pressure, pulse pressure, and serum C-reactive protein levels observed at a general health examination in a Japanese population: a cross-sectional study. Clin Chim Acta. 2013;421:147–51. https://doi.org/10.1016/j.cca.2013.03.012.
27. Kokame K, Nobe Y, Kokubo Y, Okayama A, Miyata T. FRETS-VWF73, a first fluorogenic substrate for ADAMTS13 assay. Br J Haematol. 2005;129:93–100. https://doi.org/10.1111/j.1365-2141.2005.05420.x.
28. Kokame K, Sakata T, Kokubo Y, Miyata T. Von Willebrand factor-to-ADAMTS13 ratio increases with age in a Japanese population. J Thromb Haemost. 2011;9:1426–8. https://doi.org/10.1111/j.1538-7836.2011.04333.x.
29. Sonneveld MA, de Maat MP, Portegies ML, Kavousi M, Hofman A, Turecek PL, et al. Low ADAMTS13 activity is associated with an increased risk of ischemic stroke. Blood. 2015;126:2739–46. https://doi.org/10.1182/blood-2015-05-643338.
30. Skeppholm M, Kallner A, Kalani M, Jorneskog G, Blomback M, Wallen HN. ADAMTS13 and von Willebrand factor concentrations in patients with diabetes mellitus. Blood Coagul Fibrinolysis. 2009;20:619–26. https://doi.org/10.1097/MBC.0b013e32832da183.
31. Miura M, Kaikita K, Matsukawa M, Soejima K, Fuchigami S, Miyazaki Y, et al. Prognostic value of plasma von Willebrand factor-cleaving protease (ADAMTS13) antigen levels in patients with coronary artery disease. Thromb Haemost. 2010;103:623–9. https://doi.org/10.1160/th09-08-0568.
32. de Vries PS, van Herpt TT, Ligthart S, Hofman A, Ikram MA, van Hoek M, et al. ADAMTS13 activity as a novel risk factor for incident type 2 diabetes mellitus: a population-based cohort study. Diabetologia. 2016. doi: https://doi.org/10.1007/s00125-016-4139-5.
33. Pamukcu B, Oflaz H, Onur I, Oncul A, Ozcan M, Umman B, et al. Clinical relevance of aspirin resistance in patients with stable coronary artery disease: a prospective follow-up study (PROSPECTAR). Blood Coagul Fibrinolysis. 2007;18:187–92. https://doi.org/10.1097/MBC.0b013e328040c115.
34. Poulsen TS, Kristensen SR, Korsholm L, Haghfelt T, Jorgensen B, Licht PB, et al. Variation and importance of aspirin resistance in patients with known cardiovascular disease. Thromb Res. 2007;120:477–84. https://doi.org/10.1016/j.thromres.2006.10.022.
35. Cattaneo M, Federici AB, Lecchi A, Agati B, Lombardi R, Stabile F, et al. Evaluation of the PFA-100 system in the diagnosis and therapeutic monitoring of patients with von Willebrand disease. Thromb Haemost. 1999;82:35–9.
36. Folsom AR, KK W, Rosamond WD, Sharrett AR, Chambless LE. Prospective study of hemostatic factors and incidence of coronary heart disease: the atherosclerosis risk in communities (ARIC) study. Circulation. 1997;96:1102–8.
37. Montgomery RR, Flood VH. What have we learned from large population studies of von Willebrand disease? Hematology Am Soc Hematol Educ Program. 2016;2016:670–7. https://doi.org/10.1182/asheducation-2016.1.670.

Circulating activated protein C levels are not increased in septic patients treated with recombinant human soluble thrombomodulin

Takuro Arishima[1†], Takashi Ito[1,2*†], Tomotsugu Yasuda[1†], Nozomi Yashima[3], Hiroaki Furubeppu[1], Chinatsu Kamikokuryo[3], Takahiro Futatsuki[1], Yutaro Madokoro[1], Shotaro Miyamoto[1], Tomohiro Eguchi[1], Hiroyuki Haraura[1], Ikuro Maruyama[2] and Yasuyuki Kakihana[1,3]

Abstract

Background: Recombinant human soluble thrombomodulin (rTM) has been used for the treatment of disseminated intravascular coagulation in Japan, and an international phase III clinical trial for rTM is currently in progress. rTM mainly exerts its anticoagulant effects through an activated protein C (APC)-dependent mechanism, but the circulating APC levels after rTM treatment have not been clarified. This prospective observational study investigated plasma APC levels after rTM treatment.

Methods: Plasma levels of soluble thrombomodulin, thrombin-antithrombin complex (TAT), protein C, and APC were measured in eight septic patients treated with rTM. APC generation in vitro was assessed in the presence or absence of rTM.

Results: rTM significantly increased thrombin-mediated APC generation in vitro. In septic patients, soluble thrombomodulin levels were significantly increased during a 30–60-min period of rTM treatment and TAT levels were decreased. However, APC activity was not increased during the treatment period.

Conclusions: Plasma APC activity is not increased in septic patients treated with rTM. It is possible that APC acts locally and does not circulate systemically.

Keywords: Disseminated intravascular coagulation, Protein C, Sepsis, Thrombomodulin

Background

Thrombomodulin is an anticoagulant protein expressed on the surface of endothelial cells [1]. Thrombomodulin binds to thrombin and boosts its potential for activating protein C. Activated protein C (APC) then inactivates coagulation factors Va and VIIIa, limiting the amplification of blood coagulation [2]. In septic conditions, thrombomodulin expression can be compromised, leading to sepsis-associated disseminated intravascular coagulation (DIC) [3]. Substitution with recombinant human soluble thrombomodulin (rTM) is a therapeutic option in Japan under these conditions [4, 5], and an international phase III clinical trial for rTM is currently in progress.

Recombinant human APC (rhAPC) originally showed a significant reduction in all-cause mortality in patients with severe sepsis [6]. However, the initial success was not replicated in subsequent clinical trials involving adult patients with severe sepsis and low risk of death [7], children with severe sepsis [8], and patients with septic shock [9]. As a result, rhAPC has been withdrawn from the market. Although rTM shares its fundamental mechanism of action with rhAPC, it has several unique features. For example,

* Correspondence: takashi@m3.kufm.kagoshima-u.ac.jp
†Takuro Arishima, Takashi Ito and Tomotsugu Yasuda contributed equally to this work.
[1]Emergency and Critical Care Center, Kagoshima University Hospital, Kagoshima, Japan
[2]Department of Systems Biology in Thromboregulation, Kagoshima University Graduate School of Medical and Dental Sciences, 8-35-1 Sakuragaoka, Kagoshima 890-8544, Japan
Full list of author information is available at the end of the article

rTM did not increase the incidence of bleeding complications [10], unlike the case for rhAPC [11]. This may be because rTM preferentially exerts its APC-dependent anticoagulant effects when and where thrombin exists [1]. In this context, it is important to consider whether APC acts locally or circulates systemically after rTM treatment. However, there has been no evidence for plasma APC levels after rTM treatment.

Recently, a novel method for measurement of plasma APC levels has been developed [12]. The method employs a single-stranded DNA aptamer that captures APC with high affinity and high specificity without capturing inactive protein C. Using this aptamer-based enzyme capture assay, we examined the plasma APC levels in septic patients treated with rTM. We found that circulating APC levels were not increased in these patients even though soluble TM levels were significantly increased by rTM treatment.

Methods

In vitro APC generation assay

Pooled normal plasma (George King Bio-Medical, Overland Park, KS) was incubated with thrombin (Mochida Pharmaceutical, Tokyo, Japan) and rTM (Asahi Kasei Pharma, Tokyo, Japan) at 37 °C for 10 min. The reaction was terminated by addition of a protease inhibitor cocktail containing hirudin and aprotinin (Sekisui Medical, Tokyo, Japan). In some experiments, protein C deficient plasma (Affinity Biologicals, Ancaster, Canada), antithrombin deficient plasma (Affinity Biologicals), protein C (kindly provided by Chemo-Sero-Therapeutic Research Institute, Kumamoto, Japan), and antithrombin (Japan Blood Products Organization, Tokyo, Japan) were used for preparing plasma with various concentrations of protein C and antithrombin. For pre-analytical APC stability assays, whole blood samples from three healthy volunteers were spiked with 16.7 ng/mL equivalent activity of APC (Haematologic Technologies, Essex Junction, VT) followed by addition of the protease inhibitor cocktail. Samples were stored at − 80 °C until analysis of APC concentrations.

Patients and blood sampling

This prospective observational study conformed to the provisions of the Declaration of Helsinki and was approved by the Ethics Committee of Kagoshima University Hospital. Between May 2016 and March 2017, written informed consent was obtained from eight patients with sepsis-associated DIC prior to participation in the study. Although the number of enrolled patients did not reach the recruiting goal of this study, we decided not to extend the study period because the data of eight patients were enough to support the conclusion that plasma APC activity was not significantly increased in septic patients treated with rTM. Diagnoses of sepsis and DIC were made according to the Third International Consensus Definition for Sepsis (Sepsis-3) [13] and the diagnostic criteria established by the Japanese Association for Acute Medicine (JAAM DIC criteria) [14], respectively. Blood samples were collected from intravascular catheter in eight patients with sepsis-associated DIC before and after administration of rTM (130 or 380 U/kg, intravenous drip infusion; Asahi Kasei Pharma, Tokyo, Japan) on day 1 and day 2. The samples were immediately anticoagulated with one-tenth volume of sodium citrate and kept at 4 °C to minimize covalent inhibition of APC by plasma proteins. The samples were then centrifuged at 2000×g for 10 min at 4 °C. Part of the citrated plasma was mixed with the protease inhibitor cocktail containing hirudin and aprotinin within 15 min after blood sampling and

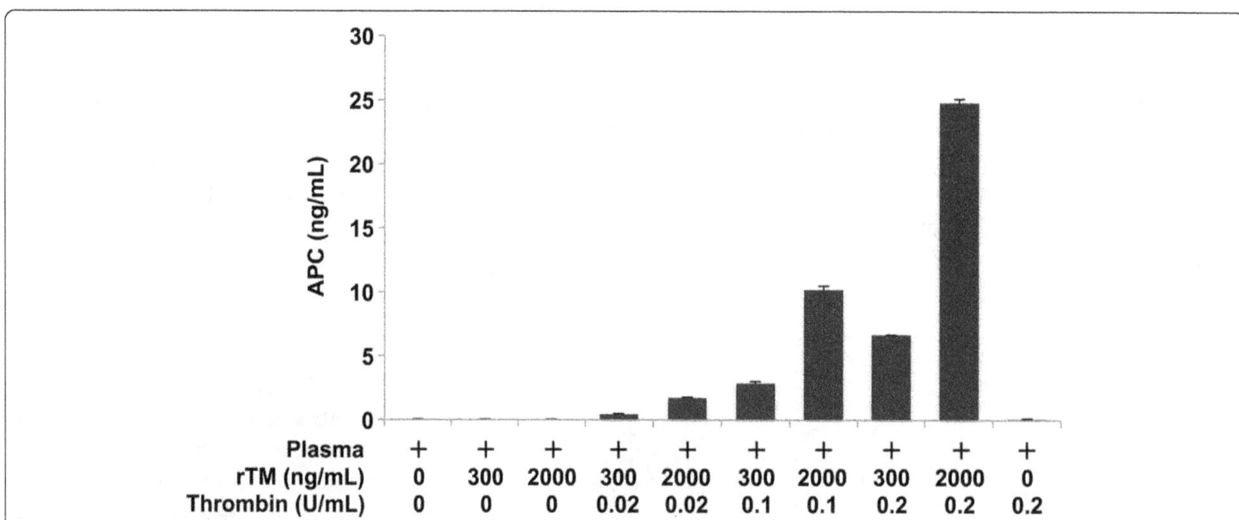

Fig. 1 rTM promotes thrombin-mediated APC generation in vitro. Pooled normal plasma was incubated with thrombin (0–0.2 U/mL) and rTM (0–2000 ng/mL) at 37 °C for 10 min. APC levels were analyzed by the OLIGOBIND APC activity assay. The data represent mean ± SD ($n = 3$). Representative data of two independent experiments are shown

stored at − 80 °C until analysis of APC concentrations. APC measurement with this protocol was comparable to the authentic protocol [12] in which aprotinin was added to blood collection tubes prior to blood sampling (data not shown).

Measurement of plasma levels of APC, soluble thrombomodulin (sTM), protein C, thrombin-antithrombin complex (TAT), and prothrombin fragment 1 + 2 (F1 + 2)

Plasma APC levels were analyzed by the OLIGOBIND APC activity assay (Sekisui Diagnostics GmbH, Pfungstadt, Germany) according to the manufacturer's instructions. Plasma sTM levels were measured by ELISA using monoclonal antibodies against thrombomodulin. The plasma sTM levels determined by this technique were well correlated with a functional assay [15]. Plasma protein C levels were measured by a synthetic chromogenic substrate method using HemosIL Protein C (Instrumentation Laboratory, Bedford, MA). Plasma TAT levels were analyzed using STACIA CLEIA TAT (LSI Medience, Tokyo, Japan) according to the manufacturer's instructions. Plasma F1 + 2 levels were analyzed using Enzygnost F1 + 2 (Siemens Healthcare Diagnostics, Tokyo, Japan) according to the manufacturer's instructions.

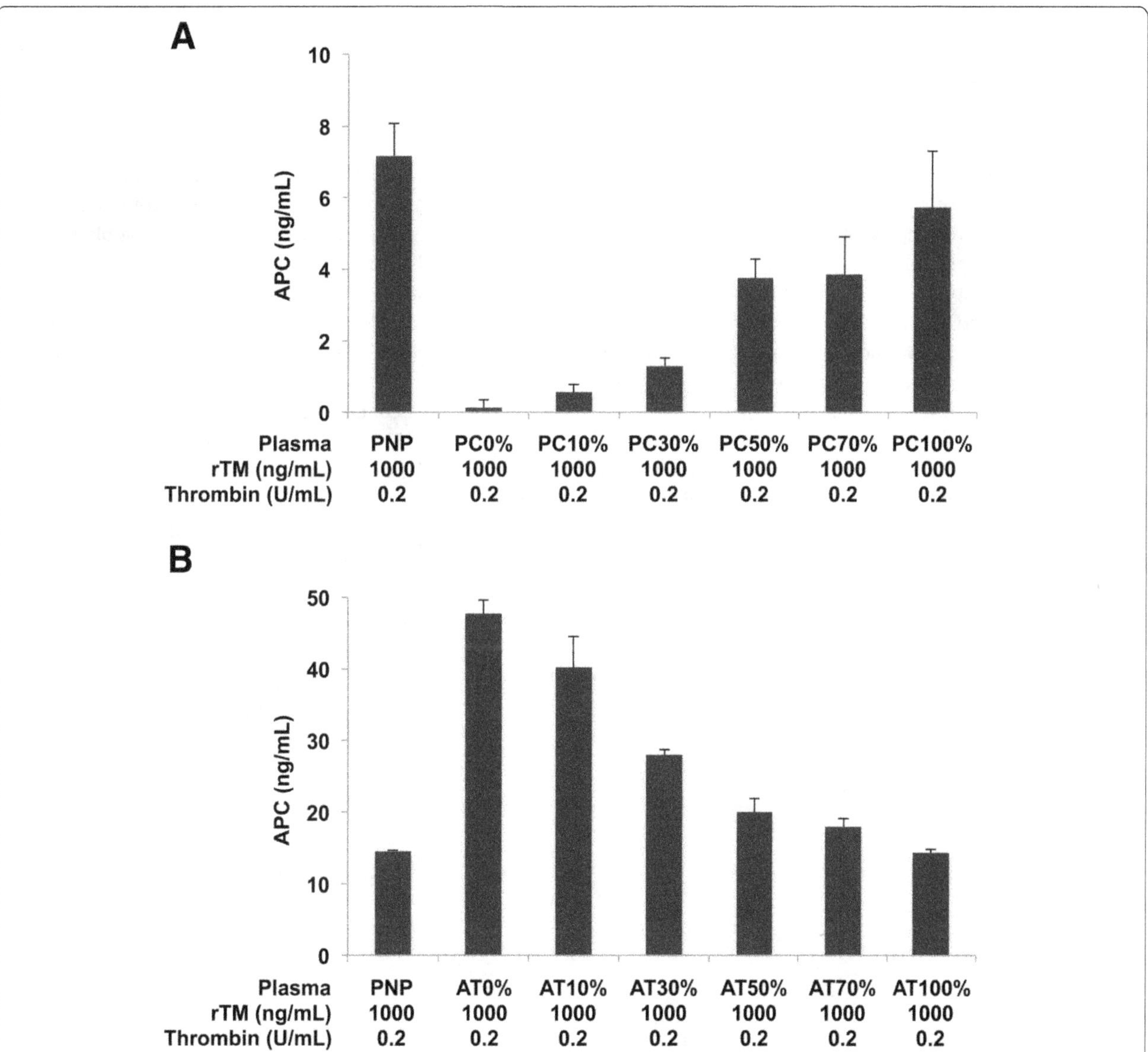

Fig. 2 Decreased concentrations of protein C and antithrombin are associated with decreased and increased APC generation, respectively. **a** Plasma samples with 0, 10, 30, 50, 70, and 100% protein C levels were prepared by the addition of vehicle, 0.36, 1.08, 1.81, 2.53, and 3.61 μg/mL of protein C, respectively, to protein C deficient plasma. **b** Plasma samples with 0, 10, 30, 50, 70, and 100% antithrombin levels were prepared by the addition of vehicle, 0.07, 0.25, 0.43, 0.61, and 0.88 U/mL of antithrombin, respectively, to antithrombin deficient plasma. These plasma samples were incubated with 0.2 U/mL of thrombin (T1063, Sigma-Aldrich, St. Louis, MO) and 1000 ng/mL of rTM at 37 °C for 10 min. APC levels were analyzed by the OLIGOBIND APC activity assay. The data represent mean ± SD (n = 3). Representative data of two independent experiments are shown. PNP: pooled normal plasma, PC: protein C, AT: antithrombin

Statistical analysis

In vitro APC generation assays were evaluated by analysis of variance followed by a Tukey–Kramer test. For assessment of clinical samples, a paired *t*-test was used for comparisons before and after rTM treatment. Data were presented as mean ± SD. A probability of < 0.05 was considered significant.

Results and discussion

First, we conducted in vitro APC generation and quantification assays to verify that rTM can promote thrombin-mediated APC generation and that the aptamer-based enzyme capture assay can detect APC quantitatively. As shown in Fig. 1, thrombin alone or rTM alone did not induce APC generation. In contrast, the combination of thrombin and rTM increased APC generation in a dose-dependent manner. The concentrations of rTM in these assays were equivalent to those detected in our clinical samples (Fig. 3a). TAT levels in our in vitro samples (Additional file 1: Figure S1) were also equivalent to those in our clinical samples (Fig. 3b), suggesting that thrombin concentrations used in our in vitro assays were reasonable. These results indicate that rTM can promote thrombin-mediated APC generation in vitro, and that the assay can detect this generation.

Next, we examined the impact of protein C and antithrombin levels on APC generation in vitro. Protein C and antithrombin are a substrate and an inhibitor of thrombin, respectively, and these levels are expected to have significant impacts on thrombin-mediated APC generation. As expected, APC generation was decreased as plasma protein C levels decreased (Fig. 2a). In contrast, APC generation was increased as plasma antithrombin levels decreased (Fig. 2b). These findings indicate that APC generation can be increased or decreased depending on the balance of antithrombin and protein C levels.

Then, we examined the plasma levels of sTM, TAT, protein C, and APC in patients with sepsis-associated DIC before and after administration of rTM. The background characteristics of the patients are summarized in Table 1. Plasma sTM levels rapidly increased during a 30–60-min period of rTM treatment on day 1 and day 2 (Fig. 3a). The detected sTM levels were essentially equivalent to those reported in previous clinical studies [16, 17] and those adopted in our in vitro assays. Plasma TAT levels were slightly, but significantly, decreased during a 30–60-min period of rTM treatment on day 2 (Fig. 3b). Plasma F1 + 2 levels remained unchanged during this treatment period (day 1 pre 557 ± 418 vs day 1 post 553 ± 415, day 2 pre 403 ± 340 vs day 2 post 395 ± 325). Plasma APC levels were not increased after rTM treatment, and instead showed a declining trend (Fig. 3c). Plasma protein C levels remained unchanged during this treatment period (Fig. 3d). These findings indicate that rTM promotes thrombin-mediated APC generation in vitro, but does not increase plasma APC levels in patients with sepsis-associated DIC.

It remains a matter of debate why rTM treatment did not increase plasma APC levels in septic patients. The anticoagulant effects of rTM treatment have been demonstrated in ex vivo settings where prothrombinase activity was attenuated in plasma containing rTM when compared to plasma without rTM [15, 18]. The anticoagulant property of rTM has also been demonstrated in clinical settings where TAT, D-dimer, or fibrin/fibrinogen degradation products (FDP) concentrations were lower in the rTM treatment group compared with the control group [10, 19, 20]. Our results also showed a decrease in the TAT concentration after rTM treatment (Fig. 3b). The anticoagulant effects of rTM appear to be mainly mediated by APC, because subjects with factor V Leiden, an APC-resistant factor V variant, showed less

Table 1 Background characteristics of the patients with sepsis-associated DIC

Case	1	2	3	4	5	6	7	8
Age	69	39	72	65	64	71	67	81
Sex	F	M	M	M	M	M	M	M
Site of infection	Abd	Pulm	Pulm	Abd	Abd	Pulm	Abd	Pulm
APACHE II	7	13	21	36	28	23	30	22
SOFA	5	7	11	13	18	12	13	9
SIRS	4	3	3	3	4	3	4	2
DIC score	5	8	5	4	8	8	5	5
AT activity	78	80	58	44	33	74	55	77
Concomitant anticoagulants		NM	AT NM	AT NM	AT NM	AT	AT NM	NM
Outcome	Alive	Alive	Dead	Alive	Dead	Alive	Alive	Dead

F female, *M* male, *Abd* abdominal, *Pulm* pulmonary, *APACHE* acute physiology and chronic health evaluation, *SOFA* sequential organ failure assessment, *SIRS* systemic inflammatory response syndrome, *DIC* disseminated intravascular coagulation, *AT* antithrombin, *NM* nafamostat mesilate

APACHE II score was evaluated on the first day of intensive care unit admission. Overall prognosis was evaluated on day 28 after rTM treatment. All other parameters, including SIRS score, SOFA score, DIC score, and AT activity, were evaluated on the first day of rTM treatment

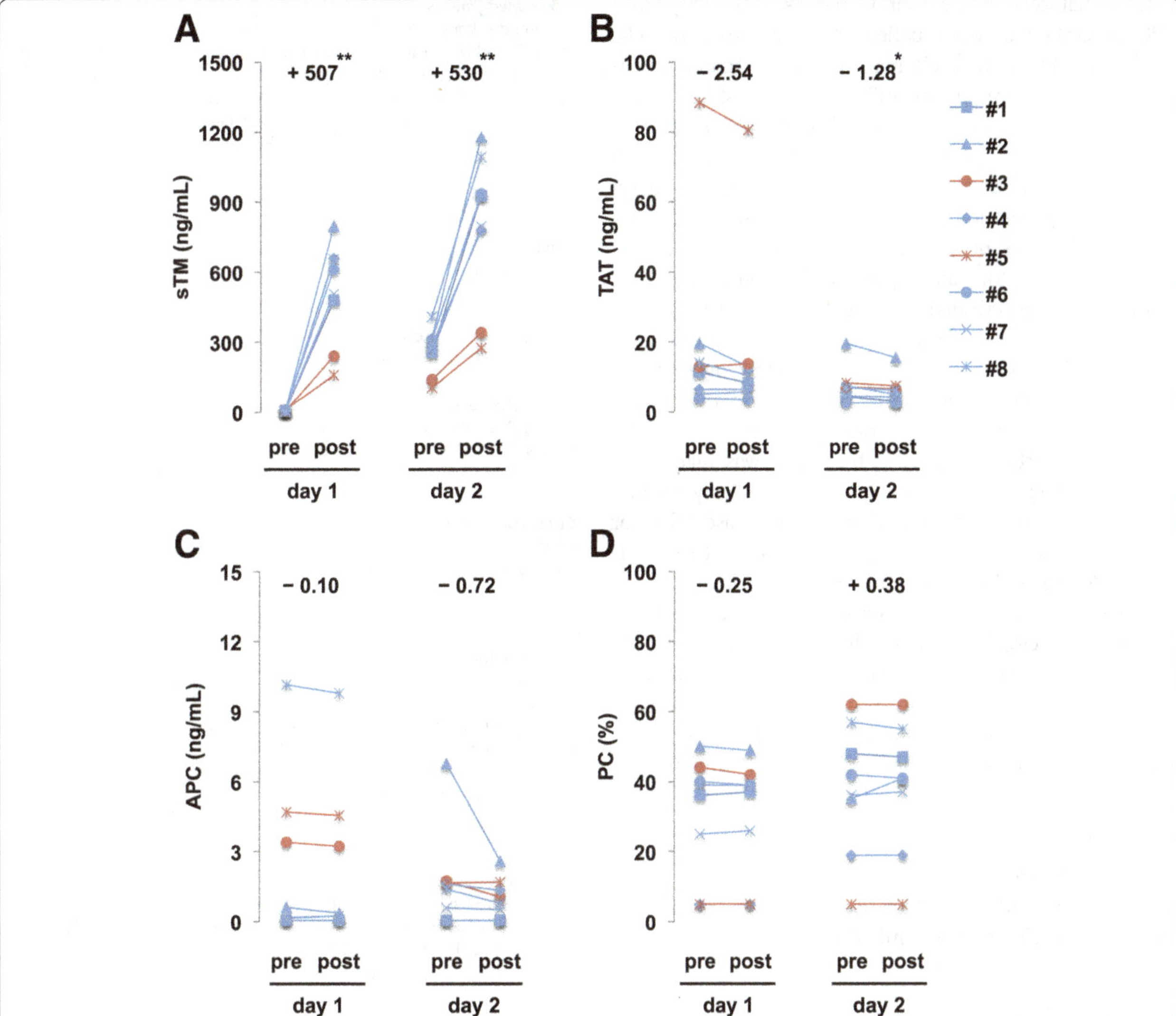

Fig. 3 Plasma APC levels are not increased in septic patients during a 30–60-min period of rTM treatment, while TAT levels are decreased during the treatment period. **a** Blood samples were collected from eight patients with sepsis-associated DIC before and after administration of rTM (130 U/kg: red symbols; 380 U/kg: blue symbols) on day 1 and day 2. Plasma sTM levels were determined by ELISA. **b** Plasma TAT levels were analyzed by STACIA CLEIA TAT. **c** Plasma APC levels were analyzed by the OLIGOBIND APC activity assay. **d** Plasma protein C levels were measured by a synthetic chromogenic substrate method using HemosIL Protein C. A paired *t*-test was used for comparisons before and after rTM treatment. $^{*}P < 0.05$, $^{**}P < 0.01$

pronounced anticoagulant effects after rTM treatment [15]. These findings indicate that the anticoagulant effects of rTM are evident in clinical settings and appear to be APC-dependent.

There could be some possible explanations for why deliverable APC was not detected in the plasma of septic patients after rTM treatment. One possibility is that APC acted locally and did not circulate systemically. APC conveys its anticoagulant activity when bound to phospholipids in the plasma membrane of activated platelets or other types of cells. APC also exerts multiple cytoprotective effects when bound to endothelial protein C receptor. Furthermore, APC in the systemic circulation can be inactivated by plasma proteins, such as protein C inhibitor, antitrypsin, and α2-macroglobulin. Thus, APC mainly acts on the surface of platelets and endothelial cells in focal coagulation sites, and a large part of APC generated in vivo may not circulate in the active form. The second possibility is that protein C levels and thrombin levels in septic patients were insufficient for APC generation. Plasma protein C levels can be decreased in septic patients in part due to decreased production of protein C in the liver and increased leakage to the extravascular space. Thrombin generation can be decreased in patients treated with rTM due to APC-mediated inactivation of the coagulation cascade. It is possible that decreased protein C and thrombin may blunt APC generation in septic patients treated with rTM. The third possibility is that plasma APC levels might be increased at other time points. rTM was administered to patients via drip infusion over a period of 30–60 min. Plasma rTM concentrations peak immediately after the completion of rTM administration [16]. In our in vitro APC generation assays, APC generation peaked within 10 min and the activity of APC was decreased over time probably because protein C inhibitor, antitrypsin, and α2-macroglobulin bound to and inactivated APC. Based on these findings, blood samples were collected immediately after the completion of rTM administration in this study. However, it is possible that APC generation in vivo requires more time, especially when APC is generated in the extravascular space. The fourth possibility is that APC was inactivated during handling of plasma samples. This is unlikely because all plasma samples were mixed with a protease inhibitor cocktail within 15 min after blood sampling and reconstituted APC was stable during this period (Additional file 2: Figure S2). Taken together, the present findings suggest that APC does not circulate systemically in the active form after rTM treatment. This may explain why bleeding complications occur infrequently after rTM treatment. However, we cannot completely exclude the possibility that rTM exerts anticoagulant effects in an APC-independent manner.

Conclusions

Plasma APC activity is not increased in septic patients treated with rTM. It is possible that APC acts locally and does not circulate systemically.

Additional files

Additional file 1: Figure S1. TAT levels in in vitro APC generation assays. Pooled normal plasma was incubated with thrombin T1063 (0–0.2 U/mL) and rTM (0–2000 ng/mL) at 37 °C for 10 min. TAT levels were analyzed by STACIA CLEIA TAT. The data represent mean ± SD. Representative data of two independent experiments are shown.

Additional file 2: Figure S2. Reconstituted APC is stable at 4 °C for 15 min before adding the protease inhibitor cocktail. For pre-analytical APC stability assays, whole blood samples from three healthy volunteers were spiked with 16.7 ng/mL equivalent activity of APC and kept at 4 °C. The protease inhibitor cocktail (PI cocktail) was added either before or 15 min after the APC spike. Plasma APC levels were analyzed by the OLIGOBIND APC activity assay. The data represent mean ± SD. Representative data of two independent experiments are shown.

Abbreviations

APACHE: Acute physiology and chronic health evaluation; APC: Activated protein C; DIC: Disseminated intravascular coagulation; ELISA: Enzyme-linked immunosorbent assay; F1 + 2: Prothrombin fragment 1 + 2; FDP: Fibrin/fibrinogen degradation products; rhAPC: Recombinant human activated protein C; rTM: Recombinant human soluble thrombomodulin; SIRS: Systemic inflammatory response syndrome; SOFA: Sequential organ failure assessment; sTM: Soluble thrombomodulin; TAT: Thrombin-antithrombin complex

Acknowledgments

The authors thank G. Honda (Asahi Kasei Pharma), T. Takano (Sekisui Medical), and M. Nakamura (Kagoshima University Hospital) for their expert technical assistance in performing the sTM, APC, and TAT quantification assays. The authors would also like to acknowledge the contribution of Dr. K. Yanagimoto for supporting the patient enrollment. The author would like to thank Alison Sherwin, PhD, from Edanz Group (www.edanzediting.com/ac) for editing a draft of this manuscript.

Funding

This study was supported by Asahi Kasei Pharma.

Authors' contributions

TA contributed to data analysis. TI contributed to study design and manuscript preparation. TY, HF, CK, TF, YM, SM, TE, and HH contributed to data analysis and sample collection. NY contributed to in vitro experiments. IM and YK contributed to data analysis and manuscript editing. All authors read and approved the final manuscript.

Competing interests

IM and TI have received research funding from Asahi Kasei Pharma, outside of the submitted work. All other authors state that they have no conflict of interests.

Author details

[1]Emergency and Critical Care Center, Kagoshima University Hospital, Kagoshima, Japan. [2]Department of Systems Biology in Thromboregulation, Kagoshima University Graduate School of Medical and Dental Sciences, 8-35-1 Sakuragaoka, Kagoshima 890-8544, Japan. [3]Emergency and Intensive Care Medicine, Kagoshima University Graduate School of Medical and Dental Sciences, Kagoshima, Japan.

References

1. Ito T, Kakihana Y, Maruyama I. Thrombomodulin as an intravascular safeguard against inflammatory and thrombotic diseases. Expert Opin Ther Targets. 2015;20:151–8. https://doi.org/10.1517/14728222.2016.1086750.
2. Esmon CT. The regulation of natural anticoagulant pathways. Science. 1987; 235:1348–52.
3. Faust SN, Levin M, Harrison OB, Goldin RD, Lockhart MS, Kondaveeti S, Laszik Z, Esmon CT, Heyderman RS. Dysfunction of endothelial protein C activation in severe meningococcal sepsis. N Engl J Med. 2001;345:408–16. https://doi.org/10.1056/NEJM200108093450603.
4. Saito H, Maruyama I, Shimazaki S, Yamamoto Y, Aikawa N, Ohno R, Hirayama A, Matsuda T, Asakura H, Nakashima M, Aoki N. Efficacy and safety of recombinant human soluble thrombomodulin (ART-123) in disseminated intravascular coagulation: results of a phase III, randomized, double-blind clinical trial. J Thromb Haemost. 2007;5:31–41. https://doi.org/10.1111/j.1538-7836.2006.02267.x.
5. Hayakawa M, Yamakawa K, Saito S, Uchino S, Kudo D, Iizuka Y, Sanui M, Takimoto K, Mayumi T, Ono K. Japan septic disseminated intravascular coagulation study group. Recombinant human soluble thrombomodulin and mortality in sepsis-induced disseminated intravascular coagulation A multicentre retrospective study. *Thromb Haemost*. 2016;115:1157–66. https://doi.org/10.1160/TH15-12-0987.
6. Bernard GR, Vincent J-L, Laterre P-F, LaRosa SP, Dhainaut J-F, Lopez-Rodriguez A, Steingrub JS, Garber GE, Helterbrand JD, Ely EW, Fisher CJ. Efficacy and safety of recombinant human activated protein C for severe Sepsis. N Engl J Med. 2001;344:699–709. https://doi.org/10.1056/NEJM200103083441001.
7. Abraham E, Laterre P-F, Garg R, Levy H, Talwar D, Trzaskoma BL, François B, Guy JS, Brückmann M, Rea-Neto Á, Rossaint R, Perrotin D, Sablotzki A, Arkins N, Utterback BG, Macias WL. Drotrecogin Alfa (activated) for adults with severe Sepsis and a low risk of death. N Engl J Med. 2005;353:1332–41. https://doi.org/10.1056/NEJMoa050935.
8. Nadel S, Goldstein B, Williams MD, Dalton H, Peters M, Macias WL, Abd-Allah SA, Levy H, Angle R, Wang D, Sundin DP, Giroir B. Drotrecogin alfa (activated) in children with severe sepsis: a multicentre phase III randomised controlled trial. Lancet. 2007;369:836–43.

9. Ranieri VM, Thompson BT, Barie PS, Dhainaut J-F, Douglas IS, Finfer S, Gårdlund B, Marshall JC, Rhodes A, Artigas A, Payen D, Tenhunen J, Al-Khalidi HR, Thompson V, Janes J, Macias WL, Vangerow B, Williams MD. Drotrecogin Alfa (activated) in adults with septic shock. N Engl J Med. 2012; 366:2055–64. https://doi.org/10.1056/NEJMoa1202290.
10. Vincent JL, Ramesh MK, Ernest D, Larosa SP, Pachl J, Aikawa N, Hoste E, Levy H, Hirman J, Levi M, Daga M, Kutsogiannis DJ, Crowther M, Bernard GR, Devriendt J, Puigserver JV, Blanzaco DU, Esmon CT, Parrillo JE, Guzzi L, Henderson SJ, Pothirat C, Mehta P, Fareed J, Talwar D, Tsuruta K, Gorelick KJ, Osawa Y, Kaul I. A Randomized, Double-Blind, Placebo-Controlled, Phase 2b Study to Evaluate the Safety and Efficacy of Recombinant Human Soluble Thrombomodulin, ART-123, in Patients With Sepsis and Suspected Disseminated Intravascular Coagulation. *Crit Care Med*. 2013;**41**:2069–79. https://doi.org/10.1097/CCM.0b013e31828e9b03.
11. Umemura Y, Yamakawa K, Ogura H, Yuhara H, Fujimi S. Efficacy and safety of anticoagulant therapy in three specific populations with sepsis: a meta-analysis of randomized controlled trials. J Thromb Haemost. 2016;14:518–30. https://doi.org/10.1111/jth.13230.
12. Muller J, Friedrich M, Becher T, Braunstein J, Kupper T, Berdel P, Gravius S, Rohrbach F, Oldenburg J, Mayer G, Potzsch B. Monitoring of plasma levels of activated protein C using a clinically applicable oligonucleotide-based enzyme capture assay. J Thromb Haemost. 2012;10:390–8. https://doi.org/10.1111/j.1538-7836.2012.04623.x.
13. Singer M, Deutschman CS, Seymour C, et al. The third international consensus definitions for sepsis and septic shock (sepsis-3). JAMA. 2016;315: 801–10. https://doi.org/10.1001/jama.2016.0287.
14. Gando S, Iba T, Eguchi Y, Ohtomo Y, Okamoto K, Koseki K, Mayumi T, Murata A, Ikeda T, Ishikura H, Ueyama M, Ogura H, Kushimoto S, Saitoh D, Endo S, Shimazaki S. A multicenter, prospective validation of disseminated intravascular coagulation diagnostic criteria for critically ill patients: comparing current criteria. Crit Care Med. 2006;34:625–31.
15. Moll S, Lindley C, Pescatore S, Morrison D, Tsuruta K, Mohri M, Serada M, Sata M, Shimizu H, Yamada K, White GC 2nd. Phase I study of a novel recombinant human soluble thrombomodulin, ART-123. J Thromb Haemost. 2004;2:1745–51. https://doi.org/10.1111/j.1538-7836.2004.00927.x.
16. Hayakawa M, Kushimoto S, Watanabe E, Goto K, Suzuki Y, Kotani T, Kiguchi T, Yatabe T, Tagawa J, Komatsu F, Gando S. Pharmacokinetics of recombinant human soluble thrombomodulin in disseminated intravascular coagulation patients with acute renal dysfunction. Thromb Haemost. 2017; 117:851–9. https://doi.org/10.1160/th16-07-0547.
17. Watanabe E, Yamazaki S, Setoguchi D, Sadahiro T, Tateishi Y, Suzuki T, Ishii I, Oda S. Pharmacokinetics of standard- and reduced-dose recombinant human soluble Thrombomodulin in patients with septic disseminated intravascular coagulation during continuous Hemodiafiltration. Front Med. 2017;4:15. https://doi.org/10.3389/fmed.2017.00015.
18. Hayakawa M, Yamamoto H, Honma T, Mukai N, Higashiyama A, Sugano M, Kubota N, Uegaki S, Sawamura A, Gando S. Pharmacokinetics and pharmacodynamics of recombinant soluble thrombomodulin in disseminated intravascular coagulation patients with renal impairment. Shock. 2012;37:569–73. https://doi.org/10.1097/SHK.0b013e318252bc82.
19. Yamakawa K, Fujimi S, Mohri T, Matsuda H, Nakamori Y, Hirose T, Tasaki O, Ogura H, Kuwagata Y, Hamasaki T, Shimazu T. Treatment effects of recombinant human soluble thrombomodulin in patients with severe sepsis: a historical control study. Crit Care. 2011;15:R123. https://doi.org/10.1186/cc10228.
20. Yamakawa K, Ogura H, Fujimi S, Morikawa M, Ogawa Y, Mohri T, Nakamori Y, Inoue Y, Kuwagata Y, Tanaka H, Hamasaki T, Shimazu T. Recombinant human soluble thrombomodulin in sepsis-induced disseminated intravascular coagulation: a multicenter propensity score analysis. Intensive Care Med. 2013;39:644–52. https://doi.org/10.1007/s00134-013-2822-2.

24

Differences and similarities between disseminated intravascular coagulation and thrombotic microangiopathy

Hideo Wada[1*], Takeshi Matsumoto[2], Kei Suzuki[3], Hiroshi Imai[3], Naoyuki Katayama[4], Toshiaki Iba[5] and Masanori Matsumoto[6]

Abstract

Introduction: Both disseminated intravascular coagulation (DIC) and thrombotic microangiopathy (TMA) cause microvascular thrombosis associated with thrombocytopenia, bleeding tendency and organ failure.

Reports and discussion: The frequency of DIC is higher than that of thrombotic thrombocytopenic purpura (TTP). Many patients with TMA are diagnosed with DIC, but only about 15% of DIC patients are diagnosed with TMA. Hyperfibrinolysis is observed in most patients with DIC, and microangiopathic hemolytic anemia is observed in most patients with TMA. Markedly decreased ADAMTS13 activity, the presence of Shiga-toxin-producing *Escherichia coli* (STEC) and abnormality of the complement system are useful for the diagnosis of TTP, STEC-hemolytic uremic syndrome (HUS)and atypical HUS, respectively. However, there are no specific biomarkers for the diagnosis of DIC.

Conclusion: Although DIC and TMA are similar appearances, all coagulation, fibrinolysis and platelet systems are activated in DIC, and only platelets are markedly activated in TMA.

Keywords: DIC, TMA, Microvascular thrombosis, Hyperfibrinolysis, Organ failure, Microangiopathic hemolytic anemia

Background

Disseminated intravascular coagulation (DIC) [1, 2] is a serious disease that causes microvascular thrombosis associated with thrombocytopenia, a bleeding tendency and organ failure. These symptoms and laboratory data are similar to those of thrombotic microangiopathy (TMA) [3] which includes thrombotic thrombocytopenic purpura (TTP) [4, 5], Shiga-toxin-producing *Escherichia coli* (STEC) - hemolytic uremic syndrome (HUS) [6, 7], complement-mediated TMA (also called atypical HUS; aHUS) [7, 8] and secondary TMA [3, 9]. DIC also has several clinical subtypes, including asymptomatic type, marked bleeding type, organ failure type and complication types such as TTP or heparin-induced thrombocytopenia [10]. As the treatment of DIC [11] differs from that of TMA [4, 12], it is important to perform a differential diagnosis of DIC and TMA. The differences and similarities between DIC and TMA are reviewed in this study.

* Correspondence: wadahide@clin.medic.mie-u.ac.jp
[1]Department of Molecular and Laboratory Medicine, Mie University Graduate School of Medicine, Tsu, Mie 514-8507, Japan
Full list of author information is available at the end of the article

Differences in the definition and concept of DIC and TMA

The frequency of pneumonia associated DIC was reported to be about 10,000 cases per year according to the Japanese Diagnosis Procedure Combination (DPC) database [13], suggesting that DIC due to pneumonia occurs in about $70/10^6$ populations. With the addition of other types of DIC, the frequency of all DIC is about $300/10^6$ populations. In contrast, the frequency of TTP was reported to be $2.0/10^6$ populations [3]. These reports suggest that the frequency of DIC in Japan is 150-fold higher than that of TTP (Fig. 1). According to the International Society of Thrombosis and Haemostasis (ISTH), DIC is an acquired syndrome characterized by the intravascular activation of coagulation with the loss of localization arising from different causes. It can originate from and cause damage to the microvasculature, which if sufficiently severe, can produce organ dysfunction. DIC is characterized by the generation of fibrin

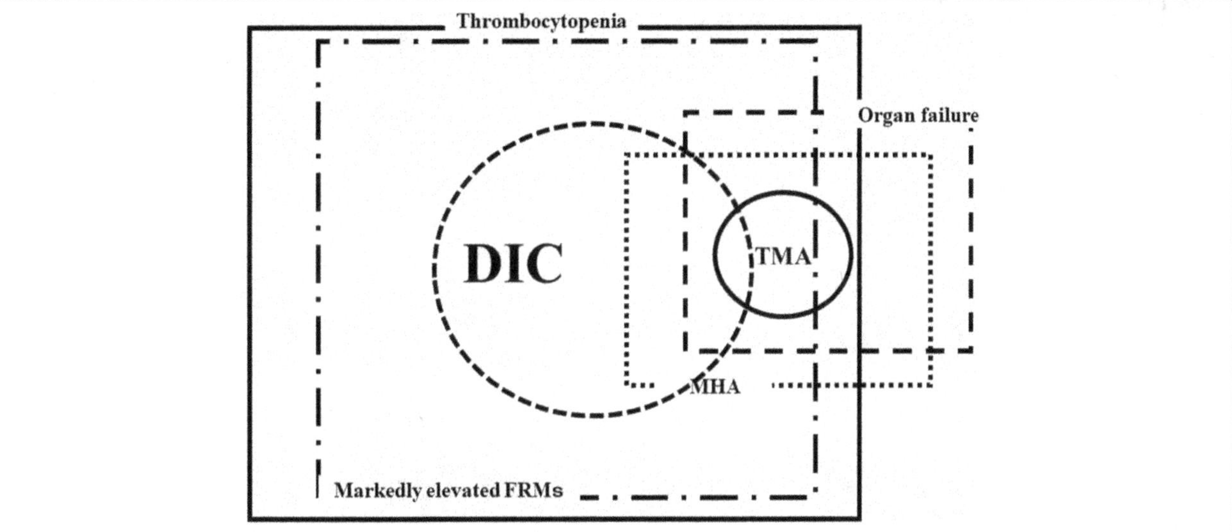

Fig. 1 Concept of DIC and TMA. DIC, disseminated intravascular coagulation; TMA, thrombotic microangiopahy; MHA, microangiopathic hemolyitc anemia; FRMs; fibrin related markers

related markers (FRMs; soluble fibrin monomers, fibrinogen and fibrin degradation products [FDPs], D-dimers, etc.) and reflects an acquired (inflammatory) or non-inflammatory disorder of the microvasculature [1]. Regarding the definition of TMA, TMA presents with microangiopathic hemolytic anemia (MHA), including hemolytic anemia, thrombocytopenia and organ failure in the kidney, central nervous system, and other organs [3, 4]. These findings suggest that marked elevation of FRMs is required in DIC while MHA is required in TMA; the diagnosis of TTP among TMA requires a markedly decreased ADAMTS13 level [14], that of STEC-HUS requires the detection of a STEC infection [15] and that of aHUS requires the detection of abnormalities in the complement system [16].

However, DIC has no specific marker for its diagnosis and is instead diagnosed by a scoring system using global coagulation tests. Furthermore, DIC is often associated with TMA, and TMA is often associated with DIC [17], suggesting that a differential diagnosis between DIC and TMA may be difficult.

DIC associated with TMA was observed in patients with bone marrow metastasis of solid cancer as gastric cancer, those with liver failure and those with group A streptococcal infection. In patients with DIC, bone marrow metastasis mainly causes MHA, liver failure mainly causes an

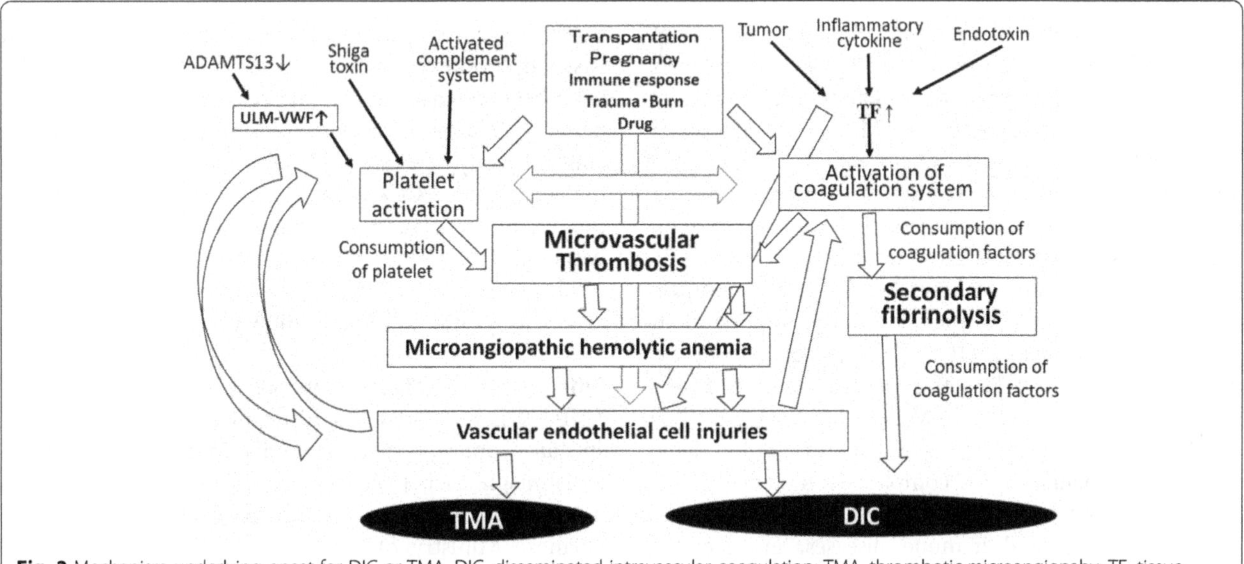

Fig. 2 Mechanism underlying onset for DIC or TMA. DIC, disseminated intravascular coagulation; TMA, thrombotic microangiopahy; TF, tissue factor; ULM-VWF, ultra-large multimers of von Willebrand factor

Table 1 Diagnostic criteria for infectious DIC

	ISTH	P	JSTH	P	JMHLW	P	JAAM	P
PLT (× 10³/μl)	100 ≧ > 50	1	120 ≧ > 80	1	120 ≧ > 80	1	120 ≧ > 8.0	1
	50 ≧	2	80 ≧ > 50	2	80 ≧ > 50	2		
			50 ≧	3	50 ≧	3	80 ≧	3
Reduction of PLT			30%	1*			30%	1*
							50%	3*
Prothrombin time ratio or Prolongation (s)	3 ≦ < 6.0	1	1.25 ≦ < 1.67	1	1.25 ≦ < 1.67	1	1.2 ≦	1
	6 ≦	2	1.67 ≦	2	1.67 ≦	2		
Fibrinogen (g/L)	1.0 ≧	1			1.5 ≧ > 1.0	1		
					1.0 ≧	2		
Fibrin related markers, FDP (μg/ml)			10 ≦ < 20	1	10 ≦ < 20	1	10 ≦ < 25	1
	Increase	2	20 ≦ < 40	2	20 ≦ < 40	2		
	Markedly increase	3	40 ≦	3	40 ≦	3	25 ≦	3
Antithrombin			< 70%	1				
TAT or SF			2 fold higher of NR					
Underlying diseases					Positive	1		
Bleeding					Positive	1		
OF due to thrombosis					Positive	1		
SIRS							Positive	1
DIC		5 ≦		5 ≦		7 ≦		4 ≦

ISTH International Society of Thrombosis and Haemostasis, *JSTH* Japanese Society of Thrombosis and Hemostasis, *JMHLW* Japanese Ministry of Health, Labor and Welfare, *JAAM* Japanese Association for Acute Medicine, *PLT* platelet count, *FDP* fibrinogen and fibrin degradation products, *TAT* thrombin antithrombin complex, *SF* soluble fibrin, *SIRS* systemic inflammatory response syndrome, *DIC* disseminated intravascular coagulation
*PLT and reduction of PLT pointes should be within 3 points

increase in the von Willebrand factor/ADAMTS13 ratio, and group A streptococcal infection mainly cause massive hemolysis. However, it would be much more important to find TMA associated with DIC.

Differences and similarities in the mechanism of onset for DIC and TMA

The basic mechanism of onset for DIC is the marked activation and consumption of coagulation system followed by the activation of secondary fibrinolysis [18]. In contrast, the basic mechanism of onset for TMA is the marked activation and consumption of platelets due to several factors followed by the activation and injury of vascular endothelial cells [19, 20] (Fig. 2). Triggers of the activation of coagulation system are reported to include tissue factor (TF) [21, 22], inflammatory cytokines [23, 24] and lipopolysaccharide (LPS) [25], the activation leukocytes [26] and abnormal delivery among others. Trigger of platelet and vascular endothelial cells activation are reported to be a marked decrease in the ADAMTS13 levels in TTP [27], the detection of STEC in STEC-HUS [15] and the detection of abnormalities in the complement system in aHUS [16], along with other factors, such as transplantation, pregnancy, drugs and immune diseases, in secondary TMA [28]. Particularly marked decreases in the ADAMS13 level result in an inability to cleave ultra-large multimers of von Willebrand factor [29, 30], thereby causing platelet aggregation. Markedly fibrinolysis is frequently observed in most patients with DIC, except for some septic DIC cases [31], while markedly fibrinolysis is not observed in patients with TMA.

Both DIC and TMA cause microvascular thrombosis, which is caused mainly by the activation of the coagulation system in DIC and by the activation of platelets and vascular endothelial cells in TMA. Several cases of TMA have been reported to be complicated with hemophilia patients treated with activated prothrombin complex concentrates (APCCs) in the clinical trial for Emicizumab [32]. As APCCs usually causes DIC but not TMA, the differential diagnosis is important in these cases [33]. Although DIC is an acquired disease, Upshaw-Schulman syndrome as familial TTP [34] and many patients with aHUS are examples of congenital TMA.

Difference in the diagnosis between DIC and TMA

As there is no gold standard for diagnosing DIC and no specific biomarker that clearly diagnoses DIC, the differential diagnosis between DIC and TMA is difficult. Four diagnostic criteria for DIC has been established by the Japanese Ministry of Health, Labor and Welfare [35], ISTH [1], Japanese Association for Acute Medicine [36] and the Japanese Society on Thrombosis and Hemostasis

Table 2 Diagnostic criteria for TMA [4, 35, 36]

	STEC-HUS	aHUS	TTP	TMA
Hemoglobin (g/dl)	10.0 ≧	10.0 ≧	Hemolysis	10.0 ≧
Platelet (× 10^4/μl)	15.0 ≧	15.0 ≧	Thrombocytopenia	15.0 ≧
Ogan failure	Renal failure Creatinine ≧1.5 folds of the standard	Renal failure Creatinine ≧1.5 folds of the standard	Neurological symptoms	?
Laboratory finding	Detection of STEC	Genetic abnormality in the complement system	ADAMTS13 < 10%	?

TMA thrombotic microangiopathy, *aHUS* atypical hemolytic uremic syndrome, *TTP* thrombotic thrombocytopenic purpura, *STEC* Shiga toxin-producing *Escherichia coli*

(JSTH) [37, 38]. These diagnostic criteria use a similar scoring system based on global coagulation tests (GLTs) such as the platelet count, prothrombin time (PT), FRMs (Table 1). Therefore, there are no significant differences in the usefulness among various diagnostic criteria for DIC [39]. The diagnosis of TMA is based on the presence of hemolytic anemia (hemoglobin < 10 g/dl), thrombocytopenia (12 × 10^9/ml) and organ failure. TMA patients with ADAMTS13 < 10%, those with STEC and those with abnormalities in the complement system can be easily diagnosed with TTP, STEC-HUS and aHUS, respectively (Table 2) [4, 40, 41]. However, markedly decreased ADAMTS13 levels have been reported in severe sepsis patients without TTP [42, 43], suggesting that platelet activation due to decreased ADAMTS13 might be observed in DIC patients with severe sepsis. The diagnosis of other TMA aside from DIC with hemolysis is difficult. Most patients with TMA can be diagnosed using several DIC diagnostic criteria to have DIC, but only 10%–15% of DIC patients can be diagnosed to have TMA (Fig. 2).

Differences and similarities between DIC and TMA

The differences and similarities between DIC and TMA are described in Table 3. Among clinical symptoms, bleeding and organ failure are frequently observed in patients with DIC as well as those with TMA, but lung or cardiovascular failures is more frequently observed only in patients with DIC [44], while renal or central nervous system failure is more frequently observed in patients with TMA [3]. Hypotension as organ failure is observed in many patients with DIC, while hypertension tend to be observed in patients with TMA [45]. Hypertension may be caused by acute kidney injury or arterial occlusion.

Table 3 Differences and similarities between TMA and DIC

		Severe DIC	Severe TMA
Symptoms	Organ failure	Often (Lung, Kidney, Shock)	Usually (Kidney, CNS)
	Bleeding and bleeding tendency	Frequent	Frequent
	Blood pressure	Low	High
	Hematuria	Sometimes	Frequent
	Anemia	Often	Usually
Laboratory data	Platelet count	Low	Low
	Hemoglobin	Often low	Low
	Fibrin related markers	Markedly high	Slightly high
	Prothrombin time	Often prolong	Normal
	Antithrombin	Often low	Normal
	Albumin	Often low	Normal
	Creatinine	Often high	High
	Total bilirubin, LDH	Often high	High
Treatments	Supportive therapy	Recommended	Recommended
	Blood transfusion (RBC, FFP)	Recommended	Recommended,
	Blood transfusion (PC)	Recommended	Not recommended
	Anticoagulant	Recommended (Japan)	Not mentioned
	PE/FFP	Not mentioned	Recommended
	Special treatment	AT, rhTM (Japan)	Hemodialysis (HUS), Eculizumab (aHUS), Rituximab (TTP)

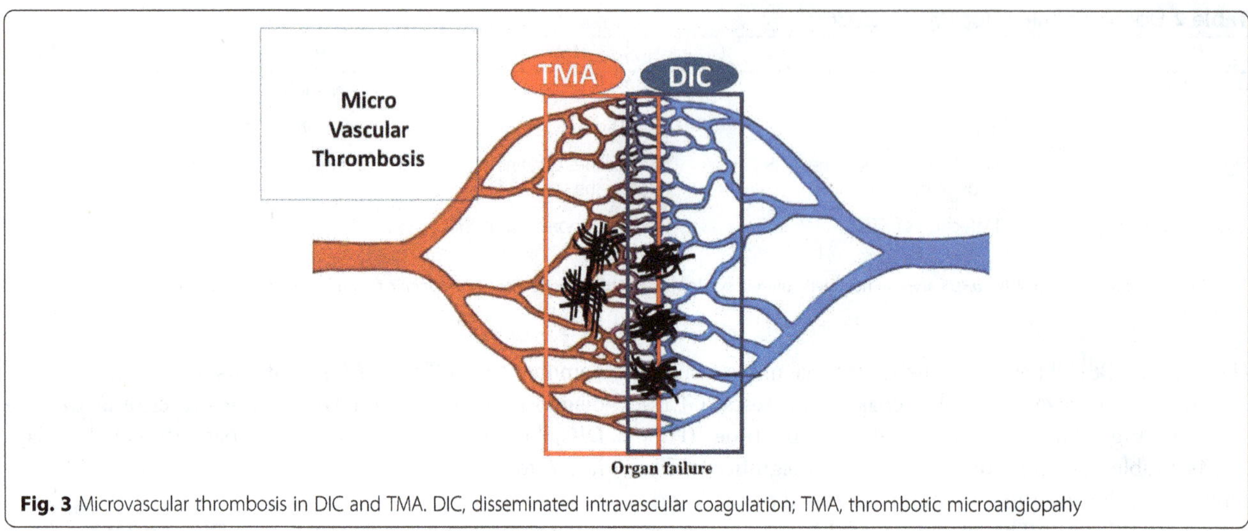

Fig. 3 Microvascular thrombosis in DIC and TMA. DIC, disseminated intravascular coagulation; TMA, thrombotic microangiopahy

Anemia is also more frequently observed in patients with TMA [20, 46] than in those with DIC. Red blood cell fragmentation may be caused by microvascular thrombosis on the arterial side which has a high blood pressure, but not on the venous side (Fig. 3). Among laboratory data, thrombocytopenia is observed in both DIC and TMA. A decreased hemoglobin level and increased levels of creatinine, total bilirubin and LDH are observed in most patients with TMA, but these abnormalities are observed in only 15% of patients with DIC. A prolonged PT and decreased AT and albumin levels are frequently (but not always) observed in patients with DIC. Markedly elevated FRMs are observed in most patients with DIC. As markedly fibrinolysis may dissolve microthromboses in patients with DIC but not in those with TMA, thrombosis of DIC is not usually detected on autopsy. Therefore, elevated FRMs and decreased platelet counts are the most useful markers for DIC [1].

In Japan, regarding the treatment of DIC and TMA, platelet transfusion is contraindicated for TMA [4], while anticoagulant therapy for DIC, but not for TMA, is recommended [10, 11]. Anti-fibrinolytic therapy is recommended for DIC patients with hyperfibrinolysis. Plasma exchange is recommended in most some cases of TMA such as TTP [47], but not for DIC. Antithrombin concentrate [48] and recombinant thrombomodulin [49] for DIC are frequently used in Japan, while eculizumab [50] has proven effective for compliment mediated TMA, such as aHUS, and rituximab [51] is effective for TTP in patients with a high titer of inhibitor for ADAMTS13.

Conclusion

DIC and TMA are similar appearances, however, all coagulation, fibrinolysis and platelet systems are activated in DIC, and only platelets are markedly activated in TMA. As treatment is different between DIC and TMA, differential diagnosis between DIC and TMA is important.

Abbreviations

aHUS: atypical HUS; DIC: Disseminated intravascular coagulation; DPC: Diagnosis Procedure Combination; FDP: fibrinogen and fibrin degradation products; FRMs: fibrin related markers; GLTs: global coagulation tests; HUS: Hemolytic uremic syndrome; ISTH: International Society of Thrombosis and Haemostasis; JSTH: Japanese Society on Thrombosis and Hemostasis; MHA: microangiopathic hemolytic anemia; PT: prothrombin time; STEC: Shiga- toxin-producing *Escherichia coli*; TMA: thrombotic microangiopathy; TTP: thrombotic thrombocytopenic purpura

Acknowledgements

None

Funding

This work was supported in part by a Grant-in-Aid from the Ministry of Health, Labour and Welfare of Japan and the Ministry of Education, Culture, Sports, Science and Technology of Japan.

Authors' contributions

WH fully wrote this manuscript. MT, SK and IH reviewed these references. KN, IT, and MM discussed and gave the suggestions for this manuscript. All authors read and approved the final manuscript.

Competing interests

The authors declare that they have no competing interests.

Author details

[1]Department of Molecular and Laboratory Medicine, Mie University Graduate School of Medicine, Tsu, Mie 514-8507, Japan. [2]Division of Blood Transfusion Medicine and Cell Therapy, Mie University Graduate School of Medicine, Tsu, Japan. [3]Emergency Critical Care Center, Mie University Graduate School of

Medicine, Tsu, Japan. [4]Department of Hematology and Oncology, Mie University Graduate School of Medicine, Tsu, Japan. [5]Department of Emergency and Disaster Medicine, Juntendo University Graduate School of Medicine, Tokyo, Japan. [6]Department of Blood Transfusion Medicine, Nara Medical University, Nara, Japan.

References

1. Taylor FB Jr, Toh CH, Hoots WK, Wada H, Levi M. Scientific subcommittee on disseminated intravascular coagulation (DIC) of the international society on thrombosis and Haemostasis (ISTH): towards definition, clinical and laboratory criteria, and a scoring system for disseminated intravascular coagulation. Thromb Haemost. 2001;86:1327–30.
2. Wada H, Matsumoto T, Yamashita Y, Hatada T. Disseminated intravascular coagulation: testing and diagnosis. Clin Chim Acta. 2014;436C:130–4.
3. Wada H, Matsumoto T, Yamashita Y. Natural history of thrombotic thrombocytopenic Purpura and hemolytic uremic syndrome. Semin Thromb Hemost. 2014;40:866–73.
4. Matsumoto M, Fujimura Y, Wada H, Kokame K, Miyakawa Y, Ueda Y, Higasa S, Moriki T, Yagi H, Miyata T, Murata M. For TTP group of blood coagulation abnormalities research team, research on rare and intractable disease supported by health, labour, and welfare sciences research grants.: Diagnostic and treatment guidelines for thrombotic thrombocytopenic purpura (TTP) 2017 in Japan. Int J Hematol. 2017;106:3–15.
5. South K, Lane DA. ADAMTS-13 and von Willebrand factor: a dynamic duo. J Thromb Haemost. 2017; in press
6. Mele C, Remuzzi G, Noris M. Hemolytic uremic syndrome. Semin Immunopathol. 2014;36:399–420.
7. Jokiranta TS. HUS and atypical HUS. Blood. 2017;129:2847–56.
8. Shen YM. Clinical evaluation of thrombotic microangiopathy: identification of patients with suspected atypical hemolytic uremic syndrome. Thromb J. 2016;14(Suppl 1):19.
9. Epperla N, Hemauer K, Hamadani M, Friedman KD, Kreuziger LB. Impact of treatment and outcomes for patients with posttransplant drug-associated thrombotic microangiopathy. Transfusion. 2017;57:2775–81.
10. Wada H, Asakura H, Okamoto K, Iba T, Uchiyama T, Kawasugi K, Koga S, Mayumi T, Koike K, Gando S, Kushimoto S, Seki Y, Madoiwa S, Maruyama I, Yoshioka A. Japanese Society of Thrombosis Hemostasis/DIC subcommittee: expert consensus for the treatment of disseminated intravascular coagulation in Japan. Thromb Res. 2010;125:6–11.
11. Wada H, Thachil J, Di Nisio M, Mathew P, Kurosawa S, Gando S, Kim HK, Nielsen JD, Dempfle CE, Levi M, Toh CH. The scientific standardization committee on DIC of the international society on thrombosis Haemostasis.: guidance for diagnosis and treatment of DIC from harmonization of the recommendations from three guidelines. J Thromb Haemost. 2013;11:761–7.
12. Scully M, Hunt BJ, Benjamin S, Liesner R, Rose P, Peyvandi F, Cheung B, Machin SJ. British Committee for Standards in Haematology: guidelines on the diagnosis and management of thrombotic thrombocytopenic purpura and other thrombotic microangiopathies. Br J Haematol. 2012;158:323–35.
13. Tagami T, Matsui H, Horiguchi H, Fushimi K, Yasunaga H. Antithrombin and mortality in severe pneumonia patients with sepsis-associated disseminated intravascular coagulation: an observational nationwide study. J Thromb Haemost. 2014;12:1470–9.
14. Yoshii Y, Fujimura Y, Bennett CL, Isonishi A, Kurumatani N, Matsumoto M. Implementation of a rapid assay of ADAMTS13 activity was associated with improved 30-day survival rate in patients with acquired primary thrombotic thrombocytopenic purpura who received platelet transfusions. Transfusion. 2017;57:2045–53.
15. Grisaru S, Xie J, Samuel S, Hartling L, Tarr PI, Schnadower D, Freedman SB, Alberta Provincial Pediatric Enteric Infection Team. Associations between hydration status, intravenous fluid administration, and outcomes of patients infected with Shiga toxin-producing Escherichia coli: a systematic review and meta-analysis. JAMA Pediatr. 2017;171:68–76.
16. Berger BE. The alternative pathway of complement and the evolving clinical-pathophysiological Spectrum of atypical hemolytic uremic syndrome. Am J Med Sci. 2016;352:177–90.
17. Schwameis M, Schörgenhofer C, Assinger A, Steiner MM, Jilma B. VWF excess and ADAMTS13 deficiency: a unifying pathomechanism linking inflammation to thrombosis in DIC, malaria, and TTP. Thromb Haemost. 2015;113:708–18.
18. Wada H. Disseminated intravascular coagulation. Clin Chim Acta. 2004;344:13–21.
19. Yamashita Y, Naitoh K, Wada H, Ikejiri M, Mastumoto T, Ohishi K, Hosaka Y, Nishikawa M, Katayama N. Elevated plasma levels of soluble platelet glycoprotein VI (GPVI) in patients with thrombotic microangiopathy. Thromb Res. 2014;133(3):440–4.
20. Ito-Habe N, Wada H, Matsumoto T, Ohishi K, Toyoda H, Ishikawa E, Nomura S, Komada Y, Ito M, Nobori T, Katayama N. Elevated Von Willebrand factor propeptide for the diagnosis of thrombotic microangiopathy and for predicting a poor outcome. Int J Hematol. 2011;93:47–52.
21. Sase T, Wada H, Nishioka J, abe Y, Gabazza EC, Shiku H, Suzuki K, Nakamura S, Nobori T. Measurement of tissue factor messenger RNA levels in leukocytes from patients in hypercoagulable state caused by several underlying diseases. Thromb Haemost. 2003;89:660–5.
22. Sase T, Wada H, Kamikura Y, Kaneko T, Abe Y, Nishioka J, Nobori T, Shiku H. Tissue factor messenger RNA levels in leukocytes compared with tissue factor antigens in plasma from patients in hypercoagulable state caused by various diseases. Thromb Haemost. 2004;92:132–9.
23. Wada H, Tamaki S, Tanigawa M, Takagi M, Deguchi A, Mori Y, Katayama N, Yamamoto T, Deguchi K, Shirakawa S. Plasma level of IL-1β in disseminated intravascular coagulation. Thrombo Haemost. 1991;65:364–8.
24. Wada H, Ohiwa M, Kaneko T, Tamaki S, Tanigawa M, Takagi M, Mori M, Shirakawa M. Plasma level of tumor necrosis factor in disseminated intravascular coagulation. Am J Hematol. 1991;37:147–51.
25. Duburcq T, Tournoys A, Gnemmi V, Hubert T, Gmyr V, Pattou F, Jourdain M. Impact of obesity on endotoxin-induced disseminated intravascular coagulation. Shock. 2015;44:341–7.
26. Matsumoto T, Kaneko T, Wada H, Kobayashi T, Abe Y, Nobori T, Shiku H, Stearns-Kurosawa DJ, Kurosawa S. Proteinase 3 expression on neutrophil membranes from patients with infectious disease. Shock. 2006;26:128–33.
27. Kobayashi T, Wada H, Nishioka J, Yamamoto M, Matsumoto T, Tamaru T, Nomura S, Masuya M, Mori Y, Nakatani K, Nishikawa M, Katayama N, Nobori T. ADAMTS13 related markers and Von Willebrand factor in plasma from patients with thrombotic Microangipathy (TMA). Thromb Res. 2008;121:849–54.
28. Franchini M, Montagnana M, Targher G, Lippi G. Reduced von Willebrand factor-cleaving protease levels in secondary thrombotic microangiopathies and other diseases. Semin Thromb Hemost. 2007;33:787–97.
29. Ruggeri ZM, Zimmerman TS. The complex multimeric composition of factor VIII/von Willebrand factor. Blood. 1981;57:1140–3.
30. Arya M, Anvari B, Romo GM, Cruz MA, Dong JF, McIntire LV, Moake JL, Lopez JA. Ultralarge multimers of von Willebrand factor form spontaneous high-strength bonds with the platelet glycoprotein Ib-IX complex: studies using optical tweezers. Blood. 2002;99:3971–7.
31. Wada T, Gando S, Maekaw K, Katabami K, Sageshima H, Hayakawa M, Sawamura A. Disseminated intravascular coagulation with increased fibrinolysis during the early phase of isolated traumatic brain injury. Crit Care. 2017;21:219.
32. Oldenburg J, Mahlangu JN, Kim B, Schmitt C, Callaghan MU, Young G, Santagostino E, Kruse-Jarres R, Negrier C, Kessler C, et al. Emicizumab prophylaxis in hemophilia a with inhibitors. N Engl J Med. 2017;377:809–18.
33. Wada H, Matsumoto T, Katayama N. Emicizumab prophylaxis in hemophilia a with inhibitors. N Engl J Med. 2017;377:2193–4.
34. Fujimura Y, Matsumoto M, Isonishi A, Yagi H, Kokame K, Soejima K, Murata M, Miyata T. Natural history of Upshaw-Schulman syndrome based on ADAMTS13 gene analysis in Japan. J Thromb Haemost. 2011;9:283–301.
35. Kobayashi N, Maekawa T, Takada M, Tanaka H, Gonmori H. Criteria for diagnosis of DIC based on the analysis of clinical and laboratory findings in 345 DIC patients collected by the research committee on DIC in Japan. Bibl Haematol. 1983;49:265–75.
36. Gando S, Saitoh D, Ogura H, Mayumi T, Koseki K, Ikeda T, et al. Japanese Association for Acute Medicine Disseminated Intravascular Coagulation (JAAM DIC) study group: natural history of disseminated intravascular coagulation diagnosed based on the newly established diagnostic criteria

for critically ill patients: results of a multicenter, prospective survey. Crit Care Med. 2008;36:145–50.
37. Asakura H, Takahashi H, Uchiyama T, Eguchi Y, Okamoto K, Kawasugi K, Madoiwa S, Wada H. DIC subcommittee of the Japanese Society on Thrombosis and Hemostasis: Proposal for new diagnostic criteria for DIC from the Japanese Society on Thrombosis and Hemostasis. Thromb J. 2016;14:42.
38. Wada H, Takahashi H, Uchiyama T, Eguchi Y, Okamoto K, Kawasugi K, Madoiwa S, Asakura H. DIC subcommittee of the Japanese Society on Thrombosis and Hemostasis: The approval of revised diagnostic criteria for DIC from the Japanese Society on Thrombosis and Hemostasis. Thromb J. 2017;15:17.
39. Takemitsu T, Wada H, Hatada T, Ohmori Y, Ishikura K, Takeda T, Sugiyama T, Yamada N, Maruyama K, Katayama N, Isaji S, Shimpo H, Kusunoki M, Nobori T. Prospective evaluation of three different diagnostic criteria for disseminated intravascular coagulation. Thromb Haemost. 2011;105:40–4.
40. Terano C, Ishikura K, Hamada R, Yoshida Y, Kubota W, Okuda Y, Shinozuka S, Harada R, Iyoda S, Fujimura Y, Hamasaki Y, Hataya H, Honda M. Practical issues in using eculizumab for children with atypical hemolytic uremic syndrome in the acute phase: a review of 4 patients. Nephrology (Carlton). 2017; in press
41. Kato H, Nangaku M, Hataya H, Sawai T, Ashida A, Fujimaru R, Hidaka Y, Kaname S, Maruyama S, Yasuda T, Yoshida Y, Ito S, Hattori M, Miyakawa Y, Fujimura Y, Okada H, Kagami S. Joint Committee for the Revision of clinical guides of atypical hemolytic uremic syndrome in Japan: clinical guides for atypical hemolytic uremic syndrome in Japan. Pediatr Int. 2016;58:549–55.
42. Ono T, Mimuro J, Madoiwa S, Soejima K, Kashiwakura Y, Ishiwata A, Takano K, Ohmori T, Sakata Y. Severe secondary deficiency of von Willebrand factor-cleaving protease (ADAMTS13) in patients with sepsis-induced disseminated intravascular coagulation: its correlation with development of renal failure. Blood. 2006;107:528–34.
43. Habe K, Wada H, Ito-Habe N, Hatada T, Matsumoto T, Ohishi K, Maruyama K, Imai H, Mizutani H, Nobori T. Plasma ADAMTS13, von Willebrand factor (VWF) and VWF propeptide profiles in patients with DIC and related diseases. Thromb Res. 2012;129:598–602.
44. Wada H, Matsumoto T, Hatada T. Diagnostic criteria and laboratory tests for disseminated intravascular coagulation. Expert Rev Hematol. 2012;5:643–52.
45. Rafiq A, Tariq H, Abbas N, Shenoy R. Atypical hemolytic-uremic syndrome: a case report and literature review. Am J Case Rep. 2015;16:109–14.
46. Ito N, Wada H, Matsumoto M, Fujimura Y, Murata M, Izuno T, Sugita M, Ikeda Y. National questionnaire survey of TMA. Int J Hematol. 2009;90:328–35.
47. Rock GA, Shumak KH, Buskard NA, Blanchette VS, Kelton JG, Nair RC, Spasoff RA, Group CAS. Comparison of plasma exchange with plasma infusion in the treatment of thrombotic thrombocytopenic purpura. N Engl J Med. 1991;325:393–7.
48. Iba T, Gando S, Saitoh D, Wada H, Di Nisio M, Thachil J. Antithrombin supplementation and risk of bleeding in patients with sepsis-associated disseminated intravascular coagulation. Thromb Res. 2016;145:46–50.
49. Hayakawa M, Yamakawa K, Saito S, Uchino S, Kudo D, Iizuka Y, Sanui M, Takimoto K, Mayumi T, Ono K. Japan septic disseminated intravascular coagulation (JSEPTIC DIC) study group: recombinant human soluble thrombomodulin and mortality in sepsis-induced disseminated intravascular coagulation. A multicentre retrospective study. Thromb Haemost. 2016;115: 1157–66.
50. Legendre CM, Licht C, Muus P, Greenbaum LA, Babu S, Bedrosian C, Bingham C, Cohen DJ, Delmas Y, Douglas K, Eitner F, Feldkamp T, Fouque D, Furman RR, Gaber O, Herthelius M, Hourmant M, Karpman D, Lebranchu Y, Mariat C, Menne J, Moulin B, Nürnberger J, Ogawa M, Remuzzi G, Richard T, Sberro-Soussan R, Severino B, Sheerin NS, Trivelli A, Zimmerhackl LB, Goodship T, Loirat C. Terminal complement inhibitor eculizumab in atypical hemolytic-uremic syndrome. N Engl J Med. 2013 Jun 6;368:2169–81.
51. George JN, Woodson RD, Kiss JE, Kojouri K, Vesely SK. Rituximab therapy for thrombotic thrombocytopenic purpura: a proposed study of the transfusion medicine/hemostasis clinical trials network with a systematic review of rituximab therapy for immune-mediated disorders. J Clin Apheresis. 2006;21:49–56.

25

Venous thromboembolism prophylaxis may cause more harm than benefit: an evidence-based analysis of Canadian and international guidelines

Andrew Kotaska[1,2,3,4]

Abstract

A majority of deep vein thromboses identified in screening studies of hospitalized patients remain clinically insignificant. Guidelines based on these studies markedly overestimate the risk of clinical venous thromboembolism (VTE) and the benefit of heparin prophylaxis. Accordingly, in 2012, the American College of Chest Physicians (ACCP) removed screening studies from the 9th edition of its Antithrombotic and Thrombolytic Therapy guideline (AT9), and downgraded recommendations. Involvement of authors of the 8th edition (AT8) was restricted due to financial and intellectual conflicts of interest. However, the first author of AT8 subsequently wrote a "Getting Started Kit," widely distributed to help Canadian hospitals develop VTE protocols. Based on screening studies reporting *asymptomatic* VTE, it lacks estimates of the magnitudes of benefit or harm from low molecular weight heparin (LMWH), yet advises prophylaxis in almost all hospitalized patients. Most Canadian hospitals have implemented guidelines based on this kit. Guidelines from the U. K National Institute for Health and Care Excellence and the U.S. Agency for Healthcare Research and Quality recommend a similar approach. However, a critical review of evidence reveals that most hospitalized patients have a risk of *clinical* VTE equal to or lower than the bleeding risk from LMWH. Most hospitalized patients should not receive LMWH until and unless randomized trials show more benefit than harm. Guidelines recommending liberal LMWH prophylaxis in hospitalized patients are not evidence based and should be critically re-examined.

Keywords: Venous thromboembolism, Prophylaxis, Guidelines, Evidence-based medicine, Conflict of interest, Deep vein thrombosis, Pulmonary embolism

Background

Venous thromboembolism (VTE) is an important clinical concern in medical and surgical patients. Up to one third of VTE are pulmonary emboli (PE), which can be rapidly fatal in up to 10% of cases; and severe post-thrombotic syndrome occurs in approximately 10% of patients after symptomatic deep vein thrombosis (DVT) [1]. High-risk patients are targeted for prophylaxis; however, myriad associated clinical factors make it difficult to identify individual patients destined to experience VTE. Scoring systems designed to identify such patients have been implemented without validation in randomized trials.

The American College of Chest Physicians (ACCP) has published an extensive series of Antithrombotic and Thrombolytic Therapy guidelines. Until and including the 8th edition (AT8), these guidelines were based on studies that screened patients for asymptomatic DVT [2]. However, few asymptomatic DVT become clinically significant, making it a poor surrogate for clinically important disease. Accordingly, the evidence was thoroughly re-evaluated in the ninth edition (AT9), published in 2012. Evidence previously rated as high quality is now moderate, and evidence previously rated

Correspondence: Andrew_kotaska@gov.nt.ca
[1]Women's & Children's Health, Northwest Territories Health and Social Services Authority, Stanton Territorial Hospital, Yellowknife, NT X1A 2N1, Canada
[2]School of Population and Public Health, University of British Columbia, Vancouver, Canada
Full list of author information is available at the end of the article

as moderate quality is now low. To a large extent, strong recommendations of AT8 have been replaced by weak recommendations in AT9 [3, 4]. Specifically:

- It is acknowledged that the use of asymptomatic, screening-detected thrombosis as an outcome substantially over-estimates the clinical benefit of prophylaxis.
- Clinically evident VTE rather than asymptomatic VTE is now used for estimates of VTE incidence and calculations of prophylaxis benefit.
- The financial and intellectual conflicts of interest of leading experts and prior authors were felt to be "highly problematic," so their involvement was restricted.

For general surgical patients, scoring systems are still advised to estimate the risk of VTE; however, bleeding risk is now acknowledged by a recommendation that the post-operative incidence of clinical VTE should exceed 3% to warrant chemo-prophylaxis [5–7]. After major orthopedic surgery, lower potency prophylaxis has been found to be effective and cause fewer wound and joint complications [8–11]. In medical patients, large randomized trials of LMWH prophylaxis demonstrate little or no benefit, calling into question the utility of poorly validated tools used to estimate risk [12–14].

This re-evaluation of the evidence and downgrading of recommendations has not been translated into corresponding changes on the front lines of clinical practice. Six years later, Canadian and international hospital VTE guidelines remain based on outdated evidence from AT8. This paper critically reviews those recommendations using an evidence-based lens and explores the role of conflict of interest in their generation and dissemination.

Main text

Accreditation Canada's required organizational practice

Accreditation Canada is a national organization that sets hospital safety standards. Required Organizational Practices (ROPs) are deemed critical to safety, and hospitals must comply or lose their accreditation. In 2011, Accreditation Canada instituted a ROP requiring hospitals identify and provide prophylaxis to admitted adult patients at elevated risk of VTE. Given a lack of clarity regarding which patients benefit from prophylaxis, Canadian hospitals needed direction. Accordingly, a "Getting Started Kit" was developed by "Safer Healthcare Now!" a self-described "flagship program of the Canadian Patient Safety Institute and a national program supporting Canadian healthcare organizations to improve safety through the use of quality improvement methods and the integration of evidence in practice" [15]. A "free resource designed to help (hospitals) implement interventions in (their) organization ... the Getting Started Kit contains clinical information, information on the science of improvement, and everything (hospitals) need to know to start using the intervention" [16, 17].

The Getting Started Kit has the same first author as AT8. Also based on studies that screened for asymptomatic DVT, it reports incidences of 10–40% for medical patients and 15–80% for surgical and trauma patients (Table 1). To an experienced clinician, these numbers are strikingly discordant from clinical practice. Although the authors state: "(Table 1) lists the DVT incidence for various hospitalized patient groups if no prophylaxis is given and screening for asymptomatic DVT is performed," they conclude "based on the significant, known rates of VTE as well as its acute and long-term consequences, it can be seen that nearly every hospitalized patient should receive thromboprophylaxis" [15].

This conclusion is highly misleading. Few patients with *asymptomatic* DVT develop clinical VTE, and the incidence of clinical DVT is an order of magnitude lower than the incidence of asymptomatic DVT [18, 19]. In the large meta-analysis of general surgical patients referenced in AT9 ($n = 5400$), the baseline risk of clinical VTE without heparin was 0.89% [20]. The pooled risk of symptomatic DVT in another large meta-analysis of mixed surgical patients was 0.6% [21]. In a retrospective cohort study used to validate a surgical risk scoring system ($N = 8216$), the baseline risk was 0.28% for moderate risk and 0.9% for high-risk patients [5]. The incidence of symptomatic VTE in surgical patients is less than one tenth that of asymptomatic DVT. In randomized studies of LMWH in more than 25,000 medical and stroke patients, the incidence of symptomatic DVT and pulmonary embolus with placebo were less than 1% each, and large randomized trials have shown no net benefit of LMWH prophylaxis [13, 14, 22].

However, none of this is mentioned in the Getting Started Kit. Alarmingly, the preferred thromboprophylaxis decision tree is one of 'opt out' (Fig. 1). Except for patients actively bleeding or at high risk of bleeding, it

Table 1 Asymptomatic VTE risk from screening studies (from the VTE Getting Started Kit, Patient Safety Institute of Canada; open source)

Patient Group	DVT Incidence (%)
Medical patients	10-26
Major gynecologic, urologic, or general surgery	15-40
Neurosurgery	15-40
Tibial fracture	20-40
Congestive heart failure	20-40
Stroke	11-75
Knee/hip arthroplasty	40-60
Hip fracture	40-60
Major trauma	40-80
Spinal cord injury	60-80
Critical care patients	15-80

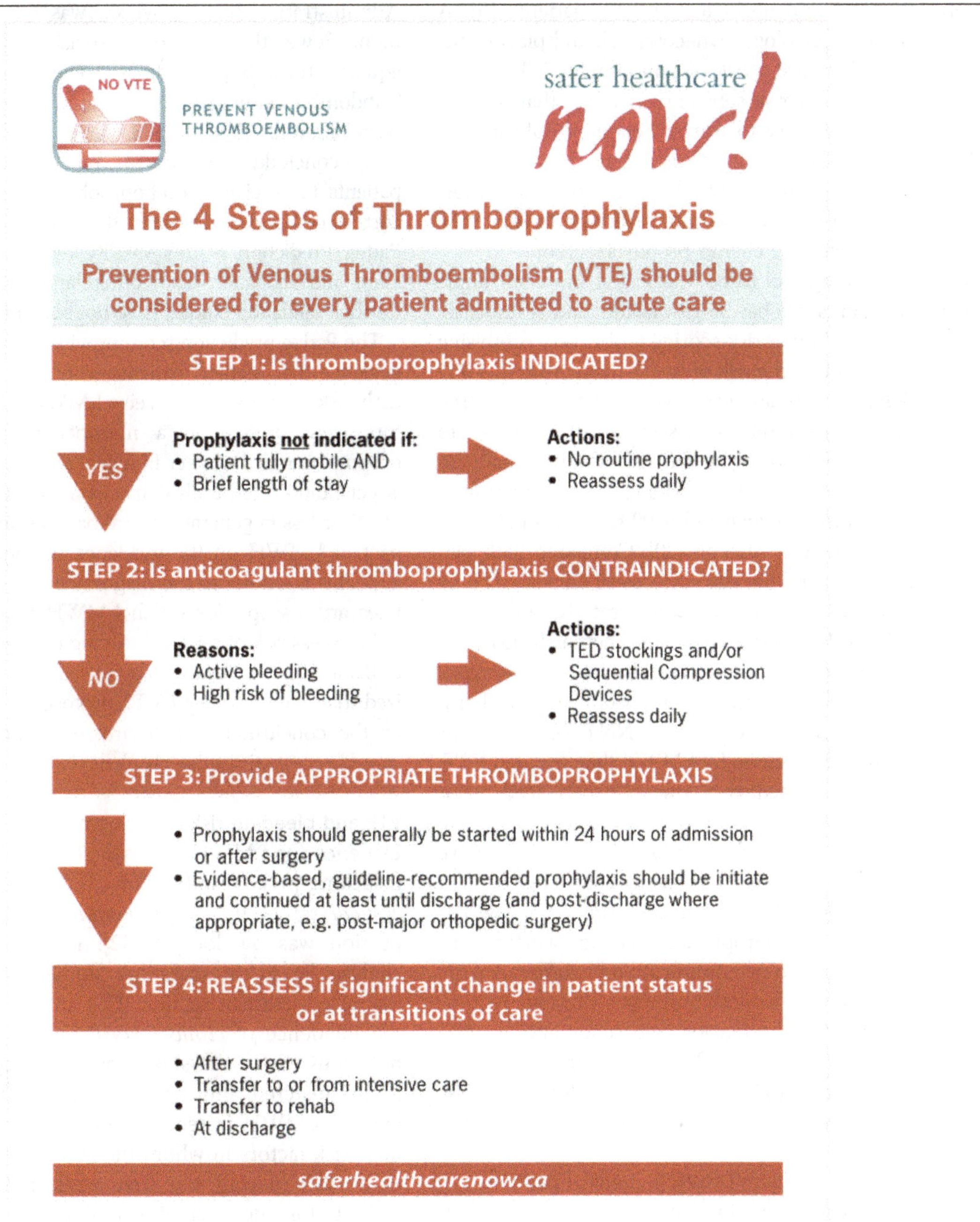

Fig. 1 Preferred 'opt-out' decision tree for VTE prophylaxis. (from the VTE Getting Started Kit, Patient Safety Institute of Canada; open source)

advises all patients receive LMWH unless fully mobile and admitted for less than 2 days. Without providing data, bleeding risk is dismissed: "Abundant data from meta-analyses and blinded, placebo controlled randomized trials have shown that clinically important bleeding secondary to prophylaxis with LDUH or LMWH is a rare event" [15]. In fact, LMWH prophylaxis causes significant increases in hemorrhage, which for many hospitalized patients likely equals or exceeds the risk of VTE prevented.

VTE incidence and bleeding risk with LMWH after surgery

The Caprini Scoring system is used to identify patients at increased postoperative risk of VTE [6]. Its scoring sheet declares *asymptomatic* VTE incidences of 10 to 80% from screening studies and recommends chemoprophylaxis in patients with a score of 2 ("moderate risk"), or greater. The Caprini score has been shown to predict which patients will experience VTE; however, in the largest validation study, the risk of symptomatic VTE was less than 1% in "moderate" and "high-risk" general, vascular and urological surgery patients [5]. A majority of otolaryngology, gynecological, and plastic surgery patients also have a risk of symptomatic VTE under 1% - a magnitude of risk substantially lower than the 3% threshold felt necessary to warrant chemoprophylaxis in AT9 [23–25]. Even in "highest-risk" general surgical patients, the VTE risk was only 2% [5]. In contrast, almost all patients requiring surgical intensive care have a VTE risk above 3%, justifying chemo-prophylaxis [26].

For a risk scoring tool to be practical, it must be simple [27]. The Caprini score has 35 risk factors and is unwieldy to administer. A simpler risk-scoring tool is very promising [28]. Recognizing that the risk of hemorrhage from LMWH is not insignificant, its authors advise that future research should provide "data on the risk-stratified response to prophylaxis side by side with the risk stratified data on bleeding complications." The meta-analysis of randomized trials referenced in AT9 included 5400 general surgical patients given LMWH or placebo [20]. Compared with placebo, LMWH reduced the absolute risk of clinical VTE by 0.68%, yielding a number needed to treat (NNT) of 147. However, LMWH increased major hemorrhages and hemorrhage requiring transfusion by absolute risk increases (ARI) of 1.5% and 3.8%, yielding numbers needed to harm (NNH) of 67 and 26 – lower than the NNT. More patients experienced bleeding caused by LMWH than avoided VTE: for every VTE prevented, two patients experienced major hemorrhage and seven received a transfusion. This data supports the AT9 recommendation that post-operative VTE risk should be at least 3% to justify LMWH [7].

The skepticism of orthopedic surgeons towards high-potency thromboprophylaxis is noteworthy. Increased wound and joint complications prompted early critical review of the evidence and more cautious recommendations [8–10]. Shorter, lower potency anticoagulation is now considered adequate after total joint replacement, with ASA 81 mg daily found to be non-inferior to rivaroxaban beyond the first 5 days [11].

VTE and bleeding risk with LMWH in medical patients

AT9 recommends LMWH in acutely ill hospitalized medical patients according to the Padua Prediction Score [29]. This risk assessment tool divides patients into low and high-risk groups based on 11 risk factors. It's validation study demonstrated clinical VTE in 11% of patients with a score of 4 or greater and 0.3% in patients with a score of less than 4 – a remarkable hazard ratio of 32 for a complex phenomenon [12]. Forty percent of all patients were deemed to be "high risk." Ninety-seven percent of those who developed VTE had at least one of four common major risk factors: prior history of VTE; active cancer; known thrombophilia; or bed rest for at least three days.

The study was not randomized and clinicians were not aware of their patients' VTE risk assessments. Administration of prophylaxis was left to clinical judgment. Fewer than 40% of high-risk patients received adequate thromboprophylaxis. The authors state that "randomization would have been unethical;" yet had patients been randomized, a full 50% would have received LMWH. They conclude "the lack of randomization of high-risk patients to receive thromboprophylaxis or not precludes a correct comparison between the two study groups ... The Padua Prediction Score's validity requires proper confirmation and validation from other large prospective studies." Further validation studies have not been published.

The Padua prediction score provides modest observational evidence that medical patients with four recognized 'very--high' risk factors should receive LMWH. However, these factors were present in a minority of patients and the proportion may be lower in a general hospital setting. Much larger randomized trials demonstrate a baseline risk of VTE of 1% or less in general medical patients, and little or no impact of LMWH on the incidence of clinical VTE [13, 14, 22]. This is similar to the magnitude of risk after outpatient knee arthroscopy, for which LMWH is not recommended [30]. Excess risk of serious bleeding in medical patients is up to 0.5% [14]. Neither the Padua prediction tool nor randomized trials support liberal VTE protocols for medical patients or the conclusion that "nearly every hospitalized patient should receive thrombo-prophylaxis" [15].

VTE and bleeding risk with postpartum LMWH

Evidence for LMWH prophylaxis in postpartum women is lacking [31]. Despite efforts to base AT9 on studies of *clinical* rather than *asymptomatic* VTE, the obstetrical portion was overlooked [32]. Drawn from a decision analysis based on screening studies, estimates of DVT risk after cesarean section (CS) are ten-fold higher than the incidence of *clinical* DVT [33]. Postpartum risk is not adjusted for the short period during which LMWH is administered, and the risks of LMWH have been overlooked. LMWH is recommended in women with common risk factors in whom the risk of clinical VTE is less than 0.1% during the first week postpartum. Giving LMWH for one week after typical CS, the NNT to prevent one VTE is 4000 [31, 34]. Approximately 1% of obstetrical VTE are fatal PE, yielding a NNT to prevent one PE-death of 400,000 [35].

Obstetrical organizations from the UK, Canada, Sweden, Australia and New Zealand have developed unvalidated guidelines based on risk factors taken from case-control studies, with little attention to the magnitude of risk [36–39]. Estimates of absolute risk reduction (ARR), NNT, ARI, and NNH are lacking. Except for women with a prior history of VTE or known thrombophilia, there is not observational or experimental evidence that LMWH prophylaxis reduces VTE after CS, even in 'high-risk' women [40–43].

However, LMWH after CS is associated with increased wound separation and re-hospitalization for wound complications, with ARIs of 3.8% and 1.3% respectively (NNH = 26 and 77) [43]. Since the NNT to prevent one VTE after typical CS is approximately 4000, some 50 women may experience wound complications from LMWH for every VTE prevented. The risk of severe hemorrhage from LMWH in postpartum patients is unknown. After CS, AT9 suggests an additional 2% risk of "major bleed" defined as "leading to death, transfusion, reoperation, or discontinuation of (heparin) therapy" [32]. In reality, birthing women are younger and healthier than most surgical patients, so the risk is likely lower. However, if the risk were only one tenth the ACCP estimate (0.2%), the NNH would be 500, and approximately eight women would experience serious hemorrhage from LMWH for each VTE prevented [30].

Canadian and international hospital VTE guidelines

In response to Accreditation Canada's ROP, most Canadian hospitals implemented VTE guidelines based on the Getting Started Kit. From a convenience sample of VTE protocols, procedures, and order sheets from 12 hospitals from 9 Provinces and Territories, all except one recommend liberal LMWH for most admitted hospitalized patients (Additional file 1). Similar to the Getting Started Kit, many recommend LMWH for all patients with an 'opt out' for very limited exclusions (Additional file 2). The remainder have adopted unvalidated risk scoring systems containing dozens of clinical factors, with a low threshold for treatment (Additional file 3). All except one lack estimates of the magnitude of benefit or harm that patients might experience from LMWH prophylaxis.

VTE guidelines for hospitalized patients from the U.K. National Institute for Health and Care Excellence (NICE) recommend a similar approach [44]. For medical and surgical patients, a link to a UK Dept. of Health VTE risk assessment tool is provided: "Any tick for thrombosis risk should prompt thromboprophylaxis according to NICE guidance ... (unless) bleeding risk is sufficient to preclude pharmacological intervention" [45]. For obstetrical patients, the unvalidated RCOG guideline is recommended [31].

The U.S. Agency for Healthcare Research and Quality (AHRQ) guideline: Preventing Hospital-Acquired Venous Thromboembolism is based on AT8. The 2008 first edition is similar to the Getting Started Kit [46]. The 2nd edition (2016) continues to recommend "... the most widely used qualitative model in the United States, the University of California San Diego model ... derived directly from tables in the AT8 guideline" [47]. All patients qualify for heparin unless they are fully mobile and remain in hospital for less than 48 h. Compared with more complicated, unpopular, individualized point-scoring systems, "this risk assessment model was considered intuitive and easy to use."

Conflicts of interest

Early ACCP guidelines fueled worldwide enthusiasm for VTE prevention and led to recommendations for liberal LMWH prophylaxis in hospitalized patients. In AT8 and guidelines based upon it, most hospitalized patients qualified for LMWH [2, 15, 45, 46]. The first author of AT8 disclosed "that he received grant monies from the Canadian Institute for Health Research, Sanofi-Aventis, and Pfizer ... consultant fees from Bayer, Eisai, Glaxo Smith Kline, Lilly, Merck, Pfizer, Roche, and Sanofi-Aventis, along with speaker's honoraria from Bayer, Calea, Oryx, Pfizer, and Sanofi-Aventis" [2]. Sanofi-Aventis, Pfizer, Bayer, GlaxoSmithKline, Lilly, and Merck produce (d) the anticoagulants enoxaparin, dalteparin, rivaroxaban, nadroparin, fondaparinux, and unfractionated heparin.

This author's involvement was restricted from AT9 because of financial and intellectual conflicts of interest; however, he is the first author of the Getting Started Kit and remains the primary consultant for Accreditation Canada regarding VTE. Published three months after AT9, the Getting Started Kit presents asymptomatic screening data that exaggerate the benefit of LMWH. However, it references both AT8 and AT9, indicating that the author was aware of the widely accepted conclusion that most asymptomatic DVT are clinically irrelevant. This conclusion is not mentioned in the Getting Started Kit. The Kit was partly funded by an "unrestricted educational grant from Pfizer." It does not contain a conflict of interest declaration.

Conflicts of interest have plagued guidelines for years [48]. With AT9, the ACCP made an unprecedented effort to address conflicts of interest, almost completely replacing authorship [4]. The presence of a conflict of interest does not necessarily mean that authors' conclusions are biased; however, transparent disclosure allows editors, guideline committees, clinicians, and patients to evaluate potential bias and adjust their decisions accordingly. Striking differences in the recommendations of AT8 and AT9 parallel a striking difference in authors' conflicts of interest. Six of seven authors of AT8 declared financial relationships to multiple companies that produce antithrombotic drugs. In contrast, one of five authors of AT9 declared any financial relationship.

Problems arise "not only from (authors') financial but equally or perhaps more importantly, their intellectual conflict of interest" [4]. In practitioners' and researchers' enthusiasm to help patients, there is a tendency to believe that our recommendations and actions are beneficial. When evidence calls previous conclusions into question, objective re-evaluation may be difficult, perhaps more so when research and commercial consulting careers are involved.

Evidence-based medicine

Enthusiasm for new cures is an essential stimulus for innovation in medicine and has driven VTE guidelines.

However, many new therapies adopted without adequate evaluation have later been found to lack benefit or even harm patients. Although all hospitalized patients are at risk of clinical VTE, for most, the magnitude of risk and our ability to prevent it have been exaggerated. Asymptomatic DVT is not a meaningful surrogate outcome for clinical VTE, and the risk of LMWH has been overlooked.

Forty years ago, Archie Cochrane challenged the medical profession to be critical of new treatments and to carefully evaluate them before widespread adoption [49]. Evidence-based medicine was our collective response [50]. Evidence-based medicine intends to balance high-quality evidence with patient values and clinical expertise to achieve optimal outcomes [51]. Critical to this effort is estimation of the absolute magnitudes of benefit and harm: the ARR, ARI, NNT, and NNH for the prevention of VTE with LMWH in medical, surgical, and postpartum patients.

Randomized controlled trials (RCTs) are the accepted gold standard for measuring benefits and harms from medical therapy. Given that the incidence of clinical VTE in most hospitalized patients is small, trials must be large to have the power to detect benefit from LMWH. The logistics are daunting; however, the imperative is great. For a majority of hospitalized patients, a low baseline risk of VTE means a greater likelihood that harm from LMWH will outweigh benefit. A large NNT also means high cost for little benefit. For these reasons, Dr. Cochrane advised that therapies' benefit be proven in adequately powered RCTs *before* their dissemination [52].

Conclusion

There is moderate evidence that patients with a prior VTE, potent thrombophilia, active cancer, prolonged bedrest, major orthopedic or abdominal-pelvic surgery, or ICU admission should receive chemoprophylaxis in hospital and for several weeks afterwards [40, 53]. For these patients, ongoing research may continue to customize the potency and duration for individual circumstances [11]. However, a majority of hospitalized medical, surgical, and postpartum patients lack these risk factors. Their risk of VTE has been exaggerated in most Canadian and major international hospital guidelines.

Admittedly, reliable estimates of VTE risk in patients with multiple medical and surgical risk factors are lacking and clinical judgment is required. However, multiple risk factors from case-control studies do not multiply VTE risk exponentially, and the absolute magnitudes of benefit and harm from LMWH must be considered [4, 54]. Low thresholds for LMWH prophylaxis may cause more harm than benefit, and the assumption that every hospitalized patient should receive LMWH unless fully mobile is oversimplified and unjustified. Protocols that recommend LMWH for surgical patients with modest risk factors such as age over 60, BMI over 30, a respiratory condition, or surgery lasting more than an hour are not evidence-based and likely cause more harm than benefit.

Pannucci and colleagues' advice that future research should provide "data on the risk-stratified response to prophylaxis side by side with the risk stratified data on bleeding complications" is a call to measure the NNT and NNH. This will particularly benefit the majority of hospitalized patients who are at modest risk of symptomatic VTE, for whom harm from LMWH may equal or exceed benefit. Only by balancing the NNT with the NNH can "physicians ... make informed decisions about the risks and benefits of prophylaxis for individual patients" [28]. Randomized trials provide direct measurement of the magnitudes of benefit and harm from LMWH and are needed to validate scoring systems for most surgical and medical patients.

Rarely, a new therapy provides such clear benefit that dissemination is justified before thorough evaluation. That is not the case here. Guidelines based on the prevention of *asymptomatic* rather than *clinical* VTE exaggerate the benefits of LMWH therapy and obscure its harms. The widespread treatment of a majority of hospitalized patients with LMWH constitutes a massive experiment: without a power calculation, ethics review, measurement of benefit and harm, or informed patient consent. In light of the advances in scientific understanding of AT9, guidelines advising liberal LMWH prophylaxis should be critically re-evaluated using the tools of evidence-based medicine. Until net benefit is proven, most hospitalized medical, surgical, and obstetrical patients should not receive LMWH prophylaxis except in the context of randomized trials.

Abbreviations

ACCP: American College of Chest Physicians; AHQR: Agency for Healthcare Research and Quality; ARI: Absolute risk increase; ARR: Absolute risk reduction; CS: Caesarean scetion; DVT: Deep vein thrombosis; LMWH: Low molecular weight heparin; NICE: National Institute for Health and Care Excellence; NNH: Number needed to harm; NNT: Number needed to treat; PE: Pulmonary embolism; RCT: Randomized controlled trial; ROP: Required organizational practice; VTE: Venous thromboembolism

Authors' contributions

Sole authorship. The author read and approved the final manuscript.

Competing interests

The author declares that he has no competing interests

Author details

[1]Women's & Children's Health, Northwest Territories Health and Social Services Authority, Stanton Territorial Hospital, Yellowknife, NT X1A 2N1, Canada. [2]School of Population and Public Health, University of British Columbia, Vancouver, Canada. [3]Department of Obstetrics and Gynaecology, University of Manitoba, Winnipeg, Canada. [4]Department of Obstetrics and Gynaecology, University of Toronto, Toronto, Canada.

References

1. Kearon C. Natural history of venous thromboembolism. Circulation. 2003; 107(23 Suppl 1):I22–30.
2. Geerts WH, Bergqvist D, Pineo GF, et al. Prevention of venous thromboembolism: American College of Chest Physicians Evidence-Based Clinical Practice Guidelines (8th edition). Chest. 2008;133(Suppl):381S–453S.
3. Guyatt GH, Akl EA, Crowther M, et al. Antithrombotic Therapy and Prevention of Thrombosis, 9th ed: American College of Chest Physicians Evidence-Based Clinical Practice Guidelines. Chest 2012;141(2) (Suppl):7S–47S.
4. Guyatt GH, Akl EA, Crowther M, et al. Introduction to the Ninth Edition, Antithrombotic Therapy and Prevention of Thrombosis, 9th ed: American College of Chest Physicians Evidence-Based Clinical Practice Guidelines. Chest 2012;141(2)(Suppl):48S–52S.
5. Bahl V, Hu HM, Henke PK, et al. A validation study of a retrospective venous thromboembolism risk scoring method. Ann Surg. 2010;251(2):344–50.
6. Caprini JA, Arcelus JI, Hasty JH, et al. Clinical assessment of venous thromboembolic risk in surgical patients. Semin Thromb Hemost. 1991; 17(suppl 3):304–12.
7. Gould MK, Garcia DA, Wren SM, et al. Prevention of VTE in Nonorthopedic Surgical Patients. Antithrombotic Therapy and Prevention of Thrombosis, 9th ed: American College of Chest Physicians Evidence-Based Clinical Practice Guidelines. Chest 2012; 141(2)(Suppl):e227S–e277S.
8. Barrack RL. Current guidelines for total joint VTE prophylaxis J Bone Joint Surg Br 2012;94-B, Supple A:3–7.
9. Cusick LA, Beverland DE. The incidence of fatal pulmonary embolism after primary hip and knee replacement in a consecutive series of 4253 patients. J Bone Joint Surg (Br). 2009;91-B:645–8.
10. Falck-Ytter Y, Francis CW, Johanson NA, Curley C, Dahl OE, Schulman S et al. Prevention of VTE in Orthopedic Surgery Patients. Antithrombotic Therapy and Prevention of Thrombosis, 9th ed: American College of Chest Physicians Evidence-Based Clinical Practice Guidelines. CHEST 2012; 141(2)(Suppl):e278S–e325S.
11. Anderson DR, Dunbar M, Murnaghan J, Kahn SR, Gross P, et al. Aspirin or rivaroxaban for VTE prophylaxis after hip or knee Arthroplasty. N Engl J Med. 2018;378:699–707.
12. Barbar S, Noventa F, Rossetto V, et al. A risk assessment model for the identification of hospitalized medical patients at risk for venous thromboembolism: the Padua prediction score. J Thromb Haemost. 2010; 8(11):2450–7.
13. Kakkar AK, Cimminiello C, Goldhaber S, et al. Low-Molecular-Weight Heparin and Mortality in Acutely Ill Medical Patients. N Engl J Med. 2011;365:2463–72.
14. Lederle F, Zylla D, MacDonald R, Wilt T. Venous Thromboembolism Prophylaxis in Hospitalized Medical Patients and Those With Stroke: A Background Review for an American College of Physicians Clinical Practice Guideline. Ann Intern Med. 2011;155:602–15.
15. Geerts W, Brown P, Diamantouros A, Budrevics G, Bartle W. Venous Thromboembolism Prevention Getting Started Kit. Safer Healthcare Now! Accessed on June 9, 2016 at http://www.patientsafetyinstitute.ca/en/toolsResources/VTE-Getting-Started-Components/Documents/VTE%20GSK%202016%20EN.pdf.
16. Patient Safety Institute Website Accessed 6 Jan 2017.
17. http://www.patientsafetyinstitute.ca/en/toolsresources/pages/vte-resources-getting-started-kit.aspx. Accessed 4 Feb 2018.
18. Guyatt GH, Eikelboom JW, Gould MK, et al. Approach to outcome measurement in the prevention of thrombosis in surgical and medical patients: antithrombotic therapy and prevention of thrombosis, 9th ed: American College of Chest Physicians evidence based clinical practice guidelines. Chest. 2012;141(2)(suppl):e185S-e194S.
19. Chan NC, Stehouwer AC, Hirsh J, Ginsberg JS, Alazzoni A, Coppens M, Guyatt GH, Eikelboom JW. Lack of consistency in the relationship between asymptomatic DVT detected by venography and symptomatic VTE in thromboprophylaxis trials. Thromb Haemost. 2015 Nov;114(5):1049–57.
20. Mismetti P, Laporte S, Darmon JY, et al. Meta-analysis of low molecular weight heparin in the prevention of venous thromboembolism in general surgery. Br J Surg. 2001;88:913–30.
21. Zareba P, Wu C, Agzarian J, et al. Meta-analysis of randomised trials comparing combined compression and anticoagulation with either modality alone for prevention of venous thromboembolism after surgery. Br J Surg. 2014;101:1053–62.
22. Samama MM, Cohen AT, Darmon JY, Desjardins L, Eldor A, Janbon C, et al. A comparison of enoxaparin with placebo for the prevention of venous thromboembolism in acutely ill medical patients. Prophylaxis in medical patients with enoxaparin study group. N Engl J Med. 1999;341:793–800.
23. Shuman AG, Hu HM, Pannucci CJ, Jackson CR, Bradford CR, Bahl V. Stratifying the risk of venous thromboembolism in otolaryngology. Otolaryngol Head Neck Surg. 2012;146(5):719–24.
24. Pannucci CJ, Bailey SH, Dreszer G, et al. Validation of the Caprini risk assessment model in plastic and reconstructive surgery patients. J Am Coll Surg. 2011;212(1):105–12.
25. Swenson CW, Berger MB, Kamdar NS, Campbell DA, Morgan DM. Risk factors for venous thromboembolism after hysterectomy. Obstet Gynecol. 2015;125:1139–44.
26. Obi AT, Pannucci CJ, Nackashi A, et al. Validation of the Caprini venous thromboembolism risk assessment model in critically ill surgical patients. JAMA Surg. 2015;150(10):941–8.
27. Pannucci CJ, Obi A, Alvare R, et al. Inadequate venous thromboembolism risk stratification predicts venous thromboembolic events in surgical intensive care unit patients. J Am Coll Surg. 2014;218:898e904.
28. Pannucci CJ, Laird S, Dimick JB, Campbell DA. PK Henke. A validated risk model to predict 90-day VTE events in postsurgical patients. Chest. 2014;145(3):567–73.
29. Kahn SR, Lim W, Dunn AS, Cushman M, Dentali F, Akl EA, et al. Prevention of VTE in Nonsurgical Patients. Antithrombotic Therapy and Prevention of Thrombosis, 9th ed: American College of Chest Physicians Evidence-Based Clinical Practice Guidelines. Chest 2012; 141(2)(Suppl):e195S–e226S.
30. van Adrichem RA, Nemeth B, Algra A, le Cessie S, Rosendaal FR, Schipper IB, Nelissen RGHH. Cannegieter SC; POT-KAST and POT-CAST group. Thromboprophylaxis after knee arthroscopy and lower-leg casting. N Engl J Med. 2017;376(6):515–25.
31. Kotaska A. Postpartum venous thromboembolism prophylaxis may cause more harm than benefit: a critical analysis of international guidelines through an evidence-based lens. BJOG. 2018; https://doi.org/10.1111/1471-0528.15150.
32. Bates SM, Greer IA, Middeldorp S, et al. VTE, Thrombophilia, Antithrombotic Therapy, and Pregnancy. Antithrombotic Therapy and Prevention of Thrombosis, 9th ed: American College of Chest Physicians Evidence-Based Clinical Practice Guidelines CHEST 2012; 141(2)(Suppl):e691S–e736S.
33. Blondon M, Perrier A, Nendaz M, et al. Thromboprophylaxis with low-molecular-weight heparin after cesarean delivery. A decision analysis. Thromb Haemost. 2010;103:129–37.
34. Sultan AA, West J, Grainge MJ, et al. Development and validation of risk prediction model for venous thromboembolism in postpartum women: multinational cohort study. BMJ. 2016;355:i6253.
35. Sibai BM, Rouse DJ. Pharmacologic Thromboprophylaxis in obstetrics: broader use demands better data. Obstet Gynecol. 2016;128(4):681–4.
36. McLintock C, Brighton T, Chunilal S, et al. Councils of the Society of Obstetric Medicine of Australia and New Zealand; Australasian Society of Thrombosis and Haemostasis. Recommendations for the prevention of pregnancy associated venous thromboembolism. Aust N Z J Obstet Gynaecol. 2012;52:3–13.
37. Nelson-Piercy C, MacCallum P, Mackillop L. Reducing the risk of thrombosis and embolism during pregnancy and the puerperium. In: Green-top guideline no. 37a. London: Royal College of Obstetricians and Gynaecologists; 2009.
38. Lindqvist PG, Hellgren M. Obstetric thromboprophylaxis: the Swedish guidelines. Adv Hematol. 2011;2011:1–6. https://doi.org/10.1155/2011/157483.
39. Chan WS, Rey E, Kent N. Society of Obstetricians & Gynaecologists of Canada clinical practice guideline #308:venous thromboembolism and antithrombotic therapy in pregnancy. J Obstet Gynaecol Can. 2014;36(6):527–53.
40. Lindqvist PG, Bremme K, Hellgren M. Swedish Society of Obstetrics and Gynecology (SFOG) Working Group on Hemostatic Disorders (Hem-ARG). Efficacy of obstetric thromboprophylaxis and long-term risk of recurrence of venous thromboembolism. Acta Obstet Gynecol Scand. 2011;90:648–53.
41. Gates S, Brocklehurst P, Ayers S, Bowler U. Thromboprophylaxis and pregnancy: two randomised controlled pilot trials that used low-molecular weight heparin. Am J Obstet Gynecol. 2004;191:1296–303.
42. Burrows RF, Gan ET, Gallus AS, et al. A randomised double-blind placebo controlled trial of low molecular weight heparin as prophylaxis in preventing venous thrombotic events after caesarean section: a pilot study. Brit J Obstet Gynaecol. 2001;108:835–9.
43. Ferres MA, Olivarez SA, Trinh V, et al. Rate of Wound Complications With Enoxaparin Use Among Women at High Risk for Postpartum Thrombosis. Obstet Gynecol. 2011;117:119–24.

44. National Institute for Health and Care Excellence. Venous thromboembolism in over 16s: reducing the risk of hospital-acquired deep vein thrombosis or pulmonary embolism. NICE guideline. March 2018; https://www.nice.org.uk/guidance/ng89.
45. https://www.nice.org.uk/guidance/ng89/resources/department-of-health-vte-risk-assessment-tool-pdf-4787149213. Accessed 29 July 2018.
46. Maynard G, Stein J. Preventing Hospital-Acquired Venous Thromboembolism: A Guide for Effective Quality Improvement. Rockville, MD: Agency for Healthcare Research and Quality. 2008. AHRQ Publication No. 08–0075.
47. Maynard G. Preventing hospital-associated venous thromboembolism: a guide for effective quality improvement, 2nd ed. Rockville, MD: Agency for Healthcare Research and Quality; August 2016. AHRQ Publication No. 16–0001-EF. https://www.ahrq.gov/sites/default/files/publications/files/vteguide.pdf.
48. Guyatt G, Akl EA, Hirsh J, et al. The vexing problem of guidelines and conflict of interest: a potential solution. Ann Intern Med. 2010;152(11):738–41.
49. Cochrane AL. 1931–1971: a critical review with particular reference to the medical profession. London: Office of Health Economics; 1979.
50. Evidence Based Medicine Working Group. Evidence based medicine. A new approach to teaching the practice of medicine. JAMA. 1992;268:2420–5.
51. Sackett DL, Rosenberg WC, Gray JAM. Evidence based medicine: what it is and what it isn't. BMJ. 1996;312:71–2.
52. Thorp J. Wooden spoons and thromboprophylaxis in obstetrics. BJOG. https://doi.org/10.1111/1471-0528.14886.
53. Rodger M. Pregnancy and venous thromboembolism: 'TIPPS' for risk stratification. Hematology Am Soc Hematol Educ Program. 2014:387–92.
54. Kotaska A. Re: postpartum venous thromboembolism prophylaxis may cause more harm than benefit: a critical analysis of international guidelines through an evidence based lens. Postpartum thromboprophylaxis is cost-effective using the Swedish thromboprophylaxis algorithm. Author's Reply BJOG. https://doi.org/10.1111/1471-0528.15267.

Design and rationale of the non-interventional, edoxaban treatment in routiNe clinical prActice in patients with venous Thromboembolism

Alexander T. Cohen[1*], Cihan Ay[2], Philippe Hainaut[3], Hervé Décousus[4], Ulrich Hoffmann[5], Sean Gaine[6], Michiel Coppens[7], Pedro Marques da Silva[8], David Jiménez[9], Beatrice Amann-Vesti[10], Bernd Brüggenjürgen[11], Pierre Levy[12], Julio Lopez Bastida[13], Eric Vicaut[14], Petra Laeis[15], Eva-Maria Fronk[15], Wolfgang Zierhut[15], Thomas Malzer[15], Peter Bramlage[16], Giancarlo Agnelli[17] and on behalf of the ETNA-VTE-Europe investigators

Abstract

Background: Venous thromboembolism (VTE, including deep vein thrombosis [DVT] and pulmonary embolism [PE]) has an annual incidence rate of 104–183 per 100,000 person-years. After a VTE episode, the two-year recurrence rate is about 17%. Consequently, effective and safe anticoagulation is paramount. Edoxaban is a direct oral anticoagulant (DOAC) approved VTE treatment. Current safety and efficacy data are derived from clinical trials, and information about treatment durations beyond 12 months are not available.

Methods: ETNA-VTE-Europe is an 18-month prospective, single-arm, non-interventional, multinational post-authorisation safety study. Approximately 310 sites across eight European countries (Austria, Belgium, Germany, Ireland, Italy, the Netherlands, Switzerland and the United Kingdom) will participate in the study, with the intention to represent the regional distributions of centres, healthcare settings and specialties. An estimated cohort of 2700 patients will be recruited, the only enrolment criteria being acute symptomatic VTE, no participation in an interventional study, and treating physician decision to prescribe edoxaban independently from the registry. Data from patient medical records and/or telephone interviews will be collected at baseline, 1, 3, 6, 12 and 18 months. The primary objective is to evaluate the 18-month rate of symptomatic VTE recurrence in patients with VTE treated with edoxaban outside a clinical trial. The co-primary objective is to evaluate the real-world rates of bleeding and adverse drug reactions. Secondary outcomes include rates of other patient-relevant safety events, adherence to and discontinuation of edoxaban. Furthermore, 12-month ETNA-VTE-Europe data will be considered in the context of those for patients receiving different anticoagulants in the PREFER in VTE registry and Hokusai-VTE clinical trial.

(Continued on next page)

* Correspondence: alexander.cohen@kcl.ac.uk
[1]Guy's and St Thomas' NHS Foundation Trust, King's College London, London, UK
Full list of author information is available at the end of the article

(Continued from previous page)

Conclusions: ETNA-VTE-Europe will allow the safety and effectiveness of edoxaban to be evaluated over an extended period in acute symptomatic VTE patients encountered in routine clinical practice. Findings will be informative for European practitioners prescribing edoxaban as part of real-world VTE treatment/prevention.

Keywords: Venous thromboembolism (VTE), Edoxaban, Direct oral anticoagulant (DOAC/NOAC), Anticoagulation, Registry

Background

Venous thromboembolism (VTE), which encompasses both deep-vein thrombosis (DVT) and pulmonary embolism (PE), has an annual incidence rate of approximately 104–183 per 100,000 person-years in individuals of European descent [1]. VTE is the third most common cardiovascular disease. The case-fatality rate is higher after PE than after DVT [2, 3]. Nevertheless, both events increase the probability of subsequent recurrent VTE, which affects approximately 17% of patients at 2 years, indicating that VTE is a chronic disease [4]. Consequently, effective anticoagulation to treat first-time VTE and prevent its recurrence is paramount.

Edoxaban is a direct oral anticoagulant (DOAC), which exerts its effects through inhibition of factor Xa. Based on results from the ENGAGE AF-TIMI 48 and Hokusai-VTE trials [5, 6], it was approved by the European Medicines Agency (EMA) regulatory for two main indications: the prevention of stroke/systemic embolism in patients with non-valvular atrial fibrillation (NVAF) with one or more risk factor, and the treatment/secondary prevention of acute VTE (DVT and/or PE) in adults [7]. However, current evidence for the safety and efficacy of edoxaban is derived from the patient populations enrolled in clinical trials. Furthermore, though current guidelines recommend that anticoagulation following VTE should be continued for at least 3 months and up to an indefinite duration, depending upon the risk of recurrence [8], no data currently exist for treatment with edoxaban beyond 12 months.

As part of an ongoing European risk-management plan, several post-authorisation safety studies (PASS) have been designed to assess the real-world outcomes of edoxaban-treated patients in the EMA-approved indications [9]. Here we describe the design and rationale for the "Edoxaban Treatment in routine cliNical prActice for patients with acute Venous ThromboEmbolism in Europe" (ETNA-VTE-Europe) PASS, the protocol for which has been reviewed and approved by the EMA's Pharmacovigilance Risk Assessment Committee (PRAC), in accordance with new regulatory requirements. The aim of this PASS is to gain further insight into the safety and effectiveness of treatment and secondary prevention of VTE with edoxaban up to 18 months in routine clinical practice. This study forms part of a global program and safety data will eventually be pooled with ETNA-AF-Europe data and with those from similar Japanese, Thai, Chinese, Taiwanese and Korean regional registries to assess the safety outcomes associated with edoxaban on a worldwide scale.

Methods

ETNA-VTE-Europe is a single-arm, multinational, prospective, non-interventional PASS, which will be conducted across approximately 310 sites in 8 European countries (Austria, Belgium, Germany, Ireland, Italy, the Netherlands, Switzerland and the United Kingdom). The registry will enrol approximately 2700 patients with acute VTE treated with edoxaban, who will be followed over the 18 months subsequent to the index VTE. Approval from the responsible ethics committees and institutional review boards will be obtained prior to protocol implementation. Informed consent will be obtained from all patients prior to enrolment and compliance with the Declaration of Helsinki will be ensured throughout the study.

Objectives and outcome measures

The primary objective of ETNA-VTE-Europe is to quantify the long-term rate of VTE recurrence in a large, real-world population of acute symptomatic VTE patients prescribed edoxaban as part of their initial treatment regimen. Accordingly, the primary outcome measure will be the proportion of such patients who experience recurrent symptomatic VTE on one or more occasions within the 18 months following their index VTE, regardless of the length of edoxaban exposure.

The co-primary objective is to collect and evaluate real-world safety data regarding adverse drug reactions (ADRs) in patients treated with edoxaban across the currently approved indications. Therefore, ETNA-VTE-Europe data will be combined with 18-month safety data from the Edoxaban Treatment in routine cliNical PrActice for patients with non-valvular Atrial Fibrillation in Europe (ETNA-AF-Europe) study, a parallel European PASS evaluating the safety and effectiveness of edoxaban in real-world treatment of atrial fibrillation (AF) [10]. The outcome measure will be the proportion of patients who experience death (all-cause, cardiovascular, and VTE-related), bleeding events (major, clinically relevant non-major [CRNM], and minor bleeding; defined according to International Society on Thrombosis and Haemostasis [ISTH] criteria [11]), hepatic events, and/or other ADRs before the 18 month time-point in the two studies.

Secondary objectives are as follows: to evaluate the effects of persistent edoxaban use and permanent discontinuation on the rate of recurrent symptomatic VTE; to assess the rates of patient-relevant safety outcomes, including bleeding, ischaemic/haemorrhagic stroke, systemic embolic events (SEE), post-thrombotic syndrome (PTS), death, and hospitalisation due to cardiovascular causes; and to characterise the extent of adherence to edoxaban, reasons for and rate of discontinuation. To evaluate the effectiveness and safety of edoxaban relative to other anticoagulants, primary and secondary ETNA-VTE outcome data will be appraised in the context of those from the PREFER in VTE real-world registry and Hokusai-VTE clinical trial [12, 13]. The influence of study setting will also be explored by considering real-world ETNA-VTE data in the context of edoxaban data from the Hokusai-VTE clinical trial [12].

Site selection

In order to represent the regional distributions of centres, healthcare settings, specialties, and approaches to VTE treatment, a sequential site selection process is underway. This involves identification of potential sites, acquisition of relevant institutional details via a feasibility questionnaire, assessment of suitability, and invitation to participate. To be considered eligible, sites are required to have access to acute VTE patients expected to receive edoxaban treatment, the ability to access the Electronic Data Capture (EDC) system and record data in English, and adequate time and staff to perform all study-related documentation activities. They must also agree to complete a screening log with the aim of maximising the potential for consecutive enrolment, and to perform follow-ups according to routine clinical practice. There is an upper limit of 100 patients per site.

Patient recruitment

The original version of the ETNA-VTE-Europe protocol was approved by the Swiss Agency for Therapeutic Products (Swissmedic) and the central Ethics Committee in Switzerland in February 2015. Accordingly, Swiss sites began enrolling patients at this time. However, protocol revision was necessary due to a change in EMA legislation and a revised PRAC process in July 2015. Upon the approval of the new protocol by the EMA's PRAC in September 2016, Swiss regulatory bodies were informed of the changes and new approval sought. Patient recruitment according to the revised protocol is now underway, taking place in two waves; the first extends from the last quarter of 2016 to the second quarter of 2018 (Switzerland and Germany) and the second from the first quarter of 2017 to the last quarter of 2018 (all other countries). In each country, the recruitment period will last 2 years, with the aim of obtaining a representative study population of approximately 2700 VTE patients from a variety of healthcare settings.

To be included in the study, patients must have been diagnosed with initial or recurrent acute VTE (distal or proximal DVT and/or PE) that occurred no more than 2 weeks prior to enrolment. In addition, the treating physician must have decided to prescribe the patient edoxaban, with indications that are in line with the edoxaban Summary of Product Characteristics (SmPC). All treatment decisions are independent of the registry and completely at the discretion of the treating physician and/or patient, with no reimbursement for any drugs or therapy received during the study. As such, any concomitant treatment is allowed and changes to medication are unrestricted. The only exclusion criteria are lack of written informed consent and participation in a simultaneous interventional study.

Documentation and assessment

Data for this study will be sourced from medical records and, when in line with routine clinical practice, from telephone calls between the patient and treating physician. As a non-interventional study, no patient contact, examinations, laboratory tests or procedures are compulsory, and will only be carried out at the discretion of the treating physician, as and when deemed appropriate and without registry influence. A standardised electronic case report form (eCRF) will be completed by the site shortly after enrolment and again after every interaction with a patient over the subsequent 18 months. The eCRFs will be uploaded to the secure, internet-based Medidata Rave EDC system.

Given that the edoxaban SmPC recommends 5 days of parenteral anticoagulation following VTE before starting edoxaban treatment [7], baseline is defined as the first day of heparin/fondaparinux administration after the index acute VTE event. The first data entry, which will be completed following enrolment and within 2 weeks of the index VTE, will include details of baseline patient characteristics, comorbidities, VTE-related parameters, past and current therapy, and other relevant assessments made according to site protocol (Table 1). Memory aids will be provided to all patients at enrolment, with space to record edoxaban-related treatment changes, use of concomitant medication, adverse events, hospitalisation, physician contact, and productivity loss. This aid can be used to assist with recall during subsequent visits/telephone calls, but are voluntary and will not be formally

Table 1 Time points for data assessment

	Baseline*	1 month	3 months	6 months	12 months	18 months	Country-specific LPO
Eligibility criteria(1)	X						
Baseline characteristics(2)	X						
VTE-related parameters(3)	X	X§	X§	X§	X§	X§	
Edoxaban therapy(4)	X	X	X	X	X	X	
Concomitant anticoagulants	X	X	X	X	X	X	
Interventions	X	X	X	X	X	X	
Adherence to VTE therapy(5)	X	X	X	X	X	X	
Recurrent VTE(6)		X	X	X	X	X	X†
Other clinical events(7)	X	X	X	X	X	X	
Hospitalisation for cardiovascular disease(8)		X	X	X	X	X	
PTS(9)	X		X		X	X	
Vital signs(10)	X	X	X	X	X	X	
Laboratory parameters(9)	X	X	X	X	X	X	
ADRs(11)	X	X	X	X	X	X	

Legend: VTE, venous thromboembolism; PTS, post-thrombotic syndrome; ADR, adverse drug reaction; LPO, last patient out. (1) Confirmed first or recurrent VTE within the 2 weeks preceding enrolment; treated with edoxaban according to Summary of Product Characteristics; written informed consent; no simultaneous interventional study participation. (2) Age and gender, alcohol consumption, smoking status, frailty, comorbidities, and medical history. (3) Details of past and current VTE risk factors, symptoms, diagnosis, interventions, treatment, and related clinical events (stroke, bleeding events, systemic embolism, non-valvular atrial fibrillation, and malignancies). (4) History and current status, including dose, prescription intervals, and any changes to edoxaban treatment since last data point (including permanent discontinuation, in which case date, reason and subsequent therapy must be provided). (5) Physician judgment only. (6) Timing, diagnosis and interventions. (7)I.e. death, stroke, bleeding events, systemic embolism, non-valvular atrial fibrillation, and malignancies. (8) Admittance and discharge dates, clinical event, and use of the emergency room and/or intensive care unit. (9) If assessed. (10) Including blood pressure, heart rate, height and weight. (11) As per the Guideline on Good Pharmacovigilance Practices (GVP) Module VI (Management and reporting of adverse reactions to medicinal products; EMA/873138/2011 Rev. 1) [16]; coding according to the standardised Medical Dictionary for Regulatory Activities (MedDRA).*Defined as the first day of heparin administration after the index acute VTE event. †Since 18-month time point. §Changes in symptoms/diagnosis and any other VTE-relevant information

assessed. In each country, all patients will be followed until the last patient for that particular country has completed the 18-month documentation period, in line with EMA requirements. At this point, a last-patient-out (LPO) questionnaire, requesting a minimum of vital status, will be issued for each patient enrolled in the respective country.

Upon completion of the ETNA-VTE-Europe registry, data will be extracted for the following time points: baseline, 1, 3, 6, 12 and 18 months. Details of the parameters to be evaluated at each time point are outlined in Table 1. The current status, change/events since baseline and change/events since the previous time point will be assessed for each parameter, as appropriate. In addition, recurrence of symptomatic VTE and death since the 18-month time point will be retrospectively documented at the time of LPO per country.

Definitions

All variables in the ETNA-VTE-Europe study are defined as similarly as possible to those in the PREFER in VTE and Hokusai-VTE studies to permit close comparison of results [6, 13–15]. However, the feasibility of this is somewhat limited by the non-interventional setting. A comparison of the most important variable definitions is provided in Table 2. Permanent edoxaban discontinuation is defined as cessation of edoxaban treatment within the follow-up period.

Quality control

ETNA-VTE-Europe will be conducted in accordance with the Guidelines for Good Pharmacoepidemiology Practice (GPP) and the EMA Guideline on Good Pharmacovigilance Practices (GVP) Module VIII (management and reporting of adverse reactions to medicinal products; EMA/813938/2011 rev 1) [16, 17]. Automated checks for plausibility and integrity will be carried out at data entry to permit correction or confirmation by the site. Furthermore, approximately 30% of sites will be randomly selected to undergo on-site monitoring, during which random source data verification will be performed. In particular, monitoring activities will closely assess the completeness and correctness of safety data. Patients with missing observations for a particular time point and/or parameter will be omitted from the corresponding analyses.

Sample size calculations

Assuming an overall 18-month symptomatic VTE recurrence rate [12, 13] of 8.0% in patients who receive

Table 2 Definitions of VTE and bleeding events in ETNA-VTE-Europe, PREFER in VTE and Hokusai-VTE studies

	ETNA-VTE-Europe	PREFER in VTE [13, 14]	Hokusai-VTE [6, 15]
VTE			
Baseline	Confirmed first time/recurrent distal/proximal acute symptomatic DVT and/or PE	Confirmed first time/recurrent distal/proximal acute symptomatic DVT and/or PE	Confirmed first time/recurrent **proximal** acute symptomatic DVT and/or PE
Recurrent (during study)	VTE, as adjudicated by an independent CEC	DVT or PE, **as diagnosed by investigator (not adjudicated)**	DVT, new non-fatal symptomatic/fatal PE, as adjudicated by an independent CEC[a]
Bleeding			
Major	Overt: fatal, symptomatic in a critical area/organ, causing a ≥ 2 g/dL fall in haemoglobin and/or ≥6.0% fall in haematocrit[b]	Overt: fatal, symptomatic in a critical area/organ, causing a ≥ 20 g L^{-1} fall in haemoglobin or **transfusion of ≥ 2 units of whole blood or red cells[b]**	Overt: fatal, occurs in a critical site, associated with a ≥ 2 g/dL decrease in haemoglobin or requires a **transfusion of ≥ 2 units of blood**
Life-threatening	Major: intracranial or associated with haemodynamic compromise requiring intervention	**Not specified**	**Not specified**
CRNM	Overt: requires medical attention but does not fulfil major bleeding criteria[b]	Overt: does not meet major bleeding criteria but prompts a clinical response (**hospital admission/physician-guided treatment/change in antithrombotic therapy**)[b]	Overt: associated with the need for medical intervention, **contact with a physician, interruption of study drug, or discomfort/impairment of ADL,** but does not fulfil major bleeding criteria
Minor	Overt: other; does not fulfil the criteria for major/CRNM[b]	Overt: other; does not fulfil the criteria for major/CRNM[b]	**Not specified**

Legend: DVT, deep-vein thrombosis; PE, pulmonary embolism; VTE, venous thromboembolism; CRNM, clinically relevant non-major; CEC, clinical events committee; ADL, activities of daily living. [a]Members unaware of treatment allocation. [b]As defined by the International Society of Thrombosis and Haemostasis (2005) [11]. Items in **bold** reflect differences compared to ETNA-VTE-Europe

edoxaban (regardless of treatment discontinuation) and a relative precision of 15% for a two-sided 95% confidence interval (95% CI), data for 1964 patients will be required to assess with sufficient accuracy the primary outcome. Given an expected dropout rate of 25%, enrolment of 2700 patients should result in an adequate sample size for evaluation at 18 months.

In order to obtain a dataset as large as possible for co-primary outcome assessment, safety data from ETNA-VTE-Europe will be combined with 18-month safety data from ETNA-AF-Europe, a sister European PASS study of edoxaban in approximately 13,100 patients with NVAF [10]. Together, these studies will enrol approximately 15,800 patients, with an overall expected 18-month dropout rate of 20%. Consequently, data for approximately 12,640 patients should be available at 18 months to assess the incidence rates of interest and their 95% CIs. A key aim of this combined analysis is to provide sufficient statistical power to capture uncommon ADRs with low incidence rates; for those that occur at rates of 0.1–1.0%, the corresponding precision of 95% CIs will range from ±0.06% to 0.17%.

Statistical analysis

Owing to the non-interventional study design, all ETNA-VTE-Europe data analysis will be explorative and descriptive only. In addition to the Europe-wide analysis, safety and effectiveness data will be presented for each individual country and region (Austria, Switzerland and Germany [DACH]; the United Kingdom and Ireland [UK/IE]; Belgium and the Netherlands [BE/NL]; and Italy). Comparisons between patients in particular edoxaban exposure categories (current use, recent use [within the last 3 days], and past use [> 3 days ago], as well as use within the last 30 days) will also be performed, with outcome data additionally presented for all patients permanently discontinuing edoxaban. Furthermore, subgroup analyses comparing patients with/without the following baseline characteristics are planned: renal impairment, hepatic impairment, DVT only (vs. PE with/without DVT), age ≥ 75 years, male gender, initial 30 mg edoxaban dose (vs. 60 mg), and active cancer.

To provide context to our results, the outcomes of ETNA-VTE patients will be appraised relative to those of PREFER in VTE patients treated with a DOAC, PREFER in VTE patients treated with a vitamin-K antagonist (VKA), Hokusai-VTE patients treated with edoxaban, and Hokusai-VTE patients treated with warfarin. These evaluations will be performed on an entirely visual basis, with no joint statistical models planned. Given the one-year follow up of the PREFER in VTE and Hokusai-VTE studies, only 12-month data from ETNA-VTE-Europe will be considered for these purposes [12, 13].

Data will be analysed and presented using descriptive statistics. Categorical variables will be reported as absolute numbers and percentages, and continuous variables will be presented as means with standard deviations or medians with interquartile ranges and minimum/maximum values, alongside the number of missing and non-missing observations. For select variables, 95% CIs will be provided. Where applicable, Kaplan-Meier analysis will be performed to illustrate risk over time. Time-to-event variables will be analysed using Cox proportional hazard regression and presented as hazard ratios with 95% CIs and *p*-values. The type of VTE (DVT only vs. PE ± DVT) will be included in all Cox models as an additional covariate. Based on the results of the Hokusai-VTE and the PREFER in VTE studies [6, 13], no further confounders will be considered at this stage, but any other relevant differences at baseline will be retrospectively added to the model.

A separate analysis combining 18-month safety data from ETNA-VTE-Europe and ETNA-AF-Europe will address the co-primary objective. Data will be presented as absolute and relative frequencies with 95% CIs, overall and for each aforementioned exposure category and subgroup. All statistical analyses will be performed using SAS® version 9.3 or higher (SAS Institute, Cary, NC, USA).

Discussion

The real-world management of acute VTE has been studied by a number of registries on a national (MASTER and SWIVTER II [18, 19]), European (PREFER in VTE [13]) and global (RIETE, GARFIELD-VTE, RECOVERY and XALIA [20–23]) scale. Such registries are important because they include patients who are usually omitted from clinical trials due to strict inclusion and exclusion criteria, allowing appraisal of treatment regimes in patients with particular characteristics. Furthermore, large-scale, non-interventional studies permit real-world comparisons across a range of healthcare settings and geographical locations, which may be helpful for evaluating the relative efficiency of national healthcare services and identifying potential improvement strategies. In this sense, ETNA-VTE Europe is similar to existing registries; however, it is different in that it focuses on patients receiving edoxaban, a drug that more recently been approved and is therefore not represented in previous real-world studies. The EMA has reviewed and approved its study protocol. Accordingly, the present registry will add value by providing an as-yet-unexplored insight into the use and associated outcomes of this agent in clinical practice. A comparison between the design of ETNA-VTE Europe and other large-scale VTE-patient registries can be found in Table 3.

Current evidence for the safety and efficacy of edoxaban largely emanates from the phase III Hokusai-VTE

Table 3 Differences in design between ETNA-VTE Europe and other important European and global observational acute VTE registries

	Study design	Geographical scope	Patients	Agents of interest	Primary objective	Enrolment period	Key outcome measures	Status
ETNA-VTE Europe	Prospective, **single-arm**, observational PASS; **18-M FU**	310 sites across 8 European countries	2700 **edoxaban-treated** acute DVT and/or PE in/outpatients across multiple healthcare settings	**Edoxaban**	To **quantify the real-world, long-term rate of VTE recurrence in patients prescribed edoxaban** as part of acute VTE treatment	**Q4 2016**[a] – **Q4 2018**	Mortality, recurrent VTE, bleeding events, **hepatic events,** ADRs, hospitalisation for CV causes**, edoxaban adherence/discontinuation**	O
RIETE [21]	Prospective, observational study; **3-M FU**	192 sites across 19 countries worldwide (**78% of data from weSpain**)	6855 acute DVT and/or PE in/outpatients across a range of healthcare settings	**Standard therapy (pre-DOACs)**	To improve physician knowledge of the natural history of thromboembolic disease and **develop scores to identify patients at high risk of complications**	**March 2001 – Feb 2004**	Mortality, recurrent VTE, bleeding events	C
XALIA [22, 24]	Prospective, observational PASS; **12-M FU**	Multiple sites[b] in 21 countries **worldwide**	5142 **acute DVT (±PE)** patients at hospitals or community care centres	**Rivaroxaban and standard therapy**	To assess the **safety and effectiveness of rivaroxaban** for the treatment of symptomatic DVT	**June 2012 – March 2014**	Mortality, recurrent VTE, bleeding events, CV events, treatment satisfaction/ adherence/discontinuation, healthcare resource utilisation, TEAEs	C
PREFER in VTE [13, 14]	Prospective, observational study; **12-M FU**	381 sites across 7 European countries	3455 acute DVT and/or PE in/outpatients across a range of healthcare settings	**DOACs (pre-edoxaban)**	To explore patient characteristics, VTE management strategies, **healthcare resource usage and associated costs**	**Jan 2013 – Jan 2014**	Mortality, recurrent VTE, bleeding events, MI, stroke, SE, post-thrombotic syndrome, CV events	C
GARFIELD-VTE [20, 25]	Prospective, observational study; **two sequential cohorts; 3-Y FU**	415 sites across 28 countries **worldwide**	10,878 acute DVT and/ or PE in/outpatients across a range of healthcare settings	**Standard therapy and DOACs**	To identify **regional/ temporal treatment variations** and **assess their impact on** clinical/ **economic** outcomes	**July 2014 – Sept 2016**	Mortality, recurrent VTE, bleeding events, post-thrombotic syndrome, chronic thromboembolic pulmonary hypertension, healthcare resource utilisation	O
RE-COVERY [23, 26]	Prospective, observational PASS; **12-M FU**	~17[b] sites in 5 countries **worldwide**	~ 8000 acute DVT and/or PE patients	**Dabigatran and VKA**	To characterise the VTE patient population and **compare the safety and effectiveness of dabigatran to VKA**	Nov 2015 – Dec 2018	Mortality, recurrent VTE, bleeding events	O

Legend: Y, year; M, month; DVT, deep vein thrombosis; FU, follow-up; PE, pulmonary embolism; DOAC, direct oral anticoagulant; VTE, venous thromboembolism; TIA, transient ischaemic attack; PASS, post-authorisation safety study; Q4, fourth quarter; MI, myocardial infarction; SE, systemic embolism; CV, cardiovascular; VKA, vitamin-K antagonist, C, completed; O, ongoing, TEAE, treatment-emergent adverse events. Important differences are highlighted in **bold**. [a]Swiss sites: February 2015. [b]Precise number unknown

clinical trial [6]. A key limitation of this study was the exclusion of patients with characteristics encountered in routine clinical practice, such as those with isolated distal symptomatic DVT, a creatinine clearance of < 30 mL/min, and significant liver disease. Consequently, the effectiveness and safety in some clinical subgroups to edoxaban remain unrepresented and uncharacterised. Data gathered from the ETNA-VTE-Europe study with minimal selection criteria will address this knowledge gap, with several pertinent subgroup analyses already planned. The gathered data will also provide a snapshot of the types of patients being prescribed edoxaban, the doses used, and the durations of treatment in a real-life setting. This will permit appraisal of the appropriateness of such therapeutic decisions as well as acting as a marker for evaluation of subsequent trends of prescription.

An additional limitation of current studies is that data are only available for up to 12 months of edoxaban therapy [6]. Considering that a number of patients will require longer-term anticoagulation in clinical practice [8], those continuing edoxaban dosing beyond 12 months will find themselves in uncharted waters. The 18-month follow-up period planned for ETNA-VTE-Europe patients will provide clinicians and patients with valuable information regarding the safety and net clinical benefit of extended treatment. In particular, trends in rare ADRs such as liver events and major bleeding will be of interest, given their low frequency in the Hokusai-VTE trial [6]. Combination of ETNA-VTE-Europe data with those from the ETNA-AF-Europe sister study will provide an even larger population from which to assess these safety outcomes [10]. Thus, the present PASS is a responsible and important part of the early post-marketing phase, designed to address several of the knowledge gaps highlighted in the EMA risk-management plan for edoxaban [9].

The single-arm design of the ETNA-VTE-Europe study reflects its key aim of characterising the real-world safety and effectiveness of edoxaban. However, visually comparing our results to those from similar studies with different anticoagulants will help to provide perspective. To these ends, data from the recent PREFER in VTE real-world registry will be used to contextualise data from ETNA-VTE-Europe, selected for its comparable bleeding definitions, coinciding data assessment time points, and high patient numbers (3545 patients) [14]. This will allow us to gain an idea of the real-world safety and effectiveness of edoxaban relative to agents such as VKAs and other DOACs, not only in the overall population, but also in specific patient subsets, such as those with renal or hepatic impairment. Furthermore, several of the countries and regional delineations in ETNA-VTE-Europe (such as Italy, DACH and UK/IE) also feature in the PREFER in VTE study, enabling various approximate geographical comparisons [13]. A further evaluation of ETNA-VTE-Europe real-world results in the context of those from the Hokusai-VTE clinical trial will provide insight into the influence of stringent enrolment criteria and closer monitoring on edoxaban-related outcomes. This will indicate to what extent the encouraging findings from phase III studies can be expected to translate into clinical practice.

Potential limitations

As a prospective, non-interventional registry that aims to represent everyday occurrence and management of VTE, the stringent inclusion/exclusion criteria, physician/patient blinding, and site/protocol standardisation that typify RTCs do not apply. This introduces the possibility for biases that are difficult to avoid, measure or correct for. In particular, heterogeneous timing and length of edoxaban exposure may prove problematic for the interpretation of results, thought this will be taken into consideration at data analysis. Furthermore, in such a large-scale study, some incompleteness, insufficient detail, or inaccuracy of patient data is unavoidable; however, measures such as the careful design of case report forms and data monitoring/verification aim to minimise such occurrences. Despite the inherent limitations associated with observational registries, the all-inclusive nature of ETNA-VTE Europe may be seen as an advantage for obtaining a realistic snapshot of the clinical climate, with two-wave recruitment potentially allowing changes in treatment behaviour over time to be elucidated. Finally, while the single-arm nature of the study means that direct comparisons with other anticoagulants will not be possible, close accordance between the designs of PREFER in VTE and ETNA-VTE Europe should permit a reasonable appraisal of outcome differences.

Conclusions

The international, observational ETNA-VTE-Europe registry will allow the safety and effectiveness of edoxaban in the general population of acute symptomatic VTE patients to be assessed over an extended time period. The planned series of explorative analyses will provide essential information regarding edoxaban treatment in a range of as-yet-unrepresented patient subsets, the effect of treatment duration and discontinuation on outcomes, and the relative costs/benefits associated with edoxaban use compared to that of other commercially available anticoagulants. Findings will help to elucidate whether the good safety profile observed in the Hokusai-VTE clinical trial can be extrapolated to the real-world population, as well as providing a wealth of valuable information for European practitioners prescribing or contemplating the use of edoxaban as part of VTE treatment/secondary prevention.

Appendix

List of ETNA in VTE investigators

Austria

Cihan Ay, Allgemeines Krankenhaus Medizinische Universität Wien, Wien; Matthias Hoke, AKH - Medizinische Universität Wien, Wien; Marianne Brodmann, LKH - Universitätsklinikum Graz, Graz; Rudolf Kirchmair, Medizinische Universität Innsbruck, Innsbruck; Rainer Mathies, Landeskrankenhaus Feldkirch, Feldkirch; Markus Rauter, Klinikum Klagenfurt am Wörthersee, Klagenfurt; Klemens Reinberg, Gemeinschaftspraxis Wachau, Weißenkirchen in der Wachau; Vinzenz Stepan, Krankenhaus der Elisabethinen Graz, Graz; Thomas Maca, Ordination Dr. Maca, Wien; Hans Domanovits, AKH - Medizinische Universität Wien, Vienna; Wolfgang Salmhofer, Landeskrakenhaus - Universitaetsklinikum Graz, Graz; Thomas Weiss, Wilhelminenspital der Stadt Wien, Wien; Walter Klimscha, Sozialmedizinisches Zentrum Ost - Donauspital, Vienna; Alexander Kober, Ordination, Sankt Aegyd am Neuwalde; Franz Hinterreiter, Konventhospital Barmherzige Brüder, Linz; Johann Auer, KH St. Josef Braunau, Braunau; Armaghan Gomari-Grisar, Krankenhaus Barmherzige Schwestern Wien, Wien; Joeg Jabkowski, Krankenhaus der Elisabethinen Linz, Linz; Paul Pinter, Wahlarzt Ordination, Dr. Paul Pinter, Altenmarkt an der Triesting

Belgium

Philippe Hainaut, Cliniques Universitaires Saint-Luc, Bruxelles; Laure Gilis, CHC - Clinique St-Jospeh, Liège; Herman Schroe, Ziekenhuis Oost-Limburg, Genk; Jos Vandekerkhof, Jessa Ziekenhuis - Campus Virga Jesse, Hasselt; Pascal Vranckx, Jessa Ziekenhuis Hospital, Hasselt; Peter Verhamme, UZ Leuven, Leuven; Mikhael Janssen, AZ Groeninge - Kennedylaan, Kortrijk; Guy Vereecken, Vereecken Guy, Halen; Luc De Munck, De Munck, Vilvoorde; Bernard Vandooren, Algemeen Ziekenhuis West, Veurne; Johan Duchateau, AZ Sint-Maarten, Duffel; Jan De Letter, AZ Sint-Jan Brugge, Brugge; Muriel Lins, AZ Sint-Maarten, Duffel; Jean-Claude Wautrecht, ULB Hopital Erasme, Bruxelles; Marc Delforge, CHR de Huy, Huy; Philippe Hermans, CHU Saint-Pierre, Bruxelles; Philippe Borgoens, CHR Citadelle, Liege; Jean-Baptiste Nicolas, CHU UCL Namur, Yvoir; Geoffrey Debonnaire, Sint-Elisabeth Ziekenhuis, Zottegem; Marion Delcroix, UZ Leuven, Leuven; Stéphane Vanden Bemden, bvba Medisch Kabinet Dr. Vanden Bemden, Steenokkerzeel; Jaak Mortelmans, Mortelmans, Jaak, Oostham; Muriel Sprynger, CHU de Liege, Liège; Yohan Balthazar, SPRL MG Balthazar & Ballard, Natoye; Geert Vileyn, Huisartsenpraktijk Vileyn bvba, Blankenberge; Michel Goetinck, Huisartsenpraktijk De Stoute, Brugge; Bart Segers, Wichelen; Philippe De Vleeschauwer, Heilige Hart Ziekenhuis Lier, Lier; Michel De Pauw, Universitair Ziekenhuis Gent, Gent; Karen Wustenberghs, GZA Ziekenhuizen - Campus Sint-Augustinus, Wilrijk; Roeland Dierickx, Huisartsen Dierickx, Westouter

Germany

Dirk Härtel, Klinikum Lippe GmbH, Detmold; Gunter Hergdt, Praxis Dr. med. Gunter Hergdt, Obermichelbach; Holger Michel, Gemeinschaftspraxis Michel und Leffler, Lutherstadt Eisleben; Annegret Otto, Gemeinschaftspraxis Dres. med. Stenzel, Ebert & Otto, Riesa; Andreas Rieker, Facharztpraxis Rieker Dr. med. Andreas Rieker - Venenpraxis im "Gesundheitszentrum Südstraße", Lauffen am Neckar; Toralf Schwarz, INFO-MED Leipzig GmbH, Markkleeberg; Jens Taggeselle, Kardiologische Praxis Dr. Jens Taggeselle, Markkleeberg; Oliver Gastmann, Ilm-Kreis-Kliniken Arnstadt-Ilmenau gGmbH, Arnstadt; Diana Razavi, Praxis Diana Razavi, Steinau; Petra Herrmann, Praxis Dipl.- Med. Petra Herrmann, Eisenach; Dag-Alexander Keilhau, Medizinisches Versorgungszentrum für Innere Medizin, Hamburg; Bernd-Thomas Kellner, Gemeinschaftspraxis Dres. Niels Erhardt und Bernd-Thomas Kellner, Dornburg-Camburg; Diethard Predel, Praxis für Gefäßmedizin, Nordhausen; Rainer Rippert, Praxis Dr. Rippert, Wiesbaden; Reinhardt Sternitzky, Zentrum für klinische Prüfungen in der Facharztzentrum Dresden-Neustadt GbR, Dresden; Andor Schmidt, Omdas GmbH and Praxis Dr. med. Andor Schmidt, Offenbach; Matthias Schulze, Asklepios Klinikum Schwalmstadt, Schwalmstadt; Heiko Schneider, Medigra - Gemeinschaftspraxis Dres. Heiko Schneider & Peter Rostock, Apolda; Franz Wolf, Praxis Dres. Wolf, Straubing; Andreas Greve, Innere Medizin im Gesundheitszentrum, Ahrensburg; Matthias Ulrich, Angiologie am Coppiplatz, Leipzig; Norbert Schön, Kardiologie Mühldorf am Inn, Mühldorf; Günter Rehling, Gemeinschaftspraxis Dres. Michael Eis und Günter Rehling, Sand am Main; Bernhard Witzenbichler, HELIOS Amper-Klinikum Dachau, Dachau; Bernadett Brado, Praxis für Angiologie, Hämatologie, Innere Medizin Dr. med. Bernadett Brado, Heidelberg-Neuenheim; Thomas N. Abahji, Ärztehaus GerMedicum, Germering; Johannes Brachmann, Klinikum Coburg GmbH, Coburg; Hans-Walter Bindig, Praxis Dr. Bindig, Georgensgmünd; Siamak Pourhassan, Gemeinschaftspraxis für Gefäßchirurgie/Gefäßmedizin - Drs. Heim & Pourhassan, Oberhausen; Tobias Geisler, Deutsches Herzkompetenzzentrum am Universitätsklinikum Tübingen, Tübingen; Berthold Amann, Franziskus-Krankenhaus Berlin, Akademisches Lehrkrankenhaus der Charité, Berlin; Svetlana Tlechas-Tkatsch, Praxis S. Tlechas-Tkatsch, Potsdam; Markus Stücker, St. Maria-Hilf-Krankenhaus, Bochum-Gerthe; Rainer Schmiedel, Praxis Dr. med. Rainer Schmiedel, Kaiserslautern; Ernst G. Vester, Evangelisches Krankenhaus Düsseldorf, Düsseldorf; Janna Dshabrailov, Praxis Dr. Dshabrailov, Osnabrück; Ayham Al-Zoebi, Kardiologische

Praxis Dr. Al-Zoebi, Wermsdorf; Sylvia Baumbach, Gemeinschaftspraxis Dr. med. Sylvia Baumbach und Dr. Elke Reichelt, Apolda; Wilma Grosskopf, Gemeinschaftspraxis Dres. Josef Anton Großkopf und Wilma Großkopf, Wallerfing; Michael Czihal, Klinikum der Universität München, München; Christoph Hehrlein, Universitäts-Herzzentrum Freiburg Bad Krozingen GmbH, Freiburg; Thomas Ludwig, Praxis Dr. med. Thomas Ludwig, Farchant; Daniel Kretzschmar, Universitätsklinikum Jena, Jena; Teja Müller, Praxis Innere Medizin Dr. Teja Müller, Wehrheim; Harriet Simone Werno, Parcside medical center, Nuernberg; Julio Perez-Delgado, Arberlandklinik Viechtach, Viechtach; Edelgard Lindhoff-Last, CCB - Cardioangiologisches Centrum Bethanien, Frankfurt; Thomas Schmitz-Rixen, Universitätsklinikum Frankfurt, Frankfurt am Main; Oliver Ritter, Städtisches Klinikum Brandenburg, Brandenburg an der Havel; Thomas May, Krankenhaus Porz am Rhein gGmbH, Köln; Enno Eißfeller, Praxis Dr. med. Eißfeller, Woellstein; Klaus Fenchel, MVZ MP Saaletal, Saalfeld; Marcus Thieme, MEDINOS Kliniken des Landkreises Sonneberg GmbH, Sonneberg; Christian Heiß, Universitätsklinikum Düsseldorf, Düsseldorf; Thomas Bader, Praxis Dr. med. Bader, Heilbronn-Biberach; Rainer J. Zotz, Marienhausklinikum Eifel Bitburg, Bitburg; Christoph Kalka, Marienhospital Brühl GmbH, Brühl; Johannes Haas, CIMS UG mbh, Bamberg; Andreas Hagenow, Praxis Dr. med. Andreas Hagenow, Elsterwerda; Karl-Heinz Binias, AMEOS Klinikum Schönebeck, Schönebeck; Jan Beyer-Westendorf, Universitätsklinikum Carl Gustav Carus TU Dresden, Dresden; Veselin Mitrovic, Kerckhoff-Klinik Forschungsgesellschaft mbH, Bad Nauheim; Wolfram Oettler, Praxis für Gefäßmedizin, Görlitz; Claudia Zemmrich, MVZ Dres. Ramdohr - Praxis für Cardiovascular und Ultraschalldiagnostik, Berlin; Jaswant Singh, St. Elisabeth-Krankenhaus, Jülich; Matthias Leschke, Klinikum Esslingen GmbH, Esslingen a. N.; Thomas Herrmann, Fachinternistische Gemeinschaftspraxis Weinheim, Weinheim; Stefan Hetzel, Gemeinschaftspraxis Dres. Hetzel & Grewe-Kemper, Greven; Frank Hamann, Klinikum Konstanz, Konstanz; Christina Hart, Universitätsklinikum Regensburg, Regensburg; Matthias Tenholt, Theresienkrankenhaus und St. Hedwig-Klinik GmbH, Mannheim; Martin Andrassy, Fürst-Stirum-Klinik Bruchsal, Bruchsal; Andreas Wilke, Kardiologische Praxis Papenburg Dr. Hans-Jürgen Stühn-Pfeifer und Dr. Andreas Wilke, Papenburg; Friederike Baron-Gielnik, CardioMed an der Alster, Hamburg; Muwafeg Abdel-Qader, Praxis Dr. med. Abdel-Qader, Winsen; Rainer Hennecke, Dres. Rolf Schenk und Rainer Hennecke, Winsen; Birgit Gerecke, MVZ Ambulantes Kardiologisches Zentrum Peine, Peine; Uwe Gremmler, MVZ Ambulantes Kardiologisches Zentrum Peine, Peine; Volker Eissing, MVZ Birkenallee GmbH, Papenburg; Nikolaos Proskynitopoulos, Kardiologische Gemeinschaftspraxis, Nienburg; Stefan Regner, Gemeinschaftspraxis Mainz Mitte am Gesundheitscentrum Mainz, Mainz; Heiner Müller Heiner, Berufsausübungsgemeinschaft Dres. med. Kolitsch/Müller, Katzhütte; Stephan Lüders, St. Josefs-Hospital, Cloppenburg; Elvira Maria Lembens, Praxis Dres. Christoph Lembens und Elvira Maria Lembens, Mainz; Werner Jung Werner, Schwarzwald-Baar Klinikum Villingen-Schwenningen GmbH, Villingen-Schwenningen; Frank Heckmann, Gefäßzentrum Dr. Heckmann und Kollegen, Neckargemuend; Kurt Jocham, Dialysezentrum Memmingen - Internistisches Facharztzentrum, Memmingen; Ralf Berg, Praxis im alten Rathaus, Einzelpraxis Dr. med. R. Berg, Ühlingen-Birkendorf; Thomas Dengler, Kreiskrankenaus am Plattenwald, Bad Friedrichshall; Uwe Zwettler, Atos clinic Heidelberg, Dres. Heckmann/ Rieger, Heidelberg; Martin Rieger, Zentrum für Gefäßerkrankungen und Präventivmedizin, Neckargemünd; Pascal Bauer, UKGM - Universitätsklinikum Gießen und Marburg GmbH, Gießen; Mirko Böhme, Praxis Dr. Mirko Böhme, Sulzberg; Christian Loges, Drs. Haney/Gehrig/ Loges, Mosbach; Sebastian Kruse, Gemeinschaftspraxis Kruse / Kuth, Aachen-Walheim; Clemens Tebbe, Marien-Hospital Euskirchen, Euskirchen; Oliver Bruder, Elisabeth Krankenhaus Essen, Essen; Dietrich Gulba, St. Marien Hospital, Oberhausen; Norbert Ludwig, Gemeinschaftspraxis Prof.Dr. Ludwig, Dr. Honl, Willich; Christoph Nielen, Gemeinschaftspraxis für Gefäßmedizin GbR, Mönchengladbach; Ulrich Overhoff, Zentrum fuer Praevention und Rehabilitation, Siegen; Helmut Renz, Gemeinschaftspraxis Vogelstang, Mannheim; Holger Lawall, Gemeinschaftspraxis Prof. Dr. med. Curt Diehm und Dr. med. Holger Lawall, Ettlingen; Sabine Genth-Zotz, Katholisches Klinikum Mainz, Caritas Werk St. Martin Gem. Träger und Betriebsf. GmbH, Mainz; Peter Wirtz, Kreiskrankenhaus Mechernich GmbH, Mechernich; Dirk Henning Walter, Kardiologie am Tibarg, Hamburg; Astrid Schmidt-Reinwald, Praxis Dr. med. Astrid Schmidt-Reinwald, Trier

Ireland

Brian McCullagh, Mater Private Hospital, Dublin; Mike Watts, University Hospital Limerick, Limerick; Azhar Bhatti, Connolly Hospital, Dublin; Peter Branagan, Beaumont Hospital,Dublin; Stuart Carr, Blackrock Clinic, Dublin

Italy

Michele Dalla Vestra, Ospedale dell'Angelo, Mestre; Crisitiano Bortoluzzi, Ospedale civile SS. Giovanni e Paolo, Venezia; David Imberti, Presidio Ospedaliero di Piacenza Ospedale "Guglielmo Da Saliceto", Piacenza; Domenico Prisco, Azienda Ospedaliera Universitaria Careggi, Firenze; Serena Rupoli, Azienda Ospedaliero Universitaria Ospedali Riuniti di Ancona "Umberto I, G.M. Lancisi, G. Salesi", Ancona; Maria Amitrano, Azienda Ospedaliera San Giuseppe Moscati, Avellino; Crisitiana D'Amrosio, Ospedale Ferdinando Veneziale,

Isernia; Angelo Ghirarduzzi, Azienda Ospedaliera Arcispedale Santa Maria Nuova - IRCCS, Reggio Emilia; Giovanni Di Minno, Azienda Ospedaliera Universitaria Federico II, Napoli; Andrea Fontanella, Ospedale Buonconsiglio - Fondazione Fatebenefratelli, Napoli; Maria Teresa De Denato, Azienda Ospedaliera Universitaria S. Giovanni di Dio - Ruggi D'Aragona, Salerno; Sophie Testa, ASST di Cremona - Ospedale di Cremona, Cremona; Lorenzo Malatino, Azienda Ospedaliera per l'emergenza "Canizzaro", Catania; Francesca Corsini, Ospedale Sant'Andrea, La Spezia; Rodolfo Tassara, Presidio Ospedaliero di Savona - Cairo Montenotte Ospedale San Paolo, Savona; Gabriele Giordano, Villa dei Fiori - Casa di cura privata, Acerra; Anita Carlizza, Azienda Ospedaliera San Giovanni Addolorata, Roma; Riccardo Margheriti, Presidio Ospedaliero Giovan Battista Grassi, Roma; Fausto Marrocco, Presidio Ospedaliero Santa Scolastica, Cassino; Raffaele Landolfi, Fondazione Policlinico Universitaria "A.Gemelli", Roma; Sabina Villalta, Ospedale di Treviso, Treviso; Adriana Visona, Presidio Ospedaliero San Giacomo Apostolo, Castelfranco Veneto; Egidio Imbalzano, Azienda Ospedaliera Universitaria Policlinico "G. Martino", Messina; Maurilio Cirrito, Fondazione Istituto "G. Giglio", Cefalù; Massimo Arquati, Presidio Ospedaliero Sacco, Milano; Giampiero Avruscio, Azienda Ospedaliera di Padova - Policlinico, Padova; Ginacarlo Agnelli, Azienda Ospedaliera di Perugia, Perugia; Lucia Anna Mameli, Ospedale Civile SS Annunziata A.S.L.1 Sassari, Sassari; Armando D'Angelo, Ospedale San Raffaele IRCCS, Milano; Roberta Risso, Ospedale Santo Spirito di Bra, Cuneo; Alessandro Celi, Azienda Ospedaliera Universitaria Pisana - Ospedale di Cisanello, Pisa; Vieri Vannucchi, Presidio Ospedaliero Santa Maria Nuova, Firenze; Fernando Parente, Ospedale Vito Fazzi, Lecce; Francesco Ventrella, Presidio Ospedaliero G. Tatarella, Cerignola; Francesco Dentali, Ospedale di Circolo e Fondazione Macchi, Varese; Pietro Tropeano, Ospedale Santa Maria degli Angeli, Pordenone; Pasquale Morella, Azienda Ospedaliera A. CARDARELLI, Napoli; Aldo Salvi, Ospedali Riuniti Ancona, Ancona; Gabriele Frausini, Azienda Ospedaliera MARCHE NORD Presidio Ospedaliero Santa Croce, Fano; Roberto Catalini, Ospedale Generale Provinciale, Macerata; Mauro Campanini, Azienda Ospedaliera Universitaria Maggiore della Carità, Novara; Corrado Amato, Policlinico Universitario Palermo, Palermo; Monica Demarco, Humanitas Mater Domini, Castellanza; Iolanda Enea, Ospedale S. Anna e S. Sebastiano, Caserta; Nello Zanatta, Ospedale S. Maria dei Battuti, Conegliano Veneto; Rita Pepe, Ospedale S. Eugenio, Roma; Roberto Cappelli, Azienda Ospedaliera Universitaria Senese, Siena; Stefano Barolo, Ospedale S. Lazzaro, Alba; Giuseppe Guigliano, Azienda Ospedaliera Universitaria Federico II, Napoli; Beilde Cosmi, Ospedale Sant'Orsola - Malpighi, Bologna; Domenic Blasis, Ospedale SS Filippo e Nicola, Avezzano; Jeness Simona Campodonico, Centro Cardiologico Monzino, Milano; Franco Spangaro, Ospedale Cattinara, Trieste

Netherlands

Michiel Coppens, Academisch Medisch Centrum, Amsterdam; Albert Mairuhu, HagaZiekenhuis, Den Haag; Wim Boersma, Noordwest Ziekenhuisgroep, Alkmaar; Marije ten Wolde, Flevoziekenhuis, Almere; Houshang Monajemi, Rijnstate, Arnhem; Heike Noordzij-Nooteboom, Van Weel-Bethesda Ziekenhuis, Dirksland; Gert-Jan Braunstahl, Franciscus Gasthuis, Rotterdam; Ragnar Lunde, Laurentius Ziekenhuis, Roermond; Sanne van Wissen, Onze Lieve Vrouwe Gasthuis, Locatie Oost, Amsterdam; Adriaan Dees, Ikazia Ziekenhuis, Rotterdam

Switzerland

Marc Righini, Hopital Universitaire Geneve, Geneva; Lucia Mazzolai, Centre Hospitalier Universitaire Vaudois, Lausanne; Frederic Baumann, Universitaetsspital Zuerich, Zuerich; Marc Schindewolf, University of Bern, Bern; Daniel Staub, Universitaetsspital Basel, Basel; Juerg H. Beer, Kantonsspital Baden AG, Baden; Martin Banyai, Cantonal hospital Lucerne, Luzern; Stefan Kradolfer, Facharzt FMH ALLG. Medizin, Basel; Daniel Erni, Schwanenpraxis, Luzern

United Kingdom

Karen Breen, Guy's Hospital, London; Ewart Jackson-Voyzey, Axbridge and Wedmore Medical Practice, Axbridge; Piers Clifford, Wycombe Hospital, High Wycombe; Peter MacCallum, Barts Health NHS Trust, London; Azhar Zafar, Danes Camp Medical Practice, Northampton; Anja Drebes, Royal Free London NHS Foundation Trust, London; Asok Venkataraman, George Eliot Hospital, Nuneaton; Gunaratnam Gunathilagan, Queen Elizabeth the Queen Mother Hospital, Margate; Salah Matti, Basingstoke and North Hampshire Hospital, Basingstoke; Nicola Stevenson, Arrowe Park Hospital, Wirral; Tamara Everington, Salisbury District Hospital, Salisbury; James Uprichard, St George's Hospital, London; Anand Dixit, Royal Victoria Infirmary, Newcastle upon Tyne; Piers Clifford, Hammersmith Hospital, London; Tina Dutt, Royal Liverpool University Hospital, Liverpool; Jeremy Platt, The Binfield Surgery, Binfield; Mark Richardson, Lindum Medical Practice, Lincoln; Paul Gilbert Conn, Ballygomartin Group Practice, Belfast; Charalampos Kartsios, Birmingham Heartlands Hospital, Birmingham; Muhsin Almusawy, Bedford Hospital, Bedford; Margaret Bowers, Ulster Hospital South Eastern Health and Social Care Trust, Belfast.

Abbreviations

ADR: Adverse drug reaction; BE/NL: BELGIUM/the Netherlands; CI: Confidence interval; CRNM: Clinically relevant non-major bleeding; DACH: Austria, Switzerland and Germany; DOAC: Direct oral anticoagulant; DVT: Deep vein thrombosis; eCRF: Electronic case report form; EDC: Electronic data capture; EMA: European Medicines Agency; GPP: Good Pharmacoepidemiology Practice; GVP: Good Pharmacovigilance Practices; LPO: Last patient out; NVAF: Non-valvular atrial fibrillation; PASS: Post-authorisation safety study; PE: Pulmonary embolism; PTS: Post-thrombotic syndrome; SEE: Systemic embolic events; UK/IE: United Kingdom/Ireland; VTE: Venous thromboembolism

Acknowledgements

We are indebted to all investigators across Austria, Germany, Belgium, Italy, Switzerland, the Netherlands and the UK who have made this registry possible. See Appendix for list of Investigators.

Funding

Daiichi Sankyo Europe GmbH, Munich, Germany.

Authors' contributions

All authors have contributed to the design of the registry and/or the preparation of the manuscript. EMF was responsible for the analysis of data. ATC and PB drafted the first version of the manuscript and the remaining authors made substantial revisions to the manuscript. All authors have approved the version to be published. Apart from the selection of the countries, all design aspects were decided by the scientific Steering Committee and executed by independent Contract Research organizations. All authors read and approved the final manuscript.

Competing interests

The members of the Steering Committee received honoraria for their advice in the planning of the Registry. They also received honoraria and travel reimbursements from Daiichi Sankyo Europe GmbH for their participation in Steering Committee Meetings.

Alexander T. Cohen, Hervé Décousus, Pedro Marques da Silva, David Jimenez Castro, Beatrice Amann-Vesti, Bernd Brüggenjürgen, Eric Vicaut and Giancarlo Agnelli have received research support and/or honoraria for lectures from a number of pharmaceutical companies including Daiichi Sankyo, the sponsor of the registry.

Cihan Ay received honoraria for lectures from Sanofi, Pfizer/BMS, Daiichi-Sankyo, Boehringer Ingelheim, and Bayer. Advisory board membership for Pfizer/BMS, Daiichi-Sankyo, Boehringer Ingelheim, and Bayer.

Philippe Hainaut received honoraria from Daiichi Sankyo Europe GmbH for lectures and advisory board membership.

Ulrich Hoffmann received honoraria for lectures from Bayer, Daiichi-Sankyo, Leo Pharma, Pfizer, Bristol-Meyers, Aspen, Sanofi-Aventis, Amgen. Advisory board membership for Bayer, Daiichi-Sankyo, Leo Pharma, Sanofi-Aventis, and Amgen.

Sean Gaine received honoraria for lectures from Actelion Pharmaceuticals Ltd., Bayer, GlaxoSmithKline, Merck Sharpe & Dohme, and has received advisory and/or drug safety board fees from Astra Zeneca, Actelion Pharmaceuticals Ltd., Bayer, GlaxoSmithKline, Novartis, Pfizer and Daiichi-Sankyo, Menerini, and United Therapeutics.

Michiel Coppens has received research funding and honoraria for consultancy or lecturing from Daiichi Sankyo, Boehringer Ingelheim, Bayer, Bristol-Myers Squibb and Pfizer.

Pierre Levy received honoraria for lectures from AbbVie, Amgen, Gilead, GSK, Novo Nordisk, ViiV. Advisory board membership for AbbVie, Actelion, Amgen, Astellas, Bayer, Biogen, Boehringer Ingelheim, Celgène, Daiichi Sankyo, Eli Lilly, EOS, GSK, Janssen, MSD, Mundipharma, Novartis, Pfizer, Roche, Shire, Vertex.

Julio Lopez Bastida received honoraria from Daiichi Sankyo.

Petra Laeis, Eva-Maria Fronk, Wolfgang Zierhut, and Thomas Malzer are employees of Daiichi Sankyo Europe GmbH.

Peter Bramlage received research funding and consultancy honoraria from Daiichi Sankyo Europe GmbH. He further received funding for drafting the manuscript.

The members of the Steering Committee received honoraria and travel reimbursements from Daiichi Sankyo Europe GmbH for their participation in Steering Committee Meetings.

Author details

[1]Guy's and St Thomas' NHS Foundation Trust, King's College London, London, UK. [2]Clinical Division of Haematology and Haemostaseology, Department of Medicine I, Medical University of Vienna, Vienna, Austria. [3]Department of General Internal Medicine, Cliniques Universitaires Saint Luc, UCL, Bruxelles, Belgium. [4]Centre Hospitalier Universitaire de Saint-Etienne, Saint-Priest En Jarez, France. [5]Division of Angiology, Medical Clinic IV, University Hospital, Ludwig-Maximilians-University, Munich, Germany. [6]National Pulmonary Hypertension Unit, Mater Misericordiae University Hospital, Dublin, Ireland. [7]Department of Vascular Medicine, Academic Medical Center, Amsterdam, The Netherlands. [8]Department of Internal Medicine, Arterial Investigation Unit, Hospital de Santa Marta, Lisbon, Portugal. [9]Respiratory Department, Ramón y Cajal Hospital, Madrid, Spain. [10]Division of Angiology, University Hospital Zurich, Zurich, Switzerland. [11]Institute for Health Economics, Steinbeis-University, Berlin, Germany. [12]LEGOS, Université Paris – Dauphine, Paris, France. [13]University of Castilla-La Mancha, Talavera de la Reina, Toledo, Spain. [14]Department of Medicine, Université Paris Descartes, Paris, France. [15]Daiichi Sankyo Europe GmbH, Munich, Germany. [16]Institute for Pharmacology and Preventive Medicine, Berlin, Germany. [17]Internal and Cardiovascular Medicine-Stroke Unit, University of Perugia, Perugia, Italy.

References

1. Heit JA. Epidemiology of venous thromboembolism. Nat Rev Cardiol. 2015; 12:464–74.
2. Goldhaber SZ, Bounameaux H. Pulmonary embolism and deep vein thrombosis. Lancet. 2012;379:1835–46.
3. Cushman M, Tsai AW, White RH, Heckbert SR, Rosamond WD, Enright P, Folsom AR. Deep vein thrombosis and pulmonary embolism in two cohorts: the longitudinal investigation of thromboembolism etiology. Am J Med. 2004;117:19–25.
4. Heit JA. Predicting the risk of venous thromboembolism recurrence. Am J Hematol. 2012;87(Suppl 1):S63–7.
5. Giugliano RP, Ruff CT, Braunwald E, Murphy SA, Wiviott SD, Halperin JL, Waldo AL, Ezekowitz MD, Weitz JI, Špinar J, et al. Edoxaban versus warfarin in patients with atrial fibrillation. N Engl J Med. 2013;369:2093–104.
6. Buller HR, Decousus H, Grosso MA, Mercuri M, Middeldorp S, Prins MH, Raskob GE, Schellong SM, Schwocho L, Segers A, et al. Edoxaban versus warfarin for the treatment of symptomatic venous thromboembolism. N Engl J Med. 2013;369:1406–15.
7. Lixiana (edoxaban): Summary of Product Characteristics [http://www.ema.europa.eu/docs/en_GB/document_library/EPAR_-_Product_Information/human/002629/WC500189045.pdf]. Accessed 2017.
8. Konstantinides SV, Torbicki A, Agnelli G, Danchin N, Fitzmaurice D, Galie N, Gibbs JS, Huisman MV, Humbert M, Kucher N, et al: 2014 ESC guidelines on the diagnosis and management of acute pulmonary embolism. Eur Heart J 2014, 35:3033–3069, 3069a-3069k.
9. Summary of the risk management plan (RMP) for Lixiana (edoxaban) [http://www.ema.europa.eu/docs/en_GB/document_library/EPAR_-_Risk-management-plan_summary/human/002629/WC500186050.pdf]. Accessed 2017.
10. Edoxaban Treatment in Routine Clinical Practice for Patients With Non Valvular Atrial Fibrillation (ETNA-AF-EU: NCT02944019) [https://clinicaltrials.gov/ct2/show/NCT02944019]. Accessed 2017.
11. Schulman S, Kearon C, the SOCOAOTS, Standardization Committee Of The International Society On T, Haemostasis. Definition of major bleeding in clinical investigations of antihemostatic medicinal products in non-surgical patients. J Thromb Haemost. 2005;3:692–4.
12. Investigators TH-V. Edoxaban versus warfarin for the treatment of symptomatic venous thromboembolism. N Engl J Med. 2013;369:1406–15.
13. Cohen AT, Gitt AK, Bauersachs R, Fronk EM, Laeis P, Mismetti P, Monreal M, Willich SN, Bramlage P, Agnelli G, et al. The management of acute venous thromboembolism in clinical practice. Results from the European PREFER in VTE registry. Thromb Haemost. 2017;117:1326–37.
14. Agnelli G, Gitt AK, Bauersachs R, Fronk EM, Laeis P, Mismetti P, Monreal M, Willich SN, Wolf WP, Cohen AT. The management of acute venous thromboembolism in clinical practice - study rationale and protocol of the European PREFER in VTE registry. Thromb J. 2015;13:41.

15. Raskob G, Buller H, Prins M, Segers A, Shi M, Schwocho L, van Kranen R, Mercuri M. Edoxaban for the long-term treatment of venous thromboembolism: rationale and design of the Hokusai-venous thromboembolism study–methodological implications for clinical trials. J Thromb Haemost. 2013;11:1287–94.
16. Guideline on good pharmacovigilance practices (GVP) Module VI – Management and reporting of adverse reactions to medicinal products (Rev 1) [http://www.ema.europa.eu/docs/en_GB/document_library/Scientific_guideline/2014/09/WC500172402.pdf]. Accessed 2017.
17. Public Policy Committee ISoP. Guidelines for good pharmacoepidemiology practice (GPP). Pharmacoepidemiol Drug Saf. 2016;25:2–10.
18. Verso M, Agnelli G, Ageno W, Imberti D, Moia M, Palareti G, Pistelli R, Cantone V. Long-term death and recurrence in patients with acute venous thromboembolism: the MASTER registry. Thromb Res. 2012;130:369–73.
19. Spirk D, Ugi J, Korte W, Husmann M, Hayoz D, Baldi T, Frauchiger B, Banyai M, Aujesky D, Baumgartner I, Kucher N. Long-term anticoagulation treatment for acute venous thromboembolism in patients with and without cancer. The SWIss venous ThromboEmbolism registry (SWIVTER) II. Thromb Haemost. 2011;105:962–7.
20. Weitz JI, Haas S, Ageno W, Angchaisuksiri P, Bounameaux H, Nielsen JD, Goldhaber SZ, Goto S, Kayani G, Mantovani L, et al. Global anticoagulant registry in the field - venous thromboembolism (GARFIELD-VTE). Rationale and design. Thromb Haemost. 2016;116:1172–9.
21. Monreal M, Suarez C, Fajardo JA, Barba R, Uresandi F, Valle R, Rondon P. Management of patients with acute venous thromboembolism: findings from the RIETE registry. Pathophysiol Haemost Thromb. 2003;33:330–4.
22. Ageno W, Mantovani LG, Haas S, Kreutz R, Monje D, Schneider J, van Eickels M, Gebel M, Zell E, Turpie AG. Safety and effectiveness of oral rivaroxaban versus standard anticoagulation for the treatment of symptomatic deep-vein thrombosis (XALIA): an international, prospective, non-interventional study. Lancet Haematol. 2016;3:e12–21.
23. Ageno W, Casella IB, Han CK, Raskob GE, Schellong S, Schulman S, Singer DE, Kimura K, Tang W, Desch M, Goldhaber SZ, RE-COVERY DVT. PE: rationale and design of a prospective observational study of acute venous thromboembolism with a focus on dabigatran etexilate. Thromb Haemost. 2017;117:415–21.
24. Ageno W, Mantovani LG, Haas S, Kreutz R, Haupt V, Schneider J, Turpie AG. XALIA: rationale and design of a non-interventional study of rivaroxaban compared with standard therapy for initial and long-term anticoagulation in deep vein thrombosis. Thromb J. 2014;12:16.
25. About GARFIELD-VTE [http://vte.garfieldregistry.org/about/about-garfield-vte]. Accessed 2017.
26. RE-COVERY DVT/PE: Global Study on Treatment Secondary Prevention of Acute Venous Thromboembolism. https://clinicaltrials.gov/ct2/show/NCT02596230.

27

Treatment with direct oral anticoagulants in patients with upper extremity deep vein thrombosis

Francisco Sánchez Montiel, Raein Ghazvinian, Anders Gottsäter and Johan Elf*

Abstract

Background: Upper extremity deep vein thrombosis (UEDVT) constitutes around 10% of all DVT, and can cause both pulmonary embolism (PE) and postthrombotic syndrome (PTS) in the arm. The incidence of secondary UEDVT is increasing due to widespread use of central venous catheters in patients with cancer and other chronic diseases. The safety and efficacy of using new direct acting oral anti coagulants (DOAC) in the treatment of UEDVT has not been systematically evaluated. Our aims were to evaulate efficacy, safety, and risk of recurrence of venous thromboembolism (VTE) during DOAC treatment in UEDVT patients.

Methods: Data from the Swedish national anticoagulation registry (AuriculA) was retrospectively evaluated for all 55 patients (27 men aged 23–86 years, and 28 women aged 18–75 years) treated with DOAC because of UEDVT between 2012 and 2015 in the southernmost hospital region of Sweden with 1.3 million inhabitants in 2016. Patients were followed for 6 months.

Results: During 6 months after institution of DOAC treatment there was one recurrence (2%) of DVT during treatment and two (4%) recurrences after cessation of treatment. No patient died, whereas one (2%) suffered a clinically relevant nonmajor bleeding.

Conclusion: DOAC can be used in the treatment of UEDVT patients with acceptable efficacy and safety.

Keywords: Venous thromboembolism, Upper extremity deep vein thrombosis, Direct acting oral anti coagulants

Background

Venous thromboembolism (VTE), including deep vein thrombosis (DVT) and pulmonary embolism (PE) affects ≈5% of the population during life [1]. VTE is treated with anticoagulant (AC) therapy for a minimun of 3 months to prevent thrombus extension or embolization, recurrences, and posttrombotic syndromes (PTS) [2]. Hereafter, the decision to stop or continue treatment depends on the balance between the risk of recurrence (1–10%/year) and bleeding (2–4%/year) [1].

Upper extremity DVT (UEDVT) constitutes around 10% of all DVT, and can cause both PE and PTS in the arm [3, 4]. The incidence of secondary UEDVT is increasing due to widespread use of central venous catheters (CVC) in patients with cancer and other chronic diseases [3, 4].

During recent years novel direct acting oral anticoagulants (DOAC) with a favorable risk profile have been increasingly used as an alternative to warfarin for VTE treament [5, 6]. Furthermore, the need for monintoring of DOAC treatment is less than for warfarin, simplifying outpatient treatment of VTE [6]. Whereas DOAC are nowadays considered as first alternative for treatment of PE and DVT in the lower extremities [7], the safety and efficacy of using DOAC for treatment of UEDVT has not been systematically evaluated.

The Swedish quality registry for patients treated with AC, AuriculA [8], includes data on patient characteristics, treatment, and complications for patients on different kinds of oral AC. AuriculA currently holds data on >25,000 patients from the southernmost hospital region in

* Correspondence: johan.elf@skane.se
Department of Vascular Diseases, Lund University, Skåne University Hospital, S-205 02 Malmö, Sweden

Sweden, about 15–20% of whom currently use DOAC, the indication being VTE in 15–20%.

Real life data are valuable for clinical decisions upon AC treatment. AuriculA offers ample opportunities for collection of such data, which can be related to clinical outcomes obtained through prospective follow up of registries and patient files. We therefore used AuriculA data to clarify risks for VTE recurrence, death, and bleeding during 6 months in 55 consecutively registered patients with UEDVT treated with DOAC.

Methods

Patients

We extracted data from AuriculA [8] for all 55 patients in the southernmost hospital region in Sweden (1.3 million inhabitants) that had been treated with DOAC for UEDVT between 2012, when DOAC were first introduced in Sweden, and 2015.

The following risk factors for UEDVT were recorded and reviewed in digital medical charts and imaging databases: malignancies diagnosed prior to or at diagnosis of UEDVT, peripheral vein catheter (PVC) inserted <1 week of diagnosis, use of CVC, cardiac pacemaker or oral contraceptives (OC), pregnancy or postpartum period (defined as the first 6 weeks after delivery), family history of VTE defined as a history of VTE in first-degree relatives and thrombophilia work up (except analysis of lupus anticoagulant due to the risk of false positive results during treatment with DOAC), immobilization defined as ≥3 days of bedrest, trauma to the upper limb or major surgery within the previous 3 months and reported recent strenuous activity of the affected arm (effort thrombosis). Data on symptomatic recurrent VTE (all locations), mortality, bleeding complications and a diagnosis of post thrombotic syndrome (PTS), during 180 days (6 months) after diagnosis were obtained from review of hospital records and imaging databases.

Statistical analysis

Descriptive statistics were used to outline patient characteristics. Results are expressed as mean ± SD or n (%). Excel® 2013 (Microsoft® Office Professional Plus) was used for all analyses.

Results

Baseline data and are available in Table 1. Symptoms reported by the 55 patients were either acute discomfort or swelling of the arm. At least one injection of low molecular weight heparin (LMWH) had initially been given to 38 (69%) patients, whereafter DOAC therapy had been prescribed for 3–6 months or indefinitely. The duration of treatment was 3–6 months if the patient had a UEDVT provoked by transient factors, and indefinite in patients with recurrent unprovoked VTE or strong permanent risk factors. The majority (37[67%]) of patients were treated in hospital (admitted to the hospital >24 h), whereas 18(33%) were treated at an outpatient basis (discharged directly from the emergency unit or admitted to the hospital <24 h). The vast majority (46[84%]) were treated with rivaroxaban, whereas 7(13%) and 2(4%) got apixaban and dabigatran, respectively. Fourty-four (80%) patients started DOAC treatment within 7 days of diagnosis.

Table 1 Baseline characteristics in 55 patients with upper extremity deep vein thrombosis (UEDVT) treated with direct oral anticoagulants (DOAC)

Average age (SD)	49 ± 16,9
Male/Female gender	27/ 28
Ongoing tobacco use	26(47)
Malignancy	10(18)
Surgery within 3 months	13(24)
Immobilisation within 3 months	8(15)
Trauma within 3 months	10(18)
Ongoing pregnancy or postpartum period	0(0)
Oral contraception (females)	7(25)
Acute concomitant medical illness	4(7)
Inpatient treatment for UEDVT	37(67)
Central venous catheter	4(7)
Cardiac pacemaker	1(2)
Peripheral venous catheter	15(27)
Trombophilia (among tested)	15(44)
Effort trombosis	3(5)

N(%)

During 6 months, one (2%) 45 year old male patient experienced recurrence of UEDVT. He was heterozygous for factor V Leiden, had BeÇhet's disease, and had previously been treated with endovascular coiling of a small cerebral aneurysm, His index UEDVT was diagnosed shortly after removal of a CVC from the left jugular vein. After 3 months of rivaroxaban (15 mg BID for 3 weeks followed by 20 mg OD) treatment he once again experienced that his left arm and was more swollen and he also had signs of superior vena caval syndrome. CT-scan showed thrombus in the left brachiocephalic vein and superior vena cava. Treatment was then switched to LMWH bridged to permanent warfarin treatment.

During the 6 months of follow-up, but after cessation of DOAC treatment, two other young male patients (4%) developed recurrent episodes of ipsilateral UEDVT. One was a current smoker and was homozygous for factor V Leiden, the other patient had a positive family history of VTE but was considered to have a primary UEDVT.

No patient died during 6 months of follow-up, whereas one patient (2%) suffered an epistaxis in need for medical attention, classified as a clinically relevant nonmajor bleeding (Table 2).

The type of DOAC treatment was changed only in one (2%) female patient, from rivaroxaban to dabigatran due to a suspected allergic reaction. After 6 months of follow-up, 6(11%) patients had been prescribed permanent DOAC treatment because of estimated high risk of VTE recurrence.

Discussion

DOAC are shown to be both effective [9–14] and safe [9–14] for VTE treatment, and are therefore recommended as first treatment option [7] both in patients treated for DVT in the lower limb and in patients with PE. Furthermore, our study confirms that DOAC are instituted in clinical practise also in many UEDVT patients, despite the lack of evidence from randomized studies and specific recommendations for this patient group. In this context, it should be noted that we studied patients treated with DOAC already from 2012, when these compounds first became available in our country for VTE treatment. Physicians have herafter become more experienced with the use of DOAC for VTE treatment; the proportion of DVT patients receiving DOAC has increased substantially and is now around 25% in a large European registry based material [15]. The same increasing use of DOAC treatment has presumably also occurred among UEDVT patients. As no systematic evaluation has been done in patients with UEDVT on DOAC treatment, however, the increasing popularity of DOAC made it even more important to evaluate the outcome for 55 patients treated with DOAC for UEDVT and consecutively registered in our quality registry.

We found that only one patient (2%) had recurrence of DVT during treatment, a recurrence rate comparable with randomized controlled trials for the treatment of DVT in the lower limb, as summarized in meta-analysis [16]. The two VTE recurrences occurring after cessation of DOAC therapy cannot be attributed to therapy failure, but instead reflect the innate risk of recurrence that these patients have, although this risk is considered lower compared to patients with DVT in the lower extremity [3]. Furthermore, no major bleedings occurred and only one patient experienced a nonmajor bleeding, figures comparing favorably with bleeding rates in previous large randomized study materials [16], from which patients perceived as having increasing bleeding risk are often excluded.

It is important to note that patients with UEDVT differ from those with DVT in the lower limb and PE, as they more often have secondary thromboses caused by for example CVC and cancer [3, 4]. The recommended treatment in patients with VTE and cancer is LMWH [1, 7], and oral anticoagulation is therefore avoided in a large proportion of UEDVT patients. The 10 patients with a diagnosis of cancer in our study either had strong personal objections to daily LMWH injections or warfarin therapy, or were without active ongoing cancer therapy.

It is also important to note that 20 of our 55 patients had either a PVC, a CVC, or a cardiac pacemaker with intravenous leads inserted in the affected region, and that this implantation had often occurred shortly before the diagnosis of UEDVT. This indicates that our patients have a fairly high rate of concomitant illness, which might also have excluded many of them from entry into randomized studies of VTE treatment. The concept of DOAC treatment of cancer-associated VTE is currently under debate [17, 18], but when rivaroxaban was recently evaluated in 70 cancer patients with UEDVT related to CVC, 13% experienced bleeding complications and one case of fatal pulmonary embolism occurred [19].

Due to logistic reasons, objective verification of a VTE diagnosis with imaging is often postponed to office hours. As in the randomized studies [9–13], many of our patient therefore recieved at least one injection of LMH before imaging and establishment of diagnosis. Hereafter, it is important to note that one third of our patients were treated as outpatients, however, enabling potential savings in addition to the gains offered by DOAC due to the lower need for surveillance in comparison to warfarin [20]. Assessment of the number of days in hospital is essential when evaluating true cost-benefit of the new anticoagulants.

Our study has several limitations, the most important is the fact that is a retrospective clinical follow-up and not a randomized prospective study with a relevant control group. A comparison with UEDVT patients treated with warfarin or LMWH would have suffered from severe inclusion bias, however; warfarin treated patients would probably more often have renal failure, and LMWH treated patients more often cancer or ongoing pregnancy. Furthermore, even if we studied all UEDVT patients treated with DOAC in an area with 1.3 million inhabitants, the material is small in comparison to

Table 2 Six months follow-up of 55 patients with upper extremity deep vein thrombosis (UEDVT) treated with direct oral anticoagulants (DOAC), N(%)

Death	0(0)
DVT recurrence on treatment	1(2)
DVT recurrence after cessation	2(4)
Major bleeding	0(0)
Clinically relevant nonmajor bleeding	1(2)
Treatment change	1(2)
Post thrombotic syndrome	6(11)
Prescribed permanent anticoagulation at 6 months	6(11)

international registry data [15]. Nevertheless, our data enable the below conclusion.

Conclusion

DOAC can be used for treatment of patients with UEDVT with acceptable recurrence and bleeding rates.

Acknowledgements
None.

Funding
No funding was obtained for this article.

Authors' contributions
FSM, AG, and JE contributed to the study concept and design, and acquisition of data. FSM, RG, AG, and JE all contributed to data analysis and interpretation, drafting and, critical revision of the manuscript. Statistical analysis was performed by FSM. All authors read and approved the final manuscript.

Competing interests
The authors state that they have no conflicts of interests.

References

1. Guyatt GH, Akl EA, Crowther M, et al. Antithrombotic therapy and prevention of thrombosis (9th edition). American College of Chest Physicians Evidence-Based Clinical Practice Guidelines. Chest. 2012;141(2Suppl):7S–47S.
2. Yeh CH, Gross P, Weitz J. Evolving use of new oral anticoagulants for treatment of venous thromboembolism. Blood. 2014;124:1020–8.
3. Munoz FJ, Mismetti P, Poggio R, Valle R, Baron M, Guil M, Monreal M. Clinical outcome of patients with upper extremity deep vein thrombosis: results from the REITE registry. Chest. 2008;133:143–8.
4. Isma N, Svensson PJ, Gottsäter A, Lindblad B. Upper extremity deep venous thrombosis in the population-based Malmö thrombophilia study (MATS). Epidemiology, risk factors, recurrence risk, and mortality. Thromb Res. 2010;125:e335–8.
5. Comerota AJ, Ramacciotti E. A comprehensive overview of direct oral anticoagulants for the management of venous thromboembolism. Am J Med Sci. 2016;352:92–106.
6. Piran S, Schulman S. Management of venous thromboembolism: an update. Thromb J. 2016;14(Suppl 1):23.
7. Kearon C, Akl EA, Ornelas J, Blaivas A, Jimenez D, Bounameaux H, Huisman M, King CS, Morris TA, Sood N, Stevens SM, Vintch JRE, Wells P, Woller SC, Moores L. Antithrombotic therapy for VTE disease CHEST guideline and expert panel report. Chest. 2016;149(2):315–52.
8. Wieloch M, Själander A, Frykman V, Rosenqvist M, Eriksson N, Svensson PJ. Anticoagulation control in Sweden: reports of time in therapeutic range, major bleeding, and thrombo-embolic complications from the national quality registry AuriculA. Eur Heart J. 2011;32:2282–9.
9. Schulman S, Kearon C, Kakkar AK, et al. Dabigatran versus warfarin in the treatment of acute venous thromboembolism. N Engl J Med. 2009;361(24): 2342–52.
10. Bauersachs R, Berkowitz SD, Brenner B, et al. Oral rivaroxaban for symptomatic venous thromboembolism. N Engl J Med. 2010;363(26):2499–510.
11. Investigators H-VTE, Buller HR, Decousus H, et al. Edoxaban versus warfarin for the treatment of symptomatic venous thromboembolism. N Engl J Med. 2013;369(15):1406–15.
12. Agnelli G, Buller HR, Cohen A, et al. Oral apixaban for the treatment of acute venous thromboembolism. N Engl J Med. 2013;369(9):799–808.
13. Investigators EINSTEIN-EP, Buller HR, Prins MH, et al. Oral rivaroxaban for the treatment of symptomatic pulmonary embolism. N Engl J Med. 2012; 366(14):1287–97.
14. van Es N, Coppens M, Schulman S, Middeldorp S, Buller HR. Direct oral anticoagulants compared with vitamin K antagonists for acute venous thromboembolism: evidence from phase 3 trials. Blood. 2014;124(12):1968–75.
15. Cohen AT, Gitt AK, Bauersachs R, Fronk EM, Laeis P, Mismetti P, Monreal M, Willich SN, Bramlage P, Agnelli G; PREFER in VTE Scientific Steering Committee and the PREFER in VTE Investigators. The management of acute venous thromboembolism in clinical practice. Results from the European PREFER in VTE Registry. Thromb Haemost. 2017 Apr 13. doi: https://doi.org/10.1160/TH16-10-0793. [Epub ahead of print].
16. Castellucci LA, Cameron C, Le Gal G, et al. Clinical and safety outcomes associated with treatment of acute venous thromboembolism: a systematic review and meta-analysis. JAMA. 2014;312(11):1122–35.
17. Alberio L. The new direct oral anticoagulants in special indications: rationale and preliminary data in cancer, mechanical heart valves, anti-phospholipid syndrome, and heparin-induced thrombocytopenia and beyond. Semin Hematol. 2014;51:152–6.
18. Ross JA, Miller M, Hernandez CR. OC-13 - safe and effective use of direct oral anticoagulants (DOAC) versus conventional anticoagulation for the treatment of cancer-related venous thromboembolism. Thromb Res. 2016;140(Suppl 1):S173–4.
19. Davies GA, Lazo-Langner A, Gandara E, Rodger M, Tagalakis V, Louzada M, Corpuz R, Kovacs MJ. A prospective study of Rivaroxaban for central venous catheter associated upper extremity deep vein thrombosis in cancer patients (Catheter 2). Thromb Res. 2017 Apr 6. pii: S0049–3848(17)30257–8. doi: https://doi.org/10.1016/j.thromres.2017.04.003. [Epub ahead of print].
20. Deitelzweig S, Amin A, Jing Y, Makenbaeva D, Wiederkehr D, Lin J, Graham J. Medical costs in the US of clinical events associated with oral anticoagulant (OAC) use compared to warfarin among non-valvular atrial fibrillation patients ≥75 and <75 years of age, based on the ARISTOTLE, RE-LY, and ROCKET-AF trials. J Med Econ. 2013;16:1163–8.

Permissions

All chapters in this book were first published in TJ, by BioMed Central; hereby published with permission under the Creative Commons Attribution License or equivalent. Every chapter published in this book has been scrutinized by our experts. Their significance has been extensively debated. The topics covered herein carry significant findings which will fuel the growth of the discipline. They may even be implemented as practical applications or may be referred to as a beginning point for another development.

The contributors of this book come from diverse backgrounds, making this book a truly international effort. This book will bring forth new frontiers with its revolutionizing research information and detailed analysis of the nascent developments around the world.

We would like to thank all the contributing authors for lending their expertise to make the book truly unique. They have played a crucial role in the development of this book. Without their invaluable contributions this book wouldn't have been possible. They have made vital efforts to compile up to date information on the varied aspects of this subject to make this book a valuable addition to the collection of many professionals and students.

This book was conceptualized with the vision of imparting up-to-date information and advanced data in this field. To ensure the same, a matchless editorial board was set up. Every individual on the board went through rigorous rounds of assessment to prove their worth. After which they invested a large part of their time researching and compiling the most relevant data for our readers.

The editorial board has been involved in producing this book since its inception. They have spent rigorous hours researching and exploring the diverse topics which have resulted in the successful publishing of this book. They have passed on their knowledge of decades through this book. To expedite this challenging task, the publisher supported the team at every step. A small team of assistant editors was also appointed to further simplify the editing procedure and attain best results for the readers.

Apart from the editorial board, the designing team has also invested a significant amount of their time in understanding the subject and creating the most relevant covers. They scrutinized every image to scout for the most suitable representation of the subject and create an appropriate cover for the book.

The publishing team has been an ardent support to the editorial, designing and production team. Their endless efforts to recruit the best for this project, has resulted in the accomplishment of this book. They are a veteran in the field of academics and their pool of knowledge is as vast as their experience in printing. Their expertise and guidance has proved useful at every step. Their uncompromising quality standards have made this book an exceptional effort. Their encouragement from time to time has been an inspiration for everyone.

The publisher and the editorial board hope that this book will prove to be a valuable piece of knowledge for researchers, students, practitioners and scholars across the globe.

List of Contributors

Luigi Brunetti
Department of Pharmacy Practice and Administration, Ernest Mario School of Pharmacy, Rutgers, The State University of New Jersey, Piscataway, USA

Betty Sanchez-Catanese
Department of Medicine, Robert Wood Johnson University Hospital-Somerset, Somerville, USA

Leonid Kagan
Department of Pharmaceutics, Ernest Mario School of Pharmacy, Rutgers, The State University of New Jersey, Piscataway, USA

Xia Wen and Lauren M. Aleksunes
Department of Pharmacology and Toxicology, Ernest Mario School of Pharmacy, Rutgers, The State University of New Jersey, Piscataway, USA

Min Liu and Brian Buckley
Chemical Analytical Core Laboratory, Environmental and Occupational Health Sciences Institute, Rutgers, The State University of New Jersey, Piscataway, USA
Pathology and Diagnostic Inv., Michigan State University, East Lansing, USA

W. Bouida, H. Baccouche and S. Nouira
Emergency Department, Fattouma Bourguiba University Hospital, 5000 Monastir, Tunisia

M. Sassi
Laboratory of Biology, Maternity and Neonatal Medicine Center, 5000 Monastir, Tunisia

Z. Dridi
Cardiology Department, Fattouma Bourguiba University Hospital, 5000 Monastir, Tunisia

T. Chakroun
Regional Blood Transfusion Center, Farhat Hached University Hospital, 4004 Sousse, Tunisia

I. Hellara
Hematology Department, Fattouma Bourguiba University Hospital, 5000 Monasitr, Tunisia

R. Boukef
Emergency Department, Sahloul University Hospital, 4011 Sousse, Tunisia

F. Added
Cardiology Department, Abderrahman Mami University Hospital, 1080 Ariana, Tunisia

I. Khochtali
Endocrinology and Internal Medicine Department, Fattouma Bourguiba University Hospital, 5000 Monastir, Tunisia

R. Razgallah
Medis Laboratories, 1053 Tunis, Tunisia

W. Bouida, H. Baccouche, M. Sassi, I. Hellara, R. Boukef, M. Hassine, F. Added, I. Khochtali and S. Nouira
Research Laboratory (LR12SP18), University of Monastir, 5000 Monastir, Tunisia

Ming-Ching Shen and Cheng-Shyong Chang
Department of Internal Medicine, Changhua Christian Hospital, Changhua, Taiwan

Wan-Ju Wu and Ming Chen
Department of Obstetrics and Gynecology, Changhua Christian Hospital, Changhua, Taiwan

Wan-Ju Wu, Gwo-Chin Ma, Wen-Hsiang Lin and Ming Chen
Department of Genomic Medicine, Changhua Christian Hospital, 500 Changhua, Taiwan

Po-Jen Cheng
Department of Obstetrics and Gynecology, Chang-Gung Memorial Hospital Linkou Medical Center and Chang-Gung University, Taoyuan, Taiwan

Wen-Chu Li
Department of Obstetrics and Gynecology, Puli Christian Hospital, Nantou, Taiwan

Jui-Der Liou
Department of Obstetrics and Gynecology, Taipei Chang-Gung Memorial Hospital, Taipei, Taiwan

Ming Chen
Department of Obstetrics and Gynecology, and Department of Medical Genetics, College of Medicine, and Hospital, National Taiwan University, Taipei, Taiwan
Department of Life Science, Tunghai University, Taichung, Taiwan

Yohko Kawai
International University of Health and Welfare, 8-10-16 Akasaka, Minato-ku, Tokyo 107-0052, Japan

Takeshi Fuji
Department of Orthopaedic Surgery, Japan Community Healthcare Organization Osaka Hospital, 4-2-78, Fukushima, Fukushima-ku, Osaka 553-0003, Japan

Satoru Fujita
Department of Orthopaedic Surgery, Satoru Fujita3Takarazuka Daiichi Hospital, 19-5 Kogetsu-cho, Takarazuka 665-0832, Japan

Tetsuya Kimura and Kei Ibusuki
Daiichi Sankyo Co., Ltd, 3-5-1, Nihonbashi Honcho, Chuo-ku, Tokyo 103-8426, Japan

Kenji Abe
Clinical Data and Biostatistics Department, Daiichi Sankyo Co. Ltd, 1-2-58, Hiromachi, Shinagawa-ku, Tokyo 140-8710, Japan

Shintaro Tachibana
Department of Orthopaedic Surgery, Mishuku Hospital, 5-33-12 Shimomeguro, Meguro-ku, Tokyo 153-0051, Japan

A. Magnette, M. Chatelain, B. Chatelain and F. Mullier
1Université catholique de Louvain, CHU UCL Namur, Namur Thrombosis and Hemostasis Center (NTHC), NARILIS, Haematology Laboratory, B-5530 Yvoir, Belgium

H. Ten Cate
Maastricht University Medical Centre and Cardiovascular Research Institute (CARIM), Department of Internal Medicine, Maastricht, The Netherlands

Yukio Ozaki
Fuefuki Central Hospital, 47-1 Yokkaichiba, Isawa, Fuefuki 406-0032, Yamanashi, Japan

Shogo Tamura and Katsue Suzuki-Inoue
Department of Laboratory Medicine, University of Yamanashi, 1110 Shimokato, Chuo, Yamanashi 409-3898, Japan

Shogo Tamura
Department of Pathophysiological Laboratory Sciences, Nagoya University Graduate School of Medicine, 1-1-20, Oosachi Minami, Higashi, Nagoya 461-8673, Aichi, Japan
Viktor Hamrefors, Artur Fedorowski and Nazim Isma
Department of Clinical Sciences Malmö, Lund University, SE 205-02 Malmö, Sweden

Viktor Hamrefors
Department of Internal Medicine, Skåne University Hospital, SE 205-02 Malmö, Sweden
Department of Medical Imaging and Physiology, Skåne University Hospital, SE 205-02 Malmö, Sweden

Artur Fedorowski
Department of Cardiology, Skåne University Hospital, Inga Marie Nilssons gata 46, SE 205-02 Malmö, Sweden

Karin Strandberg
Centre for Thrombosis and Haemostasis, Skåne University Hospital, SE 205-02 Malmö, Sweden

Richard Sutton
National Heart and Lung Institute, Imperial College, Hammersmith Hospital Campus, Ducane Road, London W12 0NN, UK

Nazim Isma
Department of Cardiology, Skåne University Hospital, SE 221-85 Lund, Sweden

Eiji Furukoji
Department of Radiology, Faculty of Medicine, University of Miyazaki, 5200 Kihara, Kiyotake, Miyazaki 889-1692, Japan

Toshihiro Gi, Atsushi Yamashita, Mio Kojima and Yujiro Asada
Department of Pathology, Faculty of Medicine, University of Miyazaki, 5200 Kihara, Kiyotake, Miyazaki 889-1692, Japan

Sayaka Moriguchi-Goto and Yuichiro Sato
Department of Diagnostic Pathology, Miyazaki University Hospital, University of Miyazaki, 5200 Kihara, Kiyotake, Miyazaki 889-1692, Japan

Chihiro Sugita
Department of Biochemistry and Microbiology, Faculty of Pharmaceutical Sciences, Kyusyu University of Health and Welfare, 1714-1 Yoshinomachi, Nobeoka 882-0072, Japan

Marjorie Paris Colombini, Priscilla Bento Matos Cruz Derogis, Valdir Fernandes de Aranda, João Carlos de Campos Guerra and Cristóvão Luis Pitangueiras Mangueira
Department of Diagnostic and Preventive Medicine and Clinical Laboratory, Hospital Israelita Albert Einstein, São Paulo, Brazil

Nelson Hamerschlak
Department of Hematology, Hospital Israelita Albert Einstein, São Paulo, Brazil

Valentina Scalise, Cristina Balia, Silvana Cianchetti, Tommaso Neri, Vittoria Carnicelli, Riccardo Zucchi, Alessandro Celi and Roberto Pedrinelli
Dipartimento di Patologia Chirurgica, Medica, Molecolare e dell'Area Critica, Università di Pisa, Pisa, Italy

Maria Franzini, Alessandro Corti and Aldo Paolicchi
Dipartimento di Ricerca Traslazionale e delle Nuove Tecnologie in Medicina e Chirurgia, Università di Pisa, Pisa, Italy

R. Ghazvinian, A. Gottsäter and J. Elf
Lund University, Division of Vascular Medicine, Skåne University Hospital, Ruth Lundskogs Gata 10, S-205 02 Malmö, Sweden

Arshi Naz, Tehmina Nafees Khan, Shariq Ahmed and Tahir S Shamsi
National Institute of Blood Diseases and Bone Marrow Transplantation, Karachi University of Bonn, ST 2/A, Block-17, Gulshan-e-Iqbal KDA scheme, 24, Karachi, Pakistan

Arijit Biswas and Johannes Oldenburg
Institute of Experimental Hematology and Transfusion Medicine, Bonn, Germany

Anne Goodeve
University of Shieffield, Shiefield, United Kingdom

Nisar Ahmed and Nazish Saqlain
Children's Hospital, Resident, Paediatric hematology, Main Ferozpur Road, Lahore, Pakistan

Ikram Din Ujjan
Liaquat university of medical and health sciences, Jamshoro, Pakistan

Arijit Biswas
Institute of Experimental Hematology and Transfusion Medicine, AG, FXIII Room No. 2.308 Sigmund Freud Street-25, 53127 Bonn, Germany

Tehmina Nafees Khan and Tahir S Shamsi
National Institute of blood diseases and bone marrow transplantation, ST 2/A, Block-17, Gulshan-e-Iqbal KDA scheme, 24, Karachi, Pakistan

Anne Goodeve
Clinical Scientist and Professor of Molecular Medicine, Sheffield Diagnostic Genetics Service, Sheffield Children's NHS Foundation Trust, Western Bank, Sheffield S10 2TH, UK

Johannes Oldenburg
Institute of Experimental Hematology and Transfusion Medicine, Sigmund Freud Street-25, 53127 Bonn, Germany

Robin Condliffe
Pulmonary Vascular Disease Unit, Sheffield Teaching Hospitals NHS Foundation Trust, Sheffield, UK

Xiaohong Ruby Xu and Heyu Ni
Department of Laboratory Medicine and Pathobiology, University of Toronto, Toronto, ON, Canada

Xiaohong Ruby Xu, Naadiya Carrim, Miguel Antonio Dias Neves, Thomas McKeown, Tyler W. Stratton, Rodrigo Matos Pinto Coelho, Xi Lei, Pingguo Chen and Heyu Ni
Department of Laboratory Medicine, Keenan Research Centre for Biomedical Science, St. Michael's Hospital, Toronto, ON, Canada

Xiaohong Ruby Xu
Guangdong Provincial Hospital of Chinese Medicine, Guangzhou University of Chinese Medicine, Guangzhou, Guangdong, People's Republic of China

Naadiya Carrim, Pingguo Chen and Heyu Ni
Canadian Blood Services, Toronto, ON, Canada

Jianhua Xu and Heyu Ni
CCOA Therapeutics Inc, Toronto, ON, Canada

Xiangrong Dai and Benjamin Xiaoyi Li
Lee's Pharmaceutical holdings limited, Shatin, Hong Kong, China
Zhaoke Pharmaceutical co. limited, Hefei, Anhui, China

Benjamin Xiaoyi
Hong Kong University of Science and technology, Hong Kong, China

Heyu Ni
Department of Medicine and Department of Physiology, University of Toronto, Toronto, ON, Canada

Virginie Dubois, Anne-Sophie Dincq, Maximilien Gourdin and Sarah Lessire
Université catholique de Louvain, CHU UCL Namur, Department of Anesthesiology, Yvoir, Belgium

Anne-Sophie Dincq, Jonathan Douxfils, Jean-Michel Dogné, Maximilien Gourdin, Bernard Chatelain, François Mullier and Sarah Lessire
Namur Thrombosis and Hemostasis Center (NTHC), NAmur Research Institute of LIfe Sciences (NARILIS), Namur, Belgium

Jonathan Douxfils and Jean-Michel Dogné
Université de Namur, Department of Pharmacy, Faculty of Medecine, Namur, Belgium

Brigitte Ickx
Université Libre de Bruxelles, Erasme University Hospital, Department of Anesthesiology, Brussels, Belgium

Charles-Marc Samama
Université Paris Descartes, Cochin University Hospital, Department of Anesthesiology and Intensive Care, Paris, France

Bernard Chatelain and François Mullier
Université catholique de Louvain, CHU UCL Namur, Hematology Laboratory, Yvoir, Belgium

Takeshi Wada, Satoshi Gando, Yuichi Ono, Kunihiko Maekawa, Kenichi Katabami, Mineji Hayakawa and Atsushi Sawamura
Division of Acute and Critical Care Medicine, Department of Anesthesiology and Critical Care Medicine, Hokkaido University Graduate School of Medicine, N15W7, Kita-ku, Sapporo 060-8638, Japan

Weiyi Feng, Manojkumar Valiyaveettil, Tejasvi Dudiki, Ganapati H. Mahabeleshwar, Eugene A. Podrez and Tatiana V. Byzova
Department of Molecular Cardiology, The Cleveland Clinic Foundation, Cleveland 44195, OH, USA

Patrick Andre
Plaint Therapeutics, Redwood City, CA, USA

Weiyi Feng
The First Affiliated Hospital, School of Medicine, Xi'an Jiaotong University, Xi'an, Shaanxi 710061, China

Manojkumar Valiyaveettil
US Army Medical Materiel Development Activity, 1430 Veterans Drive, Fort Detrick, Frederick, MD 21702, USA

Eyob Alemayehu Gebreyohannes, Akshaya Srikanth Bhagavathula and Henok Getachew Tegegn
Department of Clinical Pharmacy, University of Gondar, Gondar, Ethiopia

J. M. van den Heuvel, A. M. Hövels, A. K. Mantel-Teeuwisse, A. de Boer and A. H. Maitland-van der Zee
Utrecht Institute for Pharmaceutical Sciences (UIPS), Division of Pharmacoepidemiology and Clinical Pharmacology, Utrecht University, Utrecht, The Netherlands

J. M. van den Heuvel and A. H. Maitland-van der Zee
Department of Respiratory Medicine, Academic Medical Center, University of Amsterdam, Amsterdam, The Netherlands

H. R. Büller
Department of Vascular Medicine, Academic Medical Center, University of Amsterdam, Amsterdam, The Netherlands

Richard G. Jung, Pouya Motazedian, F. Daniel Ramirez, Trevor Simard, Pietro Di Santo, Mohammad Ali Faraz, Alisha Labinaz and Benjamin Hibbert
CAPITAL Research Group, University of Ottawa Heart Institute, 40 Ruskin
Street, H-4238, Ottawa, ON K1Y 4W7, Canada

Richard G. Jung, Trevor Simard and Benjamin Hibbert
Department of Cellular and Molecular Medicine, University of Ottawa, Ottawa, ON, Canada.

Richard G. Jung, Trevor Simard and Benjamin Hibbert
Vascular Biology and Experimental Medicine Laboratory, University of Ottawa Heart Institute, Ottawa, ON, Canada

F. Daniel Ramirez, Trevor Simard, Pietro Di Santo and Benjamin Hibbert
Division of Cardiology, University of Ottawa Heart Institute, Ottawa, ON, Canada

F. Daniel Ramirez
School of Epidemiology, Public Health and Preventive Medicine, University of Ottawa, Ottawa, ON, Canada

Sarah Visintini
Berkman Library, University of Ottawa Heart Institute, Ottawa, ON, Canada

Young Jung
Department of Health Research Methods, Evidence, and Impact, McMaster University, Hamilton, ON, Canada

Hironori Matsumoto, Jun Takeba, Kensuke Umakoshi, Satoshi Kikuchi, Muneaki Ohshita, Suguru Annen, Naoki Moriyama, Yuki Nakabayashi, Norio Sato and Mayuki Aibiki
Department of Emergency and Critical Care Medicine, Ehime University, Graduate School of Medicine, Shitsukawa 454, Toon City, Ehime 791-0295, Japan

Ellen M. K. Warlo, Alf-Åge R. Pettersen, Harald Arnesen and Ingebjørg Seljeflot
Center for Clinical Heart Research, Department of Cardiology, Oslo University Hospital, Ullevaal, Pb 4956 Nydalen, 0424 Oslo, Norway

Ellen M. K. Warlo, Harald Arnesen and Ingebjørg Seljeflot
Faculty of Medicine, University of Oslo, Oslo, Norway

Ellen M. K. Warlo, Alf-Åge R. Pettersen, Harald Arnesen and Ingebjørg Seljeflot
Center for Heart Failure Research, University of Oslo, Oslo, Norway

Alf-Åge R. Pettersen
Department of Medicine, Vestre Viken HF, Ringerike Hospital, Hønefoss, Norway

Takuro Arishima, Takashi Ito, Tomotsugu Yasuda, Hiroaki Furubeppu, Takahiro Futatsuki, Yutaro Madokoro, Shotaro Miyamoto, Tomohiro Eguchi, Hiroyuki Haraura and Yasuyuki Kakihana
Emergency and Critical Care Center, Kagoshima University Hospital, Kagoshima, Japan

Takashi Ito and Ikuro Maruyama
Department of Systems Biology in Thromboregulation, Kagoshima University Graduate School of Medical and Dental Sciences, 8-35-1 Sakuragaoka, Kagoshima 890-8544, Japan

Nozomi Yashima, Chinatsu Kamikokuryo and Yasuyuki Kakihana
Emergency and Intensive Care Medicine, Kagoshima University Graduate School of Medical and Dental Sciences, Kagoshima, Japan

Hideo Wada
Department of Molecular and Laboratory Medicine, Mie University Graduate School of Medicine, Tsu, Mie 514-8507, Japan

Takeshi Matsumoto
Division of Blood Transfusion Medicine and Cell Therapy, Mie University Graduate School of Medicine, Tsu, Japan

Kei Suzuki and Hiroshi Imai
Emergency Critical Care Center, Mie University Graduate School of Medicine, Tsu, Japan

Naoyuki Katayama
Department of Hematology and Oncology, Mie University Graduate School of Medicine, Tsu, Japan

Toshiaki Iba
Department of Emergency and Disaster Medicine, Juntendo University Graduate School of Medicine, Tokyo, Japan

Masanori Matsumoto
Department of Blood Transfusion Medicine, Nara Medical University, Nara, Japan

Andrew Kotaska
Women's and Children's Health, Northwest Territories Health and Social Services Authority, Stanton Territorial Hospital, Yellowknife, NT X1A 2N1, Canada
School of Population and Public Health, University of British Columbia, Vancouver, Canada
Department of Obstetrics and Gynaecology, University of Manitoba, Winnipeg, Canada
Department of Obstetrics and Gynaecology, University of Toronto, Toronto, Canada

Alexander T. Cohen
Guy's and St Thomas' NHS Foundation Trust, King's College London, London, UK

Cihan Ay
Clinical Division of Haematology and Haemostaseology, Department of Medicine I, Medical University of Vienna, Vienna, Austria

Philippe Hainaut
Department of General Internal Medicine, Cliniques Universitaires Saint Luc, UCL, Bruxelles, Belgium

Hervé Décousus
Centre Hospitalier Universitaire de Saint-Etienne, Saint-Priest En Jarez, France

Ulrich Hoffmann
Division of Angiology, Medical Clinic IV, University Hospital, Ludwig-Maximilians-University, Munich, Germany

Sean Gaine
National Pulmonary Hypertension Unit, Mater Misericordiae University Hospital, Dublin, Ireland

Michiel Coppens
Department of Vascular Medicine, Academic Medical Center, Amsterdam, The Netherlands

Pedro Marques da Silva
Department of Internal Medicine, Arterial Investigation Unit, Hospital de Santa Marta, Lisbon, Portugal

David Jiménez
Respiratory Department, Ramón y Cajal Hospital, Madrid, Spain

Beatrice Amann-Vesti
Division of Angiology, University Hospital Zurich, Zurich, Switzerland

Bernd Brüggenjürgen
Institute for Health Economics, Steinbeis-University, Berlin, Germany

Pierre Levy
LEGOS, Université Paris - Dauphine, Paris, France
Julio Lopez Bastida
University of Castilla-La Mancha, Talavera de la Reina, Toledo, Spain

Eric Vicaut
Department of Medicine, Université Paris Descartes, Paris, France

Petra Laeis, Eva-Maria Fronk, Wolfgang Zierhut and Thomas Malzer
Daiichi Sankyo Europe GmbH, Munich, Germany

Peter Bramlage
Institute for Pharmacology and Preventive Medicine, Berlin, Germany

Giancarlo Agnelli
Internal and Cardiovascular Medicine-Stroke Unit, University of Perugia, Perugia, Italy

Francisco Sánchez Montiel, Raein Ghazvinian, Anders Gottsäter and Johan Elf
Department of Vascular Diseases, Lund University, Skåne University Hospital,
S-205 02 Malmö, Sweden

Index

www.ingramcontent.com/pod-product-compliance
Lightning Source LLC
Chambersburg PA
CBHW080248230326
41458CB00097B/4120
9781632426741